D0168361

# Delmar's

# Dental

# Drug Reference

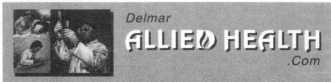

# Delmar's Dental Drug Reference

**Elena Bablenis Haveles, PharmD**
Clinical Associate Professor of Pharmacology
School of Dental Hygiene
College of Health Sciences
Old Dominion University
Norfolk, Virginia

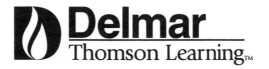

Albany • Bonn • Boston • Cincinnati • Detroit • London • Madrid
Melbourne • Mexico City • New York • Pacific Grove • Paris • San Francisco
Singapore • Tokyo • Toronto • Washington

# NOTICE TO THE READER

**Delmar Staff:**

Business Unit Director: William Brottmiller
Acquisitions Editor: Marlene Pratt
Development Editor: Melissa Riveglia
Editorial Assistant: Maria Perretta
Executive Marketing Manager: Dawn F. Gerrain
Marketing Coordinator: Nina Lontrato
Project Editor: Elizabeth B. Keller
Production Coordinator: Barbara A. Bullock
Art/Design Coordinator: Rich Killar
Technology Manager: Lisa Santy
Database Program Manager: Linda Helfrich
Cover Design: Susan Schoonmaker

COPYRIGHT © 2000

Delmar is a division of Thomson Learning. The Thomson Learning logo is a registered trademark used herein under license.

Printed in Canada
1 2 3 4 5 6 7 8 9 10 XXX 05 04 03 02 01 00 99

For more information, contact Delmar, 3 Columbia Circle, PO Box 15015, Albany, NY 12212-0515; or find us on the World Wide Web at http://www.delmar.com

Library of Congress Cataloging-in-Publication Data

Haveles, Elena B.
    Delmar's dental drug reference / Elena Bablenis Haveles.
    Includes index.
    ISBN 0-7668-0115-2
    1. Dental pharmacology Handbooks, manuals, etc. I. Title. II. Title: Dental drug reference
    RK701 .H377 2000
    615'.1'0246176—dc21

99-30080
CIP

# Notice to the Reader

The publisher and the author do not warrant or guarantee any of the products described herein or perform any independent analysis in connection with any of the product information contained herein. The publisher and the author do not assume and expressly disclaim any obligation to obtain and include information other than that provided by the manufacturer.

The reader is expressly warned to consider and adopt all safety precautions that might be indicated by the activities described herein and to avoid all potential hazards. By following the instructions contained herein, the reader willingly assumes all risks in connection with such instructions.

The publisher and the authors make no representations or warranties of any kind, including but not limited to the warranties of fitness for a particular purpose or merchantability nor are any such representations implied with respect to the material set forth herein, and the publisher and the author take no responsibility with respect to such material. The publisher and the author shall not be liable for any special, consequential, or exemplary damages resulting, in whole or in part, from the reader's use of, or reliance upon, this material.

The author and publisher have made a conscientious effort to ensure that the drug information and recommended dosages in this book are accurate and in accord with accepted standards at the time of publication. However, typographical errors can occur and pharmacology and therapeutics are rapidly changing sciences, so readers are advised to check the package insert provided by the manufacturer for the recommended dose, for contraindications, side effects, and for any added warnings and precautions. This recommendation is especially important for new, infrequently used, or highly toxic drugs.

# Preface

*Delmar's Dental Drug Reference* provides up-to-date information on drugs of particular interest to the dental care practitioner. These drugs are presented alphabetically in Chapter 3.

Chapter 1 and the "Quick Guide to the Use of *Delmar's Dental Drug Reference* should be consulted first because they outline how to use the text. General information on drug classes, including dental concerns, is found in Chapter 2. This information is easy to locate and use and prevents lengthy repetitions throughout the text. A list of drugs that are in that drug class appears at the beginning of each class discussed.

Trade names of drugs marketed in the United States and Canada are listed; trade names of drugs marketed only in Canada are designated by a maple leaf ✹. For ease of location, the FDA pregnancy category immediately follows the pronunciation of the drug at the beginning of the information for each drug in Chapter 3.

One of the important features of *Delmar's Dental Drug Reference* is the format whereby dosage information is presented. The dosage form and/or route of administration are clearly delineated and are often correlated with the disease state(s) for which the dosage is used. This makes finding dosage information easy. Another important feature is the designation in boldface italics of life-threatening side effects. The section entitled *Special Concerns* provides information of special note to the practitioner, including safety and efficacy considerations for use of the drug in certain disease states, in children, during lactation, during pregnancy, and in the geriatric client.

The presentation of *Dental Concerns* and *Client/Family Teaching* are two of the most important features of the text. Such information provides the practitioner with a mechanism to assess the client before and after oral health care, prescribed drug therapy, to obtain and review specific items (assessments, labs) related to the drug being administered or prescribed, to initiate appropriate interventions, and to incorporate appropriate client/family teaching to ensure proper drug therapy. Chapter 1 should be consulted for a more thorough discussion of how dental concerns are presented.

Appendices include a definition and listing of drugs controlled either by the United States Controlled Substances Act of the Canadian Controlled Substances Law (Appendix 1); information on the elements and interpretation of a prescription (Appendix 2); definitions of FDA pregnancy categories (Appendix 3); drugs causing dry mouth by class (Appendix 4); classes of drugs altering sense of taste (Appendix 5); common drug-drug and drug-food interactions of concern to dental health (Appendix 6); list of antibiotics used to treat periodontal disease (Appendix 7); prophylactic regimens for bacterial endocarditis for dental procedures (Appendix 8); example calculations—drug administered per dental cartridge (Appendix 9); typical local anesthetic and vasoconstrictor concentrations (Appendix 10). The index is extensively cross-referenced and facilitates locating drugs by pairing generic and trade names.

The information provided and the format used for *Delmar's Dental Drug Reference* makes the book an easy-to-use and valuable text and reference for the latest information on drugs and the proper monitoring of drug therapy by the practitioner.

# Acknowledgments

I would like to extend my thanks to the Delmar team: Lisa Santy, Barb Bullock, Melissa Riveglia, Marlene Pratt, Linda Helfrich, Bill Trudell, Rich Killar, Maria Peretta, and Nina Lontrato.

Thank you to my husband Paul and my sons Andrew and Harry for your patience, love, and understanding throughout this project—I love you all.

Delmar and the author would like to recognize the following individuals who reviewed the manuscript and made valuable suggestions:

Lori Burch, RDA
Dental Program Director'
Corinthian College
Reseda, California

Thomas A. French, PhD
Instructor of Pharmacology
Department of Pharmacology, School of Medicine
University of Health Sciences Center
Denver, Colorado

Debbie Reynon, CDA, RDA, AA, AS
Dental Assisting Instructor
Santa Cruz County Regional Occupational Program
Santa Cruz, California

Marianne Watts, CDA
Dental Instructor
Tarrant County Junior College
Hurst, Texas

Mea Weinberg, DMD, MSD, RPh
Clinical Associate Professor of Periodontics
New York University College of Dentistry
New York, New York

# Quick Guide to the Use of *Delmar's Dental Drug Reference*

An understanding of the format of *Delmar's Dental Drug Reference* will help you reference information quickly.

- There are three chapters:
    1. Detailed information on "How to Use *Delmar's Dental Drug Reference*"
    2. Alphabetical listing of therapeutic/chemical drug classes with general information for the class, plus a listing of drugs in the class covered in Chapter 3.
    3. Alphabetical listing of drugs by generic name.

- Each entry in Chapter 3 consists of two parts: general drug information and dental concerns

**General drug information** (similar in format to Chapter 2) includes the following categories (not all categories may be provided for each drug):

- **Combination Drug** heading indicates two or more drugs are combined in the same product.
- **Generic name** of drug with simplified **phonetic pronunciation**
- **FDA pregnancy category**
- **Trade name(s)** by which drug is marketed; a maple leaf (✸) indicates trade names available only in Canada
- **Drug schedule** if drug is controlled by U.S. Federal Controlled Substances Act (such as C-II, C-III)
- **Rx** = prescription drug; **OTC** = nonprescription, over-the-counter drug
- See also reference to classification in Chapter 2, if applicable
- **Classification** is the chemical or pharmacologic class to which the drug has been assigned.
- **Content** (for combination drugs) is the generic name and amount of each drug in the combination product.
- **General Statement:** General information and/or specific aspects of drugs in a class; also diseases for which drugs may be used
- **Action/Kinetics:** Mechanism(s) by which drug achieves therapeutic effect, rate of absorption, distribution, minimum effective serum or plasma level, half-life (time for half the drug to be removed from blood), duration of action, metabolism, excretion routes, and other pertinent information
- **Uses:** Therapeutic indications, including investigational uses for the drug
- **Contraindications:** Diseases or conditions for which drug should not be used
- **Special Concerns:** Considerations for use in pediatric, geriatric, pregnant, or lactating clients. Also situations or disease states when the drug should be used with caution.
- **Side Effects:** Undesired or bothersome effects in some clients, listed by

body organ or system affected. Life-threatening side effects are designated in boldface italics

– **Drug Interactions:** Drugs that may interact with one another resulting in an increase or decrease in effect of drug; when listed for a class of drugs, are likely to apply to all drugs in the class

– **Dosage:** Recommended adult and pediatric dosages for designated disease states, dosing intervals, and available dosage forms

– **Dental Concerns:** Provides general information to the practitioner regarding drug therapy and suggestions for consultation with the appropriate health care provider in order to prevent dental complications of disease

– **Client/Family Teaching:** Guidelines to promote education, active participation, understanding, precautions, and compliance with drug therapy and oral health care

• **Additional Contraindications or Additional Side Effects:** Information relevant to a specific drug but not necessarily to the class overall. More complete data can be found in the discussion of the drug class (Chapter 2).

• **Index:** Extensively cross-referenced; **boldface** = generic drug name; *italics* = therapeutic drug class; regular type = trade name; CAPITALS = combination drug names; trade name is paired with generic name to facilitate ease of locating

# Table of Contents

# Common Sound-Alike Drug Names

The following is a list of common sound-alike drug names; trade names are capitalized. In parentheses next to each drug name is the pharmacological classification/use for the drug.

Accupril (ACE inhibitor)

acetazolamide (antiglaucoma drug)

Adriamycin (antineoplastic)

albuterol (sympathomimetic)

Aldomet (antihypertensive)

allopurinol (antigout drug)

alprazolam (anti-anxiety agent)

Ambien (sedative-hypnotic)

amiloride (diuretic)

amiodarone (antiarrhythmic)

amitriptyline (antidepressant)

Apresazide (antihypertensive)

Arlidin (peripheral vasodilator)

Artane (cholinergic blocking agent)

asparaginase (antineoplastic agent)

Atarax (antianxiety agent)

atenolol (beta-blocker)

Atrovent (cholinergic blocking agent)

bacitracin (antibacterial)

Benylin (expectorant)

Brevital (barbiturate)

Bumex (diuretic)

Cafergot (analgesic)

calciferol (Vitamin D)

carboplatin (antineoplastic agent)

Cardene (calcium channel blocker)

Cataflam (NSAID)

Catapres (antihypertensive)

cefotaxime (cephalosporin)

cefuroxime (cephalosporin)

chlorpromazine (antipsychotic)

chlorpromazine (antipsychotic)

chlorpromazine (antipsychotic)

Accutane (antiacne drug)

acetohexamide (oral antidiabetic drug)

Aredia (bone growth regulator)

atenolol (beta-blocker)

Aldoril (antihypertensive)

Apresoline (antihypertensive)

lorazepam (anti-anxiety agent)

Amen (progestin)

amlodipine (calcium channel blocker)

amrinone (inotropic agent)

nortriptyline (antidepressant)

Apresoline (antihypertensive)

Aralen (antimalarial)

Altace (ACE inhibitor)

pegaspargase (antineoplastic agent)

Ativan (antianxiety agent)

timolol (beta-blocker)

Alupent (sympathomimetic)

Bactroban (anti-infective, topical)

Ventolin (sympathomimetic)

Brevibloc (beta-adrenergic blocker)

Buprenex (narcotic analgesic)

Carafate (antiulcer drug)

calcitriol (Vitamin D)

cisplatin (antineoplastic agent)

Cardizem (calcium channel blocker)

Catapres (antihypertensive)

Combipres (antihypertensive)

cefoxitin (cephalosporin)

deferoxamine (iron chelator)

chlorpropamide (oral antidiabetic)

prochlorperazine (antipsychotic)

promethazine (antihistamine)

Clinoril (NSAID) — Clozaril (antipsychotic)
clomipramine (antidepressant) — clomiphene (ovarian stimulant)
clonidine (antihypertensive) — Klonopin (anticonvulsant)
Cozaar (antihypertensive) — Zocor (antihyperlipidemic)
cyclobenzaprine (skeletal muscle relaxant) — cyproheptadine (antihistamine)

cyclophosphamide (antineoplastic) — cyclosporine (immunosuppressant)
cyclosporine (immunosuppressant) — cycloserine (antineoplastic)
Cytovene (antiviral drug) — Cytosar (antineoplastic)
Cytoxan (antineoplastic) — Cytotec (prostaglandin derivative)
Cytoxan (antineoplastic) — Cytosar (antineoplastic)
Dantrium (skeletal muscle relaxant) — danazol (gonadotropin inhibitor)
Darvocet-N (analgesic) — Darvon-N (analgesic)
daunorubicin (antineoplastic) — doxorubicin (antineoplastic)
desipramine (antidepressant) — diphenhydramine (antihistamine)
DiaBeta (oral hypoglycemic) — Zebeta (beta-adrenergic blocker)
digitoxin (cardiac glycoside) — digoxin (cardiac glycoside)
diphenhydramine (antihistamine) — dimenhydrinate (antihistamine)
dopamine (sympathomimetic) — dobutamine (sympathomimetic)
Edecrin (diuretic) — Eulexin (antineoplastic)
enalapril (ACE inhibitor) — Anafranil (antidepressant)
enalapril (ACE inhibitor) — Eldepryl (antiparkinson agent)
Eryc (erythromycin base) — Ery-Tab (erythromycin base)
etidronate (bone growth regulator) — etretinate (antipsoriatic)
etomidate (general anesthetic) — etidronate (bone growth regulator)
Fioricet (analgesic) — Fiorinal (analgesic)
flurbiprofen (NSAID) — fenoprofen (NSAID)
folinic acid (leucovorin calcium) — folic acid (vitamin B complex)
Gantrisin (sulfonamide) — Gantanol (sulfonamide)
glipizide (oral hypoglycemic) — glyburide (oral hypoglycemic)
glyburide (oral hypoglycemic) — Glucotrol (oral hypoglycemic)
Hycodan (cough preparation) — Hycomine (cough preparation)
hydralazine (antihypertensive) — hydroxyzine (antianxiety agent)
hydrocodone (narcotic analgesic) — hydrocortisone (corticosteroid)
hydromorphone (narcotic analgesic) — morphine (narcotic analgesic)
Hydropres (antihypertensive) — Diupres (antihypertensive)
Hytone (topical corticosteroid) — Vytone (topical corticosteroid)
imipramine (antidepressant) — Norpramin (antidepressant)
Inderal (beta-adrenergic blocker) — Inderide (antihypertensive)
Inderal (beta-adrenergic blocker) — Isordil (coronary vasodilator)
Indocin (NSAID) — Minocin (antibiotic)
Lanoxin (cardiac glycoside) — Lasix (diuretic)
Lioresal (muscle relaxant) — lisinopril (ACE inhibitor)
Lithostat (lithium carbonate) — Lithobid (lithium carbonate)
Lithotabs (lithium carbonate) — Lithobid (lithium carbonate)
Lodine (NSAID) — codeine (narcotic analgesic)

| | |
|---|---|
| Lopid (antihyperlipidemic) | Lorabid (beta-lactam antibiotic) |
| lovastatin (antihyperlipidemic) | Lotensin (ACE inhibitor) |
| metolazone (thiazide diuretic) | methotrexate (antineoplastic) |
| metolazone (thiazide diuretic) | metoclopramide (GI stimulant) |
| metoprolol (beta-adrenergic blocker) | misoprostol (prostaglandin derivative) |
| | |
| Monopril (ACE inhibitor) | minoxidil (antihypertensive) |
| nelfinavir (antiviral) | nevirapine (antiviral) |
| Norlutate (progestin) | Norlutin (progestin) |
| Norvasc (calcium channel blocker) | Navane (antipsychotic) |
| Ocufen (NSAID) | Ocuflox (fluoroquinolone antibiotic) |
| Orinase (oral hypoglycemic) | Ornade (upper respiratory product) |
| Percocet (narcotic analgesic) | Percodan (narcotic analgesic) |
| paroxetine (antidepressant) | paclitaxel (antineoplastic) |
| Paxil (antidepressant) | paclitaxel (antineoplastic) |
| Paxil (antidepressant) | Taxol (antineoplastic) |
| penicillamine (heavy metal antagonist) | penicillin (antibiotic) |
| pindolol (beta-adrenergic blocker) | Parlodel (inhibitor of prolactin secretion) |
| | |
| Platinol (antineoplastic) | Paraplatin (antineoplastic) |
| Pravachol (antihyperlipidemic) | Prevacid (GI drug) |
| Pravachol (antihyperlipidemic) | propranolol (beta-adrenergic blocker) |
| | |
| prednisolone (corticosteroid) | prednisone (corticosteroid) |
| Prilosec (inhibitor of gastric acid secretion) | Prozac (antidepressant) |
| | |
| Prinivil (ACE inhibitor) | Prilosec (GE drug) |
| Prinivil (ACE inhibitor) | Proventil (sympathomimetic) |
| propranolol (beta-adrenergic blocker) | Propulsid (GI drug) |
| Provera (progestin) | Premarin (estrogen) |
| Prozac (antidepressant) | Proscar (androgen hormone inhibitor) |
| | |
| quinidine (antiarrhythmic) | clonidine (antihypertensive) |
| quinidine (antiarrhythmic) | Quinamm (antimalarial) |
| quinine (antimalarial) | quinidine (antiarrhythmic) |
| Regroton (antihypertensive) | Hygroton (diuretic) |
| Rifamate (antituberculous drug) | rifampin (antituberculous drug) |
| Rimantadine (antiviral) | flutamide (antineoplastic) |
| Seldane (antihistamine) | Feldene (NSAID) |
| Stadol (narcotic analgesic) | Haldol (antipsychotic) |
| terbinafine (antifungal agent) | terfenadine (antihistamine) |
| terbutaline (sympathomimetic) | tolbutamide (oral hypoglycemic) |
| tolazamide (oral hypoglycemic) | tolbutamide (oral hypoglycemic) |
| torsemide (loop diuretic) | furosemide (loop diuretic) |
| trifluoperazine (antipsychotic) | trihexyphenidyl (antiparkinson drug) |

| | |
|---|---|
| Trimox (amoxicillin product) | Diamox (carbonic anhydrase inhibitor) |
| Vancenase (corticosteroid) | Vanceril (corticosteroid) |
| Vasosulf (sulfonamide/decongestant) | Velosef (cephalosporin) |
| Versed (benzodiazepine sedative) | Vistaril (antianxiety agent) |
| Versed (benzodiazepine sedative) | VePesid (antineoplastic) |
| Xanax (antianxiety agent) | Zantac ($H_2$ histamine blocker) |
| Zebeta (beta-blocker) | DiaBeta (oral hypoglycemic) |
| Zinacef (cephalosporin) | Zithromax (macrolide antibiotic) |
| Zocor (antihyperlipidemic) | Zoloft (antidepressant) |
| Zofran (antiemetic) | Zantac ($H_2$ histamine blocker) |
| Zosyn (penicillin antibiotic) | Zofran (antiemetic) |

# Commonly Used Abbreviations and Symbols

| | |
|---|---|
| aa, A | of each |
| a.c. | before meals |
| ACE | angiotensin-converting enzyme |
| ACLS | advanced cardiac life support |
| ACS | acute coronary syndrome |
| ACTH | adrenocorticotropic hormone |
| ad | to, up to |
| a.d. | right ear |
| ADD | attention deficit disorder |
| ad lib | as desired, at pleasure |
| ADP | adenosine diphosphate |
| ADH | antidiuretic hormone |
| ADL | activities of daily living |
| AFB | acid fast bacillus |
| AIDS | acquired immune deficiency syndrome |
| a.l. | left ear |
| a.m., A.M. | morning |
| AMI | acute myocardial infarction |
| AML | acute myeloid leukemia |
| ANS | autonomic nervous system |
| APTT | activated partial thromboplastin time |
| aq | water |
| aq dist. | distilled water |
| ARC | AIDS-related complex |
| ARDS | adult respiratory distress syndrome |
| ASA | aspirin |
| ASAP | as soon as possible |
| ASHD | arteriosclerotic heart disease |
| AST | aspartate aminotransferase |
| ATC | around the clock |
| ATS/CDC | American Thoracic Society/Centers for Disease Prevention and Control |
| ATU | antithrombin unit |
| ATX | antibiotics |
| a.u. | each ear, both ears |
| AV | atrioventricular |
| b.i.d. | two times per day |
| b.i.n. | two times per night |
| BP | blood pressure |
| BPD | bronchopulmonary dysplasia |
| BPH | benign prostatic hypertrophy |
| BS | blood sugar, bowel sounds |
| BSA | body surface area |
| BSE | breast self-exam |

| | |
|---|---|
| BSP | Bromsulphalein |
| BUN | blood urea nitrogen |
| C | Celsius/Centigrade |
| CABG | coronary artery bypass graft |
| CAD | coronary artery disease |
| caps, Caps | capsule(s) |
| CBC | complete blood count |
| CCB | calcium channel blocker |
| $C_{CR}$ | creatinine clearance |
| $CD_4$ | helper $T_4$ lymphocyte cells |
| CDC | Centers for Disease Control and Prevention |
| C&DB | cough and deep breathe |
| CF | cystic fibrosis |
| CHF | congestive heart failure |
| CHO | carbohydrate |
| CLL | chronic lymphocytic leukemia |
| cm | centimeter |
| CML | chronic myelocytic leukemia |
| CMV | cytomegalovirus |
| CNS | central nervous system |
| CO | cardiac output |
| COMT | catechol-o-methyltransferase |
| COPD | chronic obstructive pulmonary disease |
| CP | cardiopulmonary |
| CPK | creatine phosphokinase |
| CPR | cardiopulmonary resuscitation |
| CRF | chronic renal failure |
| CSF | cerebrospinal fluid |
| CSID | congenital sucrase-isomaltase deficiency |
| CT | computerized tomography |
| CTS | carpal tunnel syndrome |
| CTZ | chemoreceptor trigger zone |
| CV | cardiovascular |
| CVA | cerebrovascular accident |
| CXR | chest X ray |
| DBP | diastolic BP |
| dc | discontinue |
| DEA | Drug Enforcement Agency |
| DI | diabetes insipidus |
| dil. | dilute |
| dL | deciliter (one-tenth of a liter) |
| DM | diabetes mellitus |
| DNA | deoxyribonucleic acid |
| DOE | dyspnea on exertion |
| dr. | dram (0.0625 ounce) |
| DVT | deep vein thrombosis |
| EC | enteric-coated |
| ECG, EKG | electrocardiogram, electrocardiograph |
| EEG | electroencephalogram |
| EENT | eye, ear, nose, and throat |
| EF | ejection fraction |
| e.g. | for example |
| elix | elixir |
| emuls. | emulsion |
| ENL | erythema nodosum leprosum |
| ENT | ear, nose, throat |

| | |
|---|---|
| EPS | electrophysiologic studies, extrapyramidal symptoms |
| ER | extended release |
| ESRD | end-stage renal disease |
| ET | endotracheal |
| ETOH | alcohol |
| ext. | extract |
| F | Fahrenheit, fluoride |
| FBS | fasting blood sugar |
| FDA | Food and Drug Administration |
| FEV | forced expiratory volume |
| FOB | fecal occult blood |
| FS | finger stick |
| FSH | follicle-stimulating hormone |
| F/U | follow-up |
| FVC | forced vital capacity |
| g, gm | gram (1,000 mg) |
| GABA | gamma-aminobutyric acid |
| GERD | gastroesophageal reflux disease |
| GFR | glomerular filtration rate |
| GGT | gamma-glutamyl transferase: *syn.* gamma-glutamyl transpeptidase |
| gi, GI | gastrointestinal |
| GnRH | gonadotropin-releasing hormone |
| GP | glycoprotein |
| G6PD | glucose-6-phosphate dehydrogenase |
| gr | grain |
| gtt | a drop, drops |
| GU | genitourinary |
| h, hr | hour |
| HCG | human chorionic gonadotropin |
| HCP | health-care provider |
| HCV | hepatitis C virus |
| HDL | high density lipoprotein |
| H&H | hematocrit and hemoglobin |
| HIT | heparin-induced thrombocytopenia |
| HIV | human immunodeficiency virus |
| HMG-CoA | 3-hydroxy-3-methyl-glutaryl-coenzyme A |
| HOB | head of bed |
| HR | heart rate |
| h.s. | at bedtime |
| HSE | herpes simplex encephalitis |
| HSV | herpes simplex virus |
| 5-HT | 5-hydroxytryptamine |
| HTN | hypertension |
| IA | intra-arterial |
| IBD | inflammatory bowel disease |
| ICP | intracranial pressure |
| ICU | intensive care unit |
| Ig | immunoglobulin |
| im, IM | intramuscular |
| IOP | intraocular pressure |
| IPPB | intermittent positive pressure breathing |
| ITP | idiopathic thrombocytopenia purpura |
| IU | international units |
| iv, IV | intravenous |
| kg | kilogram (2.2 lb) |

| | |
|---|---|
| l, L | liter (1,000 mL) |
| L | left |
| LDH | lactic dehydrogenase |
| LDL | low density lipoprotein |
| LFTs | liver function tests |
| LH | luteinizing hormone |
| LHRH | luteinizing hormone-releasing hormone |
| LOC | level of consciousness |
| LV | left ventricular |
| LVFP | left ventricular function pressure |
| m | meter |
| MAC | *Mycobacterium avium* complex |
| MAO | monoamine oxidase |
| max | maximum |
| mcg | microgram |
| MDI | metered-dose inhaler |
| mEq | milliequivalent |
| mg | milligram |
| MI | myocardial infarction |
| MIC | minimum inhibitory concentration |
| min | minute, minim |
| mist, mixt | mixture |
| mL | milliliter |
| MRI | magnetic resonance imaging |
| MS | multiple sclerosis |
| NaCl | sodium chloride |
| ng | nanogram |
| NIDDM | non-insulin dependent diabetes mellitus |
| NKA | no known allergies |
| NKDA | no known drug allergies |
| noct | at night, during the night |
| non rep | do not repeat |
| NPN | nonprotein nitrogen |
| NPO | nothing by mouth |
| NR | do not refill (e.g., a prescription) |
| NSAID | nonsteroidal anti-inflammatory drug |
| NSR | normal sinus rhythm |
| NSS | normal saline solution |
| N&V | nausea and vomiting |
| $O_2$ | oxygen |
| o.d. | once a day |
| O.D. | right eye |
| OH | orthostatic hypotension |
| OOB | out of bed |
| OR | operating room |
| os | mouth |
| O.S. | left eye |
| OTC | over the counter |
| O.U. | each eye, both eyes |
| oz | ounce |
| PABA | para-aminobenzoic acid |
| p.c. | after meals |
| PCA | patient-controlled analgesia |
| PCN | penicillin |
| PCP | *Pneumocystis carinii* pneumonia |
| per | by, through |

| | |
|---|---|
| PID | pelvic inflammatory disease |
| PMH | past medical history |
| PMS | premenstrual syndrome |
| PND | paroxysmal nocturnal dyspnea |
| po, p.o., PO | by mouth |
| PR | by rectum |
| p.r.n., PRN | when needed or necessary |
| PSP | phenolsulfonphthalein |
| PT | prothrombin time |
| PTH | parathyroid hormone |
| PTSD | post traumatic stress disorder |
| PTT | partial thromboplastin time |
| PUD | peptic ulcer disease |
| PVD | peripheral vascular disease |
| q.d. | every day |
| q.h. | every hour |
| q2hr | every two hours |
| q3hr | every three hours |
| q4hr | every four hours |
| q6hr | every six hours |
| q8hr | every eight hours |
| qhs | every night |
| q.i.d. | four times a day |
| qmo | every month |
| q.o.d. | every other day |
| q.s. | as much as needed, quantity sufficient |
| RA | right atrium; rheumatoid arthritis |
| RBC | red blood cell |
| RDA | recommended daily allowance |
| REM | rapid eye movement |
| Rept. | let it be repeated |
| RNA | ribonucleic acid |
| ROS | review of systems |
| RV | right ventricular |
| RUQ | right upper quadrant |
| Rx | symbol for a prescription |
| SA | sinoatrial or sustained-action |
| SBE | subacute bacterial endocarditis |
| SBP | systolic BP |
| sc, SC, SQ | subcutaneous |
| S., Sig. | mark on the label |
| SI | sacroiliac |
| SIADH | syndrome inappropriate antidiuretic hormone |
| SL | sublingual |
| SLE | systemic lupus erythematosus |
| SOB | shortness of breath |
| sol | solution |
| sp | spirits |
| SR | sustained-release |
| ss | one-half |
| S&S | signs and symptoms |
| stat | immediately, first dose |
| STD | sexually transmitted disease |
| syr | syrup |
| tab | tablet |
| TB | tuberculosis |

| | |
|---|---|
| TCA | tricyclic antidepressant |
| TIA | transient ischemic attack |
| TIBC | total iron binding capacity |
| t.i.d. | three times per day |
| t.i.n. | three times per night |
| TKR | total knee replacement |
| TNF | tumor necrosis factor |
| T.O. | telephone order |
| TSH | thyroid stimulating hormone |
| U | unit |
| $\mu$ | micron |
| $\mu$Ci | microcurie |
| $\mu$g | microgram |
| $\mu$m | micrometer |
| UGI | upper gastrointestinal |
| ULN | upper limit of normal |
| ung | ointment |
| UO | urine output |
| URI, URTI | upper respiratory infection |
| US | ultrasound |
| USP | U. S. Pharmacopeia |
| ut dict | as directed |
| UTI | urinary tract infection |
| UV | ultraviolet |
| VAD | venous access device |
| VF | ventricular fibrillation |
| vin | wine |
| vit | vitamin |
| VLDL | very low density lipoprotein |
| VMA | vanillylmandelic acid |
| V.O. | verbal order |
| VS | vital signs |
| VT | ventricular tachycardia |
| WBC | white blood cell |
| XRT | radiation therapy |
| & | and |
| > | greater than |
| < | less than |
| ↑ | increased, higher |
| ↓ | decreased, lower |
| - | negative |
| / | per |
| % | percent |
| + | positive |
| x | times, frequency |

# CHAPTER ONE

# How To Use Delmar's Dental Drug Reference

*Delmar's Dental Drug Reference* is intended to be a quick reference to obtain useful information on drugs. An important objective is also to provide information on the proper monitoring of drug therapy and to assist practitioners in teaching clients and family members about important aspects of dental drug therapy.

Chapter 2 includes general information on important therapeutic or chemical classes of drugs. The classes of drugs are listed alphabetically. Specific drugs in therapeutic or chemical classes are found in Chapter 3 (alphabetical listing of drugs). The information on each therapeutic or chemical class in Chapter 2 begins with a list of the drugs addressed in that drug class. Information on the specific drugs is provided under that drug name in Chapter 3. Chapter 3 also includes information on many other drugs.

The format for information on individual drugs (and for drug classes when appropriate) is presented as follows:

**Drug Names:** The generic name for the drug is presented first; this is followed by the phonetic pronunciation of the generic name. The FDA pregnancy category A, B, C, D, or X (see Appendix 3 for definitions) to which the drug is assigned is also listed in this section. All trade names follow this; if the trade name is available only in Canada, the name is followed by a maple leaf ( ✽). If the drug is controlled by the U.S. Federal Controlled Substances Act, the schedule in which the drug is placed follows the trade name (e.g., C-II, C-

III, C-IV or I, II, III, IV, V). See Appendix 1 for a listing of controlled substances in both the United States and Canada. A combination drug heading indicates that two or more drugs are combined in the same product.

**Classification:** This section defines the type of drug or the class under which the drug is listed. This information is most useful in learning to categorize drugs. To minimize the need to repeat general information, a cross reference to Chapter 2 is often made for drugs listed in Chapter 3. This information should also be consulted.

**General Statement:** Information about the drug class and/or what might be specific or unusual about a particular group of drugs is presented. In addition, brief information may be presented about the disease(s) for which the drugs are indicated.

**Action/Kinetics:** The action portion describes the proposed mechanism(s) by which a drug achieves its therapeutic effect. Not all mechanisms of action are known, and some are self-evident, as when a hormone is administered as a replacement. The kinetics portion lists pertinent pharmacologic properties, if known, about rate of drug absorption, distribution, time for peak plasma levels or peak effect, minimum effective serum or plasma level, biologic half-life, duration of action, metabolism, and excretion. Metabolism and excretion routes may be important for clients with systemic liver disease, kidney disease, or both. Again, information is not available for all therapeutic agents.

The time it takes for half the drug to be excreted or removed from the blood, t½ (half-life), is important in determining how often a drug is to be administered and how long to assess for side effects. Therapeutic levels indicate the desired concentration, in serum or plasma, for the drug to exert its beneficial effect and are helpful in predicting the onset of side effects or the lack of effect. Drug therapy is often monitored in this fashion (e.g., antibiotics, theophylline, phenytoin, amiodarone).

**Uses:** Approved therapeutic use(s) for the particular drug are presented. Some investigational uses are also listed for selected drugs.

**Contraindications:** Disease states or conditions in which the drug should not be used are noted. The safe use of many of the newer pharmacologic agents during pregnancy, lactation, or childhood has not been established. As a general rule, the use of drugs during pregnancy is contraindicated unless specified by the provider where the benefits of drug therapy far outweigh the potential risks.

**Special Concerns:** This section covers considerations for use with pediatric, geriatric, pregnant, or lactating clients. Situations and disease states when the drug should be used with caution are also listed.

**Side Effects:** Undesired or bothersome effects the client *may* experience while taking a particular agent are described. Side effects are listed by the body organ or system affected and are usually presented with the most common side effects in descending order of incidence. It is important to note that nearly all of the potential side effects are listed; in any given clinical situation, however, a client may show no side effects, or one or more side effects. If potentially life threatening, the side effect is indicated by boldface italic print.

**Drug Interactions:** This is an alphabetical listing of drugs that may interact with one another. This section focuses on those drug interactions which are of particular concern to dental health and dental practitioners. The study of drug interactions is an important area of pharmacology and is changing constantly as a result of the influx of new drugs, clinical feedback, and increased client usage. The compilation of such interactions is far from complete; therefore, listings in this handbook are to be considered *only* as general cautionary guidelines.

Drug interactions may result from a number of different mechanisms (e.g., additive or inhibitory effects, interference with degradation of drug, increased rate of elimination, decreased absorption from the GI tract, and competition for or displacement from receptor sites or plasma protein binding sites). Such interactions may manifest themselves in a variety of ways; however, an attempt has been made throughout the text to describe these interactions whenever possible as an increase ($\uparrow$) or a decrease ($\downarrow$) in the effect of the drug, and a reason for the change.

It is important to realize that any side effects that accompany the administration of a particular agent also may be increased as a result of a drug interaction.

The reader should be aware that drug interactions are often listed for classes of drugs. Thus, the drug interaction is likely to occur for all drugs in a particular class. Consult this information in Chapter 2.

**How Supplied:** The various dosage form(s) available for the drug and amounts of the drug in each of the dosage forms is presented. Such information is important as one dosage form may be more appropriate for a client than another. This information also allows the user to ensure the appropriate dosage form and strength is being administered.

**Dosage:** The dosage form and route of administration is followed by the disease state or condition (in italics) for which the dosage is recommended. This is followed by the adult and pediatric doses, when available. The listed dosage is to be considered as a general guideline; the exact amount of the drug to be given is determined by the provider. However, one should question orders when dosages differ markedly from the accepted norm.

**Dental Concerns:** The dental concerns section was developed to assist the practitioner to apply the assessment process to pharmacotherapeutics. Guidelines for assessing the client before, during, and after drug therapy are identified as are interventions for the prescribed therapy.

The practitioner must also assess the client for the *Side Effects* which must be documented and reported to the provider. Severe side effects generally are cause for dosage modification or discontinuation of the drug.

**Client/Family Teaching:** Specific information for the client is provided for each drug. Client/family teaching emphasizes specifics to help the client/family recognize side effects, avoid potentially dangerous situations, and to alleviate anxiety that may result from taking a particular drug. Side effects that require medical intervention are included as well as specifics on how to minimize side effects for certain medications (i.e., take medication with food to decrease GI upset or take at bedtime to minimize daytime sedative effects).

The proper education of clients is one of the most challenging aspects of dental care. The instructions must be tailored to the needs, awareness, and sophistication of each client. For example, clients who take medication to lower BP should assume responsibility for taking their own BP or having it taken and recorded. Clients should carry identification listing the drugs currently prescribed. They should know what they are taking and why, and develop a mechanism to remind themselves to take their medication as prescribed. Clients should carry this drug list with them whenever they go for a check-up or seek medical care. The drug list should be shared with the pharmacist if there is a question concerning

drugs prescribed, if the client is considering taking an over-the-counter medication, or if the client has to change pharmacies. The records, especially BP recordings, should be shared with the health care provider to ensure accurate evaluation of the response to the prescribed drug therapy. This may also alert the provider to any medication consumption by the client that they did not prescribe, were not aware of, or that may interfere with (i.e., potentiate, antagonize) the current pharmacologic regimen. The provider may also encourage the client to call with any questions or concerns about their therapy.

Finally, when taking the dental history, emphasis should be placed on the client's ability to read and to follow directions. Clients with language barriers should be identified, and appropriate written translations should be provided. In addition, client life-style, cultural factors, and income as well as the availability of health insurance and transportation are important factors that may affect adherence with therapy and followup care. The potential for a client being/becoming pregnant, and whether a mother is breast feeding her infant should be included in assessments. The age and orientation level, whether learned from personal observation or from discussion with close friends or family members, can be critical in determining potential relationships between drug therapy and/or drug interactions. Including these factors in the dental health assessment will assist all on the dental care team to determine the type of therapy and drug delivery system best suited to a particular client and promotes the highest level of adherence.

Information that requires emphasis or is relevant to a particular drug is listed under appropriate headings, such as *Additional Contraindications* or *Additional Side Effects*. These are *in addition to* and not *instead of* the regular entry, which is referenced and must also be consulted.

The scope of drugs covered in this reference includes traditional dental drugs used in the treatment of periodontal disease, antibiotic prophylaxis, and pain management with amide local anesthetics, NSAIDs, and opioid analgesics. Also, coverage is provided for other dental related drugs that are given systemically for the treatment of anxiety and other general infections. Coverage also includes cardiovascular drugs, opioid analgesics, opioid antagonists, drugs used for smoking cessation programs, and certain other drugs of special interest to dental practitioners.

Additional information to assist in monitoring drug therapy is also included. A list of sound-alike drug names is included in the front portion of the book to alert the provider to these similarities in an effort to prevent a potential lethal error. Also helpful are the Elements of a Pre-scription (Appendix 2), Drugs Causing Dry Mouth by Class (Appendix 4), Commonly Used Abbreviations and Symbols (front portion of book).

The Index has been designed for maximum efficiency in finding a drug. Generic drug names are presented in boldface, trade names in regular type, therapeutic drug classes in italics, and combination drugs in all capital letters. In addition, each generic name is followed, in parentheses, by the most common trade name; and, each trade name is followed, in parentheses, by the generic name.

You are now ready to use *Delmar's Dental Drug Reference*. We hope that the text will be useful and assist you in your education, profession, and practice. The safe administration of drugs, assessment of potential interactions and adverse effects, as well as outcome evaluation are crucial parts of the dental health process.

# CHAPTER TWO
# Therapeutic Drug Classifications

## ALPHA-1-ADRENERGIC BLOCKING AGENTS

*See also the following individual entries:*

Doxazosin mesylate
Prazosin hydrochloride
Terazosin

See also *Beta-Adrenergic Blocking Agents.*

**Action/Kinetics:** Selectively block postsynaptic alpha-1-adrenergic receptors. Results in dilation of both arterioles and veins leading to a decrease in supine and standing BP. Diastolic BP is affected the most. Prazosin and terazosin do not produce reflex tachycardia. Terazosin also relaxes smooth muscle in the bladder neck and prostate, making it useful to treat BPH.

Adrenergic blocking agents have many undesirable effects which, although not toxic, limit their use. Always start treatment at low doses and increase gradually.

**Uses:** Alone or in combination with diuretics or beta-adrenergic blocking agents to treat hypertension. Doxazosin and terazosin are used to treat BPH. *Non-FDA Approved Uses:* Prazosin is used for refractory CHF, management of Raynaud's vasospasm, and to treat BPH. Doxazosin, along with digoxin and diuretics, is used to treat CHF.

**Contraindications:** Hypersensitivity to these drugs (i.e., quinazolines).

**Special Concerns:** The first few doses may cause postural hypotension and syncope with sudden loss of consciousness. Use with caution in lactation, with impaired hepatic function, or if receiving drugs known to influence hepatic metabolism. Safety and efficacy have not been established in children.

**Side Effects:** The following side effects are common to alpha-1-adrenergic blockers. See individual drugs as well. *Oral:* Dry mouth. *CV:* Palpitations, postural hypotension, hypotension, tachycardia, chest pain, arrhythmia. *GI:* N&V, diarrhea, constipation, abdominal discomfort or pain, flatulence. *CNS:* Dizziness, depression, decreased libido, sexual dysfunction, nervousness, paresthesia, somnolence, anxiety, insomnia, asthenia, drowsiness. *Musculoskeletal:* Pain in the shoulder, neck, or back; gout, arthritis, joint pain, arthralgia. *Respiratory:* Dyspnea, nasal congestion, sinusitis, bronchitis, **bronchospasm,** cold symptoms, epistaxis, increased cough, flu symptoms, pharyngitis, rhinitis. *Ophthalmic:* Blurred vision, abnormal vision, reddened sclera, conjunctivitis. *GU:* Impotence, urinary frequency, incontinence. *Miscellaneous:* Tinnitus, vertigo, pruritus, sweating, alopecia, lichen planus, headache, edema, weight gain, facial edema, fever.

**Drug Interactions:** See individual agents.

**Dosage** ───────────
See individual agents.

### DENTAL CONCERNS
**General**
1. Monitor vital signs at every appointment because of cardiovascular effects.

2. Have the patient sit up slowly and remain seated for at least two minutes after being supine in order to minimize the risk of orthostatic hypotension.

3. Decreased saliva flow can put the patient at risk for dental caries, periodontal disease, and candidiasis.

**Consultation with Primary Care Provider**

1. Consultation with primary care provider may be necessary to assess patient status (disease control and ability to tolerate stress).

**Client/Family Teaching**

1. Daily home fluoride treatments for persistent dry mouth.

2. Avoid alcohol-containing mouth rinses and beverages.

3. Avoid caffeine-containing beverages.

4. Dry mouth can be treated with tart, sugarless gum or candy, water, sugar-free beverages, or with saliva substitutes if dry mouth persists.

---

# AMIDE LOCAL ANESTHETIC AGENTS

*See also the following individual entries:*

  Bupivacaine hydrochloride
  Etidocaine hydrochloride
  Lidocaine hydrochloride
  Mepivacaine hydrochloride
  Prilocaine hydrochloride

**Action/Kinetics:** These drugs inhibit ion transfers across the membrane, in particular, sodium transport across the cell membrane; decrease the rise of the depolarization phase of the action potential; block nerve action potential. Pharmacokinetics: See individual drugs.

**Uses:** See individual drugs.

**Contraindications:** Hypersensitivity, severe liver disease.

**Special Concerns:** Elderly, severe drug allergies, children.

**Side Effects:** *Oral:* Numbness, tingling, trismus. *GI:* Nausea, vomiting. *CNS:* Drowsiness, disorientation, tremors, shivering, anxiety, restlessness, *seizures, loss of consciousness.*

*Cardiovascular: **Myocardial depression, cardiac arrest, dysrhythmias,*** bradycardia, hypotension, hypertension, fetal bradycardia. *Pulmonary: **status asthmaticus, respiratory arrest, anaphylaxis.*** *Skin:* Rash, urticaria, allergic reaction, edema, burning, skin discoloration at the site of injection, tissue necrosis. *Miscellaneous:* Blurred vision, tinnitus, pupil constriction.

**Drug Interactions**

*Beta-adrenergic blockers* / ↑ Risk of cardiovascular side effects with rapid intravascular administration of a local anesthetic containing a vasoconstrictor

*Cocaine* / ↑ Risk of cardiovascular side effects with rapid intravascular administration of a local anesthetic containing a vasoconstrictor

*CNS depressants* / ↑ Risk of CNS depression

*Digoxin* / ↑ Risk of cardiovascular side effects with rapid intravascular administration of a local anesthetic containing a vasoconstrictor

*Halogenated hydrocarbons* / ↑ Risk of cardiovascular side effects with rapid intravascular administration of a local anesthetic containing a vasoconstrictor

*MAOIs* / ↑ Risk of cardiovascular side effects with rapid intravascular administration of a local anesthetic containing a vasoconstrictor

*Phenothiazines* / ↑ Risk of cardiovascular side effects with rapid intravascular administration of a local anesthetic containing a vasoconstrictor

*Tricyclic antidepressants* / ↑ Risk of cardiovascular side effects with rapid intravascular administration of a local anesthetic containing a vasoconstrictor

**Dosage** —————————————
See individual agents.

---

## DENTAL CONCERNS
### General

1. Dental cartridges should not be placed in disinfectant solutions with heavy metals or surface active agents. Metal ions may be released

into the local anesthetic solution which could cause tissue irritation upon injection.

2. Excessive exposure of dental cartridges to light or heat can lead to deterioration of the vasoconstrictor. Inspect the cartridge for color changes which would indicate a breakdown.

3. Vasoconstrictors should not be used in patients with uncontrolled hypertension, angina, hyperthyroidism, or diabetes. Patients should be referred to their primary health care provider for medical evaluation before an elective procedure is performed.

4. Dry lips can be lubricated prior to injection or dental teatment as necessary.

5. Monitor vital signs at every appointment because of cardiovascular and respiratory side effects.

**Client/Family Teaching**

1. Do not eat or chew gum following dental anesthesia and use care to prevent injury while still numb.

2. The numbness will last for several hours.

3. Report any signs of infection, muscle pain, or fever when oral sensations return.

4. Report any unusual soft tissue reactions.

# AMINOGLYCOSIDES

*See also the following individual entries:*

Gentamicin sulfate

**Action/Kinetics:**  Broad-spectrum antibiotics believed to inhibit protein synthesis by binding irreversibly to ribosomes (30S subunit).

Rapidly absorbed after IM injection. **Peak plasma levels, after IM:** Usually ½–2 hr. Measurable levels persist for 8–12 hr after a single administration. **t½:** 2–3 hr (increases sharply in impaired kidney function). Ranges of t½ from 24 to 110 hr have been observed. Excreted mainly unchanged in urine. Resistance develops slowly.

**Uses:**  Are powerful antibiotics that induce serious side effects—do not use for minor infections. Gram-negative bacteria causing bone and joint infections, septicemia (including neonatal sepsis), skin and soft tissue infections (including those from burns), respiratory tract infections, postoperative infections, intra-abdominal infections (including peritonitis), UTIs. In combination with clindamycin for mixed aerobic-anaerobic infections. Also, see individual drugs.

Used for gram-positive bacteria only when other less toxic drugs are either ineffective or contraindicated. Use in CNS *Pseudomonas* infections such as meningitis or ventriculitis is questionable.

**Contraindications:**  Hypersensitivity to aminoglycosides, long-term therapy (except streptomycin for tuberculosis). Use with extreme caution with impaired renal function or preexisting hearing impairment. Safe use in pregnancy and during lactation not established.

**Special Concerns:**  Assess premature infants, neonates, and older clients closely as they are particularly sensitive to toxic effects. Considerable cross-allergenicity occurs among the aminoglycosides.

**Side Effects:** *Ototoxicity:* Both auditory and vestibular damage have been noted. The risk of ototoxicity and vestibular impairment is increased with poor renal function and in the elderly. Auditory symptoms include tinnitus and hearing impairment, while vestibular symptoms include dizziness, nystagmus, vertigo, and ataxia.

*Renal Impairment:* This may be characterized by cylindruria, oliguria, proteinuria, azotemia, hematuria, increase or decrease in frequency of urination; increased BUN, NPN, or creatinine; and increased thirst. *Neurotoxicity:* Neuromuscular blockade, headache, tremor, lethargy, paresthesia, peripheral neuritis (numbness, tingling, or burning of face/mouth), arachnoiditis, encephalopathy, acute organic brain syndrome. CNS depression, characterized by stupor, flaccidity, and rarely, **coma, and respiratory depression in infants.** Optic neuritis with blurred vision or loss of vision. *GI:* N&V, diarrhea, increased salivation, anorexia, weight loss. *Allergic:* Rash, urticaria, pruritus, burning, fever, stomatitis, eosinophilia. Rarely, **agranulocytosis and anaphylaxis.** Cross-allergy among aminoglycosides has been observed. *Miscellaneous:* Joint pain, **laryngeal edema, pulmonary fibrosis,** superinfection.

**Drug Interactions**
*Cephalosporins* / ↑ Risk of renal toxicity
*Ciprofloxacin HCl* / Additive antibacterial activity
*Methoxyflurane* / ↑ Risk of renal toxicity
*Penicillins* / ↓ Effect of aminoglycosides
*Polymyxins* / ↑ Muscle relaxation
*Skeletal muscle relaxants (surgical)* / ↑ Muscle relaxation
*Vancomycin* / Additive ototoxicity and renal toxicity

**DENTAL CONCERNS**

See also *General Dental Concerns for All Anti-Infectives.*

---

# AMPHETAMINES AND DERIVATIVES

*See also the following individual entries:*

Amphetamine sulfate
Dextroamphetamine sulfate

**Action/Kinetics:** Thought to act on the cerebral cortex and reticular activating system (including the medullary, respiratory, and vasomotor centers) by releasing norepinephrine and dopamine from central adrenergic neurons. Readily absorbed from the GI tract and distributed throughout most tissues, with the highest concentrations in the brain and CSF. Duration of anorexia (PO): 3–6 hr. Metabolized in liver and excreted by kidneys. Excreted slowly (5–7 days);

cumulative effects may occur with continued administration.

Psychic stimulation is often followed by a rebound effect manifested as fatigue. Tolerance will develop to all drugs of this class. There is a relatively wide margin of safety between the therapeutic and toxic doses of amphetamines. However, both acute and chronic toxicity can occur.

**Uses:** See individual drugs.

**Contraindications:** Hyperthyroidism, advanced arteriosclerosis, nephritis, diabetes mellitus, hypertension, narrow-angle glaucoma, angina pectoris, CV disease, and individuals with hypersensitivity to these drugs. Use in emotionally unstable persons susceptible to drug abuse and in agitated states. Psychotic children. Lactation. Appetite suppressants in children less than 12 years of age. Concurrent use or within 14 days of MAO inhibitors.

**Special Concerns:** Use with caution in clients suffering from hyperexcitability states; in elderly, debilitated, or asthenic clients; and in clients with psychopathic personality traits or a history of homicidal or suicidal tendencies.

**Side Effects:** *CNS:* Nervousness, dizziness, depression, headache, insomnia, euphoria, symptoms of excitation. Rarely, psychoses. In children, manifestation of vocal and motor tics and Tourette's syndrome. *Oral:* Dry mouth, metallic taste. *GI:* N&V, cramps, diarrhea, constipation, anorexia. *CV:* Arrhythmias, palpitations, dyspnea, pulmonary hypertension, peripheral hyper- or hypotension, precordial pain, fainting. *Dermatologic:* Symptoms of allergy including rash, urticaria, erythema, burning. Pallor. *GU:* Urinary frequency, dysuria. *Ophthalmologic:* Blurred vision, mydriasis. *Hematologic:* **Agranulocytosis,** leukopenia. *Endocrine:* Menstrual irregularities, gynecomastia, impotence, and changes in libido. *Miscellaneous:* Alopecia, increased motor activity, fever, sweating, chills, muscle pain, chest pain.

Long-term use results in psychic

dependence, as well as a high degree of tolerance.

**Drug Interactions**

*Anesthetics, general* / ↑ Risk of cardiac arrhythmias and other serious cardiovascular side effects

*Caffeine or caffeine-containing products* / ↑ Risk of insomnia and dry mouth

*MAO inhibitors* / All peripheral, metabolic, cardiac, and central effects of amphetamine are potentiated for up to 2 weeks after termination of MAO inhibitor therapy (symptoms include hypertensive crisis with possible intracranial hemorrhage, hyperthermia, convulsions, coma); death may occur. ↓ Effect of amphetamine by ↓ uptake of drug into its site of action

*Meperidine* / ↑ Risk of serious side-effects

*Phenothiazines* / ↓ Effect of amphetamine by ↓ uptake of drug at its site of action

*Propoxyphene* / ↑ Risk of serious side effects

*Sodium bicarbonate* / ↑ Effect of amphetamine by ↑ renal tubular reabsorption

*Tricyclic antidepressants* / ↓ Effect of amphetamines

**Dosage** ⎯⎯⎯⎯⎯⎯⎯⎯⎯

See individual drugs. Many compounds are timed-release preparations.

**DENTAL CONCERNS**

**General**

1. Monitor vital signs at every appointment because of cardiovascular side effects.

2. Decreased saliva flow can put the patient at risk for dental caries, periodontal disease, and candidiasis.

3. Psychological and physical dependence can occur with chronic use.

**Consultation with Primary Care Provider**

1. Consultation may be required to assess patient's health status.

**Client/Family Teaching**

1. Daily home fluoride treatment for chronic dry mouth.

2. Avoid OTC medications and ingesting large amounts of caffeine in any form. Caffeine can exacerbate dry mouth. Read labels for the detection of caffeine since this contributes to CV side effects.

3. Avoid alcohol-containing mouth rinses and beverages.

4. Dry mouth can be treated with tart, sugarless gum or candy, water, sugar-free beverages, or with saliva substitutes if dry mouth persists.

---

# ANGIOTENSIN-CONVERTING ENZYME (ACE) INHIBITORS

*See also the following individual entries:*

> Benazepril hydrochloride
> Captopril
> Enalapril maleate
> Fosinopril sodium
> Lisinopril
> Ramipril

**Action/Kinetics:** Believed to act by suppressing the renin-angiotensin-aldosterone system. The ACE inhibitors prevent the conversion of angiotensin I to angiotensin II. This results in a decrease in plasma angiotensin II and subsequently a decrease in peripheral resistance and decreased aldosterone secretion (leading to sodium and fluid loss) and therefore a decrease in BP.

**Uses:** Alone or in combination with other antihypertensive agents (especially thiazide diuretics) for the treatment of hypertension. Several are used to treat congestive heart failure. See also individual drug entries.

**Contraindications:** History of angioedema due to previous treatment with an ACE inhibitor.

**Special Concerns:** Use during the second and third trimesters of pregnancy can result in injury and even death to the developing fetus. May cause a profound drop in BP following the first dose; initiate therapy under close medical supervision. Use with caution in renal disease (especially renal artery stenosis) as increases in BUN and serum creatinine have occurred. Use with caution in clients with aortic stenosis due to possible decreased coronary perfusion following vasodilator use. With the exception of fosinopril (contraindicated), use with caution during lactation. Geriatric clients may show a greater sensitivity to the hypotensive effects of ACE inhibitors although these drugs may preserve or improve renal function and reverse LV hypertrophy. For most ACE inhibitors, safety and effectiveness have not been determined in children.

**Side Effects:** See individual entries. Side effects common to most ACE inhibitors include the following. *Oral:* Dry mouth, loss of taste, oral ulceration. *GI:* Abdominal pain, N&V, diarrhea, constipation, dry mouth. *CNS:* Sleep disturbances, insomnia, headache, dizziness, fatigue, nervousness, paresthesias. *CV:* Hypotension (especially following the first dose), palpitations, angina pectoris, **MI,** orthostatic hypotension, chest pain. *Hepatic:* Rarely, cholestatic jaundice progressing to **hepatic necrosis and death.** *Miscellaneous:* Chronic cough, dyspnea, increased sweating, diaphoresis, pruritus, rash, impotence, syncope, asthenia, arthralgia, myalgia. **Angioedema** of the face, lips, tongue, glottis, larynx, extremities, and mucous membranes. **Anaphylaxis.**

**Drug Interactions**
*Anesthetics* / ↑ Risk of hypotension if used with anesthetics that also cause hypotension
*Antacids* / Possible ↓ bioavailability of ACE inhibitors
*Indomethacin* / ↓ Hypotensive effects of ACE inhibitors, especially in low renin or volume-dependent hypertensive clients
*NSAIDS* / Possible ↓ hypotensive effects of ACE inhibitors
*Phenothiazines* / ↑ Effect of ACE inhibitors

*Sympathomimetics* / Possible ↓ hypotensive effects of ACE inhibitors

**Dosage**
See individual drugs.

## DENTAL CONCERNS
**General**
1. Monitor vital signs at every appointment because of cardiovascular and respiratory side effects.
2. Report any evidence of angioedema (swelling of face, lips, extremities, tongue, mucous membranes, glottis, or larynx) esp. after first dose (but may also be delayed response).
3. Have the patient sit up slowly and remain seated for at least two minutes after being supine in order to minimize the risk of orthostatic hypotension.
4. Decreased saliva flow can put the patient at risk for dental caries, periodontal disease, and candidiasis.
5. Dental procedures may cause the patient anxiety or place stress on the heart. Assess cardiovascular patient for this risk.
6. Early-morning and shorter appointments as well as methods for addressing anxiety levels in the patient can help to reduce the amount of stress that the patient is experiencing.
7. Patients on chronic drug therapy may develop blood dyscrasias. Symptoms include fever, sore throat, and bleeding, and poor wound healing.
8. Patients on sodium-restricted diets should receive sodium-containing fluids (i.e., saline solution) with caution.
9. Vasoconstrictors should be used with caution, in low doses, and with careful aspiration.
**Consultation with Primary Care Provider**
1. Patients with symptoms of blood dyscrasias should be referred to their primary care provider for complete blood counts. Treatment should be postponed until the results are known.
2. Consultation may be required for very anxious patients.
3. General anesthesia should be

used with caution in patients requiring dental surgery; hypotensive episode may occur.

**Client/Family Teaching**
1. Review the importance of good oral hygiene in order to prevent soft tissue inflammation.
2. Review the proper use of oral hygiene aids in order to prevent injury.
3. Daily home, fluoride treatments for persistent dry mouth.
4. Avoid alcohol-containing mouth rinses.
5. Dry mouth can be treated with tart, sugarless gum or candy, sips of water, or with saliva substitutes if dry mouth persists.

# ANTI-INFECTIVE DRUGS

*See also the following individual entries:*

Aminoglycosides
Antiviral Drugs
Butenafine hydrochloride
Cephalosporins
Clindamycin
Erythromycins
Fluoroquinolones
Fosfomycin tromethamine
Loracarbef
Penicillins
Tetracyclines

**General Statement**
The following general guidelines apply to the use of most anti-infective drugs:
1. Anti-infective drugs can be divided into those that are *bacteriostatic,* that is, arrest the multiplication and further development of the infectious agent, or *bactericidal,* that is, kill and thus eradicate all living microorganisms. Both time of administration and length of therapy may be affected by this difference.
2. Some anti-infectives halt the growth of or eradicate many different microorganisms and are termed *broad-spectrum antibiotics.* Others affect only certain specific organisms and are termed *narrow-spectrum antibiotics.*
3. Some of the anti-infectives elicit a hypersensitivity reaction in some persons. Penicillins cause more severe and more frequent hypersensitivity reactions than any other drug.
4. Because of differences in susceptibility of infectious agents to anti-infectives, the sensitivity of the microorganism to the drug ordered should be determined before treatment is initiated. Several sensitivity tests are commonly used for this purpose.
5. Certain anti-infective agents have marked side effects, some of the more serious of which are neurotoxicity, including ototoxicity, and nephrotoxicity. Care must be taken not to administer two anti-infectives with similar side effects concomitantly, or to administer these drugs to clients in whom the side effects might be damaging (e.g., a nephrotoxic drug to a client suffering from kidney disease). The choice of anti-infective also depends on its distribution in the body (i.e., whether it passes the blood-brain barrier).
6. Anti-infective drugs can also eradicate the normal intestinal flora necessary for proper digestion, synthesis of vitamin K, and control of fungi that may gain access to the GI tract (superinfection).

**Action/Kinetics:** The mechanism of action of the anti-infectives varies. The following modes of action have been identified.* Note the considerable overlap among these mechanisms:
1. Inhibition of synthesis of or activation of enzymes that disrupt bacterial cell walls leading to loss of viability and possibly cell lysis (e.g., penicillins, cephalosporins, cycloserine, bacitracin, vancomycin, miconazole, ketoconazole, clotrimazole).
2. Direct effect on the microbial cell membrane to affect permeability

---

*Chambers, H.F., Sande, M.A.: Antimicrobial agents. In *Goodman and Gilman's The Pharmacological Basis of Therapeutics,* 9th ed. Edited by Hardman, J.G., Limbud, L.E., New York, McGraw-Hill, 1996, p. 1029.

and leading to leakage of intracellular components (e.g., polymyxin, colistimethate, nystatin, amphotericin).

3. Effect on the function of 30S and 50S bacterial ribosomes to cause a reversible inhibition of protein synthesis (e.g., chloramphenicol, tetracyclines, erythromycin, clindamycin).

4. Bind to the 30S ribosomal subunit that alters protein synthesis and leads to cell death (e.g., aminoglycosides).

5. Effect on nucleic acid metabolism which inhibits DNA-dependent RNA polymerase (e.g., rifampin) or inhibition of gyrase (e.g., quinolones).

6. Antimetabolites that block specific metabolic steps essential to the life of the microorganism (e.g., trimethoprim, sulfonamides).

7. Bind to viral enzymes that are essential for DNA synthesis leading to a halt of viral replication (e.g., acyclovir, ganciclovir, vidarabine, zidovudine).

**Uses:** See individual drugs. The choice of the anti-infective depends on the nature of the illness to be treated, the sensitivity of the infecting agent, and the client's previous experience with the drug. Hypersensitivity and allergic reactions may preclude the use of the agent of choice.

**Contraindications:** Hypersensitivity or allergies to the drug.

**Side Effects:** The antibiotics and anti-infective agents have few direct toxic effects. Kidney and liver damage, deafness, and blood dyscrasias are occasionally observed.

The following undesirable manifestations, however, occur frequently:

1. Suppression of the normal flora of the body, which in turn keeps certain pathogenic microorganisms, such as *Candida albicans, Proteus,* or *Pseudomonas,* from causing infections. If the flora is altered, *superinfections* (monilial vaginitis, enteritis, UTIs), which necessitate the discontinuation of therapy or the use of other antibiotics, can result.

2. Incomplete eradication of an infectious organism. Casual use of anti-infectives favors the emergence of *resistant* strains insensitive to a particular drug.

To minimize the chances for the development of resistant strains, anti-infectives are usually given at specified doses for a prescribed length of time after acute symptoms have subsided.

**Drug Interactions**
*Oral contraceptives* / ↓ Effectiveness of OCs.
*Oral anticoagulants* / ↑ Bleeding potential

## GENERAL DENTAL CONCERNS FOR ALL ANTI-INFECTIVES
**General**
1. Document type and onset of symptoms, location and source of infection (if known).

2. Note any unusual reaction or problems with any anti-infectives (usually penicillin).

3. Conspicuously mark allergy in the chart.

4. Assess for side effects such as hives, rashes, difficulty breathing, which may indicate a hypersensitivity or allergic response; stop drug and report.

5. If drug mainly excreted by the kidneys, reduce dose with renal dysfunction. Nephrotoxic drugs are usually contraindicated with renal dysfunction because toxic levels of the drugs are rapidly attained when renal function is impaired.

6. Assess for superinfections, particularly of fungal origin, characterized by black furred tongue, nausea, and/or diarrhea.

**Client/Family Teaching**
1. Take meds at prescribed intervals; use only under medical supervision.

2. Do not share with friends or family members. Prevent recurrence by completing entire prescription, despite feeling well. This ensures that the organism is eradicated and diminishes the emergence of drug-resistant bacterial strains. Incomplete

therapy may render client unresponsive to the antibiotic with the next infection.

3. Report any unusual bruising or bleeding, e.g., bleeding gums, blood in stool, urine, or other secretions; S&S of allergic reactions, including rash, fever, pruritis, and urticaria or superinfections such as pain, swelling, redness, drainage, perineal itching, diarrhea, rash, or a change in symptoms.

4. Discard any unused drug after therapy completed.

5. Take antipyretics as prescribed RTC (q 4 hr) for fever reduction when needed.

6. Women taking OCs should use a back-up method of birth control for their current cycle of antibiotic therapy.

# ANTIANGINAL DRUGS— NITRATES/NITRITES

*See also the following individual entries:*

Isosorbide dinitrate
Isosorbide mononitrate, oral
Nitroglycerin sublingual
Nitroglycerin sustained release
Nitroglycerin transdermal system
Nitroglycerin translingual spray

**General Statement:** Three groups of drugs are currently used for the treatment of angina. These agents include the nitrates/nitrites, beta-adrenergic blocking agents, and calcium channel blocking drugs.

**Action/Kinetics:** Nitrates reduce preload and afterload leading to decreased left ventricular end diastolic pressure, systemic vascular resistance, and arterial and venous dilation. The oxygen requirements of the myocardium are reduced and there is more efficient redistribution of blood flow through collateral channels in myocardial tissue. Diastolic, systolic, and mean BP are decreased. The onset and duration depend on the product and route of administration (sublingual, topical, transdermal, parenteral, oral, and buccal).

**Onset:** Less than 1 min for amyl nitrite to 1 to 3 min for IV, sublingual, translingual, and transmucosal nitroglycerin or sublingual isosorbide dinitrate; 20 to 60 min for sustained-release, topical, and transdermal nitroglycerin or oral isosorbide dinitrate or mononitrate; and up to 4 hr for sustained-release isosorbide dinitrate.

**Duration of action:** 3 to 5 min for amyl nitrite and IV nitroglycerin; 30 to 60 min for sublingual or translingual nitroglycerin; several hours for transmucosal, sustained-release, or topical nitroglycerin and all isosorbide dinitrate products; and up to 24 hr for transdermal nitroglycerin.

**Uses:** Treatment and prophylaxis of acute angina pectoris (use sublingual, transmucosal, or translingual nitroglycerin; amyl nitrite). Nitrates are first-line therapy for unstable angina. Prophylaxis of chronic angina pectoris (topical, transdermal, translingual, transmucosal, or oral sustained-release nitroglycerin; isosorbide dinitrate and mononitrate; erythrityl tetranitrate; pentaerythritol tetranitrate). IV nitroglycerin is used to decrease BP in surgical procedures resulting in hypertension, as well as an adjunct in treating hypertension or CHF associated with MI. *Non-FDA Approved Uses:* Nitroglycerin ointment has been used as an adjunct in treating Raynaud's disease. Also, isosorbide dinitrate with prostaglandin $E_1$ for peripheral vascular disease. Sublingual and topical nitroglycerin and oral nitrates have been used to decrease cardiac workload in clients with acute MI and in CHF.

**Contraindications:** Sensitivity to nitrites, which may result in severe hypotensive reactions, MI, or tolerance to nitrites. Severe anemia, cerebral hemorrhage, recent head trauma, postural hypotension, closed angle glaucoma, impaired hepatic function, hypertrophic cardiomyopathy, hypotension, recent MI. PO dosage forms should not be used in clients

---

with GI hypermotility or with malabsorption syndrome. IV nitroglycerin should not be used in clients with hypotension, uncorrected hypovolemia, inadequate cerebral circulation, constrictive pericarditis, increased ICP, or pericardial tamponade.

**Special Concerns:** Use with caution during lactation and in glaucoma. Tolerance to the antianginal and vascular effects may occur. Safety and efficacy have not been determined during lactation and in children.

**Side Effects:** *CNS:* Headaches (most common) which may be severe and persistent, restlessness, dizziness, weakness, apprehension, vertigo, anxiety, insomnia, confusion, nightmares, hypoesthesia, hypokinesia, dyscoordination. *CV:* Postural hypotension (common) with or without paradoxical bradycardia and increased angina, tachycardia, palpitations, syncope, rebound hypertension, crescendo angina, retrosternal discomfort, **CV collapse,** atrial fibrillation, PVCs, **arrhythmias.** *Oral:* Dry mouth, burning sensation. *GI:* N&V, dyspepsia, diarrhea, abdominal pain, involuntary passing of feces and urine, tenesmus, tooth disorder. *Dermatologic:* Crusty skin lesions, pruritus, rash, exfoliative dermatitis, cutaneous vasodilation with flushing. *GU:* Urinary frequency, impotence, dysuria. *Respiratory:* Upper respiratory tract infection, bronchitis, pneumonia. *Allergic:* Itching, wheezing, tracheobronchitis. *Miscellaneous:* Perspiration, muscle twitching, methemoglobinemia, cold sweating, blurred vision, diplopia, **hemolytic anemia,** arthralgia, edema, malaise, neck stiffness, increased appetite, rigors. **Topical use:** Peripheral edema, contact dermatitis.

Tolerance can occur following chronic use. Nitrites convert hemoglobin to methemoglobin, which impairs the oxygen-carrying capacity of the blood, resulting in **anemic hypoxia.** This interaction is dangerous in clients with preexisting anemia.

**Drug Interactions**
*Acetylcholine* / Effects ↓ when used with nitrates
*Alcohol, ethyl* / Hypotension and CV collapse due to vasodilator effect of both agents
*Aspirin* / ↑ Serum levels and effects of nitrates
*Benzodiazepines* / Additive hypotensive effect
*Opioid Analgesics* / Additive hypotensive effect
*Phenothiazines* / Additive hypotensive effect
*Sildenafil citrate* / ↑ Risk for adverse cardiovascular events
*Sympathomimetics* / ↓ Effect of nitrates; also, nitrates may ↓ effect of sympathomimetics resulting in hypotension

**Dosage** ────────────
See individual agents.

## DENTAL CONCERNS
**General**
1. Assess vital signs at every appointment because of cardiovascular side effects.
2. Make sure that the patient's drug is easily accessible in case of an angina attack.
3. Early morning and shorter appointments may be of benefit for anxious patients.
4. Antianxiety drugs, such as benzodiazepines or nitrous oxide can be prescribed if the anxiety associated with a dental appointment precipitates the patient's angina attack.
5. Talk with patient about frequency of angina attacks (disease control).
6. Stress from a dental procedure may adversely affect the patient's cardiovascular status. Assess patient risk.
7. Have the patient sit up slowly and remain seated for at least two minutes after being supine in order to minimize the risk of orthostatic hypotension.
8. A semisupine position may be necessary for patients with cardiovascular disease.
9. Vasoconstrictors should be used

with caution and in low doses. Avoid epinephrine-containing gingival retraction cords.

10. Decreased saliva flow can put the patient at risk for dental caries, periodontal disease, and candidiasis.

11. Check the expiration date on the patient's prescription and the bottle in your emergency medicine kit in order to make sure that the drug is active. Opened bottles have a *three-month shelf life* or less depending on the expiration date listed on the bottle. The spray form has a three-year shelf life.

**Consultation with Primary Care Provider**

1. Medical consultation may be necessary in order to assess patient's cardiovascular status and ability to tolerate stress.

**Client/Family Teaching**

1. Review the importance of good oral hygiene in order to prevent soft tissue inflammation.

2. Review the proper use of oral hygiene aids in order to prevent injury.

3. Daily home fluoride treatments for persistent dry mouth.

4. Avoid alcohol-containing mouth rinses and beverages.

5. Avoid caffeine-containing beverages.

6. Dry mouth can be treated with tart, sugarless gum or candy, water, sugar-free beverages, or with saliva substitutes if dry mouth persists.

---

# ANTIARRHYTHMIC DRUGS

*See also the following individual entries:*

Calcium Channel Blocking Agents
Digitoxin
Digoxin
Diltiazem hydrochloride
Flecainide acetate
Lidocaine hydrochloride
Moricizine hydrochloride
Phenytoin
Phenytoin sodium
Procainamide hydrochloride
Propranolol hydrochloride
Quinidine gluconate
Tocainide hydrochloride
Verapamil

**General Statement:** Cardiac arrhythmias are altered patterns of contraction or marked increases or decreases in the rate of the heart which reduce the ability of the heart to pump blood. Some examples of cardiac arrhythmias are *premature ventricular beats, ventricular tachycardia, atrial flutter, atrial fibrillation, ventricular fibrillation,* and *atrioventricular heart block.*

**Action/Kinetics:** The various antiarrhythmic drugs are classified according to both their mechanism of action and their effects on the action potential of cardiac cells. Importantly, one drug in a particular class may be more effective and safer in an individual client. The antiarrhythmic drugs are classified as follows:

1. Group I. These drugs decrease the rate of entry of sodium into the cell during cardiac membrane depolarization which prevents depolarization and transmission of nerve impulses. Drugs classified as group I are further listed in subgroups (according to their effects on action potential duration) as follows:

• Group IA: Prolong the duration of the action potential. Examples: Disopyramide, procainamide, and quinidine.

• Group IB: Are thought to shorten the action potential. Examples: Lidocaine, phenytoin, and tocainide.

• Group IC: Significant slowing of conduction without really affecting the action potential. Examples: Flecainide, indecainide, and propafenone.

*NOTE:* Moricizine is classified as a group I agent but it has characteristics of agents in groups IA, B, and C.

2. Group II. These drugs competitively block beta-adrenergic receptors and depress phase 4 depolarization. Examples: Acebutolol, esmolol, and propranolol.

---

3. Group III. These drugs prolong the duration of the membrane action potential (relative refractory period) without changing the phase of depolarization or the resting membrane potential. Examples: Amiodarone, bretylium, and sotalol.
4. Group IV. Verapamil, a calcium channel blocker that slows conduction velocity and increases the refractoriness of the AV node.

Two other drugs, adenosine and digoxin, are also used to treat arrhythmias. Adenosine slows conduction time through the AV node and can interrupt the reentry pathways through the AV node. Digoxin causes a decrease in maximal diastolic potential and duration of the action potential; it also increases the slope of phase 4 depolarization.

**Special Concerns:** Monitor serum levels of antiarrhythmic drugs since some drugs can cause toxic side effects which can be confused with the purpose for which the drug is used. For example, toxicity from quinidine can result in cardiac arrhythmias. Antiarrhythmic drugs may cause new or worsening of arrhythmias, ranging from an increase in frequency of PVCs to severe ventricular tachycardia, ventricular fibrillation, or tachycardia that is more sustained and rapid. Such situations (called proarrhythmic effect) may make it difficult to distinguish the proarrhythmic effect from the underlying rhythm disorder.

## DENTAL CONCERNS
### General
1. Monitor vital signs at every appointment because of cardiovascular and respiratory side effects.
2. Decreased saliva flow can put the patient at risk for dental caries, periodontal disease, and candidiasis.
3. Dental procedures may cause the patient anxiety or place stress on the heart. Assess cardiovascular patient for this risk.
4. Early morning and shorter appointments as well as methods for addressing anxiety levels in the patient

can help to reduce the amount of stress that the patient is experiencing.
5. Vasoconstrictors should be used with caution and in low doses in patients with "controlled" cardiovascular status. Avoid epinephrine-containing gingival retraction cords.

**Consultation with Primary Care Provider**
1. Medical consultation may be necessary in order to assess patient's cardiovascular status and ability to tolerate stress.

**Client/Family Teaching**
1. Review the importance of good oral hygiene in order to prevent soft tissue inflammation.
2. Avoid alcohol-containing mouth rinses and beverages.
3. Avoid caffeine-containing beverages.
4. Dry mouth can be treated with tart, sugarless gum or candy, water, sugar-free beverages, or with saliva substitutes if dry mouth persists.

# ANTICOAGULANTS

*See also the following individual entries:*

> Ardeparin sodium
> Danaparoid sodium

**Action/Kinetics:** Drugs that influence blood coagulation can be divided into three classes: (1) *anticoagulants,* or drugs that prevent or slow blood coagulation; (2) *thrombolytic agents,* which increase the rate at which an existing blood clot dissolves; and (3) *hemostatics,* which prevent or stop internal bleeding. The dosage of all agents must be carefully adjusted since overdosage can have serious consequences. The major anticoagulants are warfarin, heparin, and heparin derivatives. The following considerations are pertinent to all types. Anticoagulants do not dissolve previously formed clots, but they do forestall their enlargement and prevent new clots from forming.

**Uses:** Venous thrombosis, pulmonary embolism, acute coronary occlusions with MIs, and strokes caused by emboli or cerebral thrombi. Prophylactically for rheumatic heart disease, atrial fibrillation, traumatic injuries of blood vessels, vascular surgery, major abdominal, thoracic, and pelvic surgery, prevention of strokes in clients with transient attacks of cerebral ischemia, or other signs of impending stroke.

Heparin is often used concurrently during the therapeutic initiation period. *Non-FDA Approved Uses (Warfarin):* Reduce risk of postconversion emboli; prophylaxis of recurrent, cerebral thromboembolism; prophylaxis of myocardial reinfarction; treatment of transient ischemic attacks; reduce the risk of thromboembolic complications in clients with certain types of prosthetic heart valves; reduced risk of thrombosis and/or occlusion following coronary bypass surgery.

**Contraindications:** Hemorrhagic tendencies (including hemophilia), clients with frail or weakened blood vessels, blood dyscrasias, ulcerative lesions of the GI tract (including peptic ulcer), diverticulitis, colitis, SBE, threatened abortion, recent operations on the eye, brain, or spinal cord, regional anesthesia and lumbar block, vitamin K deficiency, leukemia with bleeding tendencies, thrombocytopenic purpura, open wounds or ulcerations, acute nephritis, impaired hepatic or renal function, or severe hypertension. Hepatic and renal dysfunction. In the presence of drainage tubes in any orifice. Alcoholism.

**Special Concerns:** Use with caution in menstruation, in pregnant women (because they may cause hypoprothrombinemia in the infant), during lactation, during the postpartum period, and following cerebrovascular accidents. Geriatric clients may be more susceptible to the effects of anticoagulants.

**Side Effects:** See individual drugs.

**Dosage**
See individual drugs.

## DENTAL CONCERNS

See also *Dental Concerns* for individual agents.
**General**
1. Local hemostatic measures, such as a vasoconstrictor, may be necessary to prevent excessive bleeding during dental procedures.
2. Antibiotic prophylaxis may be necessary if the patient has a joint prosthesis. Consult 1997 ADA guidelines.
3. It may be necessary to delay dental treatment until the patient has finished drug therapy.
4. Avoid OTC drugs. Check prior to taking any nonprescription drugs that have anticoagulant-type effects such as salicylates, NSAIDs, steroids, or vitamin preparations with high levels of vitamin K, mineral preparations from health food stores, or alcohol.
**Consultation with Primary Care Provider**
1. Consultation with appropriate health care provider is necessary to determine platelet counts and bleeding times.
**Client/Family Teaching**
1. To prevent bleeding gums, use a soft bristle toothbrush and brush gently; inform dentist of drug therapy.
2. Review the importance of good oral hygiene in order to prevent soft tissue inflammation.
3. Review the proper use of oral hygiene aids in order to prevent injury.
4. Notify dentist if oral lesions, sores, or bleeding occur.

# ANTICONVULSANTS

*See also the following individual entries:*

Carbamazepine
Clonazepam
Diazepam
Felbamate

Fosphenytoin sodium
Gabapentin
Lamotrigine
Phenobarbital
Phenobarbital sodium
Phenytoin
Phenytoin sodium extended
Tiagabine hydrochloride
Topiramate
Valproic acid

**General Statement:** Therapeutic agents cannot cure convulsive disorders, but do control seizures without impairing the normal functions of the CNS.

## Dosage

Dosage is highly individualized. However, trauma or emotional stress may necessitate an increase in drug dosage requirements (e.g., if the client requires surgery and starts having seizures). For details, see individual agents.

## DENTAL CONCERNS

**General**

1. Early morning, and shorter, more frequent appointments, as well as methods for addressing anxiety levels in the patient, can help to reduce the amount of stress that the patient is experiencing.
2. Patients on chronic drug therapy may develop blood dyscrasias. Symptoms include fever, sore throat, and bleeding, and poor wound healing.
3. Place patient on frequent recall because of gingival hyperplasia.
4. Monitor vital signs at every appointment because of cardiovascular side effects.
5. Decreased saliva flow can put the patient at risk for dental caries, periodontal disease, and candidiasis.

**Consultation with Primary Care Provider**

1. Patients with symptoms of blood dyscrasias should be referred to their primary care provider for complete blood counts. Treatment should be postponed until the results are known.
2. Consultation may be required in order to assess the extent of disease

control and the patient's ability to tolerate stress.

**Client/Family Teaching**

1. Review the importance of good oral hygiene in order to prevent soft tissue inflammation.
2. Review the proper use of oral hygiene aids in order to prevent injury.
3. With gingival hyperplasia, intensify oral hygiene, use a soft tooth brush, massage the gums, use dental floss daily, and obtain routine dental checks.
4. Daily home fluoride treatments for persistent dry mouth.
5. Avoid alcohol-containing mouth rinses and beverages.
6. Avoid caffeine-containing beverages.
7. Dry mouth can be treated with tart, sugarless gum or candy, water, sugar-free beverages, or with saliva substitutes if dry mouth persists.

# ANTIDEPRESSANTS, TRICYCLIC

*See also the following individual entries:*

Amitriptyline hydrochloride
Amoxapine
Clomipramine hydrochloride
Desipramine hydrochloride
Doxepin hydrochloride
Nortriptyline hydrochloride
Trimipramine maleate

**Action/Kinetics:** It is now believed that antidepressant drugs cause adaptive changes in the serotonin and norepinephrine receptor systems, resulting in changes in the sensitivities of both presynaptic and postsynaptic receptor sites. Well absorbed from the GI tract. All have a long serum half-life. Up to 46 days may be required to reach steady plasma levels and maximum therapeutic effects may not be noted for 24 weeks. Because of the long half-life, single daily dosage may suffice. More than 90% bound to plasma protein. Partially metabolized in the liver and excreted primarily in the urine.

**Uses:** Endogenous and reactive depressions. Preferred over MAO inhibitors because they are less toxic. See also individual drugs.

**Contraindications:** Severely impaired liver function. Use during acute recovery phase from MI. Concomitant use with MAO inhibitors.

**Special Concerns:** Use with caution during lactation and with epilepsy, CV diseases, glaucoma, BPH, suicidal tendencies, a history of urinary retention, and the elderly. Use during pregnancy only when benefits clearly outweigh risks. Generally not recommended for children less than 12 years of age. Geriatric clients may be more sensitive to the anticholinergic and sedative side effects.

**Side Effects:** Most frequent side effects are sedation and atropine-like reactions. *CNS:* Confusion, anxiety, restlessness, insomnia, nightmares, hallucinations, delusions, mania or hypomania, headache, dizziness, inability to concentrate, panic reaction, worsening of psychoses, fatigue, weakness. *Oral:* Dry mouth, unpleasant taste, stomatitis, glossitis, increased salivation, black tongue. *Anticholinergic:* Blurred vision, mydriasis, constipation, paralytic ileus, urinary retention or difficulty in urination. *GI:* N&V, anorexia, gastric distress, cramps. *CV:* Fainting, tachycardia, hypo- or hypertension, arrhythmias, *heart block,* possibility of palpitations, *MI, stroke.* *Neurologic:* Paresthesias, numbness, incoordination, neuropathies, extrapyramidal symptoms including tardive dyskinesia, dysarthria, seizures. *Dermatologic:* Skin rashes, urticaria, flushing, pruritus, petechiae, photosensitivity, edema. *Endocrine:* Testicular swelling and gynecomastia in males, increase or decrease in libido, impotence, menstrual irregularities and galactorrhea in females, hypo- or hyperglycemia, changes in secretion of ADH. *Miscellaneous:* Sweating, alopecia, nasal congestion, lacrimation, increase in body temperature, chills, urinary frequency including nocturia. Bone marrow depression including thrombocytopenia, leukopenia, *agranulocytosis,* eosinophilia.

High dosage increases the frequency of seizures in epileptic clients and may cause epileptiform attacks in normal subjects.

**Drug Interactions**
*Alcohol, ethyl* / Concomitant use may lead to ↑ GI complications and ↓ performance on motor skill tests; death has been reported
*Anticholinergic drugs* / Additive anticholinergic side effects
*Anticonvulsants* / Tricyclics may ↑ incidence of epileptic seizures
*Antihistamines* / Additive anticholinergic side effects
*Barbiturates* / Additive depressant effects; also, barbiturates may ↑ breakdown of antidepressants by liver
*Benzodiazepines* / Tricyclic antidepressants ↑ effect of benzodiazepines
*Beta-adrenergic blocking agents* / Tricyclic antidepressants ↓ effect of the blocking agents
*Chlordiazepoxide* / Concomitant use may cause additive sedative effects and/or additive atropine-like side effects
*Cimetidine* / ↑ Effect of tricyclics (especially serious anticholinergic symptoms) due to ↓ breakdown by liver
*Clonidine* / Dangerous ↑ BP and hypertensive crisis
*Diazepam* / Concomitant use may cause additive sedative effects and/or additive atropine-like side effects
*Ephedrine* / Tricyclics ↓ effects of ephedrine by preventing uptake
*Ethchlorvynol* / Combination may result in transient delirium
*Fluoxetine* / Fluoxetine ↑ pharmacologic and toxic effects of tricyclic antidepressants (effect may persist for several weeks after fluoxetine is discontinued)
*Guanethidine* / Tricyclics ↓ antihypertensive effect of guanethidine by

---

preventing uptake at its site of action

*Haloperidol* / ↑ Effect of tricyclics due to ↓ breakdown by liver

*Levodopa* / ↓ Effect of levodopa due to ↓ absorption

*MAO inhibitors* / Concomitant use may result in excitation, increase in body temperature, delirium, tremors, and convulsions although combinations have been used successfully

*Meperidine* / Tricyclics enhance opioid-induced respiratory depression; also, additive anticholinergic side effects

*Methyldopa* / Tricyclics may block hypotensive effects of methyldopa

*Methylphenidate* / ↑ Effect of tricyclics due to ↓ breakdown by liver

*Opioid analgesics* / Tricyclics enhance opioid-induced respiratory depression; also, additive anticholinergic effects

*Oxazepam* / Concomitant use may cause additive sedative effects and/or atropine-like side effects

*Phenothiazines* / Additive anticholinergic side effects; also, phenothiazines ↑ effects of tricyclics due to ↓ breakdown by liver

*Sodium bicarbonate* / ↑ Effect of tricyclics by ↑ renal tubular reabsorption of the drug

*Sympathomimetics* / Potentiation of sympathomimetic effects → hypertension or cardiac arrhythmias

*Tobacco (smoking)* / ↓ Serum levels of tricyclic antidepressants due to ↑ breakdown by liver

**Dosage** ————————

See individual drugs.

Dosage levels vary greatly in effectiveness from one client to another; therefore, dosage regimens must be carefully individualized.

### DENTAL CONCERNS
**General**
1. Monitor vital signs at every appointment because of cardiovascular side effects.
2. Have the patient sit up slowly and remain seated for at least two minutes after being supine in order to

minimize the risk of orthostatic hypotension.
3. Decreased saliva flow can put the patient at risk for dental caries, periodontal disease, and candidiasis.
4. Vasoconstrictors should be used with caution and in low doses. Avoid epinephrine-containing gingival retraction cords.
5. Patients on chronic drug therapy rarely develop blood dyscrasias. Symptoms include fever, sore throat, bleeding, and poor wound healing.
6. Place patient on frequent recall because of oral adverse effects.

**Consultation with Primary Care Provider**
1. Patients with symptoms of blood dyscrasias should be referred to their primary care provider for complete blood counts. Treatment should be postponed until the results are known.
2. Consultation may be required in order to assess the extent of disease control.
3. Health care provider should be informed of the oral adverse effects of these drugs.

**Client/Family Teaching**
1. Review the importance of good oral hygiene in order to prevent soft tissue inflammation.
2. Review the proper use of oral hygiene aids in order to prevent injury.
3. Daily home fluoride treatments for persistent dry mouth.
4. Avoid alcohol-containing mouth rinses and beverages.
5. Avoid caffeine-containing beverages.
6. Dry mouth can be treated with tart, sugarless gum or candy, water, sugar-free beverages, or with saliva substitutes if dry mouth persists.

# ANTIDIABETIC AGENTS: HYPOGLYCEMIC AGENTS

See also *Antidiabetic Agents: Insulins. See also the following individual entries:*

Acarbose

Chlorpropamide
Glimepiride
Glipizide
Glyburide
Metformin hydrochloride
Miglitol
Tolazamide
Tolbutamide
Tolbutamide sodium
Troglitazone

**Action/Kinetics:** Oral hypoglycemic drugs are classified as either first or second generation. *Generation* refers to structural changes in the basic molecule. Second-generation oral hypoglycemic drugs are more lipophilic and, as such, have greater hypoglycemic potency.

The oral hypoglycemics are believed to act by one or more of the following mechanisms: (1) stimulating insulin release from pancreatic beta cells; (2) the peripheral tissues become more sensitive to insulin due to an increase in the number of insulin receptors or an increased ability of circulating insulin to combine with receptors; or (3) extrapancreatic effects, including decreased glucagon release and hepatic glucose production. To be effective, the client must have some ability for endogenous insulin production. Differences in oral hypoglycemic drugs are mainly in their pharmacokinetic properties and duration of action.

**Uses:** Non-insulin-dependent diabetes mellitus (type II) that does not respond to diet management alone. Concurrent use of insulin and an oral hypoglycemic for type II diabetics who are difficult to control with diet and sulfonylurea therapy alone.

**Contraindications:** Stress before and during surgery, ketosis, severe trauma, fever, infections, pregnancy, diabetes complicated by recurrent episodes of ketoacidosis or coma; juvenile, growth-onset, insulin-dependent, or brittle diabetes; impaired endocrine, renal, or liver function. Use in diabetics who can be controlled by diet alone. Relapse may occur with the sulfonylureas in undernourished clients. Long-acting products in geriatric clients.

**Special Concerns:** Use with caution in debilitated and malnourished clients and during lactation since hypoglycemia may occur in the infant. Safety and effectiveness in children have not been established. Geriatric clients may be more sensitive to oral hypoglycemics and hypoglycemia may be more difficult to recognize in these clients. Use of sulfonylureas has been associated with an increased risk of CV mortality compared to treatment with either diet alone or diet plus insulin. There may be loss of blood glucose control if the client experiences stress such as infection, fever, surgery, or trauma.

**Side Effects:** Hypoglycemia is the most common side effect. *GI:* Nausea, heartburn, full feeling. *CNS:* Fatigue, dizziness, fever, headache, weakness, malaise, vertigo. *Hepatic:* Cholestatic jaundice, aggravation of hepatic porphyria. *Dermatologic:* Skin rashes, urticaria, erythema, pruritus, eczema, photophobia, morbilliform or maculopapular eruptions, lichenoid reactions, porphyria cutanea tardia. *Hematologic:* Thrombocytopenia, leukopenia, ***agranulocytosis, aplastic anemia,*** pancytopenia, ***hemolytic anemia.*** *Endocrine:* Inappropriate secretion of ADH resulting in excessive water retention, hyponatremia, low serum osmolality, and high urine osmolality. *Miscellaneous:* Paresthesia, tinnitus, resistance to drug action develops in a small percentage of clients.

**Drug Interactions**
*Alcohol* / Possible Antabuse-like syndrome, especially facial flushing and SOB. Also, ↓ effect of oral hypoglycemic due to ↑ breakdown by liver
*Beta-adrenergic blocking agents* / ↓ Hypoglycemic effect; also, symptoms of hypoglycemia may be masked
*Fluconazole* / ↑ Hypoglycemic effect

---

***bold italic*** = life-threatening side effect

*Histamine $H_2$ antagonists* / ↑ Hypoglycemic effect due to ↓ breakdown by liver

*Magnesium salts* / ↑ Hypoglycemic effect

*MAO inhibitors* / ↑ Hypoglycemic effect due to ↓ breakdown by liver

*Miconazole* / ↑ Effect of oral hypoglycemics

*Nicotinic acid* / ↓ Effect of oral hypoglycemics

*NSAIDs* / ↑ Hypoglycemic effect of oral antidiabetics

*Phenobarbital* / ↓ Effect of oral hypoglycemics due to ↑ breakdown by liver

*Phenothiazines* / ↑ Requirements for sulfonylureas due to ↓ release of insulin

*Phenylbutazone* / ↑ Effect of oral hypoglycemics due to ↓ breakdown by liver, ↓ plasma protein binding, and ↓ renal excretion

*Probenecid* / ↑ Hypoglycemic effect

*Salicylates* / ↑ Effect of oral hypoglycemics by ↓ plasma protein binding

*Sulfonamides* / ↑ Effect of oral hypoglycemics by ↓ plasma protein binding and ↓ breakdown by liver

*Sympathomimetics* / ↑ Requirements for sulfonylureas

*Tricyclic antidepressants* / ↑ Hypoglycemic effect

## DENTAL CONCERNS

See also *Dental Concerns* for *Insulins*.
**General**
1. Obtain a thorough medication/health history.
2. Morning and shorter appointments may be necessary for anxious patients.
3. Patients on chronic drug therapy may develop blood dyscrasias. Symptoms include fever, sore throat, and bleeding, and poor wound healing.
4. Frequent recall may be necessary in order to evaluate healing.
5. Vital signs may be necessary with some antidiabetics because of cardiovascular side effects (i.e., glipizide, glyburide).
6. Assess patient's knowledge of diabetes; compliance with therapy and dietary regimen.
7. Patients with diabetes may be more susceptible to infection and delayed wound healing.
8. Determine if patient is self-monitoring his/her antidiabetic therapy; including blood glucose values, finger sticks, or urine glucose monitoring. Elevated blood glucose levels put the patient at risk for dental caries.
9. Avoid prescription and over-the-counter aspirin-containing products.
**Consultation with Primary Care Provider**
1. Patients with symptoms of blood dyscrasias should be referred to their primary care provider for complete blood counts. Treatment should be postponed until the results are known.
2. Consultation may be required to determine level of disease control.
3. Consultation may be necessary in order to obtain information regarding the patient's blood glucose levels including glycosolated hemoglobin (Gb) or HbA1-C testing.
**Client/Family Teaching**
1. Review the importance of good oral hygiene in order to prevent soft tissue inflammation.
2. Review the proper use of oral hygiene aids in order to prevent injury.
3. Avoid alcohol-containing mouth rinses and beverages.

# ANTIDIABETIC AGENTS: INSULINS

See also *Antidiabetic Agents: Hypoglycemic Agents. See also the following individual entries:*

> Insulin injection
> Insulin injection concentrated
> Insulin lispro injection
> Insulin zinc suspension (Lente)
> Insulin zinc suspension, Extended (Ultralente)

**General Statement:** Insulin preparations with different times of onset, peak activity, and duration of action have been developed. Such products are prepared by precipitating insulin in the presence of zinc chloride to form zinc insulin crystals and/or by combining insulin with a protein such as protamine. Based on these modifications, insulin products are classified as fast-acting, intermediate-acting, and long-acting. These preparations permit the provider to select the preparation best suited to the life-style of the client.

RAPID-ACTING INSULIN: Insulin injection (Regular Insulin, Crystalline Zinc Insulin, Unmodified Insulin)

INTERMEDIATE-ACTING INSULIN
1. Isophane insulin suspension (NPH)
2. Insulin zinc suspension (Lente)

LONG-ACTING INSULIN: Insulin zinc suspension extended (Ultralente)

*NOTE:* Insulin preparations with various times of onset and duration of action are often mixed to obtain optimum control in diabetic clients.

**Action/Kinetics:** Decreases in blood glucose. Insulin also aids in the regulation of fat and protein metabolism.

Since insulin is a protein, it is destroyed in the GI tract. Thus, it must be administered SC so that it is readily absorbed into the bloodstream and distributed throughout the extracellular fluid. Metabolized mainly by the liver.

**Uses:** Replacement therapy in type I diabetes. Diabetic ketoacidosis or diabetic coma (use regular insulin). Insulin is also indicated in type II diabetes when other measures have failed (e.g., diet, exercise, weight reduction) or with surgery, trauma, infection, fever, endocrine dysfunction, pregnancy, gangrene, Raynaud's disease, kidney or liver dysfunction.

Human insulins are used for local insulin allergy, lipodystrophy at the injection site, immunologic insulin resistance, temporary insulin use (e.g., surgery, acute stress, gestational diabetes), and newly diagnosed diabetes.

Regular insulin is used in IV HA solutions, in IV dextrose to treat severe hyperkalemia, and IV as a provocative test for growth hormone secretion.

Insulin and oral hypoglycemic drugs have been used in type II diabetics who are difficult to control with diet and PO therapy alone.

Diabetic clients should adhere to a regular meal schedule.

**Contraindications:** Hypersensitivity to insulin.

**Special Concerns:** Pregnant diabetic clients often manifest decreased insulin requirements during the first half of pregnancy and increased requirements during the latter half. Lactation may decrease insulin requirements.

**Side Effects:** *Hypoglycemia*
*Allergic:* Urticaria, angioedema, lymphadenopathy, bullae, anaphylaxis.
*At site of injection:* Swelling, stinging, redness, itching, warmth.
*Insulin resistance*
*Ophthalmologic:* Blurred vision, transient presbyopia.
*Hyperglycemic rebound (Somogyi effect).*

**Drug Interactions**
*Alcohol, ethyl* / ↑ Hypoglycemia → low blood sugar and shock
*Corticosteroids* / ↓ Effect of insulin due to corticosteroid-induced hyperglycemia
*Epinephrine* / ↓ Effect of insulin due to epinephrine-induced hyperglycemia
*Oxytetracycline* / ↑ Effect of insulin
*Phenothiazines* / ↑ Dosage of antidiabetic due to phenothiazine-induced hyperglycemia
*Phenytoin* / Phenytoin-induced hyperglycemia ↓ diabetic control
*Salicylates* / ↑ Effect of hypoglycemic effect of insulin
*Sulfinpyrazone* / ↑ Hypoglycemic effect of insulin
*Tetracyclines* / May ↑ hypoglycemic effect of insulin

---

**Dosage**
Dosage highly individualized. Usually administered SC. Insulin injection (regular insulin) is the **only** preparation that may be administered IV. Give IV only for clients with severe ketoacidosis or diabetic coma. Dosage for insulin is always expressed in USP units.

## DENTAL CONCERNS

**General**
1. Obtain a thorough medication/health history.
2. Patients may need frequent appointments to monitor healing process.
3. Decreased saliva flow can put the patient at risk for dental caries, periodontal disease, and candidiasis.
4. Assess patient's knowledge of diabetes; compliance with therapy and dietary regimen.
5. Patients with diabetes may be more susceptible to infection and delayed wound healing and may require frequent appointments 3–4 times a year.
6. Determine if patient is self-monitoring his/her antidiabetic therapy; including blood glucose values, finger sticks, or urine glucose monitoring.
7. Prophylactic antibiotics may be necessary in order to prevent infection if surgery or deep scaling is required.
8. Keep a sugar source readily available, i.e., tube of cake frosting, orange juice.

**Consultation with Primary Care Provider**
1. Consultation may be required to determine level of disease control and patient's ability to tolerate stress.
2. Consultation may be necessary in order to obtain information regarding the patient's blood glucose levels including glycosolated hemoglobin (Gb) or HbA1-C testing.

**Client/Family Teaching**
1. Review the importance of good oral hygiene in order to prevent soft tissue inflammation.
2. Review the proper use of oral hygiene aids in order to prevent injury.

3. Avoid alcohol-containing mouth rinses and beverages.

# ANTIHISTAMINES (H₁ BLOCKERS)

*See also the following individual entries:*

Astemizole
Brompheniramine maleate
Cetirizine hydrochloride
Chlorpheniramine maleate
Dimenhydrinate
Diphenhydramine hydrochloride
Fexofenadine hydrochloride
Loratidine
Olopatadine hydrochloride
Terfenadine

**Action/Kinetics:** Compete with histamine at $H_1$ histamine receptors (competitive inhibition), thus preventing or reversing the effects of histamine. First-generation antihistamines bind to central and peripheral $H_1$ receptors and can cause CNS depression or stimulation. Second-generation antihistamines are selective for peripheral $H_1$ receptors and cause less sedation. Antihistamines prevent or reduce increased capillary permeability (i.e., decrease edema, itching) and bronchospasms. Allergic reactions unrelated to histamine release are not affected by antihistamines. Certain of the first-generation antihistamines also have anticholinergic, antiemetic, antipruritic, or antiserotonin effects. Clients unresponsive to a certain antihistamine may regain sensitivity by switching to a different antihistamine.

From a chemical point of view, the antihistamines can be divided into the following classes.

**FIRST GENERATION:**
1. **Ethylenediamine Derivatives.** Moderate sedative effects; almost no anticholinergic or antiemetic activity. Frequently cause GI distress. Example: Tripelennamine.
2. **Ethanolamine Derivatives.** Moderate to high sedative effects.

Significant anticholinergic and anti-emetic effects. Low incidence of GI side effects. Examples: Clemastine, diphenhydramine.

3. **Alkylamines.** Among the most potent antihistamines. Minimal sedation, moderate anticholinergic effects, and no antiemetic effects. Paradoxical excitation may also occur. Examples: Brompheniramine, chlorpheniramine, dexchlorpheniramine.

4. **Phenothiazines.** Significant antihistaminic action and sedation; high degree of both anticholinergic and antiemetic effects. Example: Promethazine.

5. **Piperidines.** Moderate antihistaminic activity, low to moderate sedation, moderate anticholinergic activity, and no antiemetic effects. Examples: Azatadine, cyproheptadine, phenindamine.

**SECOND GENERATION:**

1. **Piperazines.** Low to no sedation or anticholinergic effects and no antiemetic activity. Example: Cetirizine.

2. **Piperidines.** Moderate to high antihistamine activity, low to no sedation and anticholinergic activity, and no antiemetic action. Examples: Astemizole, fexofenadine, loratidine, terfenadine.

The kinetics of most first-generation antihistamines are similar. **Onset:** 15–30 min; **peak:** 1–2 hr; **duration:** 4–6 hr (piperidines have a longer duration). Many antihistamines are available as timed-release preparations. Most first-generation antihistamines are metabolized by the liver and excreted in the urine. The pharmacokinetics of the second-generation antihistamines vary; consult individual drugs.

**Uses: PO:** Treatment of vasomotor, perennial, or seasonal allergic rhinitis and allergic conjunctivitis. Treatment of angioedema, urticarial transfusion reactions, urticaria, pruritus. Atopic dermatitis, contact dermatitis, pruritus ani, pruritus vulvae, insect bites. Sneezing and rhinorrhea due to the common cold. Treatment of anaphylaxis, parkinsonism, drug-induced extrapyramidal reactions, vertigo. Prophylaxis and treatment of motion sickness, including N&V. Nighttime sleep aid. See also the individual drugs.

**Contraindications:** *First-generation antihistamines.* Hypersensitivity to the drug, narrow-angle glaucoma, symptomatic prostatic hypertrophy, stenosing peptic ulcer, and pyloroduodenal or bladder neck obstruction. Use with MAO inhibitors. Pregnancy or possibility thereof (some agents), lactation, premature and newborn infants. The phenothiazine-type antihistamines are contraindicated in CNS depression from any cause, bone marrow depression, jaundice, dehydrated or acutely ill children, and in comatose clients. Use to treat lower respiratory tract symptoms such as asthma.

*Second-generation antihistamines.* Hypersensitivity. Astemizole and terfenadine use in significant hepatic dysfunction and concomitant use with clarithromycin, erythromycin, itraconazole, ketoconazole, quinine, and troleandomycin due to the possibility of serious CV effects (including torsades de pointes, prolongation of the QT interval, other ventricular arrhythmias, cardiac arrest, and death). Also terfenadine use with cisapride, HIV protease inhibitors, mibefradil, serotonin reuptake inhibitors, sparfloxacin, and zileuton.

**Special Concerns:** Administer with caution to clients with convulsive disorders and in respiratory disease. Excess dosage may cause hallucinations, convulsions, and death in infants and children. Use in geriatric clients may result in dizziness, excessive sedation, syncope, toxic confusional states, and hypotension.

**Side Effects:** *CNS:* Sedation ranging from mild drowsiness to deep sleep. Dizziness, incoordination, faintness, fatigue, confusion, lassitude, restlessnesss, excitation, nervousness, tremor, ***tonic-clonic seizures,*** head-

---

ache, irritability, insomnia, euphoria, paresthesias, oculogyric crisis, torticollis, catatonic-like states, hallucinations, disorientation, tongue protrusion (usually with IV use or overdosage), disturbing dreams, nightmares, pseudoschizophrenia, weakness, diplopia, vertigo, hysteria, neuritis, paradoxical excitation, epileptiform seizures in clients with focal lesions. Extrapyramidal reactions include opisthotonus, dystonia, akathisia, dyskinesia, and parkinsonism. *CV:* Postural hypotension, palpitations, bradycardia, tachycardia, reflex tachycardia, extrasystoles, increased or decreased BP, ECG changes (including blunting of T waves and prolongation of the Q-T interval), *cardiac arrest. Oral:* Dry mouth, stomatitis. *GI:* Epigastric distress, anorexia, increased appetite and weight gain, N&V, diarrhea, constipation, change in bowel habits. *GU:* Urinary frequency, dysuria, urinary retention, gynecomastia, inhibition of ejaculation, decreased libido, impotence, early menses, induction of lactation. *Hematologic:* Hypoplastic anemia, *aplastic anemia, hemolytic anemia,* thrombocytopenia, leukopenia, pancytopenia, *agranulocytosis,* thrombocytopenic purpura. *Respiratory:* Thickening of bronchial secretions, wheezing, nasal stuffiness, chest tightness, sore throat, *respiratory depression;* dry mouth, nose, and throat. *Ophthalmic:* Blurred vision, diplopia. *Miscellaneous:* Tinnitus, photosensitivity, acute labyrinthitis, obstructive jaundice, erythema, high or prolonged glucose tolerance curves, glycosuria, elevated spinal fluid proteins, increased plasma cholesterol, increased perspiration, chills; tingling, heaviness, and weakness of the hands.

*Topical use:* Prolonged use may result in local irritation and allergic contact dermatitis.

**Drug Interactions**

*Alcohol, ethyl* / See *CNS depressants*
*Antidepressants, tricyclic* / Additive anticholinergic side effects

*CNS depressants, antianxiety agents, barbiturates, narcotics, phenothiazines, procarbazine, sedative-hypnotics* / Potentiation or addition of CNS depressant effects. Concomitant use may lead to drowsiness, lethargy, stupor, respiratory depression, coma, and possibly death
*MAO inhibitors* / Intensification and prolongation of anticholinergic side effects; use with phenothiazine antihistamine → hypotension and extrapyramidal reactions

*NOTE:* Also see *Drug Interactions* for *Phenothiazines.*

**Dosage**
**Usually PO.** Parenteral administration is seldom used because of irritating nature of drugs. Topical usage is also limited because antihistamines often cause hypersensitivity reactions. When given for motion sickness, antihistamines are usually given 30–60 min before anticipated travel. See individual drugs.

**DENTAL CONCERNS**
**General**
1. Determine why the patient is taking the prescribed medication.
2. Decreased saliva flow can put the patient at risk for dental caries, periodontal disease, and candidiasis.
3. Patients with respiratory difficulty may require their dental chair in the semisupine position.
**Client/Family Teaching**
1. Review the importance of good oral hygiene in order to prevent soft tissue inflammation.
2. Review the proper use of oral hygiene aids in order to prevent injury.
3. Daily home fluoride treatments for persistent dry mouth.
4. Avoid alcohol-containing mouth rinses.
5. Dry mouth can be treated with tart, sugarless gum or candy, sips of water, or with saliva substitutes if dry mouth persists.
6. Avoid driving or operating heavy equipment. Sedative effects may disappear after several days or may not occur at all.

# ANTIHYPERLIPIDEMIC AGENTS—HMG-COA REDUCTASE INHIBITORS

*See also the following individual entries:*

Atorvastatin calcium
Cerivastatin sodium
Fluvastatin sodium
Lovastatin
Pravastatin sodium
Simvastatin

**General Statement:** The National Cholesterol Education Program Expert Panel on Detection, Evaluation, and Treatment of High Blood Cholesterol in Adults has developed guidelines for the treatment of high cholesterol and LDL in adults. Cholesterol levels less than 200 mg/dL are desirable. Cholesterol levels between 200 and 239 mg/dL are considered borderline-high while levels greater than 240 mg/dL are considered high. With respect to LDL, levels less than 130 mg/dL are considered desirable while levels between 130 and 159 md/dL are considered borderline-high and levels greater than 160 mg/dL are considered high. Depending on the levels of cholesterol and LDL and the number of risk factors present for CAD, the provider will develop a treatment regimen.

**Action/Kinetics:** The HMG-CoA reductase inhibitors competitively inhibit HMG-CoA reductase; this enzyme catalyzes the early rate-limiting step in the synthesis of cholesterol. HMG-CoA reductase inhibitors increase HDL cholesterol and decrease LDL cholesterol, VLDL cholesterol, and plasma triglycerides. The maximum therapeutic response is seen in 4–6 weeks.

**Uses:** Adjunct to diet to decrease elevated total LDL and cholesterol in clients with primary hypercholesterolemia (types IIa and IIb) when the response to diet and other nondrug approaches has not been adequate. See also individual drugs.

**Contraindications:** Active liver disease or unexplained persistent elevated liver function tests. Pregnancy, lactation. Use in children.

**Special Concerns:** Use with caution in those who ingest large quantities of alcohol or who have a history of liver disease. Safety and efficacy have not been established in children less than 18 years of age.

**Side Effects:** The following side effects are common to most HMG-CoA reductase inhibitors. Also see individual drugs. *GI:* N&V, diarrhea, constipation, abdominal cramps or pain, flatulence, dyspepsia, heartburn. *CNS:* Headache, dizziness, dysfunction of certain cranial nerves (e.g., alteration of taste, facial paresis, impairment of extraocular movement), tremor, vertigo, memory loss, paresthesia, anxiety, insomnia, depression. *Musculoskeletal:* Localized pain, myalgia, muscle cramps or pain, myopathy, rhabdomyolysis, arthralgia. *Respiratory:* Upper respiratory infection, rhinitis, cough. *Ophthalmic:* Progression of cataracts (lens opacities), ophthalmoplegia. *Hypersensitivity:* **Anaphylaxis, angioedema,** vasculitis, purpura, thrombocytopenia, leukopenia, **hemolytic anemia,** lupus erythematosus-like syndrome, polymyalgia rheumatica, positive ANA, ESR increase, arthritis, arthralgia, eosinophilia, urticaria, photosensitivity, fever, chills, flushing, malaise, dyspnea, **toxic dermal necrolysis, Stevens-Johnson syndrome.** *Miscellaneous:* Rash, pruritus, cardiac chest pain, fatigue, influenza, alopecia, edema, dryness of skin and mucous membranes, changes to hair and nails, skin discoloration.

**Drug Interactions**
*Cyclosporine* / ↑ Myalgia, myositis
*Erythromycin* / ↑ Myalgia, myositis

**Dosage** ————————
See individual drugs.

## DENTAL CONCERNS
**General**
1. Review lifestyle, duration of illness, and attempts made to control

---

with diet, exercise, and weight reduction.

2. Consider repositioning dental chair to semisupine posititon to reduce patient discomfort because of GI side effects.

3. Evaluate respiration rate.

**Client/Family Teaching**

1. Use UV protection (i.e., sunglasses, sunscreens, protective clothing, and hat) to prevent a photosensitivity reaction.

# ANTIHYPERTENSIVE AGENTS

*See also the following drug classes and individual drugs:*

*Agents Acting Directly on Vascular Smooth Muscle*

Hydralazine hydrochloride

*Alpha-1-Adrenergic Blocking Agents*

Doxazosin mesylate
Prazosin hydrochloride
Terazosin

*Angiotensin-II Antagonists*

Irbesartan
Losartan potassium
Valsartan

*Angiotensin-Converting Enzyme Inhibitors*

Benazepril hydrochloride
Captopril
Enalapril maleate
Fosinopril sodium

*Beta-Adrenergic Blocking Agents*

*Calcium Channel Blocking Agents*

Amlodipine
Diltiazem hydrochloride
Felodipine
Isradipine
Nicardipine hydrochloride
Nifedipine
Nimodipine
Verapamil

*Centrally-Acting Agents*

Clonidine hydrochloride
Methyldopa

*Combination Drugs Used for Hypertension*

Triamterene and
  Hydrochlorothiazide

*Miscellaneous Agents*

Carvedilol
Labetalol hydrochloride
Minoxidil, oral

**General Statement:** The Sixth Report of the Joint National Committee on Prevention, Detection, Evaluation and Treatment of High Blood Pressure classifies BP for adults aged 18 and over as follows: Optimal as <120/<80 mm Hg, Normal as <130/<85 mm Hg, High Normal as 130–139/85–89 mm Hg, Stage 1 Hypertension as 140–159/90–99 mm Hg, Stage 2 Hypertension as 160–179/100–109 mm Hg, and Stage 3 Hypertension as 180 or greater/110 or greater mm Hg. Drug therapy is recommended depending on the BP and whether certain risk factors (e.g., smoking, dyslipidemia, diabetes, age, gender, target organ damage, clinical CV disease) are present. Life-style modification is an important component of treating hypertension, including weight reduction, reduction of sodium intake, regular exercise, cessation of smoking, and moderate alcohol intake.

The goal of antihypertensive therapy is a BP of <140/90 mm Hg, except in hypertensive diabetics where the goal is <135/85 mm Hg and those with renal insufficiency where the goal is <130/85 mm Hg. Generally speaking, the primary agents for initial monotherapy to treat uncomplicated hypertension are diuretics and beta blockers. Alternative drugs include ACE inhibitors, alpha-1 blockers, alpha-beta blocker, and calcium antagonists.

**DENTAL CONCERNS**

**General**

1. Monitor vital signs at every appointment because of cardiovascular and respiratory side effects.

2. Have the patient sit up slowly and remain seated for at least two minutes after being supine in order to

minimize the risk of orthostatic hypotension.

3. Decreased saliva flow can put the patient at risk for dental caries, periodontal disease, and candidiasis.

4. Dental procedures may cause the patient anxiety or place stress on the heart. Assess cardiovascular patient for this risk.

5. Early morning and shorter appointments as well as methods for addressing anxiety levels in the patient can help to reduce the amount of stress that the patient is experiencing.

6. Vasoconstrictors should be used with caution and in low doses.

7. Calcium channel blockers have been associated with gingival hyperplasia. Have the patient perform meticulous oral hygiene.

**Client/Family Teaching**

1. Review the importance of good oral hygiene in order to prevent soft tissue inflammation and minimize the risk of gingival hyperplasia

2. Review the proper use of oral hygiene aids in order to prevent injury.

3. Daily home fluoride treatments for persistent dry mouth.

4. Avoid alcohol-containing mouth rinses and beverages.

5. Avoid caffeine-containing beverages.

6. Dry mouth can be treated with tart, sugarless gum or candy, water, sugar-free beverages, or with saliva substitutes if dry mouth persists.

7. Several antihypertensive agents cause sedation which can be intensified with the addition of an opioid analgesic or benzodiazepine. Use caution when doing anything that requires thought or concentration, such as operating heavy machinery, driving a car, or taking care of children.

8. Several antihypertensive agents can cause gastrointestinal (GI) irritation which can be intensified with the addition of a nonsteroidal anti-inflammatory drug. Take the medication with food or milk to help avoid or minimize GI discomfort.

# ANTINEOPLASTIC AGENTS

*See also the following individual entries:*

Aldesleukin
Busulfan
Cyclophosphamide
Etoposide
Fluorouracil
Flutamide
Hydroxyurea
Methotrexate
Methotrexate sodium
Paclitaxel
Tamoxifen

**General Statement:** The choice of the chemotherapeutic agent(s) depends both on the cell type of the tumor and on its site of growth. All antineoplastic agents are cytotoxic (i.e., cell poisons) and therefore interfere with normal as well as neoplastic cells. However, neoplastic cells are more active and multiply more rapidly than normal cells and are thus more affected by the antineoplastic agents. Normal, rapidly growing tissue cells, such as those of the bone marrow, the GI mucosal epithelium, and hair follicles, are particularly susceptible to antineoplastic agents. The margin between the dose of antineoplastic drug needed to destroy the neoplastic cells and that needed to cause bone marrow damage, for example, is narrow. Since WBCs or platelets show the effect of an overdose more rapidly than do erythrocytes, the platelet and WBC counts are often used as a guide to dosage. If a blood or marrow test indicates a precipitous fall in the WBC or platelet count, the antineoplastic agent may have to be discontinued or the dosage modified significantly. Drugs are frequently withheld when the WBC count falls below 2,000/mm$^3$ and the platelet count falls below 100,000/mm$^3$. With the advent of granulocyte colony-stimulating factors, providers may now utilize this to support large dosing on an aggressive cancer, thus preventing postponement of therapy until recovery of the client's hematologic parameters. Sometimes the effect of the antineoplastic drugs on the bone marrow is cumulative, with the depression of WBCs and platelets occurring weeks or months after initiation of therapy.

GI tract toxicity is manifested by development of oral ulcers, intestinal bleeding, nausea, vomiting, loss of appetite, and diarrhea. Finally, alopecia often results from antineoplastic drug therapy.

**Action/Kinetics:** During division, cells go through a number of stages during which they may be susceptible to various chemotherapeutic agents (see *Action/Kinetics* of various agents). The various cell stages are described in Figure 1.

**Uses:** Most of the drugs discussed in this section are used exclusively for neoplastic disease. A few are used on an experimental basis for some of the rheumatic diseases.

**Contraindications:** Hypersensitivity to drug. Some antineoplastic agents may be contraindicated for a period of 4 weeks after radiation therapy or chemotherapy with similar drugs. During first trimester of pregnancy.

**Special Concerns:** Use with caution, and at reduced dosages, in clients with preexisting bone marrow depression, malignant infiltration of bone marrow or kidney, liver dysfunction, or previous recent chemotherapy usage. The safe use of these drugs during pregnancy has not been established.

**Side Effects:** *Bone marrow depression* (leukopenia, thrombocytopenia, *agranulocytosis,* anemia) is the major danger of antineoplastic therapy. *Bone marrow depression can sometimes be irreversible. It is mandatory that the client have frequent total blood counts and periodic bone marrow examinations. Precipitous falls must be reported to a physician.* Other side effects include: *Oral:* Dry mouth, stomatits, mucositis. *GI:* N&V (may be severe), anorexia, diarrhea (may be hemorrhagic), stomatitis, mucositis, enteritis, abdominal cramps, intestinal ulcers. *Hepatic:* Hepatic toxicity including jaundice and changes in liver enzymes. *Dermatologic:* Dermatitis, erythema, various dermatoses including maculopapular rash, alopecia (reversible), pruritus, staining of vein path with some drugs, urticaria, cheilosis. *Immunologic:* Immunosuppression with increased susceptibility to viral, bacterial, or fungal infections. *CNS:* Depression, lethargy, confusion, dizziness, headache, fatigue, malaise, fever, weakness. *GU: Acute renal failure,* reproductive abnormalities including amenorrhea and azoospermia. *NOTE:* Alkylating agents, in particular, may be both carcinogenic and mutagenic.

## DENTAL CONCERNS
### General
1. Alternative analgesic therapy is necessary for patients requiring opioid analgesics.
2. A chlorhexidine mouth rinse before and during chemotherapy may help to reduce the severity of mucositis.
3. Palliative therapy may be necessary for the treatment of oral side effects.
4. Apply a lubricant to the patient's lips prior to the dental appointment as a comfort measure.
5. Patients who are undergoing active chemotherapy may require WBC count checks. These medications lower WBC counts and this could prove hazardous in patients requiring dental treatment that may produce wounds.
6. Monitor vital signs at every appointment because of cardiovascular side-effects.
7. Decreased saliva flow can put the patient at risk for dental caries, periodontal disease, and candidiasis.
8. Patients on chronic drug therapy may develop blood dyscrasias. Symptoms include fever, sore throat, and bleeding, and poor wound healing.
9. A semisupine position for the dental chair may be necessary to help minimize or avoid GI effects of

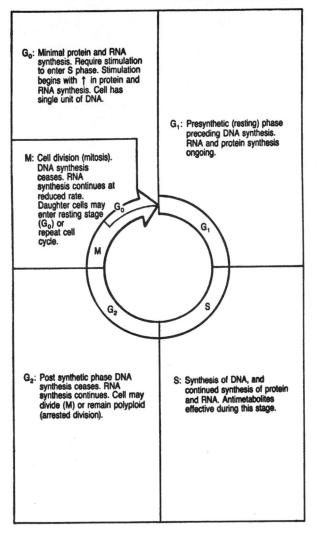

**Figure 1**   Cell stages.

the disease.

**Consultation with Primary Care Provider**

1. Consultation with the oncologist may be necessary. Prophylactic antibiotics may be necessary to prevent infection if surgery or deep scaling is required.

2. Patients with symptoms of blood dyscrasias should be referred to their primary care provider for complete blood counts. Treatment should be postponed until the results are known.

3. Consultation may be necessary in order to evaluate the patient's level of disease control.

4. Consultation may be necessary in order to determine the patient's ability to tolerate stress.

**Client/Family Teaching**

1. Report oral lesions, soreness or bleeding to the dentist.

2. Provide mouth care q 4–6 hr; otherwise mucosal deterioration occurs. Avoid lemon or glycerin; these tend to reduce saliva production and change pH of the mouth.

3. Secondary oral infections may occur. See the dentist if they should develop.

4. Review the importance of good oral hygiene in order to prevent soft tissue inflammation.

5. Review the proper use of oral hygiene aids in order to prevent injury.

6. Daily home fluoride treatments for persistent dry mouth.

7. Avoid alcohol-containing mouth rinses or beverages.

8. Avoid caffeine-containing beverages.

9. Dry mouth can be treated with tart, sugarless gum or candy, water, sugarless beverages, or with saliva substitutes if dry mouth persists.

---

# ANTIPARKINSON AGENTS

*See also the following individual entries:*

Amantadine hydrochloride
Benztropine mesylate

Biperiden hydrochloride
Bromocriptine mesylate
Carbidopa
Carbidopa/Levodopa
Diphenhydramine hydrochloride
Levodopa
Pergolide mesylate
Pramipexole
Ropinirole hydrochloride
Selegiline hydrochloride
Trihexyphenidyl hydrochloride

**General Statement:** Parkinson's disease is a progressive disorder of the nervous system, affecting mostly people over the age of 50. Parkinsonism is a frequent side effect of certain antipsychotic drugs, including prochlorperazine, chlorpromazine, and reserpine. Drug-induced symptoms usually disappear when the responsible agent is discontinued. The cause of Parkinson's disease is unknown; however, it is associated with a depletion of the neurotransmitter dopamine in the nervous system. Administration of levodopa—the precursor of dopamine—relieves symptoms in 75%–80% of the clients. Anticholinergic agents also have a beneficial effect by reducing tremors and rigidity and improving mobility, muscular coordination, and motor performance. They are often administered together with levodopa. Certain antihistamines, notably diphenhydramine (Benadryl), are also useful in the treatment of parkinsonism. Clients suffering from Parkinson's disease need emotional support and encouragement because the debilitating nature of the disorder often causes depression. Comprehensive treatment also includes physical therapy.

## DENTAL CONCERNS

See *Dental Concerns* for individual drugs.

---

# ANTIPSYCHOTIC AGENTS, PHENOTHIAZINES

*See also the following individual entries:*

Chlorpromazine
Chlorpromazine hydrochloride
Fluphenazine decanoate
Fluphenazine enanthate
Fluphenazine hydrochloride
Thioridazine hydrochloride

**General Statement:** Antipsychotic drugs do not cure mental illness, but they calm the intractable client, relieve the despondency of the severely depressed, activate the immobile and withdrawn, and make some more accessible to psychotherapy.

**Action/Kinetics:** It has been postulated that excess amounts of dopamine in certain areas of the CNS cause psychoses. Phenothiazines are thought to act by blocking postsynaptic mesolimbic dopamine receptors, leading to a reduction in psychotic symptoms. Phenothiazines block both $D_1$ and $D_2$ dopamine receptors. Alpha-adrenergic blockade produces sedation. In addition, these drugs produce anticholinergic and antihistaminic effects and depress the release of hypothalamic and hypophyseal hormones. Peripheral effects include anticholinergic and alpha-adrenergic blocking properties.

**Peak plasma levels:** 2–4 hr after PO administration. Widely distributed throughout the body. **t½ (average):** 10–20 hr. Most metabolized in the liver and excreted by the kidney.

**Uses:** Psychoses, especially if excessive psychomotor activity manifested. Involutional, toxic, or senile psychoses. Used in combination with MAO inhibitors in depressed clients manifesting anxiety, agitation, or panic (use with caution). With lithium in acute manic phase of manic-depressive illness. As an adjunct in alcohol withdrawal to reduce anxiety, tension, depression, nausea, and/or vomiting. For severe behavioral problems in children, manifested by hyperexcitable and/or combative behavior; also, for short-term use in hyperactive children who exhibit excess motor activity and conduct disorders.

**Contraindications:** Severe CNS depression, coma, clients with subcortical brain damage, bone marrow depression, lactation. In clients with a history of seizures and in those on anticonvulsant drugs. Geriatric or debilitated clients, hepatic or renal disease, CV disorders, glaucoma, prostatic hypertrophy. Contraindicated in children with chickenpox, CNS infections, measles, gastroenteritis, dehydration due to increased risk of extrapyramidal symptoms.

**Special Concerns:** Use with caution in clients exposed to extreme heat or cold and in those with asthma, emphysema, or acute respiratory tract infections. Use during pregnancy only when benefits outweigh risks. Children may be more sensitive to the neuromuscular or extrapyramidal effects (especially dystonias); those especially at risk include children with chickenpox, CNS infections, measles, dehydration, or gastroenteritis. Thus, generally, phenothiazines are not recommended for use in children less than 12 years of age. Geriatric clients often manifest higher plasma levels due to decreases in lean body mass, total body water, and albumin and an increase in total body fat. Also, geriatric clients may be more likely to manifest orthostatic hypotension, anticholinergic effects, sedative effects, and extrapyramidal side effects.

**Side Effects:** *CNS:* Depression, drowsiness, dizziness, lethargy, fatigue. Extrapyramidal effects, Parkinson-like symptoms including shuffling gait or tic-like movements of head and face, tardive dyskinesia (see what follows), akathisia, dystonia. *Seizures,* especially in clients with a history thereof. *Neuroleptic malignant syndrome (rare). CV:* Orthostatic hypotension, increase or decrease in BP, tachycardia, fainting. *Oral:* Dry mouth. *GI:* Anorexia, constipation, paralytic ileus, diarrhea. *Endocrine:* Breast engorgement, galactorrhea, gynecomastia, increased appetite, weight gain, hyper- or hypoglycemia, glycosuria. Delayed ejaculation, increased or decreased libido. *GU:* Menstrual irregularities, loss of bladder control, urinary difficulty. *Dermatologic:* Photosensitivity, pruritus, erythema, eczema, exfoliative dermatitis, pigment changes in skin (long-term use of high doses). *Hematologic:* **Aplastic anemia,** leukopenia, **agranulocytosis,** eosinophilia, thrombocytopenia. *Ophthalmologic:* Deposition of fine particulate matter in lens and cornea leading to blurred vision, changes in vision. *Respiratory:* **Laryngospasm, bronchospasm, laryngeal edema,** breathing difficulties. *Miscellaneous:* Fever, muscle stiffness, decreased sweating, muscle spasm of face, neck, or back, obstructive jaundice, nasal congestion, pale skin, mydriasis, systemic lupus-like syndrome.

*Tardive dyskinesia* has been observed with all classes of antipsychotic drugs, although the precise cause is not known. The syndrome is most commonly seen in older clients, especially women, and in individuals with organic brain syndrome. It is often aggravated or precipitated by the sudden discontinuance of antipsychotic drugs and may persist indefinitely after the drug is discontinued. Early signs of tardive dyskinesia include fine vermicular movements of the tongue and grimacing or tic-like movements of the head and neck. Although there is no known cure for the syndrome, it may not progress if the dosage of the drug is slowly reduced. Also, a few drug-free days may unmask the symptoms of tardive dyskinesia and help in early diagnosis.

### Drug Interactions

*Alcohol, ethyl* / Potentiation or addition of CNS depressant effects. Concomitant use may lead to drowsiness, lethargy, stupor, respiratory collapse, coma, or death

*Aluminum salts (antacids)* / ↓ Absorption from GI tract

*Amphetamine* / ↓ Effect of amphetamine by ↓ uptake of drug to the site of action

*Anesthetics, general* / See *Alcohol*

*Antacids, oral* / ↓ Effect of phenothiazines due to ↓ absorption from GI tract

*Antianxiety drugs* / See *Alcohol*

*Anticholinergic drugs* / Additive anticholinergic side effects and/or ↓ antipsychotic effect

*Antidepressants, tricyclic* / Additive anticholinergic side effects

*Barbiturate anesthetics* / ↑ Chance of tremor, involuntary muscle activity, and hypotension

*Barbiturates* / See *Alcohol;* also, barbiturates may ↓ effect due to ↑ breakdown by liver

*CNS depressants* / See *Alcohol;* also, ↓ effect of phenothiazines due to ↑ breakdown by liver

*Hydantoins* / ↑ Risk of hydantoin toxicity

*MAO inhibitors* / ↑ Effect of phenothiazines due to ↓ breakdown by liver

*Meperidine* / ↑ Risk of hypotension and sedation

*Opioid Analgesics* / See *Alcohol*

*Phenytoin* / ↑ Effect of phenytoin due to ↓ breakdown by liver

*Sedative-hypnotics, nonbarbiturate* / See *Alcohol*

*Succinylcholine* / ↑ Muscle relaxation

*Tricyclic antidepressants* / ↑ Serum levels of tricyclic antidepressant

### Dosage

See individual drugs. Effective over a wide dosage range. Dosage is usually increased gradually to minimize side effects over 7 days until the minimal effective dose is attained. Dosage is increased more gradually in elderly or debilitated clients because they are more susceptible to the effects and side effects of drugs. After symptoms are controlled, dosage is gradually reduced to maintenance levels. It is usually desirable to keep chronically ill clients on maintenance levels indefinitely. Medication, especially in clients on high dosages, should not be discontinued abruptly.

## DENTAL CONCERNS
### General
1. Monitor vital signs at every appointment because of cardiovascular side effects.
2. Have the patient sit up slowly and remain seated for at least two minutes after being supine in order to minimize the risk of orthostatic hypotension.
3. Decreased saliva flow can put the patient at risk for dental caries, periodontal disease, and candidiasis.
4. Patients on chronic drug therapy may develop blood dyscrasias. Symptoms include fever, sore throat, bleeding, and poor wound healing.
5. Place patient on frequent recall because of oral adverse effects.
6. Determine the presence of movement disorders such as extrapyramidal symptoms, tardive dyskinesia, or akathisia. They may interfere with the ability of the patient to perform oral health care or they can complicate dental treatment.
### Consultation with Primary Care Provider
1. Patients with symptoms of blood dyscrasias should be referred to their primary care provider for complete blood counts. Treatment should be postponed until the results are known.
2. Contact appropriate health care provider if the patient has akathisia or tardive dyskinesia.
3. Health care provider should be informed of the oral adverse effects of these drugs.
4. Use caution if dental surgery and anesthesia are required.
### Client/Family Teaching
1. Review the importance of good oral hygiene in order to prevent soft tissue inflammation.
2. Review the proper use of oral hygiene aids in order to prevent injury.
3. Daily home fluoride treatments for persistent dry mouth.

4. Avoid alcohol-containing mouth rinses and beverages.
5. Avoid caffeine-containing beverages.
6. Dry mouth can be treated with tart, sugarless gum or candy, water, sugar-free beverages, or with saliva substitutes if dry mouth persists.

# ANTIVIRAL DRUGS

*See also the following individual entries:*

> Acyclovir (Acycloguanosine)
> Amantadine hydrochloride
> Cidofovir
> Delavirdine mesylate
> Didanosine (ddI, Dideoxyinosine)
> Famciclovir
> Indinavir sulfate
> Lamivudine
> Lamivudine and Zidovudine
> Nelfinavir mesylate
> Nevirapine
> Penciclovir
> Ritonavir
> Saquinavir mesylate
> Zalcitabine
> Zidovudine (Azidothymidine, AZT)

**Action/Kinetics:** To maintain their growth and reproduce, viruses must enter living cells. Thus, it is difficult to find a drug that is specific for the virus and that does not interfere with the function of the host cell. However, there are enzymes and replicative mechanisms that are unique to viruses and an increasing number of drugs with specific antiviral activity have been developed. The antiviral drugs currently marketed act by one of the following mechanisms:
1. Inhibition of enzymes required for DNA synthesis. Example: Idoxuridine.
2. Inhibition of viral nucleic acid synthesis by interacting directly with herpes virus DNA polymerase or HIV reverse transcriptase. Example: Foscarnet.
3. Inhibition of viral DNA synthesis. Examples: Acyclovir, Cidofovir, Di-

danosine, Famciclovir, Ganciclovir, Penciclovir, Trifluridine, Valacyclovir, Vidarabine.

4. Prevent penetration of the virus into cells by inhibiting uncoating of the RNA virus. Examples: Amantadine, Rimantadine.

5. Protease inhibitors resulting in release of immature, noninfectious viral particles. Examples: Indinavir, Ritonavir, Nelfinavir, Saquinavir.

6. Inhibition of reverse transcriptase resulting in inhibition of replication of the virus. Examples: Lamivudine, Nevirapine, Stavudine, Zalcitabine, Zidovudine. It is becoming increasingly common to combine two antiviral drugs that have different mechanisms of action in order to treat HIV infections.

### DENTAL CONCERNS

See *General Dental Concerns For All Anti-Infectives.*

**General**

1. Document indications for therapy, type and onset of symptoms, and exposure characteristics.

2. List other agents and route prescribed to ensure none interact unfavorably.

3. Note underlying medical conditions that may preclude drug therapy.

4. Consider a semi-supine position for the dental chair to avoid or minimize GI discomfort.

**Client/Family Teaching**

1. Review method and frequency for drug administration. Take exactly as directed; do not share meds.

2. Identify specific measures necessary to decrease or halt the spread of the disease.

3. Report any rashes or unusual side effects of drug therapy.

4. If symptoms do not improve or worsen after specified time frame, report to provider.

5. Need close medical supervision and follow-up during drug therapy.

6. Flouride tablets or therapy should be administered 2 hours before aluminum hydroxide administration.

# BARBITURATES

*See also the following individual entries:*

> Pentobarbital
> Pentobarbital sodium
> Phenobarbital
> Phenobarbital sodium
> Secobarbital sodium

**Action/Kinetics:** Barbiturates produce all levels of CNS depression, ranging from mild depression (sedation) following low doses to hypnotic (sleep-inducing) effects, and even coma and death, as dosage is increased. Certain barbiturates are also effective anticonvulsants. The depressant and anticonvulsant effects may be related to their ability to increase and/or mimic the inhibitory activity of the neurotransmitter GABA on nerve synapses. Importantly, barbiturates are not analgesics and therefore should not be given to clients for the purpose of ameliorating pain. Sodium salts are readily absorbed after PO, rectal, or parenteral administration. They are distributed throughout all tissues, cross the placental barrier, and appear in breast milk. The main difference between the various barbiturates is in the onset of action, which ranges from 10 to 15 min for pentobarbital and secobarbital and 60 or more minutes for phenobarbital. Metabolized almost completely in the liver (except for phenobarbital) and are excreted in the urine.

**Uses:** Preanesthetic medication. Sedation, hypnotic, anticonvulsant (phenobarbital) and for the control of acute convulsive conditions (only phenobarbital, mephobarbital), as in epilepsy, tetanus, meningitis, eclampsia, and toxic reactions to local anesthetics or strychnine. The benzodiazepines have replaced barbiturates for the treatment of many conditions, especially daytime sedation. See also information on individual drugs.

**Contraindications:** Hypersensitivity to barbiturates, severe trauma, pulmonary disease when dyspnea or obstruction is present, edema, uncontrolled diabetes, history of porphyria, and impaired liver function and for clients in whom they produce an excitatory response. Also, clients who have been addicted previously to sedative-hypnotics.

**Special Concerns:** Use with caution during lactation and in clients with CNS depression, hypotension, marked asthenia (characteristic of Addison's disease, hypoadrenalism, and severe myxedema), porphyria, fever, anemia, hemorrhagic shock, cardiac, hepatic or renal damage, and a history of alcoholism in suicidal clients. Geriatric clients usually manifest increased sensitivity to barbiturates, as evidenced by confusion, excitement, mental depression, and hypothermia. When given in the presence of pain, restlessness, excitement, and delirium may result. Intra-arterial use may cause symptoms from transient pain to gangrene; SC use produces tissue irritation, including tenderness and redness to necrosis.

**Side Effects:** *CNS:* Sleepiness, drowsiness, agitation, confusion, hyperkinesia, ataxia, CNS depression, nightmares, nervousness, psychiatric disturbances, hallucinations, insomnia, anxiety, dizziness, headache, abnormal thinking, vertigo, lethargy, hangover, excitement, appearance of being inebriated. Irritability and hyperactivity in children. *Musculoskeletal:* Localized or diffuse myalgic, neuralgic, or arthritic pain, especially in psychoneurotic clients. Pain is often most intense in the morning and is frequently located in the neck, shoulder girdle, and arms. *Respiratory:* Hypoventilation, **apnea, respiratory depression.** *CV:* Bradycardia, hypotension, syncope, **circulatory collapse.** *GI:* N&V, constipation, liver damage (especially with chronic use of phenobarbital). *Allergic:* Skin rashes, **angioedema,** exfoliative dermatitis (including **Stevens-Johnson syndrome and toxic epidermal necrolysis**). Allergic reactions are most common in clients who have asthma, urticaria, angioedema, and similar conditions. Symptoms include localized swelling (especially of the lips, cheeks, or eyelids) and erythematous dermatitis).

*After SC use:* Tissue necrosis, pain, tenderness, redness, permanent neurologic damage if injected near peripheral nerves.

*After IV use. CV:* Circulatory depression, thrombophlebitis, **peripheral vascular collapse, seizures with cardiorespiratory arrest, myocardial depression, cardiac arrhythmias.** *Respiratory:* **Apnea, laryngospasm, bronchospasm,** dyspnea, rhinitis, sneezing, coughing. *CNS:* Emergence delirium, headache, anxiety, prolonged somnolence and recovery, restlessness, **seizures.** *GI:* N&V, abdominal pain, diarrhea, cramping. *Hypersensitivity:* **Acute allergic reactions, including erythema, pruritus, anaphylaxis.** *Miscellaneous:* Pain or nerve injury at injection site, salivation, hiccups, skin rashes, shivering, skeletal muscle hyperactivity, **immune hemolytic anemia with renal failure,** and radial nerve palsy.

*After IM use:* Pain at injection site. Barbiturates can induce physical and psychologic dependence if high doses are used regularly for long periods of time. Withdrawal symptoms usually begin after 12–16 hr of abstinence. Manifestations of withdrawal include anxiety, weakness, N&V, muscle cramps, delirium, and even **tonic-clonic seizures.**

**Drug Interactions**

GENERAL CONSIDERATIONS
1. Barbiturates stimulate the activity of enzymes responsible for the metabolism of a large number of other drugs by a process known as *enzyme induction*. As a result, when barbiturates are given to clients receiving such drugs, their therapeutic effectiveness is markedly reduced or even abolished.
2. The CNS depressant effect of the barbiturates is potentiated by many drugs. Concomitant administration may result in coma or fatal CNS de-

pression. Barbiturate dosage should either be reduced or eliminated when other CNS drugs are given.

3. Barbiturates also potentiate the toxic effects of many other agents.

*Acetaminophen* / ↑ Risk of hepatotoxicity when used with large or chronic doses of barbiturates

*Alcohol* / Potentiation or addition of CNS depressant effects. Concomitant use may lead to drowsiness, lethargy, stupor, respiratory collapse, coma, or death

*Anesthetics, general* / See *Alcohol*

*Antianxiety drugs* / See *Alcohol*

*Antidepressants, tricyclic* / ↓ Effect of antidepressants due to ↑ breakdown by liver

*Carbamazepine* / ↓ Serum carbazepine levels may occur

*CNS depressants* / See *Alcohol*

*Corticosteroids* / ↓ Effect of corticosteroids due to ↑ breakdown by liver

*Doxycycline* / ↓ Effect of doxycycline due to ↑ breakdown by liver (effect may last up to 2 weeks after barbiturates are discontinued)

*Fenoprofen* / ↓ Bioavailability of fenoprofen

*Haloperidol* / ↓ Effect of haloperidol due to ↑ breakdown by liver

*MAO inhibitors* / ↑ Effect of barbiturates due to ↓ breakdown by liver

*Meperidine* / CNS depressant effects may be prolonged

*Metronidazole* / ↓ Effect of metronidazole

*Opioid analgesics* / See *Alcohol*

*Phenothiazines* / ↓ Effect of phenothiazines due to ↑ breakdown by liver; also see *Alcohol*

*Phenylbutazone* / ↓ Elimination t½ of phenylbutazone

*Phenytoin* / Effect variable and unpredictable; monitor carefully

*Sedative-hypnotics, nonbarbiturate* / See *Alcohol*

**Dosage**

See individual drugs. Aim for minimum effective dosage. As hypnotics, barbiturates should be administered intermittently because tolerance develops. Elderly clients should receive one-half of the adult dose, and children should receive one-quarter to one-half the adult dose.

## DENTAL CONCERNS
### General

1. Early morning and shorter appointments as well as methods for addressing anxiety levels in the patient can help to reduce the amount of stress that the patient is experiencing.

2. Patients on chronic drug therapy may develop blood dyscrasias. Symptoms include fever, sore throat, bleeding, and poor wound healing.

3. Monitor vital signs at every appointment because of cardiovascular and respiratory side effects.

4. If the drug is used for sedation in the dental office, assess vital signs before administration and every 30 minutes thereafter.

5. Monitor respiratory function.

6. Have the patient sit up slowly and remain seated for at least two minutes after being supine in order to minimize the risk of orthostatic hypotension.

7. The patient should have someone drive him to and from the dental office if the drug is used for conscious sedation.

### Consultation with Primary Care Provider

1. Patients with symptoms of blood dyscrasias should be referred to their primary care provider for complete blood counts. Treatment should be postponed until the results are known.

### Client/Family Teaching

1. Do not drive a car, operate other hazardous machinery after taking drug, or do anything else that requires thought or concentration.

2. Avoid OTC drugs or any other agents unless prescribed.

3. Avoid alcohol; it potentiates effects of barbiturates.

# BETA-ADRENERGIC BLOCKING AGENTS

*See also Alpha-1-Adrenergic Blocking Agents and the following individual agents:*

Acebutolol hydrochloride
Atenolol
Betaxolol hydrochloride
Carteolol hydrochloride
Metoprolol succinate
Metoprolol tartrate
Nadolol

**Action/Kinetics:** Combine reversibly with beta-adrenergic receptors to block the response to sympathetic nerve impulses, circulating catecholamines, or adrenergic drugs. Beta-adrenergic receptors have been classified as beta-1 (predominantly in the cardiac muscle) and beta-2 (mainly in the bronchi and vascular musculature). Blockade of beta-1 receptors decreases HR, myocardial contractility, and CO; in addition, AV conduction is slowed. These effects lead to a decrease in BP, as well as a reversal of cardiac arrhythmias. Blockade of beta-2 receptors increases airway resistance in the bronchioles and inhibits the vasodilating effects of catecholamines on peripheral blood vessels. The various beta-blocking agents differ in their ability to block beta-1 and beta-2 receptors (see individual drugs); also, certain of these agents have intrinsic sympathomimetic action.

Certain of these drugs (betaxolol, carteolol, levobunolol, metipranolol, and timolol) are used for glaucoma. The drugs appear to act by reducing production of aqueous humor; metipranolol and timolol may also increase outflow of aqueous humor. These drugs have little or no effect on the pupil size or on accommodation.

**Uses:** Uses vary with the individual drugs and include the treatment of hypertension, angina pectoris, cardiac arrhythmias, MI, prophylaxis of migraine, tremors (essential, lithium-induced, parkinsonism), situational anxiety, aggressive behavior, antipsychotic-induced akathisia, esophageal varices rebleeding, and alcohol withdrawal syndrome. Decrease intraocular pressure in chronic open-angle glaucoma.

**Contraindications:** Hypersensitivity to beta-blockers, cardiogenic shock, 2nd or 3rd degree heart block, sinus bradycardia, CHF, cardiac failure.

**Special Concerns:** Use with caution in diabetes, thyrotoxicosis, cerebrovascular insufficiency, and impaired hepatic and renal function. Withdrawing beta blockers before major surgery is controversial. Safe use during pregnancy and lactation and in children has not been established. May be absorbed systemically when used for glaucoma; thus, there is the potential for an additive effect with beta blockers used systemically. Certain of the products for use in glaucoma contain sulfites, which may result in an allergic reaction. Also, see individual agents.

**Side Effects:** *Oral:* dry mouth. *CV:* bradycardia, CHF, cold extremities, postural hypotension, profound hypotension, 2nd or 3rd degree heart block. *CNS:* catatonia, depression, dizziness, drowsiness, fatigue, hallucinations, insomnia, lethargy, mental changes, memory loss, strange dreams. *GI:* Diarrhea, ***ischemic colitis,*** nausea, ***mesenteric arterial thrombosis,*** vomiting. *Hematologic:* ***agranulocytosis,*** thrombocytopenia. *Allergic:* fever, sore throat, respiratory distress, rash, pharyngitis, ***laryngospasm, anaphylaxis.*** *Skin:* pruritus, rash, increased skin pigmentation, sweating, dry skin, alopecia, skin irritation, psoriasis. *Ophthalmic:* Dry, burning eyes. *GU:* dysuria, impotence, nocturia. *Other:* hypoglycemia or hyperglycemia. *Respiratory:* ***bronchospasm,*** dyspnea, wheezing. *Systemic effects due to ophthalmic beta-1 and beta-2 blockers:* Headache, depression, arrhythmia, heart block, CVA, syncope, CHF, palpitation, cerebral ischemia, nausea, localized and generalized rash, bronchospasm (especially in those with pre-existing bronchospastic disease), respiratory failure, masked symptoms of hypoglycemia in insulin-dependent diabetics, keratitis, visual

---

disturbances (including refractive changes), blepharoptosis, ptosis, diplopia.

**Drug Interactions**

*Anesthetics, general* / Additive depression of myocardium

*Anticholinergic agents* / Counteract bradycardia produced by beta-adrenergic blockers

*Epinephrine* / Beta blockers prevent beta-adrenergic action of epinephrine but not alpha-adrenergic action → ↑ systolic and diastolic BP and ↓ HR

*Fentanyl and derivatives* / ↓ Increased hypotension and cardiac depression

*Indomethacin* / ↓ Effect of beta blockers possibly due to inhibition of prostaglandin synthesis

*Lidocaine* / ↑ Effect of lidocaine due to ↓ breakdown by liver

*NSAIDs* / ↓ Effect of beta blockers, possibly due to inhibition of prostaglandin synthesis

*Salicylates* / ↓ Effect of beta blockers, possibly due to inhibition of prostaglandin synthesis

*Sympathomimetics* / Reverse effects of beta blockers

**Dosage** ———————————

See individual drugs.

## DENTAL CONCERNS

**General**

1. Monitor vital signs at every appointment because of cardiovascular and respiratory side effects.
2. Have the patient sit up slowly and remain seated for at least two minutes after being supine in order to minimize the risk of orthostatic hypotension.
3. Decreased saliva flow can put the patient at risk for dental caries, periodontal disease, and candidiasis.
4. Dental procedures may cause the patient anxiety or place stress on the heart. Assess cardiovascular patient for this risk.
5. Early-morning and shorter appointments as well as methods for addressing anxiety levels in the patient can help to reduce the amount of stress that the patient is experiencing.

6. Vasoconstrictors should be used with caution and in low doses. Avoid epinephrine-containing gingival retraction cords.
7. Patients on chronic drug therapy may develop blood dyscrasias. Symptoms include fever, sore throat, and bleeding, and poor wound healing.

OPHTHALMIC DROPS

1. Assess patient for compliance with drug regimen for glaucoma.
2. Avoid direct dental light in the patient's eyes. Keep dark glasses available for patient comfort.

**Consultation with Primary Care Provider**

1. Patients with symptoms of blood dyscrasias should be referred to their primary care provider for complete blood counts. Treatment should be postponed until the results are known.
2. Consultation with appropriate health care provider may be necessary to evaluate level of disease control.
3. General anesthesia should be used with caution in patients requiring dental surgery.

**Client/Family Teaching**

1. Review the importance of good oral hygiene in order to prevent soft tissue inflammation.
2. Review the proper use of oral hygiene aids in order to prevent injury.
3. Daily home fluoride treatments for persistent dry mouth.
4. Avoid alcohol-containing mouth rinses.
5. Dry mouth can be treated with tart, sugarless gum or candy, sips of water, or with saliva substitutes if dry mouth persists.
6. You may want to wear dark glasses in order to avoid photophobia which can occur with the dental light.

# CALCIUM CHANNEL BLOCKING AGENTS

*See also the following individual entries:*

　Amlodipine

Diltiazem hydrochloride
Felodipine
Isradipine
Nicardipine hydrochloride
Nifedipine
Nimodipine
Verapamil

**Action/Kinetics:** The calcium channel blocking agents inhibit the influx of calcium through the cell membrane, resulting in a depression of automaticity and conduction velocity in both smooth and cardiac muscle. This leads to a depression of contraction in these tissues. They also decrease total peripheral resistance by causing relaxation of vascular smooth muscle, thus reducing energy and oxygen requirements of the heart. Also effective against certain cardiac arrhythmias by slowing AV conduction and prolonging repolarization. In addition, they depress the amplitude, rate of depolarization, and conduction in atria.

**Uses:** See individual drugs.

**Contraindications:** Sick sinus syndrome, second- or third-degree AV block (except with a functioning pacemakcr). Use of bepridil, diltiazem, or verapamil for hypotension (<90 mm Hg systolic pressure). Lactation.

**Special Concerns:** Abrupt withdrawal may result in increased frequency and duration of chest pain. Hypertensive clients treated with immediate-release dose forms of calcium channel blockers have a higher risk of heart attack than clients treated with diuretics or beta-adrenergic blockers. Safety and effectiveness of bepridil, diltiazem, felodipine, and isradipine have not been established in children.

**Side Effects:** Side effects vary from one calcium channel blocker to another; refer to individual drugs.

**Drug Interactions**
*Fentanyl* / Severe hypotension or increased fluid volume requirements

**Dosage** ─────────────
See individual drugs.

─────────────────────────

## DENTAL CONCERNS
### General
1. Assess vital signs at every appointment because of cardiovascular side effects.
2. Early morning and shorter appointments may be of benefit for anxious patients.
3. Antianxiety drugs, such as benzodiazepines or nitrous oxide, can be prescribed if the anxiety associated with a dental appointment precipitates the patient's angina attack.
4. Talk with patient about frequency of angina attacks (disease control).
5. Stress from a dental procedure may adversely affect the patient's cardiovascular status. Assess patient risk.
6. Have the patient sit up slowly and remain seated for at least two minutes after being supine in order to minimize the risk of orthostatic hypotension.
7. Decreased saliva flow can put the patient at risk for dental caries, periodontal disease, and candidiasis.
8. Patients on sodium restricted diets should receive sodium-containing fluids (i.e., saline solution) with caution.

### Consultation with Primary Care Provider
1. Medical consultation may be necessary in order to assess patient's cardiovascular status and ability to tolerate stress.

### Client/Family Teaching
1. Daily home fluoride treatments for persistent dry mouth.
2. Avoid alcohol-containing mouth rinses and beverages.
3. Dry mouth can be treated with tart, sugarless gum or candy, water, sugar-free beverages, or with saliva substitutes if dry mouth persists.
4. Avoid caffeine-containing beverages.
5. May cause ginigival hyperplasia. Frequent oral prophylaxis in order to minimize overgrowth.

─────────────────────────

# CARDIAC GLYCOSIDES

*See also the following individual entries:*

Digitoxin
Digoxin

**Action/Kinetics:** Cardiac glycosides increase the force and velocity of myocardial contraction (positive inotropic effect) by increasing the refractory period of the AV node and decreasing total peripheral resistance. This effect is due to inhibition of sodium/potassium–ATPase which results in an increase of calcium influx and an increased release of free calcium ions within the myocardial cells. Clinical effects are not seen until steady-state plasma levels are reached. The initial dose of digitalis glycosides is larger (loading dose) and is traditionally referred to as the *digitalizing dose;* subsequent doses are referred to as *maintenance doses.*

**Uses:** All types of CHF, including that due to venous congestion, edema, dyspnea, orthopnea, and cardiac arrhythmia. Control of rapid ventricular contraction rate in clients with atrial fibrillation or flutter. Slow HR in sinus tachycardia due to CHF. Supraventricular tachycardia. Prophylaxis and treatment of recurrent paroxysmal atrial tachycardia with paroxysmal AV junctional rhythm. Cardiogenic shock (value not established).

**Contraindications:** Ventricular fibrillation or tachycardia (unless congestive failure supervenes after protracted episode not due to digitalis), in presence of digitalis toxicity, hypersensitivity to cardiac glycosides, beriberi heart disease, certain cases of hypersensitive carotid sinus syndrome, 2nd or 3rd degree heart block.

**Special Concerns:** Use with caution in clients with ischemic heart disease, acute myocarditis, hypertrophic subaortic stenosis, hypoxic or myxedemic states, Adams-Stokes or carotid sinus syndromes, cardiac amyloidosis, or cyanotic heart and lung disease, including emphysema and partial heart block. Those with carditis associated with rheumatic fever or viral myocarditis are especially sensitive to digoxin-induced disturbances in rhythm. Electric pacemakers may sensitize the myocardium to cardiac glycosides. Also use with caution and at reduced dosage in elderly, debilitated clients, pregnant women and nursing mothers, and newborn, term, or premature infants who have immature renal and hepatic function and in reduced renal and/or hepatic function.

**Side Effects:** Cardiac glycosides are extremely toxic and have caused death even in clients who have received the drugs for long periods of time. There is a narrow margin of safety between an effective therapeutic dose and a toxic dose. Overdosage caused by the cumulative effects of the drug is a constant danger in therapy with cardiac glycosides. Digitalis toxicity is characterized by a wide variety of symptoms, which are hard to differentiate from those of the cardiac disease itself.

*CV:* Changes in the rate, rhythm, and irritability of the heart and the mechanism of the heartbeat. Extrasystoles, bigeminal pulse, coupled rhythm, ectopic beat, and other forms of arrhythmias have been noted. ***Death most often results from ventricular fibrillation.*** Cardiac glycosides should be discontinued in adults when pulse rate falls below 60 beats/min. All cardiac changes are best detected by the ECG, which is also most useful in clients suffering from intoxication. *Acute hemorrhage. Oral:* Excessive salivation, sensitive gag reflex. *GI:* Anorexia, N&V, epigastric distress, abdominal pain, diarrhea, bowel necrosis. Clients on digitalis therapy may experience two vomiting stages. The first is an early sign of toxicity and is a direct effect of digitalis on the GI tract. Late vomiting indicates stimulation of the vomiting center of the brain, which occurs after the heart muscle has been saturated with digitalis. *CNS:* Headaches, fatigue, lassitude, irritability, malaise, muscle weakness, insomnia, stupor. Psychotomimetic effects (especially in elderly or arteriosclerotic clients or neonates) including disorientation, confusion, depression, aphasia, delirium, hallucinations, and, rarely, *convulsions.* *Neuromuscular:* Neurologic pain involving the lower third of the face and lumbar areas, paresthesia. *Visual disturbances:* Blurred vision, flickering dots, white halos, borders around dark objects, diplopia, amblyopia, color perception changes. *Hypersensitivity (5–7 days after starting therapy):* Skin reactions (urticaria, fever, pruritus, facial and *angioneurotic edema*). *Other:* Chest pain, coldness of extremities.

**Drug Interactions**
*Aminosalicylic acid* / ↓ Effect of digitalis glycosides due to ↓ absorption from GI tract
*Antacids* / ↓ Effect of digitalis glycosides due to ↓ absorption from GI tract
*Corticosteroids* / Can cause hypokalemia.
*Epinephrine* / ↑ Chance of cardiac arrhythmias
*Erythromycin* / ↑ Digoxin blood levels.
*Muscle relaxants, nondepolarizing* / ↑ Risk of cardiac arrhythmias
*Sympathomimetics* / ↑ Chance of cardiac arrhythmias
*Succinylcholine* / ↑ Chance of cardiac arrhythmias

**Dosage**
**PO, IM, or IV.** *Highly individualized.* See individual drugs: digitoxin, digoxin. The rates at which clients become digitalized vary considerably. Clients with mild signs of congestion can often be digitalized gradually over a period of several days. Clients suffering from more serious congestion, for example, those showing signs of acute LV failure, dyspnea, or lung edema, can be digitalized more rapidly by parenteral administration of a fast-acting cardiac glycoside. Once digitalization has been attained (pulse 68–80 beats/min) and symptoms of CHF

have subsided, the client is put on maintenance dosage. Depending on the drug and the age of the client, the daily maintenance dose is often approximately 10% of the digitalizing dose.

**DENTAL CONCERNS**
**General**
1. Monitor vital signs at every appointment because of cardiovascular and respiratory side effects.
2. Have the patient sit up slowly and remain seated for at least two minutes after being supine in order to minimize the risk of orthostatic hypotension.
3. Avoid direct dental light in the patient's eyes. Keep dark glasses available for patient comfort.
4. Dental procedures, such as radiographs or impressions, may be difficult because of an increased gag reflex.
5. Vasoconstrictors should be used with caution, in low doses, and with careful aspiration. Use of gingival retraction cords with epinephrine should be avoided.

**Consultation with Primary Care Provider**
1. Consultation with primary care provider may be necessary to assess patient status (disease control and ability to tolerate stress).
2. Dental procedures may compromise the patient's cardiovascular status. Assess patient risk.

# CEPHALOSPORINS

*See also the following individual entries:*

Cefaclor
Cefadroxil monohydrate
Cefixime oral
Cefpodoxime proxetil
Cefprozil
Ceftibuten
Cefuroxime axetil
Cephalexin hydrochloride
    monohydrate
Cephalexin monohydrate

---

Cephradine
Loracarbef

**General Statement:** Cephalosporins are broad-spectrum antibiotics classified as first-, second-, and third-generation drugs. The difference among generations is based on pharmacokinetics and antibacterial spectra. Generally, third-generation cephalosporins have more activity against gram-negative organisms and resistant organisms and less activity against gram-positive organisms than first-generation drugs. Third-generation cephalosporins are also stable against beta-lactamases. Cephalosporins can be destroyed by cephalosporinase. Also, the cost increases from first- to third-generation cephalosporins.

**Action/Kinetics:** The cephalosporins interfere with a final step in the formation of the bacterial cell wall (inhibition of mucopeptide biosynthesis), resulting in unstable cell membranes that undergo lysis (same mechanism of actions as penicillins). Also, cell division and growth are inhibited. The cephalosporins are most effective against young, rapidly dividing organisms and are considered bactericidal. Cephalosporins are widely distributed to most tissues and fluids. First- and second-generation drugs do not enter the CSF well but third-generation drugs enter inflamed meninges readily. Rapidly excreted by the kidneys.

**Uses:** See individual drugs. Cephalosporins are effective against infections of the biliary tract, GI tract, GU system, bones, joints, upper and lower respiratory tract, skin, and skin structures. Also, gynecologic infections, meningitis, osteomyelitis, endocarditis, intra-abdominal infections, peritonitis, otitis media, gonorrhea, septicemia, and prophylaxis prior to surgery. A listing of the drugs in each generation follows:

**First-Generation Cephalosporins:** Cefadroxil, cefazolin, cephalexin, cephalothin, cephapirin, cephradine.

**Second-Generation Cephalosporins:** Cefaclor, cefamandole, cefmetazole, cefonicid, cefotetan, cefoxitin, cefprozil, cefuroxime, and loracarbef.

**Third-Generation Cephalosporins:** Cefepime, cefixime, cefoperazone, cefotaxime, cefpodoxime, ceftazidime, ceftibuten, ceftizoxime, ceftriaxone.

**Contraindications:** Hypersensitivity to cephalosporins or related antibiotics.

**Special Concerns:** Safe use in pregnancy and lactation has not been established. Use with caution in the presence of impaired renal or hepatic function, together with other nephrotoxic drugs, and in clients over 50 years of age. Perform $C_{cr}$ on all clients with impaired renal function who receive cephalosporins. If hypersensitive to penicillin, may occasionally cross-react to cephalosporins.

**Side Effects:** *Oral:* Sore mouth or tongue, dysgeusia, candidiasis, glossitis. *GI:* N&V, diarrhea, abdominal cramps or pain, dyspepsia, glossitis, heartburn, anorexia, flatulence, cholestasis. Pseudomembranous colitis. *Allergic:* Urticaria, rashes (maculopapular, morbilliform, or erythematous), pruritus (including anal and genital areas), fever, chills, erythema, **angioedema,** serum sickness, joint pain, exfoliative dermatitis, chest tightness, myalgia, erythema multiforme, edema, itching, numbness, chills, **Stevens-Johnson syndrome, anaphylaxis.** *NOTE: Cross-allergy may be manifested between cephalosporins and penicillins.* *Hematologic:* Leukopenia, leukocytosis, lymphocytosis, neutropenia (transient), eosinophilia, thrombocytopenia, thrombocythemia, **agranulocytosis,** granulocytopenia, bone marrow depression, **hemolytic anemia,** pancytopenia, decreased platelet function, **aplastic anemia,** hypoprothrombinemia (may lead to bleeding), thrombocytosis (transient). *CNS:* Headache, malaise, fatigue, vertigo, dizziness, lethargy, confusion, paresthesia, precipitation of **seizures** (especially in clients with impaired renal function). *Hepatic:* Hepatomegaly, hepatitis. Intrathecal use may result in hallucinations, nystagmus, or **seizures**. *Miscellaneous:* Superinfection including oral candidiasis and enterococcal infections, hypotension, sweating, flushing, dyspnea, interstitial pneumonitis.

IV or IM use may result in local swelling, inflammation, cellulitis, paresthesia, burning, phlebitis, thrombophlebitis. IM use may also cause pain and induration, tenderness, increased temperature. Sterile abscesses have been observed following SC use. Nephrotoxicity (↑ BUN with and without ↑ serum creatinine) may occur in clients over 50 and in young children.

**Drug Interactions**
*Bacteriostatic agents* (i.e., Tetracyclines, erythromycin) / ↓ Effect of cephalosporins
*Oral Contraceptives* /↓ Effects of oral contraceptives
*Polymyxin B* / ↑ Risk of renal toxicity
*Probenecid* / ↑ Effect of cephalosporins by ↓ excretion by kidneys

**Dosage**
See individual drugs.

**DENTAL CONCERNS**

See also *General Dental Concerns for All Anti-Infectives.*
**General**
1. *With hypersensitivity reactions to penicillin, assess for cross-sensitivity to cephalosporins.*
2. Many agents in this group of antibiotics are quite expensive. Clients on fixed incomes with limited health benefits may be unable to afford the prescription expense.
3. Document indications for therapy and symptoms of infection.
4. With renal impairment reduce dose; for dialysis clients, administer after treatment.
**Client/Family Teaching**
1. Oral meds should be taken on an empty stomach but, if GI upset occurs, may be administered with meals.
2. Report any symptoms that may necessitate drug withdrawal such as

vaginal itching or drainage, fever, or diarrhea.
3. Yogurt or buttermilk (4 oz) may be prescribed daily for diarrhea related to intestinal superinfections (to restore intestinal flora).
4. Report signs of superinfection (black furry tongue, vaginal itching or discharge, and loose, foul-smelling stools). Nystatin may be ordered for secondary infections.
5. Take meds as ordered; report side effects so appropriate therapy may be initiated.
6. Immediately report any abnormal bleeding or bruising.
7. Avoid alcohol and alcohol-containing products, as a disulfiram-type reaction may occur with some of the cephalosporins.
8. Stress the importance of good oral hygiene in order to prevent or minimize soft tissue inflammation.

# CHOLINERGIC BLOCKING AGENTS

*See also the following individual entries:*

Atropine sulfate
Benztropine mesylate
Biperiden hydrochloride
Dicyclomine hydrochloride
Ipratropium bromide
Trihexyphenidyl hydrochloride
**Action/Kinetics:** The cholinergic blocking agents prevent the neurotransmitter acetylcholine from combining with receptors on the postganglionic parasympathetic nerve terminal (muscarinic site). Effects include reduction of smooth muscle spasms, blockade of vagal impulses to the heart, decreased secretions (e.g., gastric, salivation, bronchial mucus, sweat glands), production of mydriasis and cycloplegia, and various CNS effects. Several anticholinergic drugs abolish or reduce the S&S of Parkinson's disease, such as tremors and rigidity, and result in some improvement in mobility, muscular coordi-

nation, and motor performance. These effects may be due to blockade of the effects of acetylcholine in the CNS.

**Uses:** See individual drugs.

**Contraindications:** Glaucoma, adhesions between iris and lens of the eye, tachycardia, myocardial ischemia, unstable CV state in acute hemorrhage, partial obstruction of the GI and biliary tracts, prostatic hypertrophy, renal disease, myasthenia gravis, hepatic disease, paralytic ileus, pyloroduodenal stenosis, pyloric obstruction, intestinal atony, ulcerative colitis, obstructive uropathy. Cardiac clients, especially when there is danger of tachycardia; older persons suffering from atherosclerosis or mental impairment. Lactation.

**Special Concerns:** Use with caution in pregnancy. Infants and young children are more susceptible to the toxic side effects of anticholinergic drugs. Use in children when the ambient temperature is high may cause a rapid increase in body temperature due to suppression of sweat glands. Geriatric clients are particularly likely to manifest anticholinergic side effects and CNS effects, including agitation, confusion, drowsiness, excitement, glaucoma, and impaired memory. Use with caution in hyperthyroidism, CHF, cardiac arrhythmias, hypertension, Down syndrome, asthma, spastic paralysis, blonde individuals, allergies, and chronic lung disease.

**Side Effects:** These are desirable in some conditions and undesirable in others. Thus, the anticholinergics have an antisalivary effect that is useful in parkinsonism. This same effect is unpleasant when the drug is used for spastic conditions of the GI tract. Most side effects are dose-related and decrease when dosage decreases. *Oral:* Dry mouth, change in taste perception. *GI:* N&V, dysphagia, constipation, heartburn, bloated feeling, paralytic ileus. *CNS:* Dizziness, drowsiness, nervousness, disorientation, headache, weakness, insomnia, fever (especially in children). Large doses may produce CNS stimulation including tremor and restlessness. Anticholinergic psychoses: ataxia, euphoria, confusion, disorientation, loss of short-term memory, decreased anxiety, fatigue, insomnia, hallucinations, dysarthria, agitation. *CV:* Palpitations. *GU:* Urinary retention or hesitancy, impotence. *Ophthalmologic:* Blurred vision, dilated pupils, photophobia, cycloplegia, precipitation of acute glaucoma. *Allergic:* Urticaria, skin rashes, **anaphylaxis.** *Other:* Flushing, decreased sweating, nasal congestion, suppression of glandular secretions including lactation. Heat prostration (fever and heat stroke) in presence of high environmental temperatures due to decreased sweating.

**Drug Interactions**

*Amantadine* / Additive anticholinergic side effects

*Antacids* / ↓ Absorption of anticholinergics from GI tract

*Antidepressants, tricyclic* / Additive anticholinergic side effects

*Benzodiazepines* / Additive anticholinergic side effects

*Corticosteroids* / Additive ↑ intraocular pressure

*Cyclopropane* / ↑ Chance of ventricular arrhythmias

*Haloperidol* / Additive ↑ intraocular pressure

*MAO inhibitors* / ↑ Effect of anticholinergics due to ↓ breakdown by liver

*Meperidine* / Additive anticholinergic side effects

*Nitrates, nitrites* / Potentiation of anticholinergic side effects

*Phenothiazines* / Additive anticholinergic side effects; also, effects of phenothiazines may ↓

*Sympathomimetics* / ↑ Bronchial relaxation

**Dosage** ──────────────
See individual drugs.

**DENTAL CONCERNS**
**General**
1. Monitor vital signs at every appointment because of cardiovascular side effects.

2. Have the patient sit up slowly and remain seated for at least two minutes after being supine in order to minimize the risk of orthostatic hypotension.

3. Decreased saliva flow can put the patient at risk for dental caries, periodontal disease, and candidiasis.

4. Dark glasses may be necessary because of irritation from dental lamp.

5. Place patient on frequent recall because of oral adverse effects.

**Consultation with Primary Care Provider**

1. Consultation may be required in order to assess extent of disease control and patient's ability to tolerate stress.

2. Health care provider should be informed of the oral adverse effects of these drugs.

**Client/Family Teaching**

1. Review the importance of good oral hygiene in order to prevent soft tissue inflammation.

2. Review the proper use of oral hygiene aids in order to prevent injury.

3. Daily home fluoride treatments for persistent dry mouth.

4. Avoid alcohol-containing mouth rinses.

5. Dry mouth can be treated with tart, sugarless gum or candy, sips of water, or with saliva substitutes if dry mouth persists.

---

# CORTICOSTEROIDS

*See also the following individual entries:*

Beclomethasone dipropionate
Fluticasone propionate
Hydrocortisone
Hydrocortisone acetate
Prednisone
Triamcinolone acetonide
Triamcinolone diacetate

**Action/Kinetics:** The hormones of the adrenal gland influence many metabolic pathways and all organ systems and are essential for survival. These processes include carbohydrate metabolism, protein metabolism, fat metabolism), and water and electrolyte balance.

According to their chemical structure and chief physiologic effect, the corticosteroids fall into two subgroups, which have considerable functional overlap. First are those, like cortisone and hydrocortisone, that mainly regulate the metabolic pathways involving protein, carbohydrate, and fat. This group is often referred to as *glucocorticoids.* In the second group are those, like aldosterone and desoxycorticosterone, that are more specifically involved in electrolyte and water balance. These are often referred to as *mineralocorticoids.* Hormones, such as cortisone and hydrocortisone, although classified as glucocorticoids, possess significant mineralocorticoid activity. Therapeutically, a distinction must be made between physiologic doses used for replacement therapy and pharmacologic doses used to treat inflammatory and other disease states.

The hormones also have a marked anti-inflammatory effect and immunosuppresant effects.

**Uses**

1. **Replacement therapy.** Acute and chronic adrenal insufficiency, including Addison's disease. For replacement therapy, drugs must possess both glucocorticoid and mineralocorticoid effects.

2. **Rheumatic disorders,** including rheumatoid arthritis (including juveniles), other types of arthritis, ankylosing spondylitis, acute and subacute bursitis.

3. **Collagen diseases,** including SLE.

4. **Allergic diseases,** including control of severe allergic conditions as serum sickness, drug hypersensitivity reactions, anaphylaxis.

5. **Respiratory diseases,** including prophylaxis and treatment of bronchial asthma (and status asthmaticus), seasonal or perennial rhinitis.

6. **Ocular diseases,** including se-

---

vere acute and chronic allergic and inflammatory conditions.

7. **Dermatologic diseases,** including angioedema or urticaria, contact dermatitis, atopic dermatitis, severe erythema multiforme (Stevens-Johnson syndrome).

8. **Diseases of the intestinal tract,** including chronic ulcerative colitis, regional enteritis.

9. **Nervous system,** including acute exacerbations of multiple sclerosis, optic neuritis.

10. **Malignancies,** including leukemias and lymphomas in adults and acute leukemia in children.

11. **Nephrotic syndrome,** including that due to lupus erythematosus or of the idiopathic type.

12. **Hematologic diseases,** including acquired hemolytic anemia, RBC anemia, idiopathic and secondary thrombocytopenic purpura in adults, congenital hypoplastic anemia.

13. **Intra-articular or soft tissue administration,** including acute episodes of synovitis osteoarthritis, rheumatoid arthritis, acute gouty arthritis, bursitis.

14. **Intralesional administration,** including keloids, psoriatic plaques, discoid lupus erythematosus.

**Contraindications:** Suspected infection as these drugs may mask infections. Also peptic ulcer, psychoses, acute glomerulonephritis, herpes simplex infections of the eye, vaccinia or varicella, the exanthematous diseases, Cushing's syndrome, active tuberculosis, myasthenia gravis. Recent intestinal anastomoses, CHF or other cardiac disease, hypertension, systemic fungal infections, open-angle glaucoma. Also, hyperlipidemia, hyperthyroidism or hypothyroidism, osteoporosis, tuberculosis. Lactation (if high doses are used). Inhalation products to relieve acute bronchospasms.

Topically in the eye for dendritic keratitis, vaccinia, chickenpox, other viral disease that may involve the conjunctiva or cornea, and tuberculosis and fungal or acute purulent infections of the eye. Topically in the ear in aural fungal infections and perfo-

rated eardrum. Topically in tuberculosis of the skin, herpes simplex, vaccinia, varicella, and infectious conditions in the absence of anti-infective agents.

**Special Concerns:** Use with caution in diabetes mellitus, hypertension, chronic nephritis, thrombophlebitis, convulsive disorders, infectious diseases, renal or hepatic insufficiency, pregnancy. Chronic use may inhibit the growth and development of children or adolescents. Pediatric clients are also at greater risk for developing cataracts, osteoporosis, avascular necrosis of the femoral heads, and glaucoma. Geriatric clients are more likely to develop hypertension and osteoporosis (especially postmenopausal women).

**Side Effects:** Small physiologic doses given as replacement therapy or short-term high-dosage therapy during emergencies rarely cause side effects. Prolonged therapy may cause a Cushing-like syndrome with atrophy of the adrenal cortex and subsequent adrenocortical insufficiency. A steroid withdrawal syndrome may occur following prolonged use; symptoms include anorexia, N&V, lethargy, headache, fever, joint pain, desquamation, myalgia, weight loss, hypotension.

SYSTEMIC: *Fluid and electrolyte:* Edema, hypokalemic alkalosis, hypokalemia, hypocalcemia, hypotension or shock-like reaction, hypertension, CHF. *Musculoskeletal:* Muscle wasting, muscle pain or weakness, osteoporosis, spontaneous fractures including vertebral compression fractures and fractures of long bones, tendon rupture, aseptic necrosis of femoral and humeral heads. *Oral:* Dry mouth, candidiasis, poor wound healing, osteoporosis. *GI:* N&V, anorexia or increased appetite, diarrhea or constipation, abdominal distention, pancreatitis, gastric irritation, ulcerative esophagitis. ***Development or exacerbation of peptic ulcers with the possibility of perforation and hemorrhage; perforation of the small and large bowel,*** especially in inflammatory bowel disease. *Endocrine:* Cushing's syndrome (e.g., central obesity, moonface, buffalo hump, enlargement of supraclavicular fat pads), amenorrhea, postmenopausal bleeding, menstrual irregularities, decreased glucose tolerance, hyperglycemia, glycosuria, increased insulin or sulfonylurea requirement in diabetics, development of diabetes mellitus, negative nitrogen balance due to protein catabolism, suppression of growth in children, secondary adrenocortical and pituitary unresponsiveness (especially during periods of stress). *CNS/Neurologic:* Headache, vertigo, insomnia, restlessness, increased motor activity, ischemic neuropathy, EEG abnormalities, **seizures,** pseudotumor cerebri. Also, euphoria, mood swings, depression, anxiety, personality changes, psychoses. *CV:* Thromboembolism, thrombophlebitis, ECG changes (due to potassium deficiency), fat embolism, necrotizing angiitis, cardiac arrhythmias, **myocardial rupture following recent MI,** syncopal episodes. *Dermatologic:* Impaired wound healing, skin atrophy and thinning, petechiae, ecchymoses, erythema, purpura, striae, hirsutism, urticaria, **angioneurotic edema,** acneiform eruptions, allergic dermatitis, lupus erythematosus-like lesions, suppression of skin test reactions, perineal irritation. *Ophthalmic:* Glaucoma, posterior subcapsular cataracts, increased intraocular pressure, exophthalmos. *Miscellaneous:* Hypercholesterolemia, atherosclerosis, aggravation or masking of infections, leukocytosis, increased or decreased motility and number of spermatozoa. **In children:** Suppression of linear growth; reversible pseudobrain tumor syndrome characterized by papilledema, oculomotor or abducens nerve paralysis, visual loss, or headache.

### Drug Interactions

*Acetaminophen* / ↑ Risk of hepatotoxicity due to ↑ rate of formation of hepatotoxic acetaminophen metabolite

*Alcohol* / ↑ Risk of GI ulceration or hemorrhage

*Anabolic steroids* / ↑ Risk of edema

*Antacids* / ↓ Effect of corticosteroids due to ↓ absorption from GI tract

*Antibiotics, broad-spectrum* / Concomitant use may result in emergence of resistant strains, leading to severe infection

*Anticholinergics* / Combination ↑ intraocular pressure; will aggravate glaucoma

*Barbiturates* / ↓ Effect of corticosteroids due to ↑ breakdown by liver

*Ephedrine* / ↓ Effect of corticosteroids due to ↑ breakdown by liver

*Immunosuppressant drugs* / ↑ Risk of infection

*Indomethacin* / ↑ Chance of GI ulceration

*Ketoconazole* / ↓ Effect of corticosteroids due to ↑ rate of clearance

*Muscle relaxants, nondepolarizing* / ↓ Effect of muscle relaxants

*Neuromuscular blocking agents* / ↑ Risk of prolonged respiratory depression or paralysis

*NSAIDs* / ↑ Risk of GI hemorrhage or ulceration

*Phenobarbital* / ↓ Effect of corticosteroids due to ↑ breakdown by liver

*Phenytoin* / ↓ Effect of corticosteroids due to ↑ breakdown by liver

*Rifampin* / ↓ Effect of corticosteroids due to ↑ breakdown by liver

*Salicylates* / Both are ulcerogenic; also, corticosteroids may ↓ blood salicylate levels

*Streptozocin* / ↑ Risk of hyperglycemia

*Tricyclic antidepressants* / ↑ Risk of mental disturbances

### Dosage

Highly individualized, according to both the condition being treated and the client's response. Therapy must not be discontinued abruptly. Except for replacement therapy, treatment should always involve the minimum effective dose and the shortest period of time. If corticosteroids are used for replacement therapy or high doses are used for prolonged periods of time, the dose must be *increased* if surgery is required.

Lotions are considered best for weeping eruptions, especially in areas subject to chafing (axilla, feet, and groin). Creams are suitable for most inflammations; ointments are preferred for dry, scaly lesions.

## DENTAL CONCERNS
### General
1. Monitor vital signs at every appointment because of cardiovascular side effects.
2. Decreased saliva flow can put the patient at risk for dental caries, periodontal disease, and candidiasis.
3. Patients on chronic drug therapy may develop blood dyscrasias. Symptoms include fever, sore throat, bleeding, and poor wound healing.
4. Oral inhalers can cause oral candidiasis. Place patient on frequent recall because of oral adverse effects.
5. Avoid prescription and over-the-counter aspirin-containing products.
6. Observe for signs of oral infections because corticosteroids tend to mask them.
7. Prophylactic antibiotic therapy may be necessary if surgery or deep scaling is necessary. Steroids can delay the healing process and mask signs of infection.
8. Steroids can cause immunosuppression. Determine the patient's steroid dose and assess for risk of stress tolerance and immunosuppression.
9. Patients receiving chronic steroid therapy (> 2 weeks) may require a temporary increase in their dose for dental treatment.
10. Determine the reason for steroid use.

### Consultation with Primary Care Provider
1. Patients with symptoms of blood dyscrasias should be referred to their primary care provider for complete blood counts. Treatment

should be postponed until the results are known.
2. Consultation may be required in order to assess the extent of disease control.
3. Consultation may be necessary to determine the correct steroid dose and duration of therapy.
### Client/Family Teaching
1. Review the importance of good oral hygiene in order to prevent soft tissue inflammation.
2. Review the proper use of oral hygiene aids in order to prevent injury.
3. Daily home fluoride treatments for persistent dry mouth.
4. Avoid alcohol-containing mouth rinses or beverages.
5. Avoid caffeine-containing beverages.
6. Dry mouth can be treated with tart, sugarless gum or candy, water, sugar-free beverages, or with saliva substitutes if dry mouth persists.

# DIURETICS, LOOP

*See also the following individual entries:*

Furosemide

See also *Diuretics, Thiazides*.
**Action/Kinetics:** Loop diuretics inhibit reabsorption of sodium and chloride in the loop of Henle. Metabolized in the liver and excreted primarily through the urine. Significantly bound to plasma protein.
**Uses:** See individual drugs.
**Contraindications:** Hypersensitivity to loop diruetics or to sulfonylureas. In hepatic coma or severe electrolyte depletion (until condition improves or is corrected). Lactation.
**Special Concerns:** Sudden alterations of electrolytes in hepatic cirrhosis and ascites may precipitate hepatic encephalopathy and coma. SLE may be activated or worsened. Ototoxicity is most common with rapid injection, in severe renal impairment, with doses several times the usual dose, and with concurrent use of other ototoxic drugs. Safety and efficacy of most loop diuretics

have not been determined in children or infants.

**Side Effects:** See individual drugs. Excessive diuresis may cause dehydration with the possibility of ***circulatory collapse and vascular thrombosis or embolism.*** Ototoxicity including tinnitus, hearing impairment, deafness (usually reversible), and vertigo with a sense of fullness are possible. Electrolyte imbalance, especially in clients with restricted salt intake. Photosensitivity. Changes include hypokalemia, hypomagnesemia, and hypocalcemia.

**Drug Interactions**

*Aminoglycosides* / ↑ Ototoxicity with hearing loss

*Chloral hydrate* / Transient diaphoresis, hot flashes, hypertension, tachycardia, weakness and nausea

*Corticosteroids* / ↑ Electrolyte imbalance

*Muscle relaxants, nondepolarizing* / Effect of muscle relaxants may be either ↑ or ↓, depending on the dose of diuretic

*Nonsteroidal anti-inflammatory drugs* / ↓ Effect of loop diuretics

*Phenothiazines* / Masked ototoxicity

*Salicylates* / Diuretic effect may be ↓ in clients with cirrhosis and ascites

**Dosage** ───────────────

See individual drugs.

## DENTAL CONCERNS

See also *Diuretics, Thiazides.*

**General**

1. Monitor vital signs at every appointment because of cardiovascular and respiratory side effects.

2. Have the patient sit up slowly and remain seated for at least two minutes after being supine in order to minimize the risk of orthostatic hypotension.

3. Decreased saliva flow can put the patient at risk for dental caries, periodontal disease, and candidiasis.

4. Dental procedures may cause the patient anxiety or place stress on the heart. Assess cardiovascular patient for this risk.

5. Early morning and shorter appointments, as well as methods for addressing anxiety levels in the patient, can help to reduce the amount of stress that the patient is experiencing.

6. Vasoconstrictors should be used with caution and in low doses.

7. Patients on chronic drug therapy may develop blood dyscrasias. Symptoms include fever, sore throat, bleeding, and poor wound healing.

8. Patients on sodium restricted diets should receive sodium-containing fluids (i.e., saline solution) with caution.

9. Patients taking diuretics should have their serum potassium levels measured.

**Consultation with Primary Care Provider**

1. Patients with symptoms of blood dyscrasias should be referred to their primary care provider for complete blood counts. Treatment should be postponed until the results are known.

2. Consultation with primary care provider is recommended in order to assess disease control and patient's ability to tolerate stress.

**Client/Family Teaching**

1. Review the importance of good oral hygiene in order to prevent soft tissue inflammation and minimize the risk of gingival hyperplasia.

2. Review the proper use of oral hygiene aids in order to prevent injury.

3. Daily home fluoride treatments for persistent dry mouth.

4. Avoid alcohol-containing mouth rinses and beverages.

5. Avoid caffeine-containing beverages.

6. Dry mouth can be treated with tart, sugarless gum or candy, water, sugar-free beverages, or with saliva substitutes if dry mouth persists.

# DIURETICS, THIAZIDES

*See also the following individual entries:*

Hydrochlorothiazide
Indapamide

**Action/Kinetics:** Thiazides promote diuresis by decreasing the rate at which sodium and chloride are reabsorbed by the distal convoluted renal tubules of the kidney. A large fraction is excreted unchanged in urine.

**Uses:** Edema, CHF, hypertension, pregnancy, and premenstrual tension. Thiazides are used for edema due to CHF, nephrosis, nephritis, renal failure, PMS, hepatic cirrhosis, corticosteroid or estrogen therapy. Hypertension. *Investigational:* Thiazides are used alone or in combination with allopurinol (or amiloride) for prophylaxis of calcium nephrolithiasis. Nephrogenic diabetes insipidus.

**Contraindications:** Hypersensitivity to drug, anuria, renal decompensation. Impaired renal function and advanced hepatic cirrhosis. Do not use indiscriminately in clients with edema and toxemia of pregnancy, even though they may be therapeutically useful, because the thiazides may have adverse effects on the newborn (thrombocytopenia and jaundice).

**Special Concerns:** Geriatric clients may manifest an increased risk of hypotension and changes in electrolyte levels. Administer with caution to debilitated clients or to those with a history of hepatic coma or precoma, gout, diabetes mellitus, or during pregnancy and lactation. Particular care must be exercised when thiazides are administered concomitantly with drugs that also cause potassium loss, such as digitalis, corticosteroids, and some estrogens. Clients with advanced heart failure, renal disease, or hepatic cirrhosis are most likely to develop hypokalemia. May activate or worsen SLE.

**Side Effects:** The following side effects may be observed with most thiazides. See also individual drugs.

*Electrolyte imbalance:* Hypokalemia (most frequent) characterized by cardiac arrhythmias. Hyponatremia characterized by weakness, lethargy, epigastric distress, N&V. Hypokalemic alkalosis. *GI:* Anorexia, epigastric distress or irritation, N&V, cramping, bloating, abdominal pain, diarrhea, constipation, jaundice, pancreatitis. *CNS:* Dizziness, lightheadedness, headache, vertigo, xanthopsia, paresthesias, weakness, insomnia, restlessness. *CV:* Orthostatic hypotension, MIs in elderly clients with advanced arteriosclerosis, especially if the client is also receiving therapy with other antihypertensive agents. *Hematologic: Agranulocytosis, aplastic or hypoplastic anemia, hemolytic anemia,* leukopenia, thrombocytopenia. *Dermatologic:* Purpura, photosensitivity, photosensitivity dermatitis, rash, urticaria, necrotizing angiitis, vasculitis, cutaneous vasculitis. *Metabolic:* neutropenia, hemolytic anemia. *Endocrine:* Hyperglycemia, glycosuria, hyperuricemia. *Miscellaneous:* Blurred vision, impotence, reduced libido, fever, muscle cramps, muscle spasm, respiratory distress.

**Drug Interactions**

*Anesthetics* / Thiazides may ↑ effects of anesthetics

*Anticholinergic agents* / ↑ Effect of thiazides due to ↑ amount absorbed from GI tract

*Corticosteroids* / Enhanced potassium loss due to potassium-losing properties of both drugs

*Ethanol* / Additive orthostatic hypotension

*Indomethacin* / ↓ Effect of thiazides, possibly by inhibition of prostaglandins

*Muscle relaxants, nondepolarizing* / ↑ Effect of muscle relaxants due to hypokalemia

*Norepinephrine* / Thiazides ↓ arterial response to norepinephrine

*Sulfonamides* / ↑ Effect of thiazides due to ↓ plasma protein binding

*Tetracyclines* / ↑ Risk of azotemia

*Tubocurarine* / ↑ Muscle relaxation and ↑ hypokalemia

*Vasopressors (sympathomimetics) /* Thiazides ↓ responsiveness of arterioles to vasopressors

**Dosage**

See individual drugs.

## DENTAL CONCERNS
### General
1. Monitor vital signs at every appointment because of cardiovascular and respiratory side effects.
2. Have the patient sit up slowly and remain seated for at least two minutes after being supine in order to minimize the risk of orthostatic hypotension.
3. Decreased saliva flow can put the patient at risk for dental caries, periodontal disease, and candidiasis.
4. Dental procedures may cause the patient anxiety or place stress on the heart. Assess cardiovascular patient for this risk.
5. Early morning and shorter appointments as well as methods for addressing anxiety levels in the patient can help to reduce the amount of stress that the patient is experiencing.
6. Vasoconstrictors should be used with caution and in low doses.
7. Patients on chronic drug therapy may develop blood dyscrasias. Symptoms include fever, sore throat, bleeding, and poor wound healing.
8. Patients on sodium restricted diets should receive sodium-containing fluids (i.e., saline solution) with caution.
9. Patients taking diuretics should have their serum potassium levels measured.

### Consultation with Primary Care Provider
1. Patients with symptoms of blood dyscrasias should be referred to their primary care provider for complete blood counts. Treatment should be postponed until the results are known.
2. Consultation with primary care provider is recommended in order to assess disease control and patient's ability to tolerate stress.

### Client/Family Teaching
1. Review the importance of good oral hygiene in order to prevent soft tissue inflammation.
2. Review the proper use of oral hygiene aids in order to prevent injury.
3. Daily home fluoride treatments for persistent dry mouth.
4. Avoid alcohol-containing mouth rinses and beverages.
5. Avoid caffeine-containing beverages.
6. Dry mouth can be treated with tart, sugarless gum or candy, water, sugar-free beverages, or with saliva substitutes if dry mouth persists.

# ERYTHROMYCINS

*See also the following individual entries:*

Erythromycin base
Erythromycin estolate
Erythromycin ethylsuccinate
Erythromycin lactobionate
Erythromycin stearate

**Action/Kinetics:** Erythromycins are considered to be macrolide antibiotics. They inhibit protein synthesis of microorganisms by binding reversibly to a ribosomal subunit (50S), thus interfering with the transmission of genetic information and inhibiting protein synthesis. The drugs are effective only against rapidly multiplying organisms. Absorbed from the upper part of the small intestine. Those for PO use are manufactured in enteric-coated or film-coated forms to prevent destruction by gastric acid. Erythromycin is approximately 70% bound to plasma proteins and achieves concentrations in body tissues about 40% of those in the plasma. Diffuses into body tissues; peritoneal, pleural, ascitic, and amniotic fluids; saliva; through the placental circulation; and across the mucous membrane of the tracheobronchial tree. Diffuses poorly into spinal fluid, although penetration is increased in meningitis. Alkalinization of the urine (to pH 8.5) increases the gram-

---

negative antibacterial action. **Peak serum levels: PO,** 1–4 hr. **t½:** 1.5–2 hr, *but prolonged in clients with renal impairment.* Partially metabolized by the liver and primarily excreted in bile. Also excreted in breast milk.

**Uses**

1. Upper respiratory tract infections due to *Streptococcus pyogenes* (group a beta-hemolytic streptococci), *Streptococcus pneumoniae,* and *Haemophilus influenzae* (combined with sulfonamides).

2. Mild to moderate lower respiratory tract infections due to *S. pyogenes* and *S. pneumoniae.* Respiratory tract infections due to *Mycoplasma pneumoniae.*

3. Pertussis (whooping cough) caused by *Bordetella pertussis;* may also be used as prophylaxis of pertussis in exposed individuals.

4. Mild to moderate skin and skin structure infections due to *S. pyogenes* and *Staphylococcus aureus.*

5. As an adjunct to antitoxin in diphtheria (caused by *Corynebacterium diphtheriae*), to prevent carriers, and to eradicate the organism in carriers.

6. Intestinal amebiasis due to *Entamoeba histolytica* (PO erythromycin only).

7. Acute pelvic inflammatory disease due to *Neisseria gonorrhoeae.*

8. Erythrasma due to *Corynebacterium minutissimum.*

9. *Chlamydia trachomatis* infections causing urogenital infections during pregnancy, conjunctivitis in the newborn, or pneumonia during infancy. Also, uncomplicated chlamydial infections of the urethra, endocervix, or rectum in adults (when tetracyclines are contraindicated or not tolerated).

10. Nongonococcal urethritis caused by *Ureaplasma urealyticum* when tetracyclines are contraindicated or not tolerated.

11. Legionnaires' disease due to *Legionella pneumophilia.*

12. As an alternative to penicillin (in penicillin-sensitive clients) to treat primary syphilis caused by *Treponema pallidum.*

13. Prophylaxis of initial or recurrent attacks of rheumatic fever in clients allergic to penicillin or sulfonamides.

14. Infections due to *Listeria monocytogenes.*

15. Bacterial endocarditis due to alpha-hemolytic streptococci, Viridans group, in clients allergic to penicillins.

*Non-FDA Approved:* Infections due to *N. gonorrhoeae,* including uncomplicated urethral, rectal, or endocervical infections and disseminated gonococcal infections (including use in pregnancy). Severe or prolonged diarrhea due to *Campylobacter jejuni.* Genital, inguinal, or anorectal infections due to *Lymphogranuloma venereum.* Chancroid due to *Haemophilus ducreyi.* Primary, secondary, or early latent syphilis due to *T. pallidum.* Erythromycin base used with PO neomycin prior to elective colorectal surgery to reduce wound complications. As an alternative to penicillin to treat anthrax, Vincent's gingivitis, erysipeloid, actinomycosis, tetanus, with a sulfonamide to treat *Nocardia* infections, infections due to *Eikenella corrodens,* and *Borrelia* infections (including early Lyme disease).

**Contraindications:** Hypersensitivity to erythromycin; in utero syphilis.

**Special Concerns:** Use with caution in liver disease and during lactation. Use may result in bacterial and fungal overgrowth (i.e., superinfection).

**Side Effects:** Erythromycins have a low incidence of side effects (except for the estolate salt). *GI* (most common): N&V, diarrhea, cramping, abdominal pain, stomatitis, anorexia, melena, heartburn, pruritus ani, pseudomembranous colitis. *Allergic:* Skin rashes with or without pruritus, bullous fixed eruptions, urticaria, eczema, *anaphylaxis* (rare). *CNS:* Fear, confusion, altered thinking, uncontrollable crying or hysterical laughter, feeling of impending loss of consciousness. *CV:* Rarely, ventricular arrhythmias, including ***ventricular tachycardia and torsades de pointes in***

**clients with prolonged QT intervals.**
*Miscellaneous:* Superinfection, hepatotoxicity, ototoxicity. *Following topical use:* Itching, burning, irritation, or stinging of skin. Dry, scaly skin.

IV use may result in venous irritation and thrombophlebitis; IM use produces pain at the injection site, with development of necrosis or sterile abscesses.

**Drug Interactions**

*Alfentanil* / ↓ Excretion of alfentanil → ↑ effect

*Astemizole* / Serious CV side effects, including torsades de pointes and other ventricular arrhythmias (including QT interval prolongation), cardiac arrest, and death

*Carbamazepine* / ↑ Effect (and toxicity requiring hospitalization and resuscitation) of carbamazepine due to ↓ breakdown by liver

*Lincosamides* / Drugs antagonize each other

*Methylprednisolone* / ↑ Effect of methylprednisolone due to ↓ breakdown by liver

*Penicillin* / Erythromycins either ↓ or ↑ effect of penicillins

*Sodium bicarbonate* / ↑ Effect of erythromycin in urine due to alkalinization

*Terfenadine* / Serious CV side effects, including torsades de pointes and other ventricular arrhythmias (including QT interval prolongation), cardiac arrest, and death

*Triazolam* / ↑ Bioavailability of triazolam → ↑ CNS depression

**Dosage** ─────────────
See individual drugs.

## DENTAL CONCERNS

See also *General Dental Concerns* for *All Anti-Infectives.*
**General**
1. Identify allergy to any antibiotics; note allergens.
2. Document type, onset, and characteristics of symptoms, other agents used, and the outcome.
3. Avoid if also prescribed astemi-

zole, Seldane, digoxin, and theophyllines, because erythromycins can inhibit cytochrome P-450 and enhance effects of these drugs or cause lethal arrhythmias.

**Client/Family Teaching**
1. Do not administer with or immediately prior to ingestion of fruit juice or other acidic drinks; acidity may decrease drug activity. Consume up to 8 oz of water with each dose and a fluid intake of 2.5 L/day.
2. May take with food to diminish GI upset; however, food decreases the absorption of most erythromycins. Take only as directed and complete entire prescription despite feeling better.
3. If tablets are not coated, take them 2 hr after meals. Stomach acid destroys the erythromycin base thus it must be administered with an enteric coating.
4. Doses of erythromycins should be evenly spaced throughout a 24-hr period.
5. If nausea is intolerable, notify provider so the prescription can be changed to coated tablets that can be taken with meals.
6. Report symptoms of superinfection, i.e., furry tongue, vaginal itching, rectal itching, or diarrhea.
7. Any rash, yellow discoloration of skin or eyes, or irritation of the mouth or tongue should be reported.

# FLUOROQUINOLONES

*See also the following individual entries:*

Ciprofloxacin hydrochloride
Enoxacin
Lomefloxacin hydrochloride
Norfloxacin
Ofloxacin
Sparfloxacin

**Action/Kinetics:** Synthetic, broad-spectrum antibacterial agents. Are bactericidal agents by interfering with DNA gyrase, an enzyme needed for the synthesis of bacterial DNA. Food may delay the absorption of ciprofloxacin, lomefloxacin, and norfloxacin. Ciprofloxacin, levofloxacin, ofloxacin, and trovafloxacin may be given IV; all fluoroquinolones may be given PO.

**Uses:** See individual drugs; these drugs are used for a large number of gram-positive and gram-negative infections.

**Contraindications:** Hypersensitivity to the quinolone group of antibiotics, including cinoxacin and nalidixic acid. Lactation. Use in children less than 18 years of age.

**Special Concerns:** Use lower doses in impaired renal function. There may be differences in CNS toxicity between the various fluoroquinolones. Use may increase the risk of Achilles and other tendon inflammation and rupture.

**Side Effects:** See individual drugs. The following side effects are common to each of the fluoroquinolone antibiotics. *Oral:* Dry or painful mouth. *GI:* N&V, diarrhea, abdominal pain or discomfort, heartburn, dyspepsia, flatulence, constipation, pseudomembranous colitis. *CNS:* Headache, dizziness, malaise, lethargy, fatigue, drowsiness, somnolence, depression, insomnia, **seizures,** paresthesia. *Dermatologic:* Rash, photosensitivity, pruritus (except for ciprofloxacin). *Hypersensitivity reactions:* Facial or **pharyngeal edema,** dyspnea, urticaria, itching, tingling, loss of consciousness, *CV collapse.* *Other:* Visual disturbances and ophthalmologic abnormalities, hearing loss, superinfection, phototoxicity, eosinophilia, crystalluria, Achilles and other tendon inflammation and rupture. Fluoroquinolones, except norfloxacin, may also cause vaginitis, syncope, chills, and edema.

**Drug Interactions**

*Antacids* / ↓ Serum levels of fluoroquinolones due to ↓ absorption from the GI tract

*Cimetidine* / ↓ Elimination of fluoroquinolones

*Probenecid* / ↑ Serum levels of fluoroquinolones due to ↓ renal clearance

*Sucralfate* / ↓ Serum levels of fluoroquinolones due to ↓ absorption from the GI tract

*Zinc salts* / ↓ Serum levels of fluoroquinolones due to ↓ absorption from the GI tract

**Dosage**

See individual drugs.

## DENTAL CONCERNS

See also *General Dental Concerns for All Anti-Infectives.*

**General**

1. Document type, onset, and characteristics of symptoms.

2. Note any previous experiences with these antibiotics. Discontinue at the first sign of skin rash or other allergic manifestations. Hypersensitivity reactions may occur even following the first dose

3. Assess for soft tissue or extremity injury; note any instability, pain, or swelling.

4. If receiving anticoagulants and theophyllines, monitor closely as quinolones can cause increased drug levels with toxic drug effects, including increased bleeding or seizures.

**Client/Family Teaching**

1. Take only as directed. Do not take ofloxacin with food; take enoxacin and norfloxacin 1 hr before or 2 hr after meals; ciprofloxacin, lomefloxacin, and sparfloxacin may be taken without regard to meals.

2. Consume liberal amounts of fluids (>2.5 L/day).

3. Do not take any mineral supplements (i.e., iron or zinc) or antacids containing magnesium or aluminum simultaneously or 4 hr before or 2 hr after dosing with fluoroquinolones.

4. Do not perform hazardous tasks until drug effects realized; dizziness may be experienced.

5. Report any persistent, bothersome symptoms. The most frequently reported side effects include N&V and diarrhea.

6. Report symptoms of superinfection (furry tongue, vaginal or rectal itching, diarrhea).

7. Stop drug and report any new onset tendon pain or inflammation as tendon rupture may occur.

8. Wear protective clothing and sunscreens; avoid excessive sunlight or artificial ultraviolet light. Photosensitivity reactions may occur up to several weeks after stopping fluoroquinolone therapy.

# HISTAMINE H$_2$ ANTAGONISTS

*See also the following individual entries:*

Cimetidine
Famotidine
Nizatidine
Ranitidine hydrochloride

**Action/Kinetics:** Histamine H$_2$ antagonists are competitive blockers of histamine and inhibit all phases of gastric acid secretion. Cimetidine is known to affect the cytochrome P-450 drug metabolizing system for other drugs. Ranitidine also affects the P-450 enzyme system, but its effect on elimination of other drugs is not significant. Neither famotidine nor nizatidine affects the P-450 enzyme system.

**Uses:** See individual drugs. Also, these drugs are used as part of combination therapy to treat *Helicobacter pylori*–associated duodenal ulcer and maintenance therapy after healing of the active ulcer.

**Contraindications:** Hypersensitivity.

**Special Concerns:** Use with caution in impaired hepatic and renal function. Symptomatic response to these drugs does not preclude gastric malignancy. Do not use cimetidine, famotidine, and nizatidine during lactation; use ranitidine with caution. Safety and effectiveness have not been established for use in children; use of cimetidine is not recommended in children less than 16 years of age unless benefits outweigh risks.

**Side Effects:** The following side effects are common to all or most of the H$_2$-histamine antagonists. See individual drugs for complete listing. *GI:* N&V, abdominal discomfort, diarrhea, constipation, hepatocellular effects. *CNS:* Headache, fatigue, somnolence, dizziness, confusion, hallucinations, insomnia. *Dermatologic:* Rash, urticaria, pruritus, alopecia (rare), erythema multiforme (rare). *Hematologic:* Rarely, thrombocytopenia, agranulocytosis, granulocytopenia. *Other:* Gynecomastia, impotence, loss of libido, arthralgia, bronchospasm, transient pain at injection site, cardiac arrhythmias following rapid IV use (rare), arthralgia (rare), **anaphylaxis** (rare).

**Dosage**
See individual drugs.

## DENTAL CONCERNS
### General
1. Monitor vital signs at every appointment because of cardiovascular side effects.
2. A semisupine position for the dental chair may be necessary to help minimize or avoid GI adverse effects.
3. Antacids must be taken as prescribed; do not take within 1 hr of the histamine H$_2$ antagonist.
4. Avoid alcohol, caffeine, and aspirin-containing prescription and nonprescription drugs.

### Client/Family Teaching
1. Review the importance of good oral hygiene in order to prevent soft tissue inflammation.
2. Review the proper use of oral hygiene aids in order to prevent injury.

# NASAL DECONGESTANTS

*See also the following individual entries:*

Ephedrine sulfate
Epinephrine hydrochloride
Phenylephrine hydrochloride

---

Pseudoephedrine hydrochloride

**Action/Kinetics:** The most commonly used agents for relief of nasal congestion are the adrenergic drugs. They act by stimulating alpha-adrenergic receptors, thereby constricting the arterioles in the nasal mucosa; this reduces blood flow to the area, decreasing congestion. However, drugs such as ephedrine and pseudoephedrine also have beta-adrenergic effects. Both topical (sprays, drops) and oral agents may be used, although oral agents are not as effective. **Uses: PO.** Nasal congestion due to hay fever, common cold, allergies, or sinusitis. To help sinus or nasal drainage. To relieve congestion of eustachian tubes. **Topical.** Nasal and nasopharyngeal mucosal congestion due to hay fever, common cold, allergies, or sinusitis. With other therapy to decrease congestion around the eustachian tubes. Relieve ear block and pressure pain during air travel.

**Contraindications:** Oral use in severe hypertension or CAD. Use with MAO inhibitors. Oral use of pseudoephedrine and phenylpropanolamine during lactation.

**Special Concerns:** Use with caution in hyperthyroidism, arteriosclerosis, increased intraocular pressure, prostatic hypertrophy, angina, diabetes, ischemic heart disease, hypertension. Also, clients receiving MAO inhibitors may manifest hypertensive crisis following the use of oral nasal decongestants. Use with caution in geriatric clients and during pregnancy and lactation. Rebound congestion may occur after topical use. OTC products containing ephedrine have been abused.

**Side Effects:** *Topical use:* Stinging and burning, mucosal dryness, sneezing, local irritation, rebound congestion (rhinitis medicamentosa). Systemic use may produce the following symptoms. *CV:* **CV collapse with hypotension,** arrhythmias, palpitations, precordial pain, tachycardia, transient hypertension, bradycardia. *CNS:* Anxiety, dizziness, headache, fear, restlessness, tremors, insomnia, tenseness, lightheadedness, drowsiness, psychologic disturbances, weakness, psychoses, hallucinations, *seizures,* depression. *Oral:* Dry mouth, bitter taste. *GI:* N&V, anorexia. *Ophthalmologic:* Irritation, photophobia, tearing, blurred vision, blepharospasm. *Other:* Dysuria, sweating, pallor, breathing difficulties, orofacial dystonia.

*NOTE:* Ephedrine may also produce anorexia and urinary retention in men with prostatic hypertrophy.

**Drug Interactions**

*MAO inhibitors* / Use with mixed-acting drugs (e.g., ephedrine) → severe headache, hypertension, hyperpyrexia, and possibly hypertensive crisis

*Phenothiazines* / May ↓ or reverse action of nasal decongestants

*Tricyclic antidepressants* / ↑ Pressor effect of direct-acting agents → possibility of dysrhythmias; ↓ pressor effect of mixed-acting drugs

**Dosage**
See individual drugs.

## DENTAL CONCERNS

**General**

1. The patient may require a semisupine position in the dental chair to help with breathing.
2. Decreased saliva flow can put the patient at risk for dental caries, periodontal disease, and candidiasis.
3. Severe nasal congestion may prohibit the use of nitrous oxide/oxygen inhalation.

**Client/Family Teaching**

1. Overuse or misuse of nasal sprays may cause significant medical problems, i.e., a nasal spray used regularly for more than 3 or 4 days may precipitate rebound congestion.

# NONSTEROIDAL ANTI-INFLAMMATORY DRUGS

*See also the following individual entries:*

Ibuprofen

Indomethacin
Ketoprofen
Ketorolac tromethamine
Nabumetone
Naproxen
Naproxen sodium

**Action/Kinetics:** The anti-inflammatory effect is believed to result from the inhibition of the enzyme cyclooxygenase, resulting in decreased prostaglandin synthesis. The agents are effective in reducing joint swelling, pain, and morning stiffness, as well as in increasing mobility in individuals with inflammatory disease. They do not alter the course of the disease, however. Their anti-inflammatory activity is comparable to that of aspirin. The analgesic activity is due, in part, to relief of inflammation. Also, the drugs may inhibit lipoxygenase, inhibit synthesis of leukotrienes, inhibit release of lysosomal enzymes, and inhibit neutrophil aggregation. Rheumatoid factor production may also be inhibited. The antipyretic action occurs by decreasing prostaglandin synthesis in the hypothalamus, resulting in an increase in peripheral blood flow and heat loss as well as promoting sweating. NSAIDs also inhibit miosis induced by prostaglandins during the course of cataract surgery; thus, these drugs are useful for a number of ophthalmic inflammatory conditions.

The NSAIDs differ from one another with respect to their rate of absorption, length of action, anti-inflammatory activity, and effect on the GI mucosa. Most are rapidly and completely absorbed from the GI tract; food delays the rate, but not the total amount, of drug absorbed. These drugs are metabolized in the kidney and are excreted through the urine, mainly as metabolites.

**Uses:** See individual drugs. Generally are used to treat inflammatory disease, including rheumatoid arthritis, osteoarthritis, ankylosing spondylitis, gout, and other musculoskeletal diseases. Treatment of nonrheumatic inflammatory conditions including bursitis, acute painful shoulder, synovitis, tendinitis, or tenosynovitis. Mild to moderate pain including primary dysmenorrhea, episiotomy pain, strains and sprains, postextraction dental pain. Primary dysmenorrhea. Ophthalmically to inhibit intraoperative miosis, for postoperative inflammation after cataract surgery, and for relief of ocular itching due to seasonal allergic conjunctivitis.

**Contraindications:** Most for children under 14 years of age. Lactation. Individuals in whom aspirin, NSAIDs, or iodides have caused hypersensitivity, including acute asthma, rhinitis, urticaria, nasal polyps, bronchospasm, angioedema or other symptoms of allergy or anaphylaxis.

**Special Concerns:** Clients intolerant to one of the NSAIDs may be intolerant to others in this group. Use with caution in clients with a history of GI disease, reduced renal function, in geriatric clients, in clients with intrinsic coagulation defects or those on anticoagulant therapy, in compromised cardiac function, in hypertension, in conditions predisposing to fluid retention, and in the presence of existing controlled infection. The safety and efficacy of most NSAIDs have not been determined in children or in functional class IV rheumatoid arthritis (i.e., clients incapacitated, bedridden, or confined to a wheelchair).

**Side Effects:** *Oral:* Salivation, dry mouth, glossitis, gingival ulcer, sore or dry mucous membranes, stomatitis. *GI: I (most common):* Peptic or duodenal ulceration and GI bleeding, intestinal ulceration with obstruction and stenosis, reactivation of preexisting ulcers. Heartburn, dyspepsia, N&V, anorexia, diarrhea, constipation, increased or decreased appetite, indigestion, stomatitis, epigastric pain, abdominal cramps or pain, gastroenteritis, paralytic ileus, pyrosis, icterus, rectal irritation, occult blood in stool, hematemesis, gastritis, proctitis, eructation, ulcerative colitis, rectal bleeding, melena, ***perforation***

---

*and hemorrhage of esophagus, stomach, duodenum, small or large intestine.* *CNS:* Dizziness, drowsiness, vertigo, headaches, nervousness, migraine, anxiety, mental confusion, aggravation of parkinsonism and epilepsy, lightheadedness, paresthesia, peripheral neuropathy, akathisia, excitation, tremor, *seizures,* myalgia, asthenia, malaise, insomnia, fatigue, drowsiness, confusion, emotional lability, depression, inability to concentrate, psychoses, hallucinations, depersonalization, amnesia, *coma,* syncope. *CV:* CHF, hypotension, hypertension, arrhythmias, peripheral edema and fluid retention, vasodilation, exacerbation of angiitis, palpitations, tachycardia, chest pain, sinus bradycardia, peripheral vascular disease, peripheral edema. *Respiratory:* *Bronchospasm, laryngeal edema,* rhinitis, dyspnea, pharyngitis, hemoptysis, SOB, eosinophilic pneumonitis. *Hematologic:* Bone marrow depression, neutropenia, leukopenia, pancytopenia, eosinophila, thrombocytopenia, granulocytopenia, *agranulocytosis, aplastic anemia, hemolytic anemia,* decreased H&H, hypocoagulability, epistaxis. *Ophthalmologic:* Amblyopia, visual disturbances, corneal deposits, retinal hemorrhage, scotomata, retinal pigmentation changes or degeneration, blurred vision, photophobia, diplopia, iritis, loss of color vision (reversible), optic neuritis, cataracts, swollen, dry, or irritated eyes. *Dermatologic:* Pruritus, skin eruptions, sweating, erythema, eczema, hyperpigmentation, ecchymoses, petechiae, rashes, urticaria, purpura, onycholysis, vesiculobullous eruptions, cutaneous vasculitis, *toxic epidermal necrolysis, angioneurotic edema,* erythema nodosum, *Stevens-Johnson syndrome,* exfoliative dermatitis, photosensitivity, alopecia, skin irritation, peeling, erythema multiforme, desquamation, skin discoloration. *GU:* Menometrorrhagia, menorrhagia, impotence, menstrual disorders, hematuria, cystitis, azotemia, nocturia, proteinuria, UTIs, polyuria, dysuria, urinary frequency, oliguria, pyuria, anuria, renal insufficiency, nephrosis, nephrotic syndrome, glomerular and interstitial nephritis, urinary casts, acute renal failure in clients with impaired renal function, renal papillary necrosis *Metabolic:* Hyperglycemia, hypoglycemia, glycosuria, hyperkalemia, hyponatremia, diabetes mellitus. *Other:* Tinnitus, hearing loss or disturbances, ear pain, deafness, metallic or bitter taste in mouth, thirst, chills, fever, flushing, jaundice, sweating, breast changes, gynecomastia, muscle cramps, dyspnea, involuntary muscle movements, muscle weakness, facial edema, pain, serum sickness, aseptic meningitis, hypersensitivity reactions including asthma, acute respiratory distress, *shock-like syndrome, angioedema,* angiitis, dyspnea, *anaphylaxis.*

*Following ophthalmic use:* Transient burning and stinging upon installation, ocular irritation.

## Drug Interactions

*Anticoagulants* / Concomitant use results in ↑ PT

*Aspirin* / ↓ Effect of NSAIDs due to ↓ blood levels; also, ↑ risk of adverse GI effects

*Beta-adrenergic blocking agents* / ↓ Antihypertensive effect of blocking agents

*Cimetidine* / ↑ or ↓ Plasma levels of NSAIDs

*Lithium* / ↑ Serum lithium levels

*Loop diuretics* / ↓ Effect of loop diuretics

*Methotrexate* / ↑ Risk of methotrexate toxicity (i.e., bone marrow suppression, nephrotoxicity, stomatitis)

*Phenobarbital* / ↓ Effect of NSAIDs due to ↑ breakdown by liver

*Phenytoin* / ↑ Effect of phenytoin due to ↓ plasma protein binding

*Probenecid* / ↑ Effect of NSAIDs due to ↑ plasma levels

*Salicylates* / Plasma levels of NSAIDs may be ↓ ; also, ↑ risk of GI side effects

*Sulfonamides* / ↑ Effect of sulfonamides due to ↓ plasma protein binding

*Sulfonylureas* / ↑ Effect of sulfonylureas due to ↓ plasma protein binding

**Dosage**
See individual drugs.

## DENTAL CONCERNS
**General**
1. Decreased saliva flow can put the patient at risk for dental caries, periodontal disease, and candidiasis.
2. A semisupine position for the dental chair may be necessary to help minimize or avoid GI adverse effects or for patients with rheumatoid arthritis.
3. Patients on chronic drug therapy may develop blood dyscrasias. Symptoms include fever, sore throat, bleeding, and poor wound healing.
4. The patient should avoid prescription and over-the-counter aspirin-containing drug products.

**Consultation with Primary Care Provider**
1. Patients with symptoms of blood dyscrasias should be referred to their primary care provider for complete blood counts. Treatment should be postponed until the results are known.
2. Consultation may be required in order to assess extent of disease control.

**Client/Family Teaching**
1. Take NSAIDs with a full glass of water or milk, with meals, or with a prescribed antacid and remain upright 30 min following administration to reduce gastric irritation or ulcer formation.
2. Use caution in operating machinery or in driving a car; may cause dizziness or drowsiness.
3. Avoid alcohol, aspirin, acetaminophen, and any other OTC preparations without approval because of increased risk for GI bleeding.
4. Review the importance of good oral hygiene in order to prevent soft tissue inflammation.
5. Review the proper use of oral hygiene aids in order to prevent injury.
6. Daily home fluoride treatments for persistent dry mouth.

7. Avoid alcohol-containing mouth rinses and beverages.
8. Avoid caffeine-containing beverages.
9. Dry mouth can be treated with tart, sugarless gum or candy, water, sugar-free beverages, or with saliva substitutes if dry mouth persists.

# OPIOID ANALGESICS

*See also the following individual entries:*

> Butorphanol tartrate
> Codeine phosphate
> Codeine sulfate
> Fentanyl citrate
> Fentanyl transdermal system
> Hydrocodone bitartrate and
>     Acetaminophen
> Morphine hydrochloride
> Tramadol hydrochloride
> Tylenol with Codeine

**Action/Kinetics:** The opioid analgesics attach to specific receptors located in the CNS (cortex, brain stem, and spinal cord) resulting in diminished transmission of pain impulses.
**Uses:** See individual drugs. Generally are used to treat pain due to various causes (e.g., MI, carcinoma, surgery, burns, postpartum), as preanesthetic medication, as adjuncts to anesthesia, acute vascular occlusion, diarrhea, and coughs. Methadone is used for heroin withdrawal and maintenance.
**Contraindications:** Asthma, emphysema, kyphoscoliosis, severe obesity, convulsive states as in epilepsy, delirium tremens, tetanus and strychnine poisoning, diabetic acidosis, myxedema, Addison's disease, hepatic cirrhosis, and children under 6 months.
**Special Concerns:** Use with caution in clients with head injury or after head surgery because of morphine's capacity to elevate ICP and mask the pupillary response. Use with caution in the elderly, in the debilitated, in young children, in individuals with increased ICP, in ob-

stetrics, and with clients in shock or during acute alcoholic intoxication.

**Side Effects:** *Respiratory:* **Respiratory depression, apnea.** *CNS:* Dizziness, lightheadedness, sedation, lethargy, headache, euphoria, mental clouding, fainting. Idiosyncratic effects including excitement, restlessness, tremors, delirium, insomnia. *Oral:* Dry mouth. *GI:* N&V, vomiting, constipation, increased pressure in biliary tract, anorexia. *CV:* Flushing, changes in HR and BP, circulatory collapse. *Allergic:* Skin rashes including pruritus and urticaria. Sweating, *laryngospasm*, edema. *Miscellaneous:* Urinary retention, oliguria, reduced libido, changes in body temperature. Narcotics cross the placental barrier and depress respiration of the fetus or newborn.

DEPENDENCE AND TOLERANCE: All drugs of this group are addictive. Psychologic and physical dependence and tolerance develop even when clients use clinical doses. Tolerance is characterized by the fact that the client requires shorter periods of time between doses or larger doses for relief of pain. Tolerance usually develops faster when the narcotic analgesic is administered regularly and when the dose is large.

**Drug Interactions**
*Alcohol, ethyl* / Potentiation or addition of CNS depressant effects; concomitant use may lead to drowsiness, lethargy, stupor, respiratory collapse, coma, or death
*Anesthetics, general* / See *Alcohol*
*Antianxiety drugs* / See *Alcohol*
*Antidepressants, tricyclic* / ↑ Narcotic-induced respiratory depression
*Antihistamines* / See *Alcohol*
*Barbiturates* / See *Alcohol*
*CNS depressants* / See *Alcohol*
*MAO inhibitors* / Possible potentiation of either MAO inhibitor (excitation, hypertension) or narcotic (hypotension, coma) effects; death has resulted
*Phenothiazines* / See *Alcohol*
*Sedative-hypnotics, nonbarbiturate* / See *Alcohol*

*Skeletal muscle relaxants (surgical)* / ↑ Respiratory depression and ↑ muscle relaxation

**Dosage**
See individual drugs.

## DENTAL CONCERNS
**General**
1. Document indications for therapy.
2. Note any prior experience with opioid analgesics such as an adverse reaction with the drug or category of drugs prescribed.
3. Monitor vital signs at every appointment because of cardiovascular and respiratory side effects.
4. Have the patient sit up slowly and remain seated for at least two minutes after being supine in order to minimize the risk of orthostatic hypotension.
5. Decreased saliva flow can put the patient at risk for dental caries, periodontal disease, and candidiasis.
6. When used as sedation for outpatient procedures, someone must accompany client. Expect a recovery period (to assess for any adverse side effects) of up to several hours before release.
7. Psychologic and physical dependence may occur with these medications.
8. NSAIDs may be beneficial if additional analgesia is necessary.

**Client/Family Teaching**
1. Daily home fluoride treatments for persistent dry mouth.
2. Avoid alcohol-containing mouth rinses and beverages.
3. Avoid caffeine-containing beverages.
4. Dry mouth can be treated with tart, sugarless gum or candy, water, sugar-free beverages, or with saliva substitutes if dry mouth persists.
5. Patient should use caution doing anything that requires thought or concentration (i.e., driving a car, operating heavy machinery, taking care of children) after taking this medication.

# OPIOID ANTAGONISTS

*See also the following individual entries:*

Naloxone hydrochloride
Naltrexone

**Action/Kinetics:** Opioid antagonists competitively block the action of opioid analgesics by displacing previously given opioids from their receptor sites or by preventing opioids from attaching to the opiate receptors, thereby preventing access by the analgesic. Not effective in reversing the respiratory depression induced by barbiturates, anesthetics, or other nonopioid agents. These drugs almost immediately induce withdrawal symptoms in opioid addicts and are sometimes used to unmask dependence.

## DENTAL CONCERNS

**General**

1. Determine etiology of respiratory depression. Opioid antagonists do not relieve the toxicity of nonnarcotic CNS depressants.

2. This drug is intended for acute use only. However, patients may experience side effects.

3. Dose should be carefully titrated to avoid serious cardiovascular adverse effects.

4. Note agent being reversed. If opioid is long acting or sustained release, repeated doses will be required in order to continue to counteract drug effects. Monitor VS and respirations closely after duration of action of antagonist; additional doses may be necessary.

5. Observe for symptoms of airway obstruction; if comatose, turn frequently and position on side to prevent aspiration.

6. Maintain a safe, protective environment. Use side rails, supervise ambulation, and use soft supports as needed.

7. Significant opioid depression that occurs in the dental office may require transportation of the patient to a hospital.

# ORAL CONTRACEPTIVES: ESTROGEN-PROGESTERONE COMBINATIONS

*See Table 1.*

**Action/Kinetics:** The combination oral contraceptives act by inhibiting ovulation due to an inhibition (through negative-feedback mechanism) of LH and FSH, which are required for development of ova. These products also alter the cervical mucus so that it is not conducive to sperm penetration, render the endometrium less suitable for implantation of the blastocyst should fertilization occur, and inhibit enzymes required by sperm to enter the ovum.

The estrogen used in combination oral contraceptives is either ethinyl estradiol or mestranol. Mestranol is demethylated to ethinyl estradiol in the liver. **t½:** 6–20 hr. The progestin used in combination oral contraceptives is either desogestrel, ethynodiol diacetate, levonorgestrel, norethindrone, norethindrone acetate, norgestimate, or norgestrel.

The progestin-only products do not consistently inhibit ovulation. However, these products also alter the cervical mucus and render the endometrium unsuitable for implantation. These products contain either norethindrone or norgestrel. This method of contraception is less reliable than combination therapy.

Although oral contraceptives may be associated with serious side effects, a number of noncontraceptive health benefits have been confirmed. These include increased regularity of the menstrual cycle, decreased incidence of dysmenorrhea, decreased blood loss, decreased incidence of functional ovarian cysts and ectopic pregnancies, and decreased incidence of diseases such as fibroadenomas, fibrocystic dis-

---

**Table 1  Combination Oral Contraceptive Preparations Available in the United States**

| Trade Name | Estrogen | Progestin |
|---|---|---|
| **MONOPHASIC** | | |
| Alesse 21-Day and 28-Day | Ethinyl estradiol (20 mcg) | Levonorgestrel (0.1 mg) |
| Brevicon 21-Day and 28-Day | Ethinyl estradiol (35 mcg) | Norethindrone (0.5 mg) |
| Demulen 1/35–21 and 1/35–28 | Ethinyl estradiol (35 mcg) | Ethynodiol diacetate (1 mg) |
| Demulen 1/50–21 and 1/50–28 | Ethinyl estradiol (50 mcg) | Ethynodiol diacetate (1 mg) |
| Desogen (28 day) | Ethinyl estradiol (30 mcg) | Desogestrel (0.15 mg) |
| Genora 0.5/35 21 Day and 28 Day | Ethinyl estradiol (35 mcg) | Norethindrone (0.5 mg) |
| Genora 1/35 21 Day and 28 Day | Ethinyl estradiol (35 mcg) | Norethindrone (1 mg) |
| Genora 1/50 21 Day and 28 Day | Mestranol (50 mcg) | Norethindrone (1 mg) |
| Levlen 21 and 28 | Ethinyl estradiol (30 mcg) | Levonorgestrel (0.15 mg) |
| Levora 0.15/30–21 and –28 | Ethinyl estradiol (30 mcg) | Levonorgestrel (0.15 mg) |
| Loestrin 21 1/20 | Ethinyl estradiol (20 mcg) | Norethindrone acetate (1 mg) |
| Loestrin 21 1.5/30 | Ethinyl estradiol (30 mcg) | Norethindrone acetate (1.5 mg) |
| Loestrin Fe 1/20 (28 day) | Ethinyl estradiol (20 mcg) | Norethindrone acetate (1 mg) |
| Loestrin Fe 1.5/30 (28 day) | Ethinyl estradiol (30 mcg) | Norethindrone acetate (1.5 mg) |
| Lo/Ovral-21 and -28 | Ethinyl estradiol (30 mcg) | Norgestrel (0.3 mg) |
| Modicon 21 and 28 | Ethinyl estradiol (35 mcg) | Norethindrone (0.5 mg) |
| Necon 0.5/35–21 Day and 28 Day | Ethinyl estradiol (35 mcg) | Norethindrone (0.5 mg) |
| Necon 1/35–21 Day and 28 Day | Ethinyl estradiol (35 mcg) | Norethindrone (1 mg) |
| Necon 1/50–21 Day and 28 Day | Mestranol (50 mcg) | Norethindrone (1 mg) |
| N.E.E. 1/35 21 Day and 28 Day | Ethinyl estradiol (35 mcg) | Norethindrone (1 mg) |
| Nelova 0.5/35E 21 Day and 28 Day | Ethinyl estradiol (35 mcg) | Norethindrone (0.5 mg) |
| Nelova 1/35E 21 Day and 28 Day | Ethinyl estradiol (35 mcg) | Norethindrone (1 mg) |
| Nelova 1/50M 21 Day and 28 Day | Mestranol (50 mcg) | Norethindrone (1 mg) |
| Neocon 0.5/35–21 Day and –28 Day | Ethinyl estradiol (35 mcg) | Norethindrone (0.5 mg) |
| Neocon 1/35–21 Day and –28 Day | Ethinyl estradiol (35 mcg) | Norethindrone (1 mg) |
| Neocon 1/50–21 Day and –28 Day | Ethinyl estradiol (50 mcg) | Norethindrone (1 mg) |
| Nordette-21 and -28 | Ethinyl estradiol (30 mcg) | Levonorgestrel (0.15 mg) |

| Trade Name | Estrogen | Progestin |
|---|---|---|
| **MONOPHASIC** | | |
| Norethin 1/35E 21 Day and 28 Day | Ethinyl estradiol (35 mcg) | Norethindrone (1 mg) |
| Norethin 1/50M 21 Day and 28 Day | Mestranol (50 mcg) | Norethindrone (1 mg) |
| Norinyl 1 + 35 21-Day and 28-Day | Ethinyl estradiol (35 mcg) | Norethindrone (1 mg) |
| Norinyl 1 + 50 21-Day and 28-Day | Mestranol (50 mcg) | Norethindrone (1 mg) |
| Norlestrin 1/50 21 Day and 28 Day | Ethinyl estradiol (50 mcg) | Norethindrone (1 mg) |
| Norlestrin 2.5/50 21 Day and 28 Day | Ethinyl estradiol (50 mcg) | Norethindrone (2.5 mg) |
| Ortho-Cept 21 Day and 28 Day | Ethinyl estradiol (30 mcg) | Desogestrel (0.15 mg) |
| Ortho-Cyclen-21 and -28 | Ethinyl estradiol (35 mcg) | Norgestimate (0.25 mg) |
| Ortho Novum 1/35–21 and –28 | Ethinyl estradiol (35 mcg) | Norethindrone (1 mg) |
| Ortho Novum 1/50–21 and –28 | Mestranol (50 mcg) | Norethindrone (1 mg) |
| Ovcon-35 21 Day and 28 Day | Ethinyl estradiol (35 mcg) | Norethindrone (0.4 mg) |
| Ovcon-50 21 Day and 28 Day | Ethinyl estradiol (50 mcg) | Norethindrone (1 mg) |
| Ovral 21 Day and 28 Day | Ethinyl estradiol (50 mcg) | Norgestrel (0.5 mg) |
| Zovia 1/35E-21 and -28 | Ethinyl estradiol (35 mcg) | Ethynodiol diacetate (1 mg) |
| Zovia 1/50E-21 and -28 | Ethinyl estradiol (50 mcg) | Ethynodiol diacetate (1 mg) |
| **BIPHASIC** | | |
| Jenest-28 | Ethinyl estradiol (35 mcg in each tablet) | Norethindrone (10 tablets of 0.5 mg followed by 11 tablets of 1 mg) |
| Necon 10/11 21 Day and 28 Day | Ethinyl estradiol (35 mcg in each tablet) | Norethindrone (10 tablets of 0.5 mg followed by 11 tablets of 1 mg) |
| Nelova 10/11–21 and –28 | Ethinyl estradiol (35 mcg in each tablet) | Norethindrone (10 tablets of 0.5 mg followed by 11 tablets of 1 mg) |
| Necon 10/11–21 and –28 | Ethinyl estradiol (35 mcg in each tablet) | Norethindrone (10 tablets of 0.5 mg followed by 11 tablets of 1 mg) |
| Ortho-Novum 10/11–21 and –28 | Ethinyl estradiol (35 mcg in each tablet) | Norethindrone (10 tablets of 0.5 mg followed by 11 tablets of 1 mg) |

✦ = Available in Canada

***bold italic*** = life-threatening side effect

**Table 1** (continued)

| Trade Name | Estrogen | Progestin |
|---|---|---|
| | **TRIPHASIC** | |
| Estrostep (21 or 28 days) | Ethinyl estradiol (20, 30, and 35 mcg) | Norethindrone (1 mg in each tablet) |
| Ortho-Novum 7/7/7 (21 or 28 days) | Ethinyl estradiol (35 mcg in each tablet) | Norethindrone (0.5 mg the first 7 days, 0.75 mg the next 7 days, and 1 mg the last 7 days) |
| Ortho-Tri-Cyclen (21 or 28 days) | Ethinyl estradiol (35 mcg in each tablet) | Norgestimate (0.18 mg the first 7 days, 0.215 mg the next 7 days, and 0.25 mg the last seven days) |
| Tri-Levlen 21 Day and Tri-Levlen 28 Day | First 6 days: Ethinyl estradiol (30 mcg) Next 5 days: Ethinyl estradiol (40 mcg) Last 10 days: Ethinyl estradiol (30 mcg) | Levonorgestrel (0.05 mg) Levonorgestrel (0.075 mg) Levonorgestrel (0.125 mg) |
| Tri-Norinyl (21 or 28 day) | Ethinyl estradiol (35 mcg in each tablet) | Norethindrone (0.5 mg the first 7 days, 1 mg the next 9 days, and 0.5 mg the last 5 days) |
| Triphasil 21 (21 or 28 day) | First 6 days: Ethinyl estradiol (30 mcg) Next 5 days: Ethinyl estradiol (40 mcg) Last 10 days: Ethinyl estradiol (30 mcg) | Levonorgestrel (0.05 mg) Levonorgestrel (0.075 mg) Levonorgestrel (0.125 mg) |

All combination oral contraceptives are Rx and Pregnancy category: X.

ease, acute pelvic inflammatory disease, endometrial cancer, and ovarian cancer.

**Uses:** Contraception, menstrual irregularities, menopausal symptoms. High doses are used for endometriosis and hypermenorrhea. *Non-FDA Approved Uses:* High doses of Ovral (ethinyl estradiol and norgestrel) have been used as a postcoital contraceptive.

**Contraindications:** Thrombophlebitis, history of deep-vein thrombophlebitis, thromboembolic disorders, cerebral vascular disease, CAD, MI, current or past angina, known or suspected breast cancer or estrogen-dependent neoplasm, endometrial carcinoma, hepatic adenoma or carcinoma, undiagnosed abnormal genital bleeding, known or suspected pregnancy, cholestatic jaundice of pregnancy. Smoking.

**Special Concerns:** Cigarette smoking increases the risk of cardiovascular side effects from use of oral contraceptives. Low estrogen-containing oral contraceptives do not increase the risk of stroke in women. Use with caution in clients with a history of hypertension, preexisting renal disease, hypertension-related diseases during pregnancy, familial tendency to hypertension or its consequences, a history of excessive weight gain or fluid retention during the menstrual cycle; these individuals are more likely to develop elevated BP. Use with caution in clients with asthma, epilepsy, migraine, diabetes, metabolic bone disease, renal or cardiac disease, and a history of mental depression. Use with drugs (e.g., barbiturates, hydantoins, rifampin) that increase the hepatic metabolism of oral contraceptives may result in breakthrough bleeding and an increased risk of pregnancy. Use combination products during lactation only if absolutely necessary; progestin-only products do not appear to have any adverse effects on breast-feeding performance or on the health, growth, or development of the infant.

**Side Effects:** *CV: MI, thrombophlebitis, venous thrombosis with or without embolism, pulmonary embolism, coronary thrombosis, cerebral thrombosis, arterial thromboembolism, mesenteric thrombosis, thrombotic and hemorrhagic strokes, postsurgical thromboembolism, subarachnoid hemorrhage,* elevated BP, hypertension. *CNS:* Onset or exacerbation of migraine headaches, depression. *Oral:* Hyperplasia, bleeding gums. *GI:* N&V, bloating, abdominal cramps. *Ophthalmic:* Optic neuritis, retinal thrombosis, steepening of the corneal curvature, contact lens intolerance. *Hepatic: Benign and malignant hepatic adenomas,* focal nodular hyperplasia, *hepatocellular carcinoma,* gallbladder disease, cholestatic jaundice. *GU:* Breakthrough bleeding, spotting, amenorrhea, change in menstrual flow, change in cervical erosion and cervical secretions, *invasive cervical cancer,* bleeding irregularities (more common with progestin-only products), vaginal candidiasis, *ectopic pregnancies in contraceptive failures*, breast tenderness, breast enlargement. *Miscellaneous:* Acute intermittent porphyria, photosensitivity, congenital anomalies, melasma, skin rash, edema, increase or decrease in weight, decreased carbohydrate tolerance, increased incidence of cervical *Chlamydia trachomatis,* decrease in the quantity and quality of breast milk.

**Drug Interactions**

*Acetaminophen* / ↓ Effect of acetaminophen due to ↑ breakdown by liver

*Antidepressants, tricyclic* / ↑ Effect of antidepressants due to ↓ breakdown by liver

*Benzodiazepines* / ↑ or ↓ Effect of benzodiazepines due to changes in breakdown by liver

*Carbamazepine* / ↓ Effect of oral contraceptives due to ↑ breakdown by liver

---

*Corticosteroids* / ↑ Effect of corticosteroids due to ↓ breakdown by liver

*Erythromycins* / ↓ Effect of oral contraceptives due to altered enterohepatic absorption

*Penicillins, oral* / ↓ Effect of oral contraceptives due to altered enterohepatic absorption

*Phenobarbital* / ↓ Effect of oral contraceptives due to ↑ breakdown by liver

*Phenytoin* / ↓ Effect of oral contraceptives due to ↑ breakdown by liver

*Tetracyclines* / ↓ Effect of contraceptives due to altered enterohepatic absorption

*Troleandomycin* / ↑ Chance of jaundice

**DENTAL CONCERNS**

**General**

1. Avoid prolonged immobilization and restrictions of movement as with travel due to increased risk of venous thromboembolic events.

2. It may be necessary to give the patient breaks during longer appointments so she can stretch or move her legs.

3. Shorter appointments may be necessary if procedure does not allow for breaks.

**Consultation with Primary Care Provider**

1. Consultation with the appropriate health care provider may be necessary in order to evaluate the patient's ability to tolerate stress and her level of disease control.

**Client/Family Teaching**

1. Use caution when using oral hygiene aids.

2. Brush teeth with a soft-bristle tooth brush.

3. Report any unusual bruising or bleeding; advise others esp. dentist of prescribed therapy, before surgery or new meds added.

4. Practice another form of contraception if receiving ampicillin, anticonvulsants, phenylbutazone, rifampin, or tetracycline. These may cause intermittent bleeding and the drug interactions could result in an unwanted pregnancy.

# PENICILLINS

*See also the following individual entries:*

> Amoxicillin
> Amoxicillin and Potassium clavulanate
> Ampicillin oral
> Ampicillin sodium/Sulbactam sodium
> Cloxacillin sodium
> Penicillin G benzathine, parenteral
> Penicillin V potassium

**Action/Kinetics:** The bactericidal action of penicillins depends on their ability to bind penicillin-binding proteins (PBP-1 and PBP-3) in the cytoplasmic membranes of bacteria, thus inhibiting cell wall synthesis. Some penicillins act by acylation of membrane-bound transpeptidase enzymes, thereby preventing crosslinkage of peptidoglycan chains, which are necessary for bacterial cell wall strength and rigidity. Cell division and growth are inhibited and often lysis and elongation of susceptible bacteria occur. Penicillin is most effective against young, rapidly dividing organisms and has little effect on mature resting cells. Depending on the concentration of the drug at the site of infection and the susceptibility of the infectious microorganism, penicillin is either bacteriostatic or bactericidal. Penicillins are distributed throughout most of the body and pass the placental barrier. They also pass into synovial, pleural, pericardial, peritoneal, ascitic, and spinal fluids. Although normal meninges and the eyes are relatively impermeable to penicillins, they are better absorbed by inflamed meninges and eyes. **Peak serum levels, after PO:** 1 hr. $t^{1/2}$: 30–110 min; protein binding: 20%–98% (see individual agents). Excreted largely unchanged by the urine as a result of glomerular filtration and active tubular secretion.

**Uses:** See individual drugs. Effective against a variety of gram-positive, gram-negative, and anaerobic organisms.

**Contraindications:** Hypersensitivity to penicillins, imipenem, and cephalosporins. PO use of penicillins during the acute stages of empyema, bacteremia, pneumonia, meningitis, pericarditis, and purulent or septic arthritis.

**Special Concerns:** Use of penicillins during lactation may lead to sensitization, diarrhea, candidiasis, and skin rash in the infant. Use with caution in clients with a history of asthma, hay fever, or urticaria. Clients with cystic fibrosis have a higher incidence of side effects with broad spectrum penicillins. Safety and effectiveness of the beta-lactamase inhibitor/penicillin combinations (e.g., amoxicillin/potassium clavulanate, ticarcillin/ potassium clavulanate) have not been determined in children less than 12 years of age. The incidence of resistant strains of staphylococci to penicillinase-resistant penicillins is increasing. Use of prolonged therapy may lead to superinfection (i.e., bacterial or fungal overgrowth of nonsusceptible organisms).

**Side Effects:** Penicillins are potent sensitizing agents; it is estimated that up to 10% of the US population is allergic to the antibiotic. Hypersensitivity reactions are reported to be on the increase in pediatric populations. Sensitivity reactions may be immediate (within 20 min) or delayed (as long as several days or weeks after initiation of therapy). *Allergic:* Skin rashes (including maculopapular and exanthematous), exfoliative dermatitis, erythema multiforme (rarely, *Stevens-Johnson syndrome*), hives, pruritus, wheezing, *anaphylaxis,* fever, eosinophilia, *angioedema,* serum sickness, *laryngeal edema, laryngospasm, prostration, angioneurotic edema, bronchospasm, hypotension, vascular collapse, death.* *Oral:* Bitter/unpleasant taste, glossitis, gastritis, stomatitis, dry mouth, sore mouth or tongue, furry tongue, black "hairy" tongue. *GI:* Diarrhea (may be severe), abdominal cramps or pain, N&V, bloating, flatulence, increased thirst, bloody diarrhea, rectal bleeding, enterocolitis, pseudomembranous colitis. *CNS:* Dizziness, insomnia, hyperactivity, fatigue, prolonged muscle relaxation. Neurotoxicity including lethargy, neuromuscular irritability, *seizures,* hallucinations following large IV doses (especially in clients with renal failure). *Hematologic:* Thrombocytopenia, leukopenia, *agranulocytosis,* anemia, thrombocytopenic purpura, *hemolytic anemia,* granulocytopenia, neutropenia, bone marrow depression. *Renal:* Oliguria, hematuria, hyaline casts, proteinuria, pyuria (all symptoms of interstitial nephritis), nephropathy. Electrolyte imbalance following IV use. *Miscellaneous:* Hepatotoxicity (cholestatic jaundice), superinfection, swelling of face and ankles, anorexia, hyperthermia, transient hepatitis, vaginitis, itchy eyes. IM injection may cause pain and induration at the injection site, ecchymosis, and hematomas. IV use may cause vein irritation, deep vein thrombosis, and thrombophlebitis.

**Drug Interactions**

*Antacids* / ↓ Effect of penicillins due to ↓ absorption from GI tract

*Antibiotics, Chloramphenicol, Erythromycins, Tetracyclines* / ↓ Effect of penicillins

*Anticoagulants* / Penicillins may potentiate pharmacologic effect

*Aspirin* / ↑ Effect of penicillins by ↓ plasma protein binding

*Chloramphenicol* / Either ↑ or ↓ effects

*Erythromycins* / Either ↑ or ↓ effects

*Heparin* / ↑ Risk of bleeding following parenteral penicillins

*Oral contraceptives* / ↓ Effect of oral contraceptives

*Phenylbutazone* / ↑ Effect of penicillins by ↓ plasma protein binding

---

♣ = Available in Canada          ***bold italic*** = life-threatening side effect

*Tetracyclines* / ↓ Effect of penicillins

**Dosage** ―――――――――――

See individual drugs. Penicillins are available in a variety of dosage forms for PO, parenteral, inhalation, and intrathecal administration. PO doses must be higher than IM or SC doses because a large fraction of penicillin given PO may be destroyed in the stomach.

## DENTAL CONCERNS

See also *Dental Concerns for All Anti-Infectives.*

**General**
1. Assess for allergic reactions; if reaction occurs, stop drug immediately. Allergic reactions are more likely to occur with a history of asthma, hay fever, urticaria, or allergy to cephalosporins.
2. The elderly may be more sensitive to the effects of penicillin than younger people. Use care when calculating the dose based on weight and height.
3. Most penicillins are excreted in breast milk and should be prescribed cautiously to nursing mothers.

**Client/Family Teaching**
1. Review drugs prescribed, method and frequency of administration, side effects, and expected outcome/goals of therapy.
2. Report any S&S of allergic reactions, i.e., rashes, fever, joint swelling, angioneurotic edema, intense itching, and respiratory distress (during therapy and in some cases 7–12 days after therapy). Stop medication when noted and call for help immediately.
3. Oral penicillins may cause GI upset (N&V and diarrhea). Take oral penicillin with a glass of water 1 hr before or 2 hr after meals to minimize binding to foods.
4. Complete the entire prescribed course of therapy, even if feeling well. Incomplete therapy will predispose client to development of resistant bacterial strains. With alpha-hemolytic *Streptococcus* infection, must continue with penicillin therapy for a

minimum of 10 days, and preferably 14 days, to prevent development of rheumatic fever or glomerulonephritis.
5. Report S&S of superinfections (furry tongue, vaginal or rectal itching, diarrhea).
6. Notify provider if S&S do not improve or get worse after 48–72 hr of therapy.
7. For patients taking oral contraceptives, use a back-up method of birth control for the remainder of the current cycle.

# SEDATIVE-HYPNOTICS (ANTI-ANXIETY)/ ANTIMANIC DRUGS

*See also the following individual entries:*

Alprazolam
Barbiturates
Buspirone hydrochloride
Diazepam
Flurazepam hydrochloride
Lithium carbonate
Lithium citrate
Lorazepam
Midazolam hydrochloride
Zolpidem tartrate

**Action/Kinetics:** Benzodiazepines are the major antianxiety agents. They are thought to affect the limbic system and reticular formation to reduce anxiety by increasing or facilitating the inhibitory neurotransmitter activity of GABA. When used for 3–4 weeks for sleep, certain benzodiazepines may cause REM rebound when discontinued. The benzodiazepines generally have long half-lives (1–8 days); thus cumulative effects can occur. Several of the benzodiazepines are metabolized to active metabolites in the liver, which prolongs their duration of action. Benzodiazepines are widely distributed throughout the body. Approximately 70%–99% of an administered dose is bound to plasma protein. Metabolites of benzodiazepines are excreted through the kidneys. All tranquiliz-

ers have the ability to cause psychologic and physical dependence.
**Uses:** See individual drugs. Depending on the drug, used as antianxiety agents, hypnotics, anticonvulsants, and muscle relaxants.
**Contraindications:** Hypersensitivity, acute narrow-angle glaucoma, psychoses, primary depressive disorder, psychiatric disorders in which anxiety is not a signficiant symptom.
**Special Concerns:** Use with caution in impaired hepatic or renal function and in the geriatric or debilitated client. Use during lactation may cause sedation, weight loss, and possibly feeding difficulties in the infant. Geriatric clients may be more sensitive to the effects of benzodiazepines; symptoms may include oversedation, dizziness, confusion, or ataxia. When used for insomnia, rebound sleep disorders may occur following abrupt withdrawal of certain benzodiazepines.
**Side Effects:** *CNS:* Drowsiness, fatigue, confusion, ataxia, sedation, dizziness, vertigo, depression, apathy, lightheadedness, delirium, headache, lethargy, disorientation, hypoactivity, crying, anterograde amnesia, slurred speech, stupor, *coma,* fainting, difficulty in concentration, euphoria, nervousness, irritability, akathisia, hypotonia, vivid dreams, "glassy-eyed," hysteria, *suicide attempt,* psychosis. Paradoxical excitement manifested by anxiety, acute hyperexcitability, increased muscle spasticity, insomnia, hallucinations, sleep disturbances, rage, and stimulation. *Oral:* Dry mouth, bitter or metallic taste, increased salivation, coated tongue, sore gums. *GI:* Increased appetite, constipation, diarrhea, anorexia, N&V, weight gain or loss, difficulty in swallowing, gastritis, fecal incontinence. *Respiratory:* **Respiratory depression and sleep apnea,** especially in clients with compromised respiratory function. *Dermatologic:* Urticaria, rash, pruritus, alopecia, hirsutism, dermatitis, edema of ankles and face. *Endocrine:* In-

creased or decreased libido, gynecomastia, menstrual irregularities. *GU:* Difficulty in urination, urinary retention, incontinence, dysuria, enuresis. *CV:* Hypertension, hypotension, bradycardia, tachycardia, palpitations, edema, *CV collapse.* *Hematologic:* Anemia, *agranulocytosis,* leukopenia, eosinophilia, thrombocytopenia. *Ophthalmologic:* Diplopia, conjunctivitis, nystagmus, blurred vision. *Miscellaneous:* Joint pain, lymphadenopathy, muscle cramps, paresthesia, dehydration, lupus-like symptoms, sweating, SOB, flushing, hiccoughs, fever, hepatic dysfunction. *Following IM use:* Redness, pain, burning. *Following IV use:* Thrombosis and phlebitis at site.

**Drug Interactions**
*Alcohol* / Potentiation or addition of CNS depressant effects. Concomitant use may lead to drowsiness, lethargy, stupor, respiratory collapse, coma, or death
*Anesthetics, general* / See *Alcohol*
*Antacids* / ↓ Rate of absorption of benzodiazepines
*Antidepressants, tricyclic* / Concomitant use with benzodiazepines may cause additive sedative effect and/or atropine-like side effects
*Antihistamines* / See *Alcohol*
*Barbiturates* / See *Alcohol*
*Cimetidine* / ↑ Effect of benzodiazepines by ↓ breakdown in liver
*CNS depressants* / See *Alcohol*
*Erythromycin* / ↑ Effect of benzodiazepines by ↓ breakdown in liver
*Ketoconazole* / ↑ Effect of benzodiazepines due to ↓ breakdown in liver
*Neuromuscular blocking agents* / Benzodiazepines may ↑, ↓, or have no effect on the action of neuromuscular blocking agents
*Opioids* / See *Alcohol*
*Phenothiazines* / See *Alcohol*
*Phenytoin* / Concomitant use with benzodiazepines may cause ↑ effect of phenytoin due to ↓ breakdown by liver

---

*Propoxyphene* / ↑ Effect of benzodiazepines due to ↓ breakdown by liver

*Ranitidine* / May ↓ absorption of benzodiazepines from the GI tract

*Sedative-hypnotic, nonbarbiturate* / See *Alcohol*

**Dosage**
See individual drugs.

## DENTAL CONCERNS
**General**
1. Monitor vital signs at every appointment because of cardiovascular and respiratory side effects.
2. Have the patient sit up slowly and remain seated for at least two minutes after being supine in order to minimize the risk of orthostatic hypotension.
3. Decreased saliva flow can put the patient at risk for dental caries, periodontal disease, and candidiasis.
4. Early morning and shorter appointments, as well as methods for addressing anxiety levels in the patient, can help to reduce the amount of stress that the patient is experiencing.
5. Note any evidence of physical or psychologic dependence. Assess frequency and quantity of refills.
**Consultation with Primary Care Provider**
1. Consultation may be required in order to assess level of disease control and the patient's ability to tolerate stress.
**Client/Family Teaching**
1. These drugs may reduce ability to handle potentially dangerous equipment, such as automobiles and other machinery.
2. Avoid alcohol while taking antianxiety agents. Alcohol potentiates the depressant effects of both the alcohol and the medication.
3. Do not stop taking drug suddenly. Any sudden withdrawal after prolonged therapy or after excessive use may cause a recurrence of the preexisting symptoms of anxiety. It may also cause a withdrawal syndrome, manifested by increased anxiety, anorexia, insomnia, vomiting, ataxia, muscle twitching, confusion, and hallucinations. Some clients may develop seizures and convulsions.
4. These drugs are generally for short-term therapy; follow-up is imperative to evaluate response and the need for continued therapy.
5. Daily home fluoride treatments for persistent dry mouth.
6. Avoid alcohol-containing mouth rinses and beverages.
7. Avoid caffeine-containing beverages.
8. Dry mouth can be treated with tart, sugarless gum or candy, water, sugar-free beverages or with saliva substitutes if dry mouth persists.

# SELECTIVE SEROTONIN REUPTAKE INHIBITORS

*See also the following individual entries:*

> Citalopram hydrobromide
> Fluoxetine hydrochloride
> Fluvoxamine maleate
> Paroxetine hydrochloride
> Sertraline hydrochloride

**Action/Kinetics:** Effect thought to be due to inhibition of uptake of serotonin into CNS neurons. Slight to no anticholinergic, sedative, or orthostatic hypotensive effects. Also binds to muscarinic, histaminergic, and alpha-1-adrenergic receptors, accounting for many of the side effects.

**Uses:** Citalopram, fluoxetine, paroxetine, and sertraline are used to treat depression. Fluvoxamine is only used to treat obsessive-compulsive disorder. See individual agents for other uses.

**Contraindications:** Hypersensitivity, MAOIs.

**Special Concerns:** See individual agents.

**Side Effects:** The following side effects are common to the selective serotonin reuptake inhibitors. See individual drugs as well.

*Oral:* Dry mouth, taste changes. *GI:* Nausea, diarrhea, anorexia, dyspepsia, constipation, cramps, vomiting, flatulence, decreased appetite. *CNS:* Headache, nervousness, insomnia, drowsiness, anxiety, dizziness, fatique, sedation, agitation. *CV:* Hot flashes, palpitations. *Pulmonary:* Infection, pharyngitis, nasal congestion, sinus headache, sinusitis, cough, dyspnea, bronchitis. *GU:* Decreased libido, delayed ejaculation. *Eyes:* Visual changes, eye pain, photophobia. *Miscellaneous:* Sweating, rash, pruritus, urticaria, pain, asthenia, viral infection, fever, allergy, chills.

**Drug Interactions:** See individual agents.

**Dosage** ⎯⎯⎯⎯⎯⎯⎯⎯⎯⎯⎯⎯
See individual agents.

### DENTAL CONCERNS
**General**
1. Monitor vital signs at every appointment because of cardiovascular side effects.
2. Decreased saliva flow can put the patient at risk for dental caries, periodontal disease, and candidiasis.

**Consultation with Primary Care Provider**
1. Consultation may be required in order to assess extent of disease control.
2. Health care provider should be informed of the oral adverse effects of these drugs.

**Client/Family Teaching**
1. Daily home fluoride treatments for persistent dry mouth.
2. Avoid alcohol-containing mouth rinses or beverages.
3. Avoid caffeine-containing beverages.
4. Dry mouth can be treated with tart, sugarless gum or candy, water, sugar-free beverages, or with saliva substitutes if dry mouth persists.

⎯⎯⎯⎯⎯⎯⎯⎯⎯⎯⎯⎯⎯⎯⎯⎯⎯⎯

# SYMPATHOMIMETIC DRUGS
⎯⎯⎯⎯⎯⎯⎯⎯⎯⎯⎯⎯⎯⎯⎯⎯⎯⎯
*See also the following individual entries:*

Albuterol

Bitolterol mesylate
Ephedrine sulfate
Epinephrine
Epinephrine hydrochloride
Phenylephrine hydrochloride
Pirbuterol acetate
Pseudoephedrine hydrochloride
Salmeterol xinafoate

**Action/Kinetics:** The adrenergic drugs work in two ways: (1) by mimicking the action of norepinephrine or epinephrine by combining with alpha and/or beta receptors (directly acting sympathomimetics) or (2) by causing or regulating the release of the natural neurohormones from their storage sites at the nerve terminals (indirectly acting sympathomimetics). Some drugs exhibit a combination of effects 1 and 2.

Adrenergic stimulation of receptors will manifest the following general effects:

*Alpha-1-adrenergic:* / Vasoconstriction, decongestion, constriction of the pupil of the eye, contraction of splenic capsule, contraction of the trigone-sphincter muscle of the urinary bladder.

*Alpha-2-adrenergic:* / Presynaptic to regulate amount of transmitter released; decrease tone, motility, and secretory activity of the GI tract (possibly involved in hypersecretory response also); decrease insulin secretion.

*Beta-1-adrenergic:* / Myocardial contraction (inotropic), regulation of heartbeat (chronotropic), improved impulse conduction, ↑ lipolysis.

*Beta-2-adrenergic:* / Peripheral vasodilation, bronchial dilation; ↓ tone, motility, and secretory activity of the GI tract; ↑ renin secretion.

**Uses:** See individual drugs.

**Contraindications:** Tachycardia due to arrhythmias; tachycardia or heart block caused by digitalis toxicity.

**Special Concerns:** Use with caution in hyperthyroidism, diabetes, prostatic hypertrophy, seizures, degenerative heart disease, especially

⎯⎯⎯⎯⎯⎯⎯⎯⎯⎯⎯⎯⎯⎯⎯⎯⎯⎯⎯⎯⎯⎯⎯⎯⎯⎯⎯⎯

in geriatric clients or those with asthma, emphysema, or psychoneuroses. Also, use with caution in clients with coronary insufficiency, CAD, ischemic heart disease, CHF, cardiac arrhythmias, hypertension, or history of stroke. Asthma clients who rely heavily on inhaled beta-2-agonist bronchodilators may increase their chances of death. Thus, these agents should be used to "rescue" clients but should not be prescribed for regular long-term use. Beta-2 agonists may inhibit uterine contractions.

**Side Effects:** See individual drugs; side effects common to most sympathomimetics are listed. *CV:* Tachycardia, arrhythmias, palpitations, BP changes, anginal pain, precordial pain, pallor, skipped beats, chest tightness, hypertension. *Oral:* Dry mouth, altered taste or bad taste, teeth discoloration. *GI:* N&V, heartburn, anorexia, GI distress, diarrhea. *CNS:* Restlessness, anxiety, tension, insomnia, hyperkinesis, drowsiness, weakness, vertigo, irritability, dizziness, headache, tremors, general CNS stimulation, nervousness, shakiness, hyperactivity. *Respiratory:* Cough, dyspnea, dry throat, pharyngitis, *paradoxical bronchospasm,* irritation. *Other:* Flushing, sweating, *allergic reactions.*

**Drug Interactions**
*Anesthetics* / Halogenated anesthetics sensitize heart to adrenergics—causes cardiac arrhythmias
*Anticholinergics* / Concomitant use aggravates glaucoma
*Corticosteroids* / Chronic use with sympathomimetics may result in or aggravate glaucoma; aerosols containing sympathomimetics and corticosteroids may be lethal in asthmatic children
*Phenothiazines* / ↑ Risk of cardiac arrhythmias
*Sodium bicarbonate* / ↑ Effect of sympathomimetics due to ↓ excretion by kidney
*Tricyclic antidepressants* / ↑ Effect of direct-acting sympathomimetics and ↓ effect of indirect-acting sympathomimetics

**Dosage**
See individual drugs.

## DENTAL CONCERNS
### General
1. Monitor vital signs at every appointment because of cardiovascular and respiratory side effects.
2. The patient may require a semisupine position for the dental chair to help with breathing.
3. Dental procedures may cause the patient anxiety which could result in an asthma attack. Make sure that the patient has his/her sympathomimetic inhaler present or have the inhaler from the office emergency kit present.
4. Morning and shorter appointments, as well as methods for addressing anxiety levels in the patient, can help to reduce the amount of stress that the patient is experiencing.
5. Sulfites present in vasoconstrictors can precipitate an asthma attack.
6. Decreased saliva flow can put the patient at risk for dental caries, periodontal disease, and candidiasis.

### Consultation with Primary Care Provider
1. Consultation may be necessary in order to evaluate the patient's level of disease control.
2. Consultation may be necessary in order to determine the patient's ability to tolerate stress.

### Client/Family Teaching
1. Daily home fluoride treatments for persistent dry mouth.
2. Avoid alcohol-containing mouth rinses and beverages.
3. Avoid caffeine-containing beverages.
4. Dry mouth can be treated with tart, sugarless gum or candy, water, sugar-free beverages, or with saliva substitutes if dry mouth persists.
5. Review technique for use and care of prescribed inhalers and respiratory equipment. Rinsing of equipment and of mouth after use is imperative in preventing oral fungal infections.

# TETRACYCLINES

*See also the following individual entries:*

Doxycycline calcium
Doxycycline hyclate
Tetracycline hydrochloride

**Action/Kinetics:** The tetracyclines inhibit protein synthesis by microorganisms by binding to the ribosomal 50S subunit, thereby interfering with protein synthesis. The drugs block the binding of aminoacyl transfer RNA to the messenger RNA complex. Cell wall synthesis is not inhibited. The drugs are mostly bacteriostatic and are effective only against multiplying bacteria. Well absorbed from the stomach and upper small intestine. Well distributed throughout all tissues and fluids and diffuse through noninflamed meninges and the placental barrier. They become deposited in the fetal skeleton and calcifying teeth. $t\frac{1}{2}$: 7–18.6 hr (see individual agents) and is increased in the presence of renal impairment. The drugs bind to serum protein (range: 20%–93%; see individual agents). The drugs are concentrated in the liver in the bile and are excreted mostly unchanged in the urine and feces.

**Uses:** See individual drugs. Used mainly for infections caused by *Rickettsia, Chlamydia, Actinomycosis*, and *Mycoplasma.* Due to development of resistance, tetracyclines are usually not used for infections by common gram-negative or gram-positive organisms. Atypical pneumonia caused by *Mycoplasma pneumoniae.* Adjunct in the treatment of trachoma.

As an alternative to penicillin for uncomplicated gonorrhea or disseminated gonococcal infections, especially with penicillin allergy. Acute pelvic inflammatory disease. Tetracyclines are also useful as an alternative to penicillin for early syphilis.

Although not generally used for gram-positive infections, tetracyclines may be beneficial in anthrax, *Listeria* infections, and actinomycosis. They have also been used in conjunction with quinine sulfate for chloroquine-resistant *Plasmodium falciparum* malaria and as an intracavitary injection to control pleural or pericardial effusions caused by metastatic carcinoma. As an adjunct to amebicides in acute intestinal amebiasis. Used PO to treat uncomplicated endocervical, rectal, or urethral *Chlamydia* infections.

Topical uses include skin granulomas caused by *Mycobacterium marinum;* ophthalmic bacterial infections causing blepharitis, conjunctivitis, or keratitis; and as an adjunct in the treatment of ophthalmic chlamydial infections such as trachoma or inclusion conjunctivitis. As an alternative to silver nitrate for prophylaxis of neonatal gonococcal ophthalmia. Vaginitis. Severe acne.

**Contraindications:** Hypersensitivity. Avoid drug during tooth development stage (last trimester of pregnancy, neonatal period, during breast-feeding, and during childhood up to 8 years) because tetracyclines interfere with enamel formation and dental pigmentation. Never administer intrathecally.

**Special Concerns:** Use with caution and at reduced dosage in clients with impaired kidney function and liver dysfunction.

**Side Effects:** *Oral:* Tooth discoloration in children < 8 years of age, candidiasis, black hairy tongue, glossitis, stomatitis, sore throat, hypertrophy of papilla and tongue discoloration, enamel hypoplasia, bleeding (long-term use). *GI* (most common): N&V, thirst, diarrhea, anorexia, flatulence, epigastric distress, bulky loose stools. Less commonly, dysphagia, or inflammatory lesions of the anogenital area. Rarely, pseudomembranous colitis. PO dosage forms may cause esophageal ulcers, especially in clients with esophageal obstructive element or hiatal hernia. *Allergic* (rare): Urticaria, pericarditis,

---

*bold italic* = life-threatening side effect

polyarthralgia, fever, rash, pulmonary infiltrates with eosinophilia, *angioneurotic edema,* worsening of SLE, *anaphylaxis,* purpura. *Skin:* Photosensitivity, maculopapular and erythematous rashes, exfoliative dermatitis (rare), onycholysis, discoloration of nails. *CNS:* Dizziness, lightheadedness, unsteadiness, paresthesias. *Hematologic:* Eosinophilia, *hemolytic anemia,* neutropenia, thrombocytopenia, thrombocytopenic purpura. *Hepatic:* Fatty liver, increases in liver enzymes; rarely, hepatotoxicity, hepatitis, hepatic cholestasis. *Miscellaneous:* Candidal superinfections including oral and vaginal candidiasis, discoloration of infants' and children's teeth, bone lesions, delayed bone growth, abnormal pigmentation of the conjunctiva, pseudotumor cerebri in adults and bulging fontanels in infants.

IV administration may cause thrombophlebitis; IM injections are painful and may cause induration at the injection site.

The administration of deteriorated tetracyclines may result in Fanconi-like syndrome characterized by N&V, acidosis, proteinuria, glycosuria, aminoaciduria, polydipsia, polyuria, hypokalemia.

**Drug Interactions**
*Aluminum salts* / ↓ Effect of tetracyclines due to ↓ absorption from GI tract
*Antacids, oral* / ↓ Effect of tetracyclines due to ↓ absorption from GI tract
*Bismuth salts* / ↓ Effect of tetracyclines due to ↓ absorption from GI tract
*Calcium salts* / ↓ Effect of tetracyclines due to ↓ absorption from GI tract
*Contraceptives, oral* / ↓ Effect of oral contraceptives
*Iron preparations* / ↓ Effect of tetracyclines due to ↓ absorption from GI tract
*Magnesium salts* / ↓ Effect of tetracyclines due to ↓ absorption from GI tract

*Methoxyflurane* / ↑ Risk of kidney toxicity
*Penicillins and Cephalosporins* / Tetracyclines may mask bactericidal effect of penicillins and cephalosporins
*Sodium bicarbonate* / ↓ Effect of tetracyclines due to ↓ absorption from GI tract

**Dosage**
See individual drugs.

## DENTAL CONCERNS

See also *General Dental Concerns for All Anti-Infectives.*
**General**
1. Determine why the patient is taking a tetracycline antibiotic and any drug allergens or sensitivity.
2. If pregnant, document trimester.
3. Document side effects such as sore throat, dysphagia, fever, dizziness, hoarseness, inflammation of mucous membranes, and candidal superinfections.
**Consultation with Primary Care Provider**
1. Consultation with the appropriate health care provider may be necessary to assess disease control.
**Client/Family Teaching**
1. Take on a full stomach to enhance absorption. Do not lay down after administration; may precipitate erosive esophagitis.
2. Do not take with milk, cheese, ice cream, yogurt, or other foods or drugs containing calcium. If taken with meals, avoid these foods for 2 hr after administration.
3. Zinc tablets or vitamin preparations containing zinc may interfere with drug absorption. Food sources high in zinc that should be avoided include oysters, fresh and raw; cooked lobster; dry oat flakes; steamed crabs; veal; and liver.
4. Avoid direct or artificial sunlight (i.e., dental treatment lamp), which can cause a severe sunburn-like reaction; report if erythema occurs. Wear protective clothing, sunglasses, and a sunscreen if exposed and for up to 3 weeks following therapy.

5. Tetracyclines interfere with formation of tooth enamel and dental pigmentation from the third trimester of pregnancy through age 8.

6. Use alternative method of birth control, as drug may interfere with oral contraceptives; may also cause a vaginal infection.

7. Take only as directed and complete full prescription. Discard any leftover meds to prevent reaction from deteriorated drugs.

8. Let the dentist know if the infection progresses despite tetracycline therapy.

9. Report signs and symptoms of superinfection (i.e., sore throat, oral burning sensation, fever, fatigue).

10. Stress the importance of good oral hygiene in order to prevent or minimize soft tissue damage.

11. Use caution with oral hygiene aids.

12. Take tetracycline 1 hr before or 2 hr after using air polishing device (Prophy Jet).

# THEOPHYLLINE DERIVATIVES

*See also the following individual entries:*

Theophylline

**Action/Kinetics:** Theophyllines stimulate the CNS, directly relax the smooth muscles of the bronchi and pulmonary blood vessels (relieve bronchospasms), produce diuresis, inhibit uterine contractions, stimulate gastric acid secretion, and increase the rate and force of contraction of the heart. Response to the drugs is highly individualized. Theophylline is well absorbed from uncoated plain tablets and PO liquids. *Theophylline salts:* **Onset:** 1–5 hr, depending on route and formulation. **Therapeutic plasma levels:** 10–20 mcg/mL. **t½:** 3–15 hr in nonsmoking adults, 4–5 hr in adult heavy smokers, 1–9 hr in children, and 20–30 hr for premature neo-

nates. An increased t½ may be seen in individuals with CHF, alcoholism, liver dysfunction, or respiratory infections. Because of great variations in the rate of absorption (due to dosage form, food, dose level) as well as its extremely narrow therapeutic range, theophylline therapy is best monitored by determination of the serum levels. If these determinations cannot be obtained, saliva (contains 60% of corresponding theophylline serum levels) determinations can be used. Eighty-five percent to 90% metabolized in the liver and various metabolites, including the active 3-methylxanthine. Theophylline is metabolized partially to caffeine in the neonate. The premature neonate excretes 50% unchanged theophylline and may accumulate the caffeine metabolite. Excretion is through the kidneys (about 10% unchanged in adults).

**Uses:** Prophylaxis and treatment of bronchial asthma. Reversible bronchospasms associated with chronic bronchitis, emphysema, and COPD. *Non-FDA Approved Uses:* Treatment of neonatal apnea and Cheyne-Stokes respiration.

**Contraindications:** Hypersensitivity to any xanthine, peptic ulcer, seizure disorders (unless on medication), hypotension, CAD, angina pectoris.

**Special Concerns:** Use during lactation may result in irritability, insomnia, and fretfulness in the infant. Use with caution in premature infants due to the possible accumulation of caffeine. Xanthines are not usually tolerated by small children because of excessive CNS stimulation. Geriatric clients may manifest an increased risk of toxicity. Use with caution in the presence of gastritis, alcoholism, acute cardiac diseases, hypoxemia, severe renal and hepatic disease, severe hypertension, severe myocardial damage, hyperthyroidism, glaucoma.

**Side Effects:** Side effects are uncommon at serum theophylline levels

---

less than 20 mcg/mL. At levels greater than 20 mcg/mL, 75% of individuals experience side effects including N&V, diarrhea, irritability, insomnia, and headache. At levels of 35 mcg/mL or greater, individuals may manifest *cardiac arrhythmias,* hypotension, tachycardia, hyperglycemia, *seizures, brain damage, or death. Oral:* Bitter taste, dry mouth. *GI:* N&V, diarrhea, anorexia, epigastric pain, hematemesis, dyspepsia, rectal irritation (following use of suppositories), rectal bleeding, gastroesophageal reflux during sleep or while recumbent (theophylline). *CNS:* Headache, insomnia, irritability, fever, dizziness, lightheadedness, vertigo, reflex hyperexcitability, *seizures,* depression, speech abnormalities, alternating periods of mutism and hyperactivity, *brain damage, death. CV:* Hypotension, *life-threatening ventricular arrhythmias,* palpitations, tachycardia, *peripheral vascular collapse,* extrasystoles. *Renal:* Proteinuria, excretion of erythrocytes and renal tubular cells, dehydration due to diuresis, urinary retention (men with prostatic hypertrophy). *Other:* Tachypnea, *respiratory arrest,* fever, flushing, hyperglycemia, antidiuretic hormone syndrome, leukocytosis, rash, alopecia.

**Drug Interactions**
*Barbiturates* / ↓ Theophylline levels
*Benzodiazepines* / Sedative effect may be antagonized by theophylline
*Carbamazepine* / Either ↑ or ↓ theophylline levels
*Cimetidine* / ↑ Theophylline levels
*Ciprofloxacin* / ↑ Plasma levels of theophylline with ↑ possibility of side effects
*Corticosteroids* / ↑ Theophylline levels
*Ephedrine and other sympathomimetics* / ↑ Theophylline levels
*Erythromycin* / ↑ Effect of theophylline due to ↓ breakdown by liver
*Halothane* / ↑ Risk of cardiac arrhythmias
*Ketamine* / Seizures of the extensor-type

*Ketoconazole* / ↓ Theophylline levels
*Muscle relaxants, nondepolarizing* / Theophylline ↓ effect of these drugs
*Phenytoin* / ↓ Theophylline levels
*Propofol* / Theophyllines ↓ sedative effect of propofol
*Quinolones* / ↑ Theophylline levels
*Sympathomimetics* / ↓ Theophylline levels
*Tetracyclines* / ↑ Risk of theophylline toxicity
*Troleandomycin* / ↑ Effect of theophylline due to ↓ breakdown by liver

**Dosage**
Individualized. Initially, dosage should be adjusted according to plasma level of drug. Usual: 10–20 mcg theophylline/mL plasma. The dose of the various salts should be equivalent based on the content of anhydrous theophylline. See individual agents.

## DENTAL CONCERNS
**General**
1. Monitor vital signs at every appointment because of cardiovascular and respiratory side effects.
2. The patient may require a semisupine position in the dental chair to help with breathing.
3. Dental procedures may cause the patient anxiety which could result in an asthma attack. Make sure that the patient has his/her sympathomimetic inhaler present or have the inhaler from the office emergency kit present.
4. Morning and shorter appointments as well as methods for addressing anxiety levels in the patient can help to reduce the amount of stress that the patient is experiencing.
5. Sulfites present in vasoconstrictors can precipitate an asthma attack.
6. Decreased saliva flow can put the patient at risk for dental caries, periodontal disease, and candidiasis.

**Consultation with Primary Care Provider**
1. Consultation may be necessary in

order to evaluate the patient's level of disease control.

2. Consultation may be necessary in order to determine the patient's ability to tolerate stress.

**Client/Family Teaching**

1. Daily home fluoride treatments for persistent dry mouth.

2. Avoid alcohol-containing mouth rinses and beverages.

3. Avoid caffeine-containing beverages.

4. Dry mouth can be treated with tart, sugarless gum or candy, water, sugar-free beverages, or with saliva substitutes if dry mouth persists.

---

# THYROID DRUGS

*See also the following individual entries:*

Levothyroxine sodium

**Action/Kinetics:** The thyroid manufactures two active hormones: thyroxine and triiodothyronine, both of which contain iodine. These thyroid hormones are released into the bloodstream, where they are bound to protein. Synthetic derivatives include liothyronine ($T_3$), levothyronine ($T_4$), and liotrix (a 4:1 mixture of $T_4$ and $T_3$). The thyroid hormones regulate growth by controlling protein synthesis and regulating energy metabolism by increasing the resting or basal metabolic rate. This results in increases in respiratory rate; body temperature; $CO_2$ oxygen consumption; HR; blood volume; enzyme system activity; rate of fat, carbohydrate, and protein metabolism; and growth and maturation. Excess thyroid hormone causes a decrease in TSH, and a lack of thyroid hormone causes an increase in the production and secretion of TSH. Normally, the ratio of $T_4$ to $T_3$ released from the thyroid gland is 20:1 with about 35% of $T_4$ being converted in the periphery (e.g., kidney, liver) to $T_3$.

**Uses:** Replacement or supplemental therapy in hypothyroidism due to all causes except transient hypothyroid-

ism during the recovery phase of subacute thyroiditis. To treat or prevent euthyroid goiters. With antithyroid drugs for thyrotoxicosis (to prevent goiter or hypothyroidism). Diagnostically to differentiate suspected hyperthyroidism from euthyroidism. The treatment of choice for hypothyroidism is usually $T_4$ because of its consistent potency and its prolonged duration of action although it does have a slow onset and its effects are cumulative over several weeks.

**Contraindications:** Uncorrected adrenal insufficiency, acute MI, hyperthyroidism, and thyrotoxicosis. When hypothyroidism and adrenal insufficiency coexist unless treatment with adrenocortical steroids is initiated first. To treat obesity or infertility.

**Special Concerns:** Geriatric clients may be more sensitive to the usual adult dosage of these hormones. Use with extreme caution in the presence of angina pectoris, hypertension, and other CV diseases, renal insufficiency, and ischemic states. Use with caution during lactation.

**Side Effects:** Thyroid preparations have cumulative effects, and overdosage (e.g., symptoms of hyperthyroidism) may occur. *CV:* Arrhythmias, palpitations, angina, increased HR and pulse pressure, ***cardiac arrest,*** aggravation of CHF. *GI:* Cramps, diarrhea, N&V, appetite changes. *CNS:* Headache, nervousness, mental agitation, irritability, insomnia, tremors. *Miscellaneous:* Weight loss, hyperhidrosis, excessive warmth, irregular menses, heat intolerance, fever, dyspnea, allergic skin reactions (rare). Decreased bone density in pre- and postmenopausal women following long-term use of levothyroxine.

**Drug Interactions**

*Antidepressants, tricyclic /* ↑ Effect of antidepressants and ↑ effect of thyroid

*Corticosteroids /* Thyroid preparations ↑ tissue demands for corticosteroids. Adrenal insufficiency must be corrected with corticosteroids

---

before administering thyroid hormones. In clients already treated for adrenal insufficiency, dosage of corticosteroids must be increased when initiating therapy with thyroid drug

*Epinephrine* / CV effects ↑ by thyroid preparations

*Ketamine* / Concomitant use may result in severe hypertension and tachycardia

*Levarterenol* / CV effects ↑ by thyroid preparations

*Salicylates* / Salicylates compete for thyroid-binding sites on protein

**Dosage** ————————————
See individual hormone products.

## DENTAL CONCERNS
### General
1. Patients with uncontrolled thyroid disease should be referred to their health care provider.

2. Patients who are hypothyroid may require lower doses of opioid analgesics.

### Consultation with Primary Care Provider
1. Consultation with the appropriate health care provider may be necessary in order to evaluate level of disease control and the patient's ability to handle stress.

# CHAPTER THREE
# A–Z Listing of Drugs

## A

## Acarbose
(ah-**KAR**-bohs)
**Pregnancy Category:** B
Prandase ✦, Precose **(Rx)**
**Classification:** Antidiabetic agent

**Action/Kinetics:** Acarbose delays the intestinal absorption of glucose resulting in a smaller increase in blood glucose following meals. Approximately 65% of an oral dose of acarbose remains in the GI tract, which is the site of action. Metabolized in the GI tract by both intestinal bacteria and intestinal enzymes. The acarbose and metabolites that are absorbed are excreted in the urine.

**Uses:** Used alone, with diet control, to decrease blood glucose in type 2 diabetes mellitus. Also, used with a sulfonylurea when diet plus either acarbose or a sulfonylurea alone do not control blood glucose adequately.

**Contraindications:** Diabetic ketoacidosis, cirrhosis, inflammatory bowel disease, colonic ulceration, partial intestinal obstruction or predisposition to intestinal obstruction, chronic intestinal diseases associated with marked disorders of digestion or absorption, conditions that may deteriorate as a result of increased gas formation in the intestine. In significant renal dysfunction. Severe, persistent bradycardia. Lactation.

**Special Concerns:** Safety and efficacy have not been determined in children. Acarbose does not cause hypoglycemia; however, sulfonylureas and insulin can lower blood glucose sufficiently to cause symptoms or even life-threatening hypoglycemia.

**Side Effects:** *GI:* Abdominal pain, diarrhea, flatulence. GI side effects may be severe and be confused with paralytic ileus.

**Drug Interactions**
*Charcoal* / ↓ Effect of acarbose
*Digestive enzymes* / ↓ Effect of acarbose
*Digoxin* / ↓ Serum digoxin levels
*Insulin* / ↑ Hypoglycemia which may cause severe hypoglycemia
*Sulfonylureas* / ↑ Hypoglycemia which may cause severe hypoglycemia

**How Supplied:** *Tablet:* 50 mg, 100 mg

## Dosage
• **Tablets**
*Type 2 diabetes mellitus.*
Individualized, depending on effectiveness and tolerance. **Initial:** 25 mg (one-half of a 50-mg tablet) t.i.d. with the first bite of each main meal. **Maintenance:** After the initial dose of 25 mg t.i.d., the dose can be increased to 50 mg t.i.d. Some may benefit from 100 mg t.i.d. The dosage can be adjusted at 4- to 8-week intervals. The recommended maximum daily dose is 50 mg t.i.d. for clients weighing less than 60 kg and 100 mg t.i.d. for those weighing more than 60 kg.

## DENTAL CONCERNS
### General
1. Decreased salivary flow may put the patient at risk for dental caries, periodontal disease, and candidiasis.

2. Patients with diabetes are at more risk for delayed wound healing and developing infections. Prophylactic antibiotics may be necessary if surgery or deep scaling is anticipated.
3. Bring patients in more frequently to assess healing processes.
4. Make sure that the patient is following his or her diet and medication regimen.
5. Determine if the patient is self-monitoring his or her drug's antidiabetic effect.
6. Even though this medication does not cause hypoglycemia it may be used with another antidiabetic medication that does. Therefore, monitor vital signs and assess for signs and symptoms of hypoglycemia. Keep a sugar or juice source avaliable if hypoglycemia occurs.

**Client/Family Teaching**
1. Counsel the patient about the importance of good oral hygiene.
2. Avoid mouth rinses with alcohol because alcohol can exacerbate dry mouth.
3. Counsel the patient about the importance of avoiding injury with home oral care products.

---

# Acebutolol hydrochloride
(ays-**BYOU**-toe-lohl)
**Pregnancy Category:** B
Apo-Acebutolol ✹, Monitan ✹, Novo-Acebutolol ✹, Nu-Acebutolol ✹, Rhotral ✹, Sectral **(Rx)**
**Classification:** Beta-adrenergic blocking agent

---

See also *Beta-Adrenergic Blocking Agents.*
**Action/Kinetics:** Predominantly beta-1 blocking activity but will inhibit beta-2 receptors at higher doses. Some intrinsic sympathomimetic activity. **t½:** 3–4 hr. Low lipid solubility. **Onset:** 1–1½ hr; **Peak:** 2–4 hr; **Half-life:** 3–4 hr; **Duration:** 24–30 hr. Metabolized in liver and excreted in urine and bile. Fifteen to 20% excreted unchanged.
**Uses:** Hypertension (either alone or with other antihypertensive agents

such as thiazide diuretics). Premature ventricular contractions.
**Contraindications:** Hypersensitivity to acebutolol, cardiogenic shock, 2nd or 3rd degree heart block, sinus bradycardia, congestive heart failure, cardiac failure.
**Additional Contraindications:** Severe, persistent bradycardia.
**Special Concerns:** Aortic or mitral valve disease, asthma, COPD, diabetes mellitus, major surgery, renal disease, thyroid disease, well-compensated heart failure.
**Side Effects:** *Oral:* Dry mouth. *CV: **Bradycardia, CHF, cold extremities, postural hypotension, profound hypotension, 2nd or 3rd degree heart block.** CNS:* Catatonia, depression, dizziness, drowsiness, fatigue, hallucinations, insomnia, lethargy, mental changes, memory loss, strange dreams. *GI:* Diarrhea, *ischemic colitis,* nausea, ***mesenteric arterial thrombosis,*** vomiting. *Hematologic: **Agranulocytosis,*** thrombocytopenia. *Allergic:* Fever, sore throat, respiratory distress, rash, pharyngitis, ***laryngospasm, anaphylaxis.*** *Skin:* Pruritus, rash, increased skin pigmentation, sweating, dry skin, alopecia, skin irritation, psoriasis. *Ophthalmic:* Dry, burning eyes. *GU:* Dysuria, impotence, nocturia. *Other:* Hypoglycemia or hyperglycemia. *Respiratory: **Bronchospasm,*** dyspnea, wheezing.
**Drug Interactions:** See also *Drug Interactions* for *Beta-Adrenergic Blocking Agents* and *Antihypertensive Agents.*
**How Supplied:** *Capsule:* 200 mg, 400 mg

## Dosage
• **Capsules**
*Hypertension.*
**Initial:** 400 mg/day (although 200 mg b.i.d. may be needed for optimum control; **then,** 400–800 mg/day (range: 200–1,200 mg/day).
*Premature ventricular contractions.*
**Initial:** 200 mg b.i.d.; **then,** increase dose gradually to reach 600–1,200 mg/day.

Dosage should not exceed 800 mg/day in geriatric clients. In those with impaired kidney or liver function, decrease dose by 50% when creatinine clearance is 50 mL/min/1.73 m² and by 75% when it is less than 25 mL/min/1.73 m².

## DENTAL CONCERNS

See also *Dental Concerns* for *Beta-Adrenergic Blocking Agents* and *Antihypertensive Agents*.

**Client/Family Teaching**
1. 1. Review the importance of good oral hygiene in order to prevent soft tissue inflammation.
2. Review the proper use of oral hygiene aids in order to prevent injury.
3. Daily home fluoride treatments for persistent dry mouth.
4. Avoid alcohol-containing mouth rinses and beverages.
5. Avoid caffeine-containing beverages.
6. Dry mouth can be treated with tart, sugarless gum or candy, water, sugarless beverages, or with saliva substitutes if dry mouth persists.

---

# Acetaminophen (Apap, Paracetamol)

(ah-**SEAT**-ah-**MIN**-oh-fen)

**Caplets:** Arthritis Foundation Pain Reliever Aspirin Free, Aspirin Free Pain Relief, Aspirin Free Anacid Maximum Strength, Atasol ✹, Atasol Forte ✹, Genapap Extra Strength, Genebs Extra Strength Caplets, Panadol, Panadol Junior Strength, Tapanol Extra Strength, Tylenol Caplets, Tylenol Extended Relief, **Capsules:** Dapacin, Meda Cap, **Elixir:** Aceta, Genapap Children's, Mapap Children's, Oraphen-PD, Ridenol, Silapap Children's, Tylenol Children's, **Gelcaps:** Aspirin Free Anacid Maximum Strength, Tapanol Extra Strength, Tylenol Extra Strength, **Oral Liquid/Syrup:** Atasol ✹, Children's Acetaminophen Elixir Drops ✹, Halenol Children's, Panadol Children's, Pediatrix ✹, Tempra ✹, Tempra 2 Syrup, Tempra Children's Syrup ✹, Tylenol Extra Strength, **Oral Solution:** Acetaminophen Drops, Apacet, Atasol ✹, Children's Acetaminophen Oral Solution ✹, Genapap Infants' Drops, Mapap Infant Drops, Panadol Infants' Drops, Pediatrix ✹, PMS-Acetaminophen ✹, Silapap Infants, Tempra 1, Tylenol Infants' Drops, Uni-Ace, **Oral Suspension:** Tylenol Children's Suspension ✹, Tylenol Infants' Suspension ✹, **Sprinkle Capsules:** Feverall Children's, Feverall Junior Strength, **Suppositories:** Abenol 120, 325, 650 mg ✹, Acephen, Acetaminophen Uniserts, Children's Feverall, Infant's Feverall, Junior Strength Feverall, Neopap, **Tablets:** Aceta, A.F. Anacin ✹, A.F. Anacin Extra Strength ✹, Apo-Acetaminophen ✹, Aspirin Free Pain Relief, Aspirin Free Anacin Maximum Strength, Atasol ✹, Atasol Forte ✹, Extra Strength Acetaminophen ✹, Fem-Etts, Genapap, Genapap Extra Strength, Genebs, Genebs Extra Strength, Mapap Regular Strength, Mapap Extra Strength, Maranox, Meda Tab, Panadol, Redutemp, Regular Strength Acetaminophen ✹, Tapanol Regular Strength, Tapanol Extra Strength, Tempra, Tylenol Regular Strength, Tylenol Extra Strength, Tylenol Junior Strength, Tylenol Tablets 325 mg, 500 mg ✹, **Tablets, Chewable:** Apacet, Children's Chewable Acetaminophen ✹, Children's Genapap, Children's Panadol, Children's Tylenol, Tempra 3 ✹, Tempra 3, Tylenol Chewable Tablets Fruit, Tylenol Junior Strength Chewable Tablets Fruit ✹ **(OTC)**

---

# Acetaminophen, buffered

(ah-**SEAT**-ah-**MIN**-oh-fen)

Alka-Seltzer, Bromo Seltzer **(OTC)**

**Classification:** Opioid analgesic, para-aminophenol type

---

**Action/Kinetics:** Acetaminophen decreases fever by an effect on the hypothalamus leading to sweating and vasodilation. It also inhibits the effect of pyrogens on the hypothalamic heat-regulating centers. It may cause analgesia by inhibiting CNS prostaglandin synthesis; however, due to minimal effects on peripheral prostaglandin synthesis, acetaminophen has no anti-inflammatory or uricosuric effects. It does not cause any anticoagulant effect or ulceration of the GI tract. The antipyretic

---

and analgesic effects are comparable to those of aspirin.

**Peak plasma levels:** 30–120 min. **t½:** 45 min–3 hr. **Therapeutic serum levels** (analgesia): 5–20 mcg/mL. **Plasma protein binding:** Approximately 25%. Metabolized in the liver and excreted in the urine as glucuronide and sulfate conjugates. However, an intermediate hydroxylated metabolite is hepatotoxic following large doses of acetaminophen.

Acetaminophen is often combined with other drugs, as in Darvocet-N, Parafon Forte, and Tylenol with Codeine.

The extended-relief product uses a bilayer system that allows the outer layer to release acetaminophen rapidly while the inner layer is designed to release the remainder of the dose more slowly. This allows prolonged relief of symptoms.

The buffered product is a mixture of acetaminophen, sodium bicarbonate, and citric acid that effervesces when placed in water. This product has a high sodium content (0.76 g/¾ capful).

**Uses:** Control of pain due to headache, earache, dysmenorrhea, arthralgia, myalgia, musculoskeletal pain, immunizations, teething, tonsillectomy. To reduce fever in bacterial or viral infections. As a substitute for aspirin in upper GI disease, aspirin allergy, bleeding disorders, clients on anticoagulant therapy, and gouty arthritis.

**Contraindications:** Renal insufficiency, anemia. Clients with cardiac or pulmonary disease are more susceptible to toxic effects of acetaminophen. Hypersensitivity.

**Special Concerns:** Evidence indicates that acetaminophen may have to be used with caution in pregnancy. Heavy drinking and fasting may be risk factors for acetaminophen toxicity, especially if larger than recommended doses of acetaminophen are used. As little as twice the recommended dosage, over time, can lead to serious liver damage.

**Side Effects:** Few when taken in usual therapeutic doses. Chronic and even acute toxicity can develop after long symptom-free usage. *Hematologic:* Methemoglobinemia, *hemolytic anemia*, neutropenia, thrombocytopenia, pancytopenia, leukopenia. *Allergic:* Urticarial and erythematous skin reactions, skin eruptions, fever. *Miscellaneous:* CNS stimulation, hypoglycemic coma, jaundice, drowsiness, glossitis. *GI:* Nausea, vomiting, abdominal pain, *hepatotoxicity.*

**Drug Interactions**

*Barbiturates* / ↑ Potential of hepatotoxicity due to ↑ breakdown of acetaminophen by liver

*NSAIDs* / ↑ Nephrotoxicity with concurrent, chronic high dose use

*Salicylates* / ↑ Nephrotoxicity with concurrent, chronic high dose use

*Tetracycline* / ↑ Decreased absorption due to ↑ buffer in buffered acetaminophen

*Oral anticoagulants* / ↓ Increased bleeding due to ↑ chronic, high doses (> 2 g/day of acetaminophen)

**How Supplied:** *Capsule:* 80 mg, 160 mg, 325 mg, 500 mg, 650 mg; *Chew tablet:* 80 mg, 160 mg; *Elixir:* 120 mg/5 mL, 160 mg/5 mL; *Liquid:* 80 mg/2.5 mL, 160 mg/5 mL, 325 mg/5 mL, 500 mg/15 mL, 500 mg/5 mL; *Powder for reconstitution:* 950 mg; *Solution:* 80 mg/0.8 mL, 120 mg/2.5 mL, 160 mg/mL; *Suppository:* 80 mg, 120 mg, 325 mg, 650 mg; *Suspension:* 160 mg/5 mL, 80 mg/0.8 mL; *Tablet:* 80 mg, 160 mg, 325 mg, 500 mg, 648 mg, 650 mg; *Tablet, Extended Release:* 650 mg Acetaminophen, buffered: *Granule, effervescent*

**Dosage** ────────────

• **Caplets, Capsules, Chewable Tablets, Gelcaps, Elixir, Oral Liquid, Oral Solution, Oral Suspension, Sprinkle Capsules, Syrup, Tablets**

*Analgesic, antipyretic.*

**Adults:** 325–650 mg q 4 hr; doses up to 1 g q.i.d. may be used. Daily dosage should not exceed 4 g. **Pediatric:** Doses given 4–5 times/day. **Up to 3 months:** 40 mg/dose; **4–11 months:** 80 mg/dose; **1–2 years:** 120 mg/dose; **2–3 years:** 160 mg/dose; **4–5 years:** 240 mg/dose;

**6–8 years:** 320 mg/dose; **9–10 years:** 400 mg/dose; **11 years:** 480 mg/dose. **12–14 years:** 640 mg/dose. **Over 14 years:** 650 mg/dose. *Alternative pediatric dose:* 10–15 mg/kg q 4 hr.

• **Extended Relief Caplets**
*Analgesic, antipyretic.*
**Adults:** 2 caplets (1,300 mg) q 8 hr.

• **Suppositories**
*Analgesic, antipyretic.*
**Adults:** 650 mg q 4 hr, not to exceed 4 g/day for up to 10 days. Clients on long-term therapy should not exceed 2.6 g/day. **Pediatric, 3–11 months:** 80 mg q 6 hr; **1–3 years:** 80 mg q 4 hr; **3–6 years:** 120–125 mg q 4–6 hr, with no more than 720 mg in 24 hr; **6–12 years:** 325 mg q 4–6 hr with no more than 2.6 g in 24 hr. Dosage should be given as needed while symptoms persist.

BUFFERED
*Analgesic, antipyretic.*
**Adult, usual:** 1 or 2 three-quarter capfuls are placed into an empty glass; add half a glass of cool water. May be taken while fizzing or after settling. Can be repeated q 4 hr as required or directed by provider.

## DENTAL CONCERNS

**General**
1. Avoid the prescribing of aspirin-containing pain products.
2. Assess the need for acetaminophen.
3. Patients receiving chronic acetaminophen therapy may rarely present with signs and symptoms of blood dyscrasias. They include infection, bleeding, and poor wound healing.

**Consultation with Primary Care Provider**
1. Patients with symptoms of blood dyscrasias should be referred to their primary care provider for complete blood counts. Treatment should be postponed until the results are known.

**Client/Family Teaching**
1. Take only as directed and with food or milk to minimize GI upset.

2. Read the labels on all OTC preparations consumed. Many contain acetaminophen and can produce toxic reactions if taken over time with the prescribed drug.

# Acetylcysteine

(ah-see-till-**SIS**-tay-een)
**Pregnancy Category:** B
Mucomyst, Mucosil, Parvolex **(Rx)**
**Classification:** Mucolytic

**Action/Kinetics:** Acetylcysteine reduces the viscosity of purulent and nonpurulent pulmonary secretions and facilitates their removal by splitting disulfide bonds. Action increases with increasing pH (peak: pH 7–9). **Onset, inhalation:** Within 1 min; **by direct instillation:** immediate. **Time to peak effect:** 5–10 min.
**Uses:** Adjunct in the treatment of acute and chronic bronchitis, emphysema, tuberculosis, pneumonia, bronchiectasis, atelectasis. Routine care of clients with tracheostomy, pulmonary complications after thoracic or CV surgery, or in posttraumatic chest conditions. Pulmonary complications of cystic fibrosis. Diagnostic bronchial asthma. Antidote in acetaminophen poisoning to reduce hepatotoxicity. *Non-FDA Approved Uses:* As an ophthalmic solution for dry eye.
**Contraindications:** Sensitivity to drug.
**Special Concerns:** Use with caution during lactation, in the elderly, and in clients with asthma.
**Side Effects:** *Respiratory:* Increased incidence of bronchospasm in clients with asthma. Increased amount of liquefied bronchial secretions, which must be removed by suction if cough is inadequate. Bronchial and tracheal irritation, tightness in chest, bronchoconstriction. *Oral:* Stomatitis. *GI:* N&V. *Other:* Rashes, fever, drowsiness, rhinorrhea.
**Drug Interactions:** Acetylcysteine is incompatible with antibiotics and should be administered separately.

---

✦ = Available in Canada                    ***bold italic*** = life-threatening side effect

Obstructive respiratory diseases are contraindicated with nitrous oxide.

**How Supplied:** *Solution:* 10%, 20%

**Dosage**

• **10% or 20% Solution: Nebulization, Direct Application, or Direct Intratracheal Instillation**
*Nebulization into face mask, tracheostomy, mouth piece.*
1–10 mL of 20% solution or 2–10 mL of 10% solution 3–4 times/day.
*Closed tent or croupette.*
Up to 300 mL of 10% or 20% solution/treatment.
*Direct instillation into tracheostomy.*
1–2 mL of 10%–20% solution q 1–4 hr.
*Percutaneous intratracheal catheter.*
1–2 mL of 20% solution or 2–4 mL of 10% solution q 1–4 hr by syringe attached to catheter.
*Instillation to particular portion of bronchopulmonary tree using small plastic catheter into the trachea.*
2–5 mL of 20% solution instilled into the trachea by means of a syringe connected to a catheter.
*Diagnostic procedures.*
2–3 doses of 1–2 mL of 20% or 2–4 mL of 10% solution by nebulization or intratracheal instillation before the procedure.
*Acetaminophen overdose.*
**Given PO, initial:** 140 mg/kg; **then,** 70 mg/kg q 4 hr for a total of 17 doses.

### DENTAL CONCERNS

**General**
1. Monitor vital signs at every appointment because of cardiovascular and respiratory side effects.
2. Have the patient sit upright. Also, shorter appointments may be necessary.
**Consultation with Primary Care Provider**
1. Consultation with the patient's health care provider may be necessary in order to assess level of disease control.
**Client/Family Teaching**
1. Remind the patient to avoid any triggers that may stimulate broncho-

spasm (i.e., cigarette smoke, dust, chemicals, cold air).
2. Encourage the patient to attend smoking cessation classes and support groups to help stop smoking.

# Acetylsalicylic acid (ASA, Aspirin)
(ah-**SEE**-till-sal-ih-**SILL**-ick **AH**-sid)
**Pregnancy Category:** C
Apo-Asa ✦, Asaphen ✦, Aspergum, Aspirin, Aspirin Regimen Bayer 81 mg with Calcium, Bayer Children's Aspirin, Easprin, Ecotrin Caplets and Tablets, Ecotrin Maximum Strength Caplets and Tablets, Empirin, Entrophen ✦, Excedrin Geltabs, Genprin, Genuine Bayer Aspirin Caplets and Tablets, Halfprin, 8-Hour Bayer Timed-Release Caplets, Maximum Bayer Aspirin Caplets and Tablets, MSD Enteric Coated ASA ✦, Norwich Extra Strength, Novasen ✦, St. Joseph Adult Chewable Aspirin, Therapy Bayer Caplets, ZOR-prin **(OTC)** (Easprin and ZOR-prin are Rx)

# Acetylsalicylic acid, buffered
(ah-**SEE**-till-sal-ih-**SILL**-ick **AH**-sid)
**Pregnancy Category:** C
Alka-Seltzer with Aspirin, Alka-Seltzer with Aspirin (flavored), Alka-Seltzer Extra Strength with Aspirin, Arthritis Pain Formula, Ascriptin Regular Strength, Ascriptin A/D, Bayer Buffered, Buffered Aspirin, Bufferin, Buffex, Cama Arthritis Pain Reliever, Magnaprin, Magnaprin Arthritis Strength Captabs, Tri-Buffered Bufferin Caplets and Tablets **(OTC)**
**Classification:** Opioid analgesic, antipyretic, anti-inflammatory agent

**Action/Kinetics:** Aspirin manifests antipyretic, anti-inflammatory, and analgesic effects. The antipyretic effect is due to an action on the hypothalamus, resulting in heat loss by vasodilation of peripheral blood vessels and promoting sweating. The anti-inflammatory effects are probably mediated through inhibition of cyclo-oxygenase, which results in a decrease in prostaglandin synthesis and other mediators of the pain response. The mechanism of action for the analgesic effects of aspirin is not known fully but is partly attributable to improvement of the inflammatory condition. Aspirin also produces inhibition of platelet aggregation by decreasing the synthesis of endoperoxides and thromboxanes—substances that mediate platelet aggregation.

Large doses of aspirin (5 g/day or more) increase uric acid secretion, while low doses (2 g/day or less) decrease uric acid secretion. However, aspirin antagonizes drugs used to treat gout.

Rapidly absorbed after PO administration. Is hydrolyzed to the active salicylic acid, which is 70%–90% protein bound. For arthritis and rheumatic disease, blood levels of 150–300 mcg/mL should be maintained. For analgesic and antipyretic, achieve blood levels of 25–50 mcg/mL. For acute rheumatic fever, achieve blood levels of 150–300 mcg/mL. **Therapeutic salicylic acid serum levels:** 150–300 mcg/mL, although tinnitus occurs at serum levels above 200 mcg/mL and serious toxicity above 400 mcg/mL. t½: aspirin, 15–20 min; salicylic acid, 2–20 hr, depending on the dose. Salicylic acid and metabolites are excreted by the kidney. The bioavailability of enteric-coated salicylate products may be poor. The addition of antacids (buffered aspirin) may decrease GI irritation and increase the dissolution and absorption of such products.

Aspirin is found in many combination products including Darvon Compound, Empirin Compound Plain and with Codeine, Equagesic, Fiorinal Plain and with Codeine, Norgesic and Norgesic Forte, and Synalgos DC.

**Uses:** *Analgesic:* Pain arising from integumental structures, myalgias, neuralgias, arthralgias, headache, dysmenorrhea, and similar types of pain. Antipyretic. *Anti-Inflammatory:* Arthritis, osteoarthritis, SLE, acute rheumatic fever, gout, and many other conditions. Mucocutaneous lymph node syndrome (Kawasaki disease). Reduce the risk of recurrent transient ischemic attacks and strokes in men. Decrease risk of death from nonfatal MI in clients who have a history of infarction or who manifest unstable angina; aortocoronary bypass surgery. Gout. May be effective in less severe postoperative and postpartum pain; pain secondary to trauma and cancer. *Non-FDA Approved Uses:* Chronic use to prevent cataract formation; low doses to prevent toxemia of pregnancy; in pregnant women with inadequate uteroplacental blood flow. Reduce colon cancer mortality (low doses).

**Contraindications:** Hypersensitivity to salicylates. Clients with asthma, hay fever, or nasal polyps have a higher incidence of hypersensitivity reactions. Severe anemia, history of blood coagulation defects, in conjunction with anticoagulant therapy. Salicylates can cause congestive failure when taken in the large doses used for rheumatic diseases. Vitamin K deficiency; 1 week before and after surgery. In pregnancy, especially the last trimester as the drug may cause problems in the newborn child or complications during delivery. In children or teenagers with chickenpox or flu due to possibility of development of Reye's syndrome.

Controlled-release aspirin is not recommended for use as an antipyretic or short-term analgesic because adequate blood levels may not be reached. Also, controlled-release products are not recommended for children less than 12 years of age and in children with fever accompanied by dehydration.

**Special Concerns:** Use with caution during lactation. Use with caution in the presence of gastric or peptic ulcers, in mild diabetes, erosive gastritis, or bleeding tendencies, in cardiac disease, and in liver or kidney disease. Aspirin products now carry the following labeling: "It is especially important not to use aspirin during the last three months of pregnancy unless specifically directed to do so by a doctor because it may cause problems in the newborn child or complications during delivery."

**Side Effects:** The toxic effects of the salicylates are dose-related. *Oral:* Increased bleeding (chronic use). *GI:* Dyspepsia, heartburn, anorexia, nausea, occult blood loss, epigastric discomfort, *massive GI bleeding, potentiation of peptic ulcer*. *Allergic: Bronchospasm, asthma-like symptoms, anaphylaxis,* skin rashes, angioedema, urticaria, rhinitis, nasal polyps. *Hematologic:* Prolongation of bleeding time, thrombocytopenia, leukopenia, purpura, shortened erythrocyte survival time, decreased plasma iron levels. *Miscellaneous:* Thirst, fever, dimness of vision.

*NOTE:* Use of aspirin in children and teenagers with flu or chickenpox may result in the development of *Reye's syndrome*. Also, dehydrated, febrile children are more prone to salicylate intoxication.

**Drug Interactions**
*Acetazolamide* / ↑ CNS toxicity of salicylates; also, ↑ excretion of salicylic acid if urine kept alkaline
*Alcohol, ethyl* / ↑ Chance of GI bleeding caused by salicylates
*ACE inhibitors* / ↓ Effect of ACE inhibitors possibly due to prostaglandin inhibition
*Antacids* / ↓ Salicylate levels in plasma due to ↑ rate of renal excretion
*Anticoagulants, oral* / ↑ Effect of anticoagulant by ↓ plasma protein binding and plasma prothrombin
*Antirheumatics* / Both are ulcerogenic and may cause ↑ GI bleeding
*Ascorbic acid* / ↑ Effect of salicylates by ↑ renal tubular reabsorption
*Beta-adrenergic blocking agents* / Salicylates ↓ action of beta-blockers, possibly due to prostaglandin inhibition
*Corticosteroids* / Both are ulcerogenic; also, corticosteroids may ↓ blood salicylate levels by ↑ breakdown by liver and ↑ excretion

*Dipyridamole* / Additive anticoagulant effects
*Furosemide* / ↑ Chance of salicylate toxicity due to ↓ renal excretion; also, salicylates may ↓ effect of furosemide in clients with impaired renal function or cirrhosis with ascites
*Hypoglycemics, oral* / ↑ Hypoglycemia due to ↓ plasma protein binding and ↓ excretion
*Indomethacin* / Both are ulcerogenic and may cause ↑ GI bleeding
*Insulin* / Salicylates ↑ hypoglycemic effect of insulin
*Methotrexate* / ↑ Effect of methotrexate by ↓ plasma protein binding; also, salicylates block renal excretion of methotrexate
*Nitroglycerin* / Combination may result in unexpected hypotension
*Nizatidine* / ↑ Serum levels of salicylates
*NSAIDs* / Additive ulcerogenic effects; also, aspirin may ↓ serum levels of NSAIDs
*Phenylbutazone* / Combination may produce hyperuricemia
*Phenytoin* / ↑ Effect of phenytoin by ↓ plasma protein binding
*Probenecid* / Salicylates inhibit uricosuric activity of probenecid
*Sodium bicarbonate* / ↓ Effect of salicylates by ↑ rate of excretion
*Spironolactone* / Aspirin ↓ diuretic effect of spironolactone
*Sulfinpyrazone* / Salicylates inhibit uricosuric activity of sulfinpyrazone
*Sulfonamides* / ↑ Effect of sulfonamides by ↑ blood levels of salicylates
*Valproic acid* / ↑ Effect of valproic acid due to ↓ plasma protein binding

**How Supplied:** *Chew tablet:* 80 mg, 81 mg; *Enteric coated tablet:* 81 mg, 162 mg, 324 mg, 325 mg, 500 mg, 650 mg, 975 mg; *Gum:* 227 mg; *Suppository:* 60 mg, 120 mg, 125 mg, 200 mg, 300 mg, 325 mg, 600 mg, 650 mg; *Tablet:* 81 mg, 324 mg, 325 mg, 486 mg, 500 mg, 650 mg; *Tablet, Extended Release:* 650 mg, 800 mg

**Dosage**
• **Gum, Chewable Tablets, Coat-**

ed Tablets, Effervescent Tablets, Enteric-Coated Tablets, Suppositories, Tablets, Timed (Controlled) Release Tablets

*Analgesic, antipyretic.*

**Adults:** 325–500 mg q 3 hr, 325–600 mg q 4 hr, or 650–1,000 mg q 6 hr. As an alternative, the adult chewable tablet (81 mg each) may be used in doses of 4–8 tablets q 4 hr as needed. **Pediatric:** 65 mg/kg/day (alternate dose: 1.5 g/m²/day) in divided doses q 4–6 hr, not to exceed 3.6 g/day. Alternatively, the following dosage regimen can be used: **Pediatric, 2–3 years:** 162 mg q 4 hr as needed; **4–5 years:** 243 mg q 4 hr as needed; **6–8 years:** 320–325 mg q 4 hr as needed; **9–10 years:** 405 mg q 4 hr as needed; **11 years:** 486 mg q 4 hr as needed; **12–14 years:** 648 mg q 4 hr.

*Arthritis, rheumatic diseases.*

**Adults:** 3.2–6 g/day in divided doses.

*Juvenile rheumatoid arthritis.*

60–110 mg/kg/day (alternate dose: 3 g/m²) in divided doses q 6–8 hr. When initiating therapy at 60 mg/kg/day, dose may be increased by 20 mg/kg/day after 5–7 days and by 10 mg/kg/day after another 5–7 days.

*Acute rheumatic fever.*

**Adults, initial:** 5–8 g/day. **Pediatric, initial:** 100 mg/kg/day (3 g/m²/day) for 2 weeks; **then,** decrease to 75 mg/kg/day for 4–6 weeks.

*Transient ischemic attacks in men.*

**Adults:** 650 mg b.i.d. or 325 mg q.i.d. A dose of 300 mg/day may be as effective and with fewer side effects.

*Prophylaxis of MI.*

**Adults:** 300 or 325 mg/day (both solid PO dosage forms–regular and buffered as well as buffered aspirin in solution). The adult chewable tablets may also be used.

*Kawasaki disease.*

**Adults:** 80–180 mg/kg/day during the febrile period. After the fever re-

solves, the dose may be adjusted to 10 mg/kg/day.

*NOTE:* Doses as low as 80–100 mg/day are being studied for use in unstable angina, MI, and aortocoronary bypass surgery. Aspirin Regimen Bayer 81 mg with Calcium contains 250 mg calcium carbonate (10% of RDA) and 81 mg of acetylsalicylic acid for individuals who require aspirin to prevent recurrent heart attacks and strokes.

## DENTAL CONCERNS

### General

1. Take a complete drug history and note any evidence of hypersensitivity. Individuals allergic to tartrazine should not take aspirin. Clients who have tolerated salicylates well in the past may suddenly have an allergic or anaphylactoid reaction. Note the effectiveness of aspirin if used in the past for pain control.

2. Note if client has asthma, hay fever, ulcer disease, nasal polyps, or history of allergic reaction to NSAIDs. The patient may not be able to take aspirin.

3. Aspirin may interfere with blood-clotting mechanisms (antiplatelet effects) and is usually discontinued 1 week before surgery (including oral) to prevent increased risk of bleeding.

4. Chewable aspirin dose forms should not be used for 7 days following oral surgery because of the possibility of soft tissue damage.

5. Buffered-aspirin dosage forms contain sodium and should be avoided in patients with hypertension or on a sodium-restricted diet.

6. Patients on chronic drug therapy may develop blood dyscrasias. Symptoms include fever, sore throat, bleeding, and poor wound healing.

### Consultation with Primary Care Provider

1. Patients with symptoms of blood dyscrasias should be referred to their primary care provider for complete blood counts. Treatment

---

should be postponed until the results are known.

2. Aspirin can increase the risk of bleeding and should not be prescribed prior to dental surgery. Patients on long-term aspirin therapy should be referred to their health care provider to discuss a temporary discontinuation of aspirin therapy prior to oral surgery.

3. Patients presenting with tinnitus, ringing, or roaring in the ears should be referred to their health care provider for evaluation. The patient may have salicylism (aspirin toxicity).

**Client/Family Teaching**

1. Take only as directed. To reduce gastric irritation, administer with meals, milk, a full glass of water, or crackers.

2. Do not take salicylates if product is off-color or has a strange odor. Note expiration date.

3. Report any toxic effects: ringing in the ears, difficulty hearing, dizziness or fainting spells, unusual increase in sweating, severe abdominal pain, or mental confusion.

4. Do not take with alcohol because of the potential for GI bleeding.

5. Tell the dentist and other HCPs you are taking salicylates and why.

6. Before purchasing other OTC preparations, notify provider and note the quantity used per day.

7. Sodium bicarbonate may decrease the serum level of aspirin, reducing its effectiveness.

---

# Acyclovir
# (Acycloguanosine)
(ay-**SYE**-kloh-veer, ay-**SYE**-kloh-**GWON**-oh-seen)
**Pregnancy Category:** C
Avirax ✿, Nu-Acyclovir ✿, Zovirax **(Rx)**
**Classification:** Antiviral anti-infective

See also *Antiviral Drugs.*

**Action/Kinetics:** Acyclovir is a synthetic acyclic purine nucleoside analog. It is converted by HSV-infected cells to acyclovir triphosphate, which interferes with HSV DNA polymerase, thereby inhibiting DNA replication. Systemic absorption is slow from the GI tract (although therapeutic levels are reached) and following topical administration. It is preferentially taken up and converted to the active triphosphate form by herpes virus–infected cells. Food does not affect absorption. **Peak levels after PO:** 1.5–2 hr. Widely distributed in tissues and body fluids. The half-life and total body clearance depend on renal function. **t½, PO, creatinine clearance, greater than 80 mL/min/1.73 m²:** 2.5 hr. Metabolites and unchanged drug (up to 85%) are excreted through the kidney. Reduce dosage in clients with impaired renal function. Clients who take acyclovir (600–800 mg/day) with AZT had a significantly prolonged survival rate compared with clients taking only acyclovir.

**Uses: PO.** Initial and recurrent genital herpes in immunocompromised and nonimmunocompromised clients. Prophylaxis of frequently recurrent genital herpes infections in nonimmunocompromised clients. Treatment of chickenpox in children ranging from 2 to 18 years of age. Acute treatment of herpes zoster (shingles).

**Parenteral.** Initial therapy for severe genital herpes in clients who are not immunocompromised; initial and recurrent mucosal and cutaneous HSV-1 and HSV-2 infections in immunocompromised individuals. Varicella zoster infections (shingles) in immunocompromised clients. HSE in clients over 6 months of age.

**Topical.** Acyclovir decreases healing time and duration of viral shedding in initial herpes genitalis. Limited non-life-threatening mucocutaneous HSV infections in immunocompromised clients. No beneficial effect in recurrent herpes genitalis or in herpes labialis in nonimmunocompromised clients.

*Non-FDA Approved Uses:* Cytomegalovirus and HSV infection following bone marrow or renal transplantation; herpes simplex ocular infections; herpes simplex proctitis; herpes simplex labialis; herpes simplex whitlow; herpes zoster encephalitis;

disseminated primary eczema herpeticum; herpes simplex–associated erythema multiforme; infectious mononucleosis; and varicella pneumonia.

**Contraindications:** Hypersensitivity to formulation. Use in the eye. Use to prevent recurrent HSV infections.

**Special Concerns:** Use with caution during lactation or with concomitant intrathecal methotrexate or interferon. Safety and efficacy of PO form not established in children less than 2 years of age. Prolonged or repeated doses in immunocompromised clients may result in emergence of resistant viruses. Use of oral acyclovir does not eliminate latent HSV and is not a cure.

**Side Effects: PO.** *Short-term treatment of herpes simplex. Oral:* Glossitis, taste of drug. *GI:* N&V, diarrhea, anorexia, sore throat. *CNS:* Headache, dizziness, fatigue. *Miscellaneous:* Edema, skin rashes, leg pain, inguinal adenopathy.

*Long-term treatment of herpes simplex. GI:* Nausea, diarrhea. *CNS:* Headache. *Other:* Skin rash, asthenia, paresthesia.

*Treatment of herpes zoster. GI:* N&V, diarrhea, constipation. *CNS:* Headache, malaise.

*Treatment of chickenpox. GI:* Vomiting, diarrhea, abdominal pain, flatulence. *Dermatologic:* Rash.

**Parenteral (frequency greater than 1%).** *At injection site:* Phlebitis, inflammation. *GI:* N&V. *CNS:* Encephalopathic changes, including lethargy, obtundation, tremors, agitation, confusion, hallucination, ***seizures, coma***, jitters, headache. *Miscellaneous:* Skin rashes, urticaria, itching, transient elevation of serum creatinine or BUN (most often following rapid IV infusion), elevation of transaminases.

**Topical.** Transient burning, stinging (oral application), pain. Pruritus, rash, vulvitis, local edema. *NOTE:* All of these effects have also been re-

ported with the use of a placebo preparation.

**Drug Interactions**
*Probenecid* / ↑ Bioavailability and half-life of acyclovir → ↑ effect
*Zidovudine* / Severe lethargy and drowsiness

**How Supplied:** *Capsule:* 200 mg; *Ointment:* 5%; *Powder for injection:* 500 mg, 1000 mg; *Suspension:* 200 mg/5 mL; *Tablet:* 400 mg, 800 mg

## Dosage

- **Capsules, Suspension, Tablets**
  *Initial genital herpes.*
  200 mg q 4 hr, 5 times/day for 10 days.
  *Chronic genital herpes.*
  400 mg b.i.d., 200 mg t.i.d., or 200 mg 5 times/day for up to 12 months.
  *Intermittent therapy for genital herpes.*
  200 mg q 4 hr, 5 times/day for 5 days. Start therapy at the first symptom/sign of recurrence.
  *Herpes zoster, acute treatment.*
  800 mg q 4 hr, 5 times/day for 7–10 days.
  *Chickenpox.*
  20 mg/kg (of the suspension) q.i.d. for 5 days. A single dose should not exceed 800 mg. Begin therapy at the earliest sign/symptom.
- **IV Infusion**
  *Mucosal and cutaneous herpes simplex in immunocompromised clients.*
  **Adults:** 5 mg/kg infused at a constant rate over 1 hr, q 8 hr (15 mg/kg/day) for 7 days. **Children less than 12 years of age:** 250 mg/m² infused at a constant rate over 1 hr, q 8 hr for 7 days.
  *Varicella-zoster infections (shingles) in immunocompromised clients.*
  **Adults:** 10 mg/kg infused at a constant rate over 1 hr, q 8 hr for 7 days (not to exceed 500 mg/m² q 8 hr). **Children less than 12 years of age:** 500 mg/m² infused at a constant rate over at least 1 hr, q 8 hr for 7 days.
  *Herpes simplex encephalitis.*

---

**Adults:** 10 mg/kg infused at a constant rate over at least 1 hr, q 8 hr for 10 days. **Children less than 12 years of age and greater than 6 months of age:** 500 mg/m² infused at a constant rate over at least 1 hr, q 8 hr for 10 days.

• **Topical (5% Ointment)**
**Adults and children:** Lesion should be covered with sufficient amount of ointment (0.5-in. ribbon/4 in.² of surface area) q 3 hr, 6 times/day for 7 days. Initiate treatment as soon as possible after onset of symptoms.

## DENTAL CONCERNS

See also *General Dental Concerns for All Anti-Infectives* and *Antiviral Drugs.*
**General**
1. Oral Lesions: Delay dental treatment when active oral herpetic lesions are present.
2. Patients on chronic drug therapy may develop blood dyscrasias. Symptoms include fever, sore throat, and bleeding, and poor wound healing.
**Consultation with Primary Care Provider**
1. Patients with symptoms of blood dyscrasias should be referred to their primary care provider for complete blood counts. Treatment should be postponed until the results are known.
**Client/Family Teaching**
1. Apply acyclovir ointment in the amount directed with a finger cot or rubber glove to prevent transmission of infection to other body sites.
2. Adequately cover all lesions with topical acyclovir as ordered, but do not exceed dosage or the frequency of application or the length of time for treatment.
3. Report any burning, stinging, itching, and rash if evident when applying acyclovir.
4. Dispose of toothbrush and other oral hygiene devices used during the time of active infection in order to prevent reinfection with the herpes virus.
5. Avoid mouth rinses with alcohol because of their drying effects.

# Albuterol (Salbutamol)
(al-**BYOU**-ter-ohl)
**Pregnancy Category:** C
Alti-Salbutamol Sulfate ✦, Asmavent ✦, Gen-Salbutamol Sterinebs P.F. ✦, Novo-Salmol Inhaler ✦, PMS-Salbutamol Respirator Solution ✦, Proventil, Proventil HFA—3M, Proventil Repetabs, Rho-Salbutamol ✦, Sabulin ✦, Salbutamol Nebuamp ✦, Ventodisk Disk/Diskhaler ✦, Ventolin, Ventolin Rotacaps, Volmax **(Rx)**
**Classification:** Direct-acting adrenergic (sympathomimetic) agent

See also *Sympathomimetic Drugs.*
**Action/Kinetics:** Albuterol stimulates beta-2 receptors of the bronchi, leading to bronchodilation. Has minimal beta-1 activity. Albuterol sulfate is now available as an inhaler that contains no chlorofluorocarbons (Proventil HFA–3M). **Onset, PO:** 15–30 min; **inhalation,** 5–15 min. **Peak effect, PO:** 2–3 hr; **inhalation,** 60–90 min (after 2 inhalations). **Duration, PO:** 8 hr (up to 12 hr for extended-release); **inhalation,** 3–6 hr. Metabolites and unchanged drug excreted in urine and feces. Tablets not to be used in children less than 12 years of age.
**Uses:** Bronchial asthma; bronchospasm due to bronchitis or emphysema; bronchitis; reversible obstructive pulmonary disease in those 4 years of age and older; exercise-induced bronchospasm. Prophylaxis of bronchial asthma or bronchospasms. Parenteral for treatment of status asthmaticus. *Non-FDA Approved Uses:* Nebulized albuterol may be useful as an adjunct to treat serious acute hyperkalemia in hemodialysis clients.
**Contraindications:** Aerosol for prevention of exercise-induced bronchospasm is not recommended for children less than 12 years of age. Use during lactation.
**Special Concerns:** Dosage has not been established for the syrup in children less than 2 years of age, for tablets in children less than 6 years of age, and for extended-release tablets in children less than 12 years of age. Albuterol may delay preterm labor.

**Additional Side Effects:** *Oral:* Dry mouth, teeth discoloration, oropharyngeal edema. *GI:* Diarrhea, increased appetite, epigastric pain. *CNS:* CNS stimulation, malaise, emotional lability, fatigue, lightheadedness, nightmares, disturbed sleep, aggressive behavior, irritability. *Respiratory:* Bronchitis, epistaxis, hoarseness (especially in children), nasal congestion, increase in sputum. *Hypersensitivity (may be immediate):* Urticaria, **angioedema,** rash, **bronchospasm.** *Miscellaneous:* Muscle cramps, pallor, conjunctivitis, dilated pupils, difficulty in urination, muscle spasm, voice changes.

**How Supplied:** *Metered dose inhaler:* 0.09 mg/inh; *Capsule:* 200 mcg; *Solution:* 0.083%, 0.5%; *Syrup:* 2 mg/5 mL; *Tablet:* 2 mg, 4 mg; *Tablet, Extended Release:* 4 mg, 8 mg

**Dosage** ——————————————
- **Metered Dose Inhaler**
  *Bronchodilation.*

**Adults and children over 12 years of age:** 180 mcg (2 inhalations) q 4–6 hr (Ventolin aerosol may be used in children over 4 years of age). In some clients 1 inhalation (90 mcg) q 4 hr may be sufficient.

*Prophylaxis of exercise-induced bronchospasm.*

**Adults and children over 12 years of age:** 180 mcg (2 inhalations) 15 min before exercise.
- **Solution for Inhalation**
  *Bronchodilation.*

**Adults and children over 12 years of age:** 2.5 mg t.i.d.–q.i.d. by nebulization (dilute 0.5 mL of the 0.5% solution with 2.5 mL sterile NSS and deliver over 5–15 min).
- **Capsule for Inhalation**
  *Bronchodilation.*

**Adults and children over 4 years of age:** 200 mcg q 4–6 hr using a Rotahaler inhalation device. In some clients, 400 mcg q 4–6 hr may be required.

*Prophylaxis of exercise-induced bronchospasm.*

**Adults and children over 12 years:** 200 mcg 15 min before exercise using a Rotahaler inhalation device.
- **Syrup**
  *Bronchodilation.*

**Adults and children over 14 years of age:** 2–4 mg t.i.d.–q.i.d., up to a maximum of 8 mg q.i.d. **Children, 6–14 years, initial:** 2 mg (base) t.i.d.–q.i.d.; **then,** increase as necessary to a maximum of 24 mg/day in divided doses. **Children, 2–6 years, initial:** 0.1 mg/kg t.i.d.; **then,** increase as necessary up to 0.2 mg/kg, not to exceed 4 mg t.i.d.
- **Tablets**
  *Bronchodilation.*

**Adults and children over 12 years of age, initial:** 2–4 mg (of the base) t.i.d.–q.i.d.; **then,** increase dose as needed up to a maximum of 8 mg t.i.d.–q.i.d. In geriatric clients or those sensitive to beta agonists, start with 2 mg t.i.d.–q.i.d. and then increase dose gradually, if needed, to a maximum of 8 mg t.i.d.–q.i.d. **Children, 6–12 years of age, usual, initial:** 2 mg t.i.d.–q.i.d.; **then,** if necessary, increase the dose in a stepwise fashion to a maximum of 24 mg/day in divided doses.
- **Extended-Release Tablets**
  *Bronchodilation.*

**Adults and children over 12 years of age:** 4 or 8 mg (of the base) q 12 hr up to a maximum of 32 mg/day. Clients on regular-release albuterol can be switched to the Repetabs in that a 4-mg extended-release tablet q 12 hr is equivalent to a regular 2-mg tablet q 6 hr.

## DENTAL CONCERNS

See also *Dental Concerns* for *Sympathomimetic Drugs.*

# Aldesleukin (Interleukin-2; IL-2)

(al-des-**LOO**-kin)

**Pregnancy Category:** C

**A**

Proleukin **(Rx)**
Classification: Antineoplastic, miscellaneous

See also *Antineoplastic Agents.*

**Action/Kinetics:** Aldesleukin, produced by recombinant DNA technology, is a human interleukin-2 (IL-2) product. Drug effects include activation of cellular immunity with profound lymphocytosis, eosinophilia, and thrombocytopenia; the production of cytokines, including tumor necrosis factor, IL-1, and gamma-interferon; and inhibition of tumor growth. The exact mechanism of action of aldesleukin is not known. The drug reaches high plasma levels after a short IV infusion, and it is rapidly distributed to the extravascular, extracellular space. It is rapidly cleared from the circulation by both glomerular filtration and peritubular extraction; metabolized in the kidneys with little or no active form excreted through the urine. **t½, distribution:** 13 min; **t½, elimination:** 85 min.

**Uses:** Metastatic renal cell carcinoma in adults 18 years of age and older. *Non-FDA Approved Uses:* Kaposi's sarcoma in combination with AZT, metastatic melanoma in combination with low-dose cyclophosphamide, colorectal cancer and non-Hodgkin's lymphoma often in combination with lymphokine-activated killer cells.

**Contraindications:** Hypersensitivity to IL-2 or any components of the product. Abnormal thallium stress test or pulmonary function tests. Organ allografts. Use in either men or women not practicing effective contraception. Lactation.

Retreatment is contraindicated in those who have experienced the following during a previous course of therapy: sustained ventricular tachycardia; uncontrolled or unresponsive cardiac rhythm disturbances; recurrent chest pain with ECG changes that are consistent with angina or MI; intubation required for more than 72 hr; pericardial tamponade; renal dysfunction requiring dialysis for more than 72 hr; coma or toxic psychosis lasting more than 48 hr; seizures that are repetitive or difficult to control; ischemia or perforation of the bowel; and GI bleeding requiring surgery.

**Special Concerns:** Aldesleukin may worsen symptoms in clients with unrecognized or untreated CNS metastases. Use of medications known to be nephrotoxic or hepatotoxic may further increase toxicity to the kidney and liver caused by aldesleukin. May increase the risk of allograft rejection in transplant clients. Safety and efficacy have not been established in children less than 18 years of age.

**Side Effects:** Side effects are frequent, often serious, and sometimes fatal. Most clients will experience fever, chills, rigors, pruritus, and GI side effects. The frequency and severity of side effects are usually dose-related and schedule-dependent. Incidence of side effects is greater in PS 1 clients than in PS 0 clients. The side effects listed have an incidence of 1% or greater.

*Capillary leak syndrome (CLS):* Results from extravasation of plasma proteins and fluid into the extracellular space with loss of vascular tone. This results in a drop in mean arterial BP within 2–12 hr after the start of treatment and reduced organ perfusion that may be severe and result in death. CLS causes hypotension, hypoperfusion, and extravasation that leads to edema and effusion. *CLS may be associated with supraventricular and ventricular arrhythmias, MI,* angina, respiratory insufficiency requiring intubation, GI bleeding or infarction, renal insufficiency, and changes in mental status.

*CV:* Hypotension (sometimes requiring vasopressor therapy), sinus tachycardia, *arrhythmias (atrial, junctional, supraventricular, ventricular),* bradycardia, PVCs, premature atrial contractions, myocardial ischemia, *MI, cardiac arrest, CHF,* myocarditis, endocarditis, gangrene, *stroke, pericardial effusion, thrombo-*

**sis.** *Respiratory:* Pulmonary congestion, dyspnea, pulmonary edema, **respiratory failure,** tachypnea, pleural effusion, wheezing, apnea, pneumothorax, hemoptysis. *Oral:* Stomatitis, glossitis. *GI:* N&V, diarrhea, anorexia, **GI bleeding** (sometimes requiring surgery), dyspepsia, constipation, **intestinal perforation,** intestinal ileus, pancreatitis. *CNS:* Changes in mental status (may be an early indication of bacteremia or early bacterial sepsis), dizziness, sensory dysfunction, disorders of special senses (speech, taste, vision), syncope, motor dysfunction, **coma, seizure.** *GU:* Oliguria or anuria, proteinuria, hematuria, dysuria, impaired renal function requiring dialysis, urinary retention, urinary frequency. *Hepatic:* Jaundice, ascites, hepatomegaly. *Hematologic:* Anemia, thrombocytopenia, leukopenia, coagulation disorders, leukocytosis, eosinophilia. *Dermatologic:* Pruritus, erythema, rash, dry skin, exfoliative dermatitis, purpura, petechiae, urticaria, alopecia. *Musculoskeletal:* Arthralgia, myalgia, arthritis, muscle spasm. *Electrolyte and other disturbances:* Hypomagnesemia, acidosis, hypocalcemia, hypophosphatemia, hypokalemia, hyperuricemia, hypoalbuminemia, hypoproteinemia, hyponatremia, hyperkalemia, alkalosis, hypoglycemia, hyperglycemia, hypocholesterolemia, hypercalcemia, hypernatremia, hyperphosphatemia. *Miscellaneous:* Fever, chills, pain (abdominal, chest, back), fatigue, malaise, weakness, edema, infection (including the injection site, urinary tract, catheter tip, phlebitis, sepsis), weight gain or weight loss, headache, conjunctivitis, reactions at the injection site, allergic reactions, hypothyroidism.

**Drug Interactions**

*Aminoglycosides* / ↑ Risk of kidney toxicity

*Antihypertensives* / Potentiate hypotension seen with aldesleukin

*Cardiotoxic agents* / ↑ Risk of cardiac toxicity

*Corticosteroids* / Concomitant use may ↓ the antitumor effectiveness of aldesleukin (although the corticosteroids ↓ side effects of aldesleukin)

*Indomethacin* / ↑ Risk of kidney toxicity

*Methotrexate* / ↑ Risk of hepatic toxicity

**How Supplied:** *Powder for injection:* 22 million IU

## Dosage

- **Intermittent IV Infusion**

*Metastatic renal cell carcinoma in adults.*

Each course of treatment consists of two 5-day treatment cycles separated by a rest period. **Adults:** 600,000 IU/kg (0.037 mg/kg) given q 8 hr by a 15-min IV infusion for a total of 14 doses. Following 9 days of rest, repeat schedule for another 14 doses, for a maximum of 28 doses per course. *NOTE:* Due to toxicity, clients may not be able to receive all 28 doses (median number of doses given is 20).

*Retreatment for metastatic renal cell carcinoma.*

Evaluate for a response about 4 weeks after completion of a course of therapy and again just prior to the start of the next treatment course. Give additional courses only if there is evidence of some tumor shrinkage following the last course and retreatment is not contraindicated (see preceding *Contraindications*). Separate each treatment course by at least 7 weeks from the date of hospital discharge.

## DENTAL CONCERNS

See also *Dental Concerns* for *Antineoplastic Agents.*

# Alendronate sodium

(ay-**LEN**-droh-nayt)
**Pregnancy Category:** C
Fosamax **(Rx)**
**Classification:** Bone growth regulator (biphosphonate)

---

**A**

**Action/Kinetics:** Alendronate inhibits osteoclast activity, thereby preventing bone resorption. It appears to reduce fracture risk and reverse the progression of osteoporosis. Alendronate does not inhibit bone mineralization. It is well absorbed orally and is initially distributed to soft tissues, but then quickly redistributed to bone. The drug is not metabolized and is excreted through the urine. However, the $t\frac{1}{2}$, **terminal** is believed to be more than 10 years, due to slow release from the skeleton.

**Uses:** Prevention and treatment of osteoporosis in postmenopausal women (concomitant estrogen therapy is not recommended due to lack of experience). Prevention of fractures in postmenopausal women with osteoporosis. Paget's disease of bone.

**Contraindications:** In hypocalcemia. Those with severe renal insufficiency (creatinine clearance less than 35 mL/min). Lactation.

**Special Concerns:** Use with caution in those with upper GI problems, such as dysphagia, symptomatic esophageal diseases, gastritis, duodenitis, or ulcers. Safety and effectiveness have not been determined in children or for use in male osteoporosis.

**Side Effects:** *Oral:* Taster perversion. *GI:* Abdominal pain, nausea, dyspepsia, constipation, diarrhea, flatulence, acid regurgitation, esophageal ulcer, vomiting, dysphagia, abdominal distention, gastritis. *Miscellaneous:* Musculoskeletal pain, headache, rash and erythema (rare).

**Drug Interactions**

*Antacids* / ↓ Absorption of alendronate

*Aspirin* / ↑ Risk of upper GI events

*Calcium supplements* / ↓ Absorption of alendronate

*NSAIDs* / ↑ Risk of upper GI events

*Ranitidine* / ↑ Bioavailability of alendronate (significance not known)

**How Supplied:** *Tablet:* 10 mg, 40 mg

**Dosage** —————————
• **Tablets**

*Prevention of osteoporosis in postmenopausal women.*

5 mg once a day in the morning ½ hr before the first food, beverage, or medication of the day with 6–8 oz of plain water.

*Treatment of osteoporosis or prevention of fractures in postmenopausal women with osteoporosis.*

10 mg once a day in the morning ½ hr before the first food, beverage, or medication of the day with 6–8 oz of plain water. Safety of treatment for more than 4 years has not been determined.

*Paget's disease of bone.*

40 mg once a day for 6 months taken as for osteoporosis.

## DENTAL CONCERNS

**General**

1. Consider the oral sings of Paget's disease (i.e., macrognathia, alveolar pain).

2. Consider placing the patient in a semisupine position when in the dental chair to help alleviate the pain associated with osteoporosis and possible GI side effects of the drug.

3. Shorter appointments may be necessary in order to ensure patient comfort.

**Consultation with Primary Care Provider**

1. Consultation may be required in order to assess level of disease control and the patient's ability to tolerate stress.

# Alprazolam

(al-**PRAYZ**-oh-lam)

**Pregnancy Category:** D

Alti-Alprazolam ✺, Apo-Alpraz ✺, Gen-Alprazolam ✺, Novo-Alprazol ✺, Nu-Alpraz ✺, Xanax, Xanax TS ✺ **(C-IV) (Rx)**

**Classification:** Antianxiety agent

See also *Sedative Hypnotics (Antianxiety)/Antimanic Drugs.*

**Action/Kinetics: Peak plasma levels: PO,** 8–37 ng/mL after 1–2 hr. $t\frac{1}{2}$: 12–15 hr. 80% plasma protein bound. Metabolized to alpha-hydroxyalprazolam, an active metabolite. **t½:** 12–15 hr. Excreted in urine.

**Uses:** Anxiety. Anxiety associated with depression with or without agoraphobia. *Non-FDA Approved Uses:* Agoraphobia with social phobia, depression, PMS.

**Contraindications:** Use with itraconazole or ketoconazole.

**How Supplied:** *Concentrate:* 1 mg/mL; *Solution:* 0.5 mg/5 mL; *Tablet:* 0.25 mg, 0.5 mg, 1 mg, 2 mg

**Dosage** ————————————

• **Tablets, Concentrate, Solution**
*Anxiety disorder.*
**Adults, initial:** 0.25–0.5 mg t.i.d.; **then,** titrate to needs of client, with total daily dosage not to exceed 4 mg. **In elderly or debilitated: initial;** 0.25 mg b.i.d.–t.i.d.; **then,** adjust dosage to needs of client.
*Antipanic agent.*
**Adults:** 0.5 mg t.i.d.; increase dose as needed up to a maximum of 10 mg/day.
*Agoraphobia with social phobia.*
**Adults:** 2–8 mg/day.
*PMS.*
0.25 mg t.i.d.

**DENTAL CONCERNS**

See also *Dental Concerns* for *Sedative Hypnotics (Antianxiety)/Antimanic Drugs.*

# Amantadine hydrochloride

(ah-**MAN**-tah-deen)
**Pregnancy Category:** C
Endantadine ✿, Gen-Amantadine ✿, PMS-Amantadine ✿, Symadine, Symmetrel **(Rx)**
**Classification:** Antiviral and antiparkinson agent

See also *Antiviral Drugs.*
**Action/Kinetics:** Amantadine is believed to prevent penetration of the virus into cells, possibly by inhibiting uncoating of the RNA virus. The reaction appears to be virus specific for influenza A but not host specific. It may also prevent the release of infectious viral nucleic acid into the host cell. The drug reduces symptoms of viral infections if given within 24–48 hr after onset of illness. For the treatment of parkinsonism, amantadine may increase the release of dopamine from dopaminergic nerve terminals in the substantia nigra of parkinson clients, resulting in an increase in dopamine levels in dopaminergic synapses. The drug decreases extrapyramidal symptoms, including akinesia, rigidity, tremors, excessive salivation, gait disturbances, and total functional disability. Well absorbed from GI tract. **Onset:** 48 hr. **Peak serum concentration:** 0.2 mcg/mL after 1–4 hr. **t½:** Approximately 15 hr; elimination half-life increases two- to threefold when creatinine clearance is less than 40 mL/min/1.73 m². Ninety percent excreted unchanged in urine.

**Uses:** Influenza A viral infections of the respiratory tract (prophylaxis and treatment of high-risk clients with immunodeficiency, CV, metabolic, neuromuscular, or pulmonary disease). Symptomatic treatment of idiopathic parkinsonism and parkinsonism syndrome resulting from encephalitis, carbon monoxide intoxication, drugs, or cerebral arteriosclerosis. Favorable results have been obtained in about 50% of the clients. Improvements can last for up to 30 months, although some clients report that the effect of the drug wears off in 1–3 months. A rest period or an increased dosage may reestablish effectiveness. For parkinsonism, amantadine hydrochloride is usually used concomitantly with other agents, such as levodopa and anticholinergic agents.

Amantadine is recommended for prophylaxis in the following situations:

• Short-term prophylaxis during the course of a presumed outbreak of influenza A

• Adjunct to late immunization in high-risk clients

**A**

- To reduce disruption of medical care and to decrease spread of virus in high-risk clients when influenza A virus outbreaks occur
- To supplement vaccination protection in clients with impaired immune responses
- As chemoprophylaxis during flu season for those high-risk clients for whom influenza vaccine is contraindicated due to anaphylactic response to egg protein or prior severe reactions associated with flu vaccination

**Contraindications:** Hypersensitivity to drug.

**Special Concerns:** Use with caution in clients with liver and renal disease, history of epilepsy, CHF, peripheral edema, orthostatic hypotension, recurrent eczematoid dermatitis, or severe psychosis, in clients taking CNS stimulant drugs, to those exposed to rubella, and to nursing mothers. Safe use in lactating mothers and in children less than 1 year has not been established.

**Side Effects:** *GI:* N&V, constipation, anorexia, xerostomia. *CNS:* Depression, psychosis, *convulsions,* hallucinations, lightheadedness, confusion, ataxia, irritability, anxiety, headache, dizziness, fatigue, insomnia. *CV: CHF,* orthostatic hypotension, peripheral edema. *Miscellaneous:* Urinary retention, leukopenia, neutropenia, mottling of skin of the extremities due to poor peripheral circulation (livedo reticularis), skin rashes, visual problems, slurred speech, oculogyric episodes, dyspnea, weakness, eczematoid dermatitis.

**Drug Interactions**
*Anticholinergics* / Additive anticholinergic effects (including hallucinations, confusion), especially with trihexyphenidyl and benztropine
*CNS stimulants* / May ↑ CNS and psychic effects of amantadine; use cautiously together

**How Supplied:** *Capsule:* 100 mg; *Syrup:* 50 mg/5 mL

**Dosage** ——————
- **Capsules, Syrup**

*Antiviral.*
**Adults:** 200 mg/day as a single or divided dose. **Children, 1–9 years:** 4.4–8.8 mg/kg/day up to a maximum of 150 mg/day in one or two divided doses (use syrup); **9–12 years:** 100 mg b.i.d.
*Prophylactic treatment.*
Institute before or immediately after exposure and continue for 10–21 days if used concurrently with vaccine or for 90 days without vaccine.
*Symptomatic management.*
Initiate as soon as possible and continue for 24–48 hr after disappearance of symptoms. Decrease dose in renal impairment (see package insert). Reduce dose to 100 mg/day for persons with active seizure disorders due to the increased risk of seizure frequency using daily doses of 200 mg.
*Parkinsonism.*
**Use as sole agent, usual:** 100 mg b.i.d., up to 400 mg/day in divided doses, if necesssary. **Use with other antiparkinson drugs:** 100 mg 1–2 times/day.
*Drug-induced extrapyramidal symptoms.*
100 mg b.i.d. (up to 300 mg/day may be required in some). Reduce dose in impaired renal function.

## DENTAL CONCERNS

See also *General Dental Concerns for All Anti-Infectives* and *Antiviral Drugs.*
**Client/Family Teaching**
1. Avoid alcohol-containing mouth rinses.
2. Instruct the patient to use an electric toothbrush if he or she has difficulty holding a conventional one.

# Amitriptyline hydrochloride
(ah-me-**TRIP**-tih-leen)
**Pregnancy Category:** C
Apo-Amitriptyline ✽, Elavil, Levate ✽ **(Rx)**, Novo-Tryptin ✽
**Classification:** Antidepressant, tricyclic

See also *Antidepressants, Tricyclic.*

**Action/Kinetics:** Amitriptyline is metabolized to an active metabolite, nortriptyline. Has significant anticholinergic and sedative effects with moderate orthostatic hypotension. Very high ability to block serotonin uptake and moderate activity with respect to norepinephrine uptake. **Effective plasma levels of amitriptyline and nortriptyline:** Approximately 110–250 ng/mL. **Time to reach steady state:** 4–10 days. **t½:** 31–46 hr. Up to 1 month may be required for beneficial effects to be manifested. Amitriptyline is also found in Limbritrol and Triavil.

**Uses:** Relief of symptoms of depression, including depression accompanied by anxiety and insomnia. Chronic pain due to cancer or other pain syndromes. Prophylaxis of cluster and migraine headaches. *Non-FDA Approved Uses:* Pathologic laughing and crying secondary to forebrain disease, bulimia nervosa, antiulcer agent, enuresis.

**Contraindications:** Use in children less than 12 years of age.

**How Supplied:** *Injection:* 10 mg/mL; *Tablet:* 10 mg, 25 mg, 50 mg, 75 mg, 100 mg, 150 mg

**Dosage** ————————
• **Tablets**
*Antidepressant.*
**Adults (outpatients):** 75 mg/day in divided doses; may be increased to 150 mg/day. *Alternate dosage:* **Initial,** 50–100 mg at bedtime; **then,** increase by 25–50 mg, if necessary, up to 150 mg/day. **Hospitalized clients: initial,** 100 mg/day; may be increased to 200–300 mg/day. **Maintenance: usual,** 40–100 mg/day (may be given as a single dose at bedtime). **Adolescent and geriatric:** 10 mg t.i.d. and 20 mg at bedtime up to a maximum of 100 mg/day. **Pediatric, 6–12 years:** 10–30 mg (1–5 mg/kg) daily in two divided doses.
*Chronic pain.*
50–100 mg/day.
*Enuresis.*

**Pediatric, over 6 years:** 10 mg/day as a single dose at bedtime; dose may be increased up to a maximum of 25 mg. **Less than 6 years:** 10 mg/day as a single dose at bedtime.
• **IM Only**
*Antidepressant.*
**Adults:** 20–30 mg q.i.d.; switch to **PO** therapy as soon as possible.

## DENTAL CONCERNS

See also *Dental Concerns* for *Antidepressants, Tricyclic.*

# Amlexanox
(am-**LEX**-an-ox)
**Pregnancy Category:** B
Aphthasol **(Rx)**
**Classification:** Aphthous ulcer product.

**Action/Kinetics:** Mechanism not known. May be absorbed through GI tract.
**Uses:** Treat aphthous ulcers in those with normal immune systems.
**Contraindications:** Hypersensitivity
**Special Concerns:** Use caution during lactation. Safety and efficacy in children have not been determined.
**Side Effects:** *Oral:* Transient pain, burning, or stinging at application site, contact mucositis. *GI:* Nausea, diarrhea.

**Dosage** ————————
• **Paste**
*Aphthous ulcers.*
Squeeze about 0.25 inch of paste onto fingertip and, with gentle pressure, dab onto each mouth ulcer. Apply following oral hygiene after breakfast, lunch, dinner, and at bedtime. Start as soon as possible after symptoms of aphthous ulcer noted and continue until ulcer heals.

## DENTAL CONCERNS
**General**
1. Recurrent aphthous stomatits may be indicative of a systemic infection. Patients should be evualated for

systemic conditions if the stomatitis has not healed within 10 days.

**Client/Family Teaching**

1. Apply paste as soon as ulcers appear; rinse mouth thoroughly and use after each meal and at bedtime.

2. Place a small amount of paste on fingertip and gently dab onto each oral ulcer.

3. Wash hands after applying; avoid contact with eyes and wash promptly if eye contact occurs.

4. Continue to apply paste until healing takes place. Report if pain or ulcers persist after 10 days.

---

# Amlodipine

(am-**LOH**-dih-peen)

**Pregnancy Category:** C

Norvasc **(Rx)**

**Classification:** Antihypertensive, antianginal (calcium channel blocking agent)

See also *Calcium Channel Blocking Agents.*

**Action/Kinetics:** Amlodipine decreases myocardial contractility although this effect may be counteracted by reflex activity. CO is increased and there is a pronounced decrease in peripheral vascular resistance. **Peak plasma levels:** 6–12 hr. **t½, elimination:** 30–50 hr. 90% metabolized in the liver to inactive metabolites; 10% excreted unchanged in the urine.

**Uses:** Hypertension alone or in combination with other antihypertensives. Chronic stable angina alone or in combination with other antianginal drugs. Confirmed or suspected Prinzmetal's or variant angina alone or in combination with other antianginal drugs.

**Contraindications:** Cardiogenic shock, hypotension 90 mm Hg, 2nd or 3rd degree heart block, severe CHF, sick sinus syndrome.

**Special Concerns:** Use with caution in clients with CHF and in those with impaired hepatic function or reduced hepatic blood flow. Safety and efficacy have not been determined in children.

**Side Effects:** *CNS:* Headache, fatigue, lethargy, somnolence, dizziness, lightheadedness, sleep disturbances, depression, amnesia, psychosis, hallucinations, paresthesia, asthenia, insomnia, abnormal dreams, malaise, anxiety, tremor, hand tremor, hypoesthesia, vertigo, depersonalization, migraine, apathy, agitation, amnesia. *Oral:* Dry mouth, thirst, gingival hyperplasia, altered taste. *GI:* Nausea, abdominal discomfort, cramps, dyspepsia, diarrhea, constipation, vomiting, flatulence, dysphagia, loose stools. *CV:* Peripheral edema, palpitations, hypotension, syncope, bradycardia, unspecified arrhythmias, tachycardia, ventricular extrasystoles, peripheral ischemia, *cardiac failure,* pulse irregularity, increased risk of MI. *Dermatologic:* Dermatitis, rash, pruritus, urticaria, photosensitivity, petechiae, ecchymosis, purpura, bruising, hematoma, cold/clammy skin, skin discoloration, dry skin. *Musculoskeletal:* Muscle cramps, pain, or inflammation; joint stiffness or pain, arthritis, twitching, ataxia, hypertonia. *GU:* Polyuria, dysuria, urinary frequency, nocturia, sexual difficulties. *Respiratory:* Nasal or chest congestion, sinusitis, rhinitis, SOB, dyspnea, wheezing, cough, chest pain. *Ophthalmologic:* Diplopia, abnormal vision, conjunctivitis, eye pain, abnormal visual accommodation, xerophthalmia. *Miscellaneous:* Tinnitus, flushing, sweating, weight gain, epistaxis, anorexia, increased appetite, parosmia.

**Drug Interactions**

*Barbiturates* / ↓ Effect of amlodipine

*Carbamazepine* / ↑ Amlodipine increase the effects of carbamazepine

*Indomethacin* / ↓ Effect of amlodipine

*Inhalation general anesthetics* / ↑ Effect of amlodipine

*NSAIDs* / ↓ Possible effect of amlodipine

*Parenteral general anesthetics* / ↑ Effect of amlodipine

*Other drugs with hypotensive effects* / ↑ Effect of amlodipine

**How Supplied:** *Tablet:* 2.5 mg, 5 mg, 10 mg

**Dosage** —————————
• **Tablets**
*Hypertension.*
**Adults, usual, individualized:** 5 mg/day, up to a maximum of 10 mg/day. Titrate the dose over 7–14 days.
*Chronic stable or vasospastic angina.*
**Adults:** 5–10 mg, using the lower dose for elderly clients and those with hepatic insufficiency. Most clients require 10 mg.

## DENTAL CONCERNS

See also *Dental Concerns* for *Calcium Channel Blocking Agents.*

---

# Amoxapine
(ah-**MOX**-ah-peen)
**Pregnancy Category:** C
Asendin **(Rx)**
**Classification:** Antidepressant, tricyclic

See also *Antidepressants, Tricyclic.*
**Action/Kinetics:** In addition to its effect on monoamines, this drug also blocks dopamine receptors. Significant anticholinergic effects, moderate sedation, and slight orthostatic hypotensive effect. Metabolized to the active metabolites 7-hydroxy- and 8-hydroxyamoxapine. **Peak blood levels:** 90 min. **Effective plasma levels:** 200–500 ng/mL. **Time to reach steady state:** 2–7 days. t½: 8 hr; t½ of major metabolite: 30 hr. Excreted in urine.
**Uses:** Endogenous and reactive depression. Antianxiety agent.
**Contraindications:** Avoid high dose levels in clients with a history of convulsive seizures. During acute recovery period after MI.
**Special Concerns:** Safe use in children under 16 years of age and during lactation not established.
**Additional Side Effects:** Tardive dyskinesia. *Overdosage may cause seizures (common), neuroleptic malig-*

*nant syndrome,* testicular swelling, impairment of sexual function, and breast enlargement in males and females. Also, renal failure may be seen 2–5 days after overdosage.
**How Supplied:** *Tablet:* 25 mg, 50 mg, 100 mg, 150 mg

**Dosage** —————————
• **Tablets**
*Antidepressant.*
**Adults, individualized, initial:** 50 mg t.i.d. Can be increased to 100 mg t.i.d. during first week. Do not use doses greater than 300 mg/day unless this dose has been ineffective for at least 14 days. **Maintenance:** 300 mg as a single dose at bedtime. **Hospitalized clients:** Up to 150 mg q.i.d. **Geriatric, initial:** 25 mg b.i.d.–t.i.d. If necessary, increase to 50 mg b.i.d.–t.i.d. after first week. **Maintenance:** Up to 300 mg/day at bedtime.

## DENTAL CONCERNS

See also *Dental Concerns* for *Antidepressants, Tricyclic.*

---

# Amoxicillin (amoxycillin)
(ah-mox-ih-**SILL**-in)
Amox ✹, Amoxil, Amoxil Pediatric Drops, Apo-Amoxi ✹, Biomox, Novamoxin ✹, Nu-Amoxi ✹, Polymox, Polymox Drops, Pro-Amox ✹, Trimox 125, 250, and 500, Wymox **(Rx)**

*NOTE:* Canadian products are all amoxicillin trihydrate.
**Classification:** Antibiotic, penicillin

See also *Anti-Infectives* and *Penicillins.*
**Action/Kinetics:** Semisynthetic broad-spectrum penicillin closely related to ampicillin. Destroyed by penicillinase, acid stable, and better absorbed than ampicillin. From 50% to 80% of a PO dose is absorbed from the GI tract. **Peak serum levels: PO:** 4–11 mcg/mL after 1–2 hr. t½: 60 min. Mostly excreted unchanged in urine.
**Uses:** Gram-positive streptococcal infections including *Streptococcus*

---

*faecalis, S. pneumoniae,* and non-penicillinase-producing staphylococci. Gram-negative infections due to *Hemophilus influenzae, Proteus mirabilis, Escherichia coli,* and Neisseria gonorrhoeae.

**Contraindications:** Hypersensitivity to penicillins.

**Special Concerns:** Safe use during pregnancy has not been established. Hypersensitivity to cephalosporins.

**Side Effects:** See also *Anti-Infectives* and *Penicillins.*

**Drug Interactions:** See also *Anti-Infectives* and *Penicillins.*

**How Supplied:** *Capsule:* 250 mg, 500 mg; *Chew tablet:* 125 mg, 250 mg; *Powder for reconstitution:* 50 mg/mL, 125 mg/5 mL, 250 mg/5 mL

**Dosage** —————————————
• **Capsules, Oral Suspension, Chewable Tablets**
*Susceptible infections of ear, nose, throat, GU tract, skin and soft tissues, lower respiratory tract.*
**Adults:** 250–500 mg q 8 hr; **pediatric under 20 kg:** 20–40 (or more) mg/kg/day in three equal doses. The pediatric dose should not exceed the maximum adult dose.
*Prophylaxis of bacterial endocarditis.*
**Adults:** 2 g 1 hr prior to procedure.
*Gonococcal infections.* **Children:** 50 mg/kg of body weight, not to exceed adult dose 1 hr prior to procedure.
3 g with probenecid, 1 g, given as a single dose. In addition, tetracycline, 0.5 mg, q.i.d. for 7 days.
*Gonococcal infection in pregnancy.*
3 g with probenecid, 1 g, given as a single dose. In addition, erythromycin base, 0.5 g q.i.d. for 7 days.
*Disseminated gonococcal infections.*
3 g with probenecid, 1 g, given as a single dose; **then,** 0.5 g q.i.d. for 7 days.
*Acute pelvic inflammatory disease.*
3 g with probenecid, 1 g, given as a single dose. In addition, doxycycline, 100 mg b.i.d. for 10–14 days.

*Sexually transmitted epididymo-orchitis.*
3 g with probenecid, 1 g, given as a single dose. In addition, tetracycline, 0.5 g q.i.d. for 10 days.
*Bacterial vaginosis.*
0.5 g q.i.d. for 7 days.
*Chlamydia trachomatis during pregnancy (as an alternative to erythromycin).*
0.5 g t.i.d. for 7 days.

## DENTAL CONCERNS

See also *Dental Concerns* for *Anti-Infectives* and *Penicillins.*
**Client/Family Teaching**
1. Take entire prescription; do not stop when feeling "better" as this creates antibiotic resistance.
2. With school-age child space medication evenly over the 24-hr period. Give suspension or tablet before school, upon arrival home, and at bedtime.
3. Report any unusual rash or lack of response.

————COMBINATION DRUG————
# Amoxicillin and Potassium clavulanate
(ah-mox-ih-**SILL**-in, poh-**TASS**-ee-um klav-you-**LAN**-ayt)
Pregnancy Category: B
Augmentin **(Rx)**
Classification: Antibiotic, penicillin

See also *Anti-Infectives* and *Penicillins.*
**Content:** Each '250' Tablet contains: 250 mg amoxicillin and 125 mg potassium clavulanate. Each '500' Tablet contains 500 mg amoxicillin and 125 mg potassium clavulanate.

Each '875' tablet contains: 875 mg amoxicillin, 125 mg potassium clavulanate

Each '125' Chewable Tablet contains 125 mg amoxicillin and 31.25 mg potassium clavulanate. Each 200 Chewable Tablet contains 200 mg amoxicillin and 28.5 mg potassium clavulanate. Each '250' Chewable Tablet contains 250 mg amoxicillin and 62.5 mg potassium clavulanate. Each 400 Chewable Tablet contains 400 mg amoxicillin and 57 mg potassium clavulanate.

Each 5 mL of the '125' Powder for Oral Suspension contains 125 mg amoxicillin and 31.25 mg potassium clavulanate. Each 5 mL of the 200 Powder for Oral Suspension contains 200 mg amoxicillin and 28.5 mg potassium clavulanate. Each 5 mL of the '250' Powder for Oral Suspension contains 250 mg amoxicillin and 62.5 mg potassium clavulanate. Each 5 mL of the 400 Powder or the 400 Powder for Oral Suspension contains 400 mg amoxicillin and 57 mg potassium clavulanate.

**Action/Kinetics:** *For details, see amoxicillin.* Potassium clavulanate inactivates lactamase enzymes, which are responsible for resistance to penicillins. Thus, is effective against microorganisms that have manifested resistance to amoxicillin. For potassium clavulanate: **Peak serum levels:** 1–2 hr. **t½:** 1 hr.

**Uses:** For beta-lactamase-producing strains of the following organisms: *Hemophilus influenzae* and *Moraxella catarrhalis* causing lower respiratory tract infections, otitis media, and sinusitis; *Staphylococcus aureus, Escherichia coli,* and *Klebsiella,* causing skin and skin structure infections; *E. coli, Klebsiella,* and *Enterobacter,* causing UTI. *Note:* Mixed infections caused by organisms susceptible to ampicillin and organisms susceptible to amoxicillin/potassium clavulanate should not require an additional antibiotic.

**Contraindications:** Hypersensitivity to penicillins. Clavulanate K-associated cholestatic and/or liver dysfunction.

**Special Concerns:** Hypersensitivity to cephalosporins. Liver impairment.

**Side Effects:** See also *Anti-Infectives* and *Penicillins.*

**Drug Interactions**
*Allupurinol* / ↑ Risk of skin rashes
*Probenecid* / ↑ Amoxicillin concentrations

**How Supplied:** See Content.

**Dosage** —
**• Oral Suspension, Chewable Tablets, Tablets**
*Susceptible infections.*
**Adults, usual:** One 500-mg tablet q 12 hr or one 250-mg tablet q 8 hr. Adults unable to take tablets can be given the 125-mg/5 mL or the 250-mg/5 mL suspension in place of the 500-mg tablet or the 200-mg/5 mL or 400-mg/5 mL suspension can be given in place of the 875-mg tablet. **Children less than 3 months old:** 30 mg/kg/day amoxicillin in divided doses q 12 hr. Use of the 125-mg/5 mL suspension is recommended. **Children over 3 months old:** 25 mg/kg/day in divided doses q 12 hr or 20 mg/kg/day in divided doses q 8 hr.

*Respiratory tract and severe infections.*
**Adults:** One 875-mg tablet q 12 hr or one 500-mg tablet q 8 hr. **Children over 3 months old:** 45 mg/kg/day of amoxicillin in divided doses q 12 hr or 40 mg/kg/day in divided doses q 8 hr (these doses are used in children for otitis media, lower respiratory tract infections, or sinusitis). Treatment duration for otitis media is 10 days.

*Chancroid* (Haemophilus ducreyi infection).
**Adults:** One 500-mg tablet t.i.d. for 7 days (alternative to erythromycin or ceftriaxone).

*Disseminated gonococcal infections.*
Following therapy with an appropriate cephalosporin, (ceftriaxone, ceftizoxime, or cefotaxime) uncomplicated disease therapy may be completed with one 500-mg tablet t.i.d. for 1 week.

## DENTAL CONCERNS

See also *Dental Concerns* for *Anti-Infectives* and *Penicillins.*
**Client/Family Teaching**
1. Take exactly as directed and complete entire prescription.
2. Report any rash, persistent diarrhea, lack of response or worsening

**A**

of symptoms after 48–72 hr of therapy.

3. Return as scheduled for follow-up evaluation.

# Amphetamine sulfate
(am-**FET**-ah-meen)

**Pregnancy Category:** C
Dexedrine ✸ **(C-II) (Rx)**
**Classification:** CNS stimulant

See also *Amphetamines and Derivatives.*

**Action/Kinetics:** After PO, completely absorbed in 3 hr. The peak effects of the drug are observed 2–3 hr after administration. **Duration: PO,** 4–24 hr; **t½:** 10–30 hr, depending on urinary pH. Excreted in urine. Acidification increases excretion, whereas alkalinization decreases it. For every one unit increase in pH, the plasma half-life will increase by 7 hr.

**Uses:** Attention deficit disorders in children, narcolepsy. A product containing dextroamphetamine sulfate, dextroamphetamine saccharate, amphetamine sulfate, and amphetamine aspartate is available for use in children aged three years and older who have attention deficit disorder with hyperactivity or narcolepsy.

**Special Concerns:** Use in children less than 3 years of age for attention deficit disorders and in children less than 6 years of age for narcolepsy. Not recommended as an appetite suppressant.

**How Supplied:** *Tablet:* 5 mg, 10 mg

**Dosage**
• **Tablets**
*Narcolepsy.*
**Adults:** 5–20 mg 1–3 times/day. **Children over 12 years, initial:** 5 mg b.i.d.; increase in increments of 10 mg/day at weekly intervals until optimum dose is reached. **Children, 6–12 years, initial:** 2.5 mg b.i.d.; increase in increments of 5 mg at weekly intervals until optimum dose is reached (maximum is 60 mg/day).
*Attention deficit disorders in children.*
**3–6 years, initial:** 2.5 mg/day; increase by 2.5 mg/day at weekly

intervals until optimum dose is achieved (usual range 0.1–0.5 mg/kg/dose each morning). **6 years and older, initial:** 5 mg 1–2 times/day; increase in increments of 5 mg/week until optimum dose is achieved (rarely over 40 mg/day).

## DENTAL CONCERNS

See also *Dental Concerns* for *Amphetamines and Derivatives.*

# Amphotericin B (Deoxycholate)
(am-foe-**TER**-ih-sin)

**Pregnancy Category:** B
Amphotec, Fungizone ✸, Fungizone Intravenous **(Rx)**

# Amphotericin B Lipid Complex (Amphotericin B Cholesteryl Sulfate Complex)
(am-foe-**TER**-ih-sin)

**Pregnancy Category:** B
Abelcet, AmBisome, Amphotec **(Rx)**
**Classification:** Antibiotic, antifungal

See also *Anti-Infectives.*

**Action/Kinetics:** This antibiotic is produced by *Streptomyces nodosus;* it is fungistatic or fungicidal depending on the concentration of the drug in body fluids and the susceptibility of the fungus. Amphotericin B binds to specific chemical structures—sterols—of the fungal cellular membrane, increasing cellular permeability and promoting loss of potassium and other substances. Liposomal encapsulation or incorporation in a lipid complex can significantly affect the functional properties of the drug compared with those of the unencapsulated or non-lipid-associated drug. The liposomal amphotericin B product causes less nephrotoxicity. Amphotericin B is used either IV or topically. It is highly bound to serum protein (90%) **Peak plasma levels:** 0.5–2 mcg/mL. **t½, initial:** 24 hr; **second phase:** 15 days. Slowly excreted by kidneys. The kinetics of the drug differ in adults and children.

**Uses:** The drug is toxic and should be used only for clients under close medical supervision with progressive or potentially fatal fungal infections. *Systemic: Amphotericin B deoxycholate:* Disseminated North American blastomycosis, cryptococcosis, and other systemic fungal infections, including coccidioidomycosis, histoplasmosis, mucormycosis, sporotrichosis, aspergillosis, disseminated candidiasis, and monilial overgrowth resulting from oral antibiotic therapy. Secondary therapy to treat American mucocutaneous leishmaniasis. *Liposomal Amphotericin B:* Aspergillosis in clients refractory to or intolerant of conventional amphotericin B therapy. *Non-FDA Approved Uses:* Prophylaxis of fungal infections in clients with bone marrow transplantation. *Topical:* Cutaneous and mucocutaneous infections of *Candida (Monilia)* infections, especially in children, adults, and AIDS clients with thrush.

**Contraindications:** Hypersensitivity to drug unless the condition is life-threatening and amenable only to amphotericin B therapy. Use to treat common forms of fungal diseases showing only positive skin or serologic tests. Use to treat noninvasive forms of fungal disease such as oral thrush, vaginal candidiasis, and esophageal candidiasis in clients with normal neutrophil counts. Lactation.

**Special Concerns:** The bone marrow depressant effects may result in increased incidence of microbial infection, delayed healing, and gingival bleeding. Although used in children, safety and efficacy have not been determined. Use with caution in clients receiving leukocyte transfusions.

**Side Effects: After topical use.** Irritation, pruritus, dry skin. Redness, itching, or burning especially in skin folds. **After IV use.** *Acute reactions occurring 1 to 3 hr after starting IV in-*

*fusion:* Fever, hypotension, shaking chills, hypotension, anorexia, N&V, headache, tachypnea. Rapid infusion may cause hypotension, hypokalemia, arrhythmias, and *shock. Oral:* stomatitis. *GI:* N&V, diarrhea, dyspepsia, anorexia, abdominal cramps, epigastric pain, melena; rarely, GI disorder, *GI hemorrhage,* hematemesis, dyspepsia, enlarged abdomen, hepatomegaly, cholangitis, cholecystitis, hemorrhagic gastroenteritis, acute liver failure, hepatitis, jaundice, veno-occlusive liver disease, hepatic failure. *CNS:* Fever, chills, headache, depressoin, abnormal thinking, malaise, vertigo, leukoencephalopathy; rarely, dizziness, somnolence, agitation, stupor, tremor, anxiety, paresthesia, hallucinations, *seizures,* encephalopathy, extrapyramidal symptoms, peripheral neuropathy, and other neurologic symptoms. *Respiratory:* Respiratory disorder, pneumonia, *respiratory failure.* Acute dyspnea, hypoxia, epistaxis, increased cough, lung disorder, hemoptysis, hyperventilation, hypersensitivity pneumonitis, apnea. Interstitial infiltrates seen in neutropenic clients receiving amphotericin B and leukocyte transfusions. *CV:* Thrombophlebitis, hypotension, hypertension, tachycardia, tachypnea, phlebitis. Rarely, arrhythmias, phlebitis, syncope, ventricular extrasystoles, postural hypotension, supraventricular tachycardia, thrombophlebitis, pleural effusion, hemoptysis, atrial fibrillation, bradycardia, CHF, *ventricular fibrillation, cardiac arrest, cardiac failure, shock, hemorrhage, pulmonary embolus, MI, cardiomyopathy. Renal:* Renal damage (including tubular dysfunction), azotemia, hyposthenuria, nephrocalcinosis, renal tubular acidosis, *kidney failure;* rarely, acute renal failure, decreased renal function, anuria, oliguria, hematuria, dysuria, infection. *Hematologic:* Normochromic, normocytic anemia; anemia, coagulation disorder. Rarely, *coagulation defects,* thrombocytopenia, leukopenia, ag-

---

ranulocytosis, eosinophilia, leukocytosis, hypochromic anemia, blood dyscrasias. *Dermatologic:* Maculopapular rash, pruritus, rash; rarely, exfoliative dermatitis, erythema multiforme, skin disorder. *Hypersensitvity:* Rarely, **bronchospasm, asthma, anaphylactoid reactions,** wheezing. *Ophthalmic/Otic:* Rarely, tinnitus, hearing loss, blurred vision, eye hemorrhage, diplopia, impaired vision. *At injection site:* Venous pain with phlebitis and thrombophlebitis. *Miscellaneous:* Muscle and joint pain, weight loss, infection, sweating, pain, chest pain, back pain, **multiple organ failure, sepsis, face edema, asthenia, peripheral edema, mucous membrane disorder; rarely, flushing, impotence, myasthenia, arthralgia, myalgia, After intrathecal use:** Blurred vision, changes in vision, difficulty in urination, numbness, tingling, pain, or weakness.

**Drug Interactions**
*Corticosteroids* / ↑ Potassium depletion caused by amphotericin B → cardiac dysfunction
*Skeletal muscle relaxants, surgical* (e.g., succinylcholine, *d*-tubocurarine) / ↑ Muscle relaxation due to amphotericin B–induced hypokalemia

**How Supplied:** *Cream:* 3%; *Lotion:* 3%; *Powder for injection:* 50 mg

**Dosage** ———————————
• **Amphotericin B Deoxycholate, IV**
*Test dose by slow IV infusion.*
1 mg in 20 mL of 5% dextrose injection should be infused over 20 to 30 min to determine tolerance.
*Severe and rapidly progressing fungal infection.*
**Initial:** 0.3 mg/kg over 2 to 6 hr.
*Note:* In impaired cardiorenal function or if a severe reaction to the test dose, therapy should be initiated with smaller daily doses (e.g., 5–10 mg). Depending on the status of the client, the dose may be increased gradually by 5–10 mg/day to a final daily dose of 0.5–0.7 mg/kg. The total daily dose should not exceed 1.5 mg/kg.

*Sporotrichosis.*
20 mg/injection. Therapy may be required for up to 9 months.
*Aspergillosis.*
Total dose of 3.6 g or less per day for 11 months or less.
*Rhinocerebral phycomyosis.*
A cumulative dose of 3 g/day.
*Prophylaxis of fungal infections in bone marrow transplants.*
0.1 mg/kg/day.
• **Amphotericin B Deoxycholate Suspension**
*Oral candidiasis.*
Swish the suspension in the mouth and then swallow.
• **Liposomal Amphotericin B**
*All uses.*
**Adults and children, initial:** 3–4 mg/kg/day, as required. May be increased to 6 mg/kg/day if there is no improvement or if the fungal infection has progressed.
*Aspergillosis.*
**Adults and children:** 5 mg/kg/day as a single infusion.
• **Intrathecal, Intraventricular**
*Fungal meningitis.*
**Initial:** 0.1 mg; **then,** increase gradually up to 0.5 mg q 48 to 72 hr.
• **Bladder Irritation**
*Candidal cystitis.*
5–15 mg/dL instilled periodically or continuously for 5 to 10 days.
• **Topical (Lotion, Cream, Ointment—Each 3%)**
Apply liberally to affected areas b.i.d.–q.i.d. Depending on the type of lesion, up to 4 weeks of therapy may be necessary.

## DENTAL CONCERNS

See also *General Dental Concerns* for *All Anti-Infectives.*
**Client/Family Teaching**
1. Amphotericin therapy usually requires long-term treatments (6–11 weeks) to ensure an adequate response and to prevent any relapse.

———————————————
# Ampicillin oral
(am-pih-**SILL**-in)
**Pregnancy Category:** B
Apo-Ampi ✳, Jaa Amp ✳, Novo-Ampicillin ✳, Nu-Ampi ✳, Omnipen,

Penbritin ✿, Polycillin, Polycillin Pediatric Drops, Principen, Pro-Ampi ✿, Taro-Ampicillin ✿, Totacillin **(Rx)**

*NOTE:*The following Canadian drugs are ampicillin trihydrate: Apo-Ampi, Jaa Amp, Nu-Ampi, Pro-Ampi, Taro-Ampicillin.

————COMBINATION DRUG————

# Ampicillin with Probenecid

(am-pih-**SILL**-in, proh-**BEN**-ih-sid)
Pro-Biosan ✿, Polycillin-PRB, Probampacin **(Rx)**

# Ampicillin sodium, parenteral

(am-pih-**SILL**-in)
**Pregnancy Category:** B
Ampicin ✿, Omnipen N, Polycillin-N, Totacillin-N **(Rx)**
**Classification:** Antibiotic, penicillin

See also *Anti-Infectives* and *Penicillins.*

**Content:** The Powder for Oral Suspension of Ampicillin with Probenecid contains 3.5 g ampicillin and 1 g probenecid per bottle.

**Action/Kinetics:** Synthetic, broad-spectrum antibiotic suitable for gram-negative bacteria. Acid resistant, destroyed by penicillinase. Absorbed more slowly than other penicillins. From 30% to 60% of PO dose absorbed from GI tract. **Peak serum levels: PO:** 1.8–2.9 mcg/mL after 2 hr; **IM,** 4.5–7 mcg/mL. **t½:** 80 min—range 50–110 min. Partially inactivated in liver; 25%–85% excreted unchanged in urine.

**Uses:** Infections of respiratory, GI, and GU tracts caused by *Shigella, Salmonella, Escherichia coli, Hemophilus influenzae, Proteus* strains, *Neisseria gonorrhoeae, N. meningitidis,* and *Enterococcus.* Also, otitis media in children, bronchitis, rat-bite fever, and whooping cough. Penicillin G-sensitive staphylococci, streptococci, pneumococci.

**Contraindications:** Hypersensitivity to penicillins.
**Special Concerns:** Hypersensitivity to cephalosporins. Use in neonates.
**Side Effects:** See also *Anti-Infectives* and *Penicillins.*
**Drug Interactions:** See also *Anti-Infectives* and *Penicillins.*
*Probenecid /* ↑ Ampicillin concentrations.

**How Supplied:** Ampicillin oral: *Capsule:* 250 mg, 500 mg; *Powder for reconstitution:* 125 mg/5 mL, 250 mg/5 mL.Ampicillin with Probenecid: See Content. Ampicillin sodium parenteral: *Powder for injection:* 125 mg, 250 mg, 500 mg, 1 g, 2 g, 10 g

**Dosage** ————
• **Ampicillin: Capsules, Oral Suspension; Ampicillin Sodium: IV, IM**
   *Respiratory tract and soft tissue infections.*
**PO: 20 kg or more:** 250 mg q 6 hr; **less than 20 kg:** 50 mg/kg/day in equally divided doses q 6–8 hr. **IV, IM: 40 kg or more:** 250–500 mg q 6 hr;   **less than 40 kg:** 25–50 mg/kg/day in equally divided doses q 6–8 hr.
   *Disseminated gonococcal infections.*
**PO:** 1 g q 6 hr.
   *Bacterial meningitis.*
**Adults:** A total of 8–12 g/day given in divided doses q 3–4 hr. **Pediatric:** 100–200 mg/kg/day in divided doses q 3–4 hr.
   *Bacterial endocarditis prophylaxis (upper respiratory tract procedures; GI or GU tract surgery or instrumentation).*
**Adult, IM, IV:** 1–2 g (use 2 g for GI or GU tract surgery) plus gentamicin, 1.5 mg/kg (not to exceed 80 mg) IM or IV, given 30 min before procedure followed by amoxicillin, 1.5 g, 6 hr after initial dose; or, repeat parenteral dose 8 hr after initial dose. **Pediatric:** Ampicillin, 50 mg/kg with gentamicin, 2 mg/kg 30 min prior to procedure followed by amoxicillin, 25 mg/kg, after 6 hr or a

parenteral dose of ampicillin is given after 8 hr.

*Bacterial endocarditis prophylaxis (dental or oral procedures).*
**Adult, IM, IV:** 2 g IM or IV, given 30 min before procedure. **Pediatric:** Ampicillin, 50 mg/kg 30 min prior to procedure.

*Septicemia.*
**Adults/children:** 150–200 mg/kg, IV for first 3 days, then IM q 3–4 hr.
• **Ampicillin with Probenecid: Oral Suspension**
*Urethral, endocervical, or rectal infections due to* N. gonorrhoeae.
**Adults:** 3.5 g ampicillin and 1 g probenecid as a single dose.

*Prophylaxis of infection in rape victims.*
3.5 g with 1 g probenecid.

## DENTAL CONCERNS

See also *Dental Concerns* for *Anti-Infectives* and *Penicillins*.
**Client/Family Teaching**
1. Take medication 1 hr before or 2 hr after meals.
2. Teach person administering drug the appropriate method for administration and storage.
3. Take for the prescribed number of days even if the symptoms subside to prevent drug resistance.
4. Ampicillin chewable tablets should not be swallowed whole.
5. Do not save for future use or share with family members/friends who have similar symptoms.
6. May decrease effectiveness of oral contraceptives; practice alternative method of contraception during therapy.
7. Report any "ampicillin rashes"; a dull, red, itchy, flat or raised rash occurs more often with this drug than with other penicillins and is usually benign. If a late skin rash develops with symptoms of fever, fatigue, sore throat, generalized lymphadenopathy, and enlarged spleen, a heterophil antibody test may be considered to rule out mononucleosis.
8. Notify dentist if the infection is still present after three days of therapy.

————COMBINATION DRUG————
# Ampicillin sodium/Sulbactam sodium
(am-pih-**SILL**-in/sull-**BACK**-tam)
**Pregnancy Category:** B
Unasyn **(Rx)**
**Classification:** Antibiotic, penicillin

See also *Anti-Infectives* and *Penicillins*.

**Content:** The Powder for Injection contains either 1 g ampicillin sodium and 0.5 g sulbactam sodium or 2 g ampicillin sodium and 1 g sulbactam sodium.
**Action/Kinetics:** For details, see *Ampicillin oral*. Sulbactam is present in this product because it irreversibly inhibits beta-lactamases, thus ensuring activity of ampicillin against beta-lactamase-producing microorganisms. Thus, sulbactam broadens the antibiotic spectrum of ampicillin to those bacteria normally resistant to it. **Peak serum levels, after IV infusion:** 15 min. **t½, both drugs:** about 1 hr. From 75%–85% of both drugs is excreted unchanged in the urine within 8 hr after administration.
**Uses:** Infections caused by beta-lactamase-producing strains of the following: (a) skin and skin structure infections caused by *Staphylococcus aureus, Escherichia coli, Klebsiella* species (including *K. pneumoniae*), *Proteus mirabilis, Bacteroides fragilis, Enterobacter* species, and *Acinetobacter calcoaceticus;* (b) intra-abdominal infections caused by *E. coli, Klebsiella* species (including *K. pneumoniae*), *Bacteroides* (including *B. fragilis* and *Enterobacter);* (c) gynecologic infections caused by *E. coli* and *Bacteroides* (including *B. fragilis).* NOTE: Mixed infections caused by ampicillin-susceptible organisms and beta-lactamase-producing organisms are susceptible to this product; thus, additional antibiotics do not have to be used.
**Contraindications:** Hypersensitivity to penicillins.

**Special Concerns:** Safety and efficacy in children less than 12 years of age have not been established.

**Side Effects:** *At site of injection:* Pain and thrombophlebitis. *GI:* Diarrhea, N&V, flatulence, abdominal distention, glossitis. *CNS:* Fatigue, malaise, headache. *GU:* Dysuria, urinary retention. *Miscellaneous:* Itching, chest pain, edema, facial swelling, erythema, chills, tightness in throat, epistaxis, substernal pain, mucosal bleeding, candidiasis.

**Drug Interactions:** See also *Anti-Infectives* and *Penicillins*.

**How Supplied:** See Content

**Dosage** ———————
• **IV, IM**
**Adults:** 1 g ampicillin/0.5 g sulbactam to 2 g ampicillin/1 g sulbactam q 6 hr, not to exceed 4 g sulbactam daily. Doses must be decreased in renal impairment.

---

**DENTAL CONCERNS**

See also *Dental Concerns* for *Anti-Infectives, Penicillins* and *Ampicillin.*

---

# Amrinone lactate
(**AM**-rih-nohn)
**Pregnancy Category:** C
Inocor **(Rx)**
**Classification:** Cardiac inotropic agent

**Action/Kinetics:** Amrinone causes an increase in CO by increasing the force of contraction of the heart, probably by inhibiting cyclic AMP phosphodiesterase, thereby increasing cellular levels of c-AMP. It reduces afterload and preload by directly relaxing vascular smooth muscle. **Time to peak effect:** 10 min. **t½, after rapid IV:** 3.6 hr; **after IV infusion:** 5.8 hr. **Steady-state plasma levels:** 2.4 mcg/mL by maintaining an infusion of 5–10 mcg/kg/min. **Duration:** 30 min–2 hr, depending on the dose. Excreted primarily in the urine both unchanged and as metabolites. Children have a larger volume

of distribution and a decreased elimination half-life.

**Uses:** Congestive heart failure (short-term therapy in clients unresponsive to digitalis, diuretics, and/or vasodilators). Can be used in digitalized clients.

**Contraindications:** Hypersensitivity to amrinone or bisulfites. Severe aortic or pulmonary valvular disease in lieu of surgery. Acute MI.

**Special Concerns:** Safety and efficacy not established in children. Use with caution during lactation.

**Side Effects:** *GI:* N&V, abdominal pain, anorexia. *CV:* Hypotension, *supraventricular and ventricular arrhythmias.* *Allergic:* Pericarditis, pleuritis, ascites, allergic reaction to sodium bisulfite present in the product. *Other:* Thrombocytopenia, *hepatotoxicity,* fever, chest pain, burning at site of injection.

**Drug Interactions:** Excessive hypotension when used with disopyramide.

**How Supplied:** *Injection:* 5 mg/mL

**Dosage** ———————
• **IV**
  *CHF.*
**Initial:** 0.75 mg/kg as a bolus given slowly over 2–3 min; may be repeated after 30 min if necessary. **Maintenance, IV infusion:** 5–10 mcg/kg/min. Daily dose should not exceed 10 mg/kg although up to 18 mg/kg/day has been used in some clients for short periods.

---

**DENTAL CONCERNS**

None reported.

---

# Anagrelide hydrochloride
(an-**AG**-greh-lyd)
**Pregnancy Category:** C
Agrylin **(Rx)**
**Classification:** Antiplatelet drug

**Action/Kinetics:** May act to reduce platelets by decreasing megakaryocyte hypermaturation. Does not cause significant changes in white cell counts or coagulation parame-

---

ters. Inhibits platelet aggregation at higher doses than needed to reduce platelet count. **Peak plasma levels:** 5 ng/mL at 1 hr. **t½:** 1.3 hr; **terminal t½:** About 3 days. Metabolized in liver and excreted in urine and feces. **Uses:** Reduce platelet count in essential thrombocythemia. **Contraindications:** Lactation. **Special Concerns:** Use with caution in known or suspected heart disease and in impaired renal or hepatic function. Safety and efficacy have not been determined in those less than 16 years of age. **Side Effects:** *CV:* CHF, palpitations, chest pain, tachycardia, arrhythmias, angina, postural hypotension, hypertension, cardiovascular disease, vasodilation, migraine, syncope, *MI, cardiomyopathy, complete heart block, fibrillation, CVA, pericarditis, hemorrhage, heart failure,* cardiomegaly, atrial fibrillation. *Oral:* Aphthous stomatitis. *GI:* Diarrhea, abdominal pain, pancreatitis, gastric/duodenal ulcers, N&V, flatulence, anorexia, constipation, GI distress, *GI hemorrhage,* gastritis, melena, aphthous stomatitis, eructations. *Respiratory:* Rhinitis, epistaxis, respiratory disease, sinusitis, pneumonia, bronchitis, asthma, pulmonary infiltrate, *pulmonary fibrosis, pulmonary hypertension,* dyspnea. *CNS:* Headache, *seizures,* dizziness, paresthesia, depression, somnolence, confusion, insomnia, nervousness, amnesia. *Musculoskeletal:* Arthralgia, myalgia, leg cramps. *Dermatologic:* Pruritus, skin disease, alopecia, rash, urticaria. *Hematologic:* Anemia, thrombocytopenia, ecchymosis, lymphadenoma. *Body as a whole:* Fever, flu symptoms, chills, photosensitivity, dehydration, malaise, asthenia, edema, pain. *Ophthalmic:* Amblyopia, abnormal vision, visual field abnormality, diplopia. *Miscellaneous:* Back pain, tinnitus.

**Drug Interactions**
*Aspirin* / ↑ Risk of bleeding
*NSAIDs* / ↑ Risk of bleeding

**Dosage** ————————————
- **Capsules**

*Essential thrombocythemia.*
**Initial:** 0.5 mg q.i.d. or 1 mg b.i.d. Maintain for one week or more. **Then,** adjust to lowest effective dose to maintain platelet count less than 600,000/mcL. Can increase the dose by 0.5 mg or less/day in any 1 week. **Maximum dose:** 10 mg/day or 2.5 mg in single dose. Most respond at a dose of 1.5 to 3 mg/day.

## DENTAL CONCERNS
### General
1. Laboratory studies should include CBCs and PT times.
2. Increased risk of thrombo-hemorrhagic complications including prolonged bleeding time, anemia, and splenomegaly. Thrombosis may occur in some patients.
3. Mucosal bleeding may be a symptom of essential thrombocythemia.
4. Consider repositioning dental chair to semisupine condition for patient discomfort because of GI side effects.
5. Monitor vital signs at every appointment because of cardiovascular and respiratory side effects.
### Consultation with Primary Care Provider
1. Consult with physician supervising therapy or hematologist before dental treatment.
### Client/Family Teaching
1. Inform dental personnel of unusual bleeding episodes which occur after dental procedure.
2. Update medication/health history each time the physician changes anagrelide regimen.

## Ardeparin sodium
(ar-dee-**PAH**-rin)
**Pregnancy Category:** C
Normiflo **(Rx)**
**Classification:** Anticoagulant, low molecular weight heparin

See also *Anticoagulants.*
**Action/Kinetics:** Binds to and accelerates activity of antithrombin III, thus inhibiting thrombosis by inactivating Factor Xa and thrombin. Also inhibits thrombin by binding to hep-

arin cofactor II. At usual doses, no effect on PT; APTT may not be affected or may be slightly prolonged. Plasma levels of ardeparin cannot be measured directly; rather, serine protease activity is used. Well absorbed following SC administration. **t½, disposition:** 3.3 hr (for ardeparin anti-Xa) and 1.2 hr (for ardeparin anti-IIa).

**Uses:** Prevention of deep vein thrombosis following knee replacement surgery.

**Contraindications:** Use with active major bleeding, hypersensitivity to drug or to pork products, thrombocytopenia associated with a positive *in vitro* test for anti-platelet antibodies in the presence of ardeparin. IM or IV use.

**Special Concerns:** Use with caution during lactation, in hypersensitivity to methylparaben or propylparaben, in those with bleeding diathesis, recent GI bleeding, thrombocytopenia or platelet defects, severe liver disease, hypertensive or diabetic retinopathy, in those undergoing invasive procedures (especially if they are receiving other drugs that interfere with hemostasis), or in severe renal failure. Use with extreme caution in those with a history of heparin-induced thrombocytopenia or in which there is an increased risk of hemorrhage (e.g., bacterial endocarditis, congenital or acquired bleeding disorders, active ulceration or angiodysplastic GI disease, severe uncontrolled hypertension, hemorrhagic stroke, soon after brain, spinal, or ophthalmologic surgery; or, with concomitant treatment with platelet inhibitors). Product contains metasulfite which may cause an allergic reaction in some. Safety and efficacy have not been determined in children.

**Side Effects:** *Bleeding events:* Intraoperative bleeding, postoperative surgical site or nonsurgical site hematoma or hemorrhage, bleeding requiring an invasive procedure; ecchymosis, *GI hemorrhage,* hematemesis, hematuria, melena, petechiae, *rectal hemor-*

*rhage, retroperitoneal hemorrhage, CVA,* abnormal stools. *GI:* N&V, constipation. *Allergic reaction:* Maculopapular rash, vesiculobullous rash, urticaria. *CNS:* Confusion, dizziness, headache, insomnia. *Miscellaneous:* Fever, pruritus, anemia, thrombocytopenia, arthralgia, chest pain, dyspnea, reactions at injection site (edema, hypersensitivity, inflammation, pain), peripheral edema.

**Drug Interactions:** Additive anticoagulant effects if given with other anticoagulants or platelet inhibitors (e.g., aspirin, NSAIDs).

**Dosage** ———————————
• **SC**
  *Prophylaxis of deep vein thrombosis during knee replacement surgery.*
  **Adults:** 50 anti-Xa U/kg q 12 hr. Begin treatment evening of day of surgery or following morning and continue for up to 14 days or until client is fully ambulatory, whichever is shorter.

## DENTAL CONCERNS

See also *Dental Concerns* for *Anticoagulants.*
**Client/Family Teaching**
1. Review the importance of good oral hygiene in order to prevent soft tissue inflammation.
2. Review the proper use of oral hygiene aids in order to prevent injury.
3. Notify dentist if oral lesions, sores, or bleeding occur.

# Astemizole
(ah-**STEM**-ih-zohl)
**Pregnancy Category:** C
Hismanil **(Rx)**
**Classification:** Antihistamine, miscellaneous

See also *Antihistamines.*
**Action/Kinetics:** Low to no sedative, antiemetic, or anticholinergic effects. Absorption decreased up to 60% when taken with food. Metabolized in the liver to both active and inactive metabolites and excreted through the feces. **t½:** About 1.6

days. **Onset:** 2–3 days. **Duration:** Up to several weeks. Over 95% is bound to plasma protein. Mainly excreted through the feces.

**Uses:** Allergic rhinitis, urticaria.

**Contraindications:** Impaired hepatic function.

**Special Concerns:** Safety and efficacy have not been established in children less than 12 years of age. Dose should not exceed 10 mg/day.

**Additional Side Effects:** *Serious CV side effects, including death, cardiac arrest, QT interval prolongation, torsades de pointes and other ventricular arrhythmias* have been observed in clients exceeding the recommended dose of astemizole. Syncope may precede severe arrhythmias. Overdose may be observed with doses as low as 20–30 mg/day.

**Drug Interactions:** Concomitant use of astemizole with erythromycin, itraconazole, or ketoconazole may cause serious CV effects, including death, cardiac arrest, torsades de pointes, and other ventricular arrhythmias (including QT interval prolongation).

**How Supplied:** *Tablet:* 10 mg

**Dosage** ─────────────
• **Tablets**
**Adults and children over 12 years:** 10 mg once daily. **Children, 6–12 years:** 5 mg daily; **children, less than 6 years:** 0.2 mg/kg/day.

## DENTAL CONCERNS

See also *Dental Concerns* for *Antihistamines.*

**General**

1. Monitor vital signs at every appointment because of cardiovascular side effects.

2. Decreased saliva flow can put the patient at risk for dental caries, periodontal disease, and candidiasis.

3. Patients on chronic drug therapy may develop blood dyscrasias. Symptoms include fever, sore throat, bleeding, and poor wound healing.

4. Determine why the patient is taking the medication.

**Consultation with Primary Care Provider**

1. Patients with symptoms of blood dyscrasias should be referred to their primary care provider for complete blood counts. Treatment should be postponed until the results are known.

# Atenolol
(ah-**TEN**-oh-lohl)
**Pregnancy Category:** C
Apo-Atenol ✶, Gen-Atenolol ✶, Med-Atenolol ✶, Novo-Atenol ✶, Nu-Atenol ✶, Taro-Atenolol ✶, Tenolin ✶, Tenormin **(Rx)**
**Classification:** Beta-adrenergic blocking agent

See also *Beta-Adrenergic Blocking Agents.*

**Action/Kinetics:** Predominantly beta-1 blocking activity. Has no membrane stabilizing activity or intrinsic sympathomimetic activity. Low lipid solubility. **Peak blood levels:** 2–4 hr. **t½:** 6–9 hr. 50% eliminated unchanged in the feces.

**Uses:** Hypertension (either alone or with other antihypertensives such as thiazide diuretics). Angina pectoris due to hypertension, coronary atherosclerosis, and AMI. *Non-FDA Approved Uses:* Prophylaxis of migraine, alcohol withdrawal syndrome, situational anxiety, ventricular arrhythmias, prophylactically to reduce incidence of supraventricular arrhythmias in coronary artery bypass surgery.

**Contraindications:** Hypersensitivity to atenolol, cardiogenic shock, 2nd or 3rd degree heart block, sinus bradycardia, congestive heart failure, cardiac failure.

**Special Concerns:** Aortic or mitral valve disease, asthma, COPD, diabetes mellitus, major surgery, renal disease, thyroid disease, well-compensated heart failure.

**Side Effects:** *Oral:* Dry mouth. *CV: Bradycardia, CHF, cold extremities, postural hypotension, profound hypotension, 2nd or 3rd degree heart block. CNS:* Catatonia, depression, dizziness, drowsiness, fatigue, hallucinations, insomnia, lethargy, mental changes, memory loss, strange dreams. *GI:* Diarrhea, *ischemic colitis,* nausea, *mesenteric arterial thrombosis,* vomiting. *Hematologic: Agranulocytosis,* thrombocytopenia. *Allergic:* Fever, sore throat, respiratory distress, rash, pharyngitis, *laryngospasm, anaphylaxis. Skin:* Pruritus, rash, increased skin pigmentation, sweating, dry skin, alopecia, skin irritation, psoriasis. *Ophthalmic:* Dry, burning eyes. *GU:* Dysuria, impotence, nocturia. *Other:* Hypoglycemia or hyperglycemia. *Respiratory: Bronchospasm,* dyspnea, wheezing.

**Drug Interactions:** See also *Drug Interactions* for *Beta-Adrenergic Blocking Agents* and *Antihypertensive Agents.*

**How Supplied:** *Injection:* 0.5 mg/mL; *Tablet:* 25 mg, 50 mg, 100 mg

**Dosage** ————————
• **Tablets**
  *Hypertension.*
**Initial:** 50 mg/day, either alone or with diuretics; if response is inadequate, 100 mg/day. Doses higher than 100 mg/day will not produce further beneficial effects. Maximum effects usually seen within 1–2 weeks.
  *Angina.*
**Initial:** 50 mg/day; if maximum response is not seen in 1 week, increase dose to 100 mg/day (some clients require 200 mg/day).
  *Alcohol withdrawal syndrome.*
50–100 mg/day.
  *Prophylaxis of migraine.*
50–100 mg/day.
  *Ventricular arrhythmias.*
50–100 mg/day.
  *Prior to coronary artery bypass surgery.*
50 mg/day started 72 hr prior to surgery.
  Adjust dosage in cases of renal failure to 50 mg/day if creatinine clearance is 15–35 mL/min/1.73 m² and to 50 mg every other day if crea-

tinine clearance is less than 15 mL/min/1.73 m².
• **IV**
  *Acute myocardial infarction.*
**Initial:** 5 mg over 5 min followed by a second 5-mg dose 10 min later. Begin treatment as soon as possible after client arrives at the hospital. In clients who tolerate the full 10-mg dose, give a 50-mg tablet 10 min after the last IV dose followed by another 50-mg dose 12 hr later. **Then,** 100 mg/day or 50 mg b.i.d. for 6–9 days (or until discharge from the hospital).

## DENTAL CONCERNS

See also *Dental Concerns* for *Antihypertensive Agents* and *Beta-Adrenergic Blocking Agents.*
**Client/Family Teaching**
1. Review the importance of good oral hygiene in order to prevent soft tissue inflammation.
2. Review the proper use of oral hygiene aids in order to prevent injury.
3. Daily home fluoride treatments for persistent dry mouth.
4. Avoid alcohol-containing mouth rinses and beverages.
5. Avoid caffeine-containing beverages.
6. Dry mouth can be treated with tart, sugarless gum or candy, water, sugar-free beverages, or with saliva substitutes if dry mouth persists.

## Atorvastatin calcium
(ah-**TORE**-vah-**stah**-tin)
**Pregnancy Category:** X
Lipitor **(Rx)**
**Classification:** Antihyperlipidemic, HMG–CoA reductase inhibitor

See also *Antihyperlipidemic Agents—HMG–CoA Reductase Inhibitors.*

**Action/Kinetics:** Atorvastatin undergoes first-pass metabolism. $t^1/_2$: 14 hr. The drug is over 98% bound to plasma proteins. Plasma levels are not affected by renal disease but they are markedly increased with chronic alcoholic liver disease.

**Uses:** Adjunct to diet to reduce elevated total and LDL cholesterol levels in primary hypercholesterolemia (Types IIa and IIb) when the response to diet and other nondrug measures alone have been inadequate.

**Contraindications:** Active liver disease or unexplained persistently high liver function tests. Pregnancy, lactation.

**Special Concerns:** Safety and efficacy have not been determined in children less than 18 years of age.

**Side Effects:** See also *Antihyperlipidemic Agents—HMG–CoA Reductase Inhibitors. GI:* Altered liver function tests (usually within the first 3 months of therapy). *Musculoskeletal:* Myalgia. *Miscellaneous:* Infection, hypersensitivity reactions, photosensitivity.

**Drug Interactions**
*Antacids* / ↓ Atorvastatin plasma levels
*Erythromycin* / ↑ Plasma levels of erythromycin

**How Supplied:** *Tablets:* 10 mg, 20 mg, 40 mg

**Dosage** ────────────
- **Tablets**
  *Hyperlipidemia.*
**Initial:** 10 mg/day; **then,** a dose range of 10–80 mg/day may be used.

## DENTAL CONCERNS

See also *Dental Concerns* for *Antihyperlipidemic Agents—HMG-CoA Reductase Inhibitors.*

─────────────

# Atovaquone
(ah-**TOV**-ah-kwohn)
**Pregnancy Category:** C
Mepron **(Rx)**
**Classification:** Antiprotozoal agent

**Action/Kinetics:** The mechanism of action of atovaquone against *Pneumocystis carinii* is not known. However, it may inhibit the synthesis of ATP and nucleic acids. The bioavailability of the drug is increased twofold when taken with food. The tablet formulation has been replaced by a suspension, as the latter achieves plasma levels of atovaquone that are 58% higher than those reached using tablets. Plasma levels in AIDS clients are about one-third to one-half the levels achieved in asymptomatic HIV-infected volunteers. **t½:** 2.2 days in AIDS clients due to enterohepatic cycling and eventually fecal elimination. Not metabolized in the liver; over 94% is excreted unchanged in the feces.

**Uses:** Acute oral treatment of mild to moderate *P. carinii* in clients who are intolerant to trimethoprim-sulfamethoxazole. The drug has not been evaluated as an agent for prophylaxis of *P. carinii.* Not effective for concurrent pulmonary diseases such as bacterial, viral, or fungal pneumonia or in mycobacterial diseases.

**Contraindications:** Hypersensitivity to atovaquone or any components of the formulation; potentially life-threatening allergic reactions are possible.

**Special Concerns:** Use with caution during lactation and in elderly clients. There are no efficacy studies in children. GI disorders may limit absorption of atovaquone.

**Side Effects:** Since many clients taking atovaquone have complications of HIV disease, it is often difficult to distinguish side effects caused by atovaquone from symptoms caused by the underlying medical condition. *Dermatologic:* Rash (including maculopapular), pruritus. *Oral:* Candidiasis, taste perversion. *GI:* Nausea, diarrhea, vomiting, abdominal pain, constipation, dyspepsia. *CNS:* Headache, fever, insomnia, dizziness, anxiety, anorexia. *Respiratory:* Cough, sinusitis, rhinitis. *Hematologic:* Anemia, neutropenia. *Miscellaneous:* Asthenia, pain, sweating, hypoglycemia, hypotension, hyperglycemia, hyponatremia.

**Drug Interactions:** Since atovaquone is highly bound to plasma proteins (>99.9%), caution should be exercised when giving the drug with other highly plasma protein-bound drugs with narrow therapeutic indices as competition for binding may occur. **How Supplied:** *Suspension:* 750 mg/5 mL

Dosage ――――――――――――――
• **Suspension**
**Adults:** 750 mg (5 mL) given with food b.i.d. for 21 days (total daily dose: 1,500 mg).

## DENTAL CONCERNS
**General**
1. Examine patient for oral signs and symptoms of opportunistic infection.
2. Frequent recall in order to evaluate for signs and symptoms of side effects due to drug and disease.
3. Semisupine chair position may be necessary because of GI adverse effects.
4. Semisupine chair position may be necessary for patients with respiratory disease.
5. Patients on chronic drug therapy may develop blood dyscrasias. Symptoms include fever, sore throat, bleeding, and poor wound healing.
**Consultation with Primary Care Provider**
1. Medical consultation may be necessary in order to assess patient's ability to tolerate stress.
2. Medical consultation may be necessary in order to assess patient's level of disease control.
3. Patients with symptoms of blood dyscrasias should be referred to their primary care provider for complete blood counts. Treatment should be postponed until the results are known.
4. Acute oral infection may require consultation with health care provider.
**Client/Family Teaching**
1. Review the importance of good oral hygiene in order to prevent soft tissue inflammation.
2. Review the proper use of oral hygiene aids in order to prevent injury.
3. Improved dietary measures may

help to maintain oral and systemic health
4. Report oral sores, lesions, or bleeding to the dentist.
5. Update patient's dental record (medication/health history) as needed.

―――――――――――――――――――

## Atropine sulfate
(**AH**-troh-peen)
**Pregnancy Category:** C
Atropair, Atropine-1 Ophthalmic, Atropine Sulfate Ophthalmic, Atropine-Care Ophthalmic, Atropisol Ophthalmic, Dioptic's Atropine ✷, Isopto Atropine Ophthalmic, Minims Atropine ✷ **(Rx)**
**Classification:** Cholinergic blocking agent

―――――――――――――――――――

See also *Cholinergic Blocking Agents.*
**Action/Kinetics:** Atropine blocks the action of acetylcholine on postganglionic cholinergic receptors in smooth muscle, cardiac muscle, exocrine glands, urinary bladder, and the AV and SA nodes in the heart. Ophthalmologically, atropine blocks the effect of acetylcholine on the sphincter muscle of the iris and the accommodative muscle of the ciliary body. This results in dilation of the pupil (mydriasis) and paralysis of the muscles required to accommodate for close vision (cycloplegia). **Peak effect:** M*ydriasis,* 30–40 min; *cycloplegia,* 1–3 hr. **Recovery:** Up to 12 days. **Duration, PO:** 4–6 hr. **t½:** 2.5 hr. Metabolized by the liver although 30%–50% is excreted through the kidneys unchanged.
**Uses: PO:** Adjunct in peptic ulcer treatment. Irritable bowel syndrome. Adjunct in treatment of spastic disorders of the biliary tract. Urologic disorders, urinary incontinence. During anesthesia to control salivation and bronchial secretions. Has been used for parkinsonism but more effective drugs are available.
  **Parenteral:** Antiarrhythmic, adjunct in GI radiography. Prophylaxis of arrhythmias induced by succinyl-

―――――――――――――――――――

choline or surgical procedures. Reduce sinus bradycardia (severe) and syncope in hyperactive carotid sinus reflex. Prophylaxis and treatment of toxicity due to cholinesterase inhibitors, including organophosphate pesticides. Treatment of curariform block. As a preanesthetic or in dentistry to decrease secretions.

**Ophthalmologic:** Cycloplegic refraction or pupillary dilation in acute inflammatory conditions of the iris and uveal tract. *Non-FDA Approved Uses:* Treatment and prophylaxis of posterior synechiae; pre- and postoperative mydriasis; treatment of malignant glaucoma.

**Additional    Contraindications:** Ophthalmic use: Infants less than 3 months of age, primary glaucoma or a tendency toward glaucoma, adhesions between the iris and the lens, geriatric clients and others where undiagnosed glaucoma or excessive pressure in the eye may be present, in children who have had a previous severe systemic reaction to atropine.

**Special Concerns:** Use with caution in infants, small children, geriatric clients, diabetes, hypo- or hyperthyroidism, narrow anterior chamber angle, individuals with Down syndrome.

**Additional Side Effects:** *Ophthalmologic:* Blurred vision, stinging, increased intraocular pressure, contact dermatitis. Long-term use may cause irritation, photophobia, eczematoid dermatitis, conjunctivitis, hyperemia, or edema.

**How Supplied:** *Injection:* 0.05 mg/mL, 0.1 mg/mL, 0.4 mg/mL, 0.5 mg/mL, 0.8 mg/mL, 1 mg/mL; *Ophthalmic Ointment:* 1%; *Ophthalmic Solution:* 0.5%, 1%; *Tablet:* 0.4 mg

**Dosage** —————————
• **Tablets**
*Anticholinergic or antispasmodic.*
**Adults:** 0.3–1.2 mg q 4–6 hr. **Pediatric, over 41 kg:** same as adult; **29.5–41 kg:** 0.4 mg q 4–6 hr; **18.2–29.5 kg:** 0.3 mg q 4–6 hr; **10.9–18.2 kg:** 0.2 mg q 4–6 hr; **7.3–10.9 kg:** 0.15 mg q 4–6 hr; **3.2–7.3 kg:** 0.1 mg q 4–6 hr.

*Prophylaxis of respiratory tract secretions and excess salivation during anesthesia.*
**Adults:** 2 mg.
*Parkinsonism.*
**Adults:** 0.1–0.25 mg q.i.d.
• **IM, IV, SC**
*Anticholinergic.*
**Adults, IM, IV, SC:** 0.4–0.6 mg q 4–6 hr. **Pediatric, SC:** 0.01 mg/kg, not to exceed 0.4 mg (or 0.3 mg/m²).
*To reverse curariform blockade.*
**Adults, IV:** 0.6–1.2 mg given at the same time or a few minutes before 0.5–2 mg neostigmine methylsulfate (use separate syringes).
*Treatment of toxicity from cholinesterase inhibitors.*
**Adults, IV, initial:** 2–4 mg; **then,** 2 mg repeated q 5–10 min until muscarinic symptoms disappear and signs of atropine toxicity begin to appear. **Pediatric, IM, IV, initial:** 1 mg; **then,** 0.5–1 mg q 5–10 min until muscarinic symptoms disappear and signs of atropine toxicity appear.
*Treatment of mushroom poisoning due to muscarine.*
**Adults, IM, IV:** 1–2 mg q hr until respiratory effects decrease.
*Treatment of organophosphate poisoning.*
**Adults, IM, IV, initial:** 1–2 mg; **then,** repeat in 20–30 min (as soon as cyanosis has disappeared). Dosage may be continued for up to 2 days until symptoms improve.
*Arrhythmias.*
**Pediatric, IV:** 0.01–0.03 mg/kg.
*Prophylaxis of respiratory tract secretions, excessive salivation, succinylcholine- or surgical procedure-induced arrhythmias.*
**Pediatric, up to 3 kg, SC:** 0.1 mg; **7–9 kg:** 0.2 mg; **12–16 kg:** 0.3 mg; **20–27 kg:** 0.4 mg; **32 kg:** 0.5 mg; **41 kg:** 0.6 mg.
• **Ophthalmic Solution**
*Uveitis.*
**Adults:** 1–2 gtt instilled into the eye(s) up to q.i.d. **Children:** 1–2 gtt of the 0.5% solution into the eye(s) up to t.i.d.
*Refraction.*
**Adults:** 1–2 gtt of the 1% solution into the eye(s) 1 hr before refracting.

**Children:** 1–2 gtt of the 0.5% solution into the eye(s) b.i.d. for 1–3 days before refraction.
• **Ophthalmic Ointment**
Instill a small amount into the conjunctival sac up to t.i.d.

## DENTAL CONCERNS

See also *Dental Concerns* for *Cholinergic Blocking Agents*.
**General**
1. Oral dose should be given 30 to 60 minutes prior to dental procedure for drying effects.
2. Contact lenses should be removed prior to administration of drug because of drying effects.
3. Patients may experience dry, burning sensation in throat and may experience blurred vision.
4. This drug is only intended as a single-dose treatment; therefore chronic dry mouth should not be an issue.
5. Dark glasses may be necessary because of the irritating effect of the dental light.
**Consultation with Primary Care Provider**
1. Consultation may be necessary for patients with a history of GI disease, cardiac disease, or glaucoma.

# Azithromycin
(az-**zith**-roh-**MY**-sin)
**Pregnancy Category:** B
Zithromax **(Rx)**
**Classification:** Antibiotic, macrolide

**Action/Kinetics:** Azithromycin is an azalide antibiotic (subclass of macrolides) derived from erythromycin. The drug acts by binding to the 50S ribosomal subunit of susceptible organisms, thus interfering with microbial protein synthesis. Rapidly absorbed and distributed widely throughout the body. Food decreases the absorption of azithromycin. $t\frac{1}{2}$, **terminal:** 68 hr. A loading dose will achieve steady-state levels more quickly. Elimination is by biliary excretion of unchanged drug with a small amount being excreted through the kidneys.

**Uses: Adults:** Acute bacterial exacerbations of COPD due to *Hemophilus influenzae, Moraxella catarrhalis,* or *Streptococcus pneumoniae.* Required initial IV therapy in community-acquired pneumonia due to *S. pneumoniae, H. influenzae, M. catarrhalis, Legionella pneumophila,* and *Staphylococcus aureus.* Those who can take PO therapy in community-acquired pneumonia due to *Chlamydia pneumoniae, Mycoplasma pneumoniae, S. pneumoniae, or H. influenzae.* Used alone or with rifabutin for prophylaxis of *Mycobacterium avium* complex (MAC) disease in clients with advanced HIV infections. PO for genital ulcer disease in men due to *Haemophilus ducreyi.* Initial IV therapy in pelvic inflammatory disease due to *Chlamydia trachomatis, Neisseria gonorrhoeae,* or *Mycoplasma hominis.* As an alternative to first-line therapy to treat streptococcal pharyngitis or tonsillitis due to *Streptococcus pyogenes.* PO for uncomplicated skin and skin structure infections due to *S. aureus, Staphylococcus pyogenes,* or *Streptococcus agalactiae.* Abscesses usually require surgical drainage. PO for urethritis and cervicitis due to *C. trachomatis* or *N. gonorrhoeae.*

**Children:** PO for acute otitis media due to *H. influenzae, M. catarrhalis,* or *S. pneumoniae* in children over 6 months of age. PO for community-acquired pneumonia due to *C. pneumoniae, H. influenzae, M. pneumoniae,* or *S. pneumoniae* in children over 6 months of age. Pharyngitis/tonsillitis due to *S. pyogenes* in children over 2 years of age who cannot use first-line therapy.

**Contraindications:** Hypersensitivity to azithromycin, any macrolide antibiotic, or erythromycin. In clients who are not eligible for outpatient PO therapy (e.g., known or suspected bacteremia, immunodeficiency, functional asplenia, nosocomially acquired infections, geriatric or debilitated clients).

**Special Concerns:** Use with caution in clients with impaired hepatic or renal function and during lactation. Safety and efficacy for acute otitis media have not been determined in children less than 6 months of age or for pharyngitis/tonsillits in children less than 2 years of age. Recommended doses should not be relied upon to treat gonorrhea or syphilis.

**Side Effects:** *Oral:* Oral candidiasis, stomatitis. *GI:* N&V, diarrhea, loose stools, abdominal pain, dyspepsia, flatulence, melena, cholestatic jaundice, pseudomembranous colitis. In children, gastritis, constipation, and anorexia have also been noted. *CNS:* Dizziness, headache, somnolence, fatigue, vertigo. In children, hyperkinesia, agitation, nervousness, insomnia, fever, and malaise have also been noted. *CV:* Chest pain, palpitations, **ventricular arrhythmias (including ventricular tachycardia and torsades de pointes in clients with prolonged QT intervals observed with other macrolides).** *GU:* Monilia, nephritis, vaginitis. *Allergic:* Angioedema, photosensitivity, rash, **anaphylaxis.** *Hematologic:* Leukopenia, neutropenia, decreased platelet count. *Miscellaneous:* Superinfection, local IV site reactions. In children, rash, conjunctivitis, and chest pain have also been noted.

**Drug Interactions:** See also *Drug Interactions* for *Erythromycins.*
*Aluminum- and magnesium-containing antacids /* ↑ Peak serum levels of azithromycin but not the total amount absorbed
*Carbamazepine /* ↑ Serum levels of carbamazepine due to ↓ metabolism
*Cyclosporine /* ↑ Serum levels of cyclosporine due to ↓ metabolism
*Digoxin /* ↑ Digoxin levels
*Ergot alkaloids /* Acute ergot toxicity, including severe peripheral vasospasm and dysesthesia
*Phenytoin /* ↑ Serum levels of phenytoin due to ↓ metabolism

*Tacrolimus /* Azithromycin may ↑ plasma levels of tacrolimus → ↑ risk of toxicity
*Terfenadine /* ↑ Serum levels of terfenadine due to ↓ metabolism
*Triazolam /* ↓ Clearance of triazolam → ↑ effect

**How Supplied:** *Capsule:* 250 mg; *Powder for Reconstitution:* 100 mg/5 mL, 200 mg/5 mL, 1 gm/packet; *Tablet:* 600 mg

**Dosage** ─────────────

• **Capsules, Suspension, Tablets**
*Adults: Mild to moderate acute bacterial exacerbations of COPD, mild community-acquired pneumonia, second-line therapy for pharyngitis/tonsillitis; uncomplicated skin and skin structure infections, prophylaxis of bacterial endocarditis.*
**Adults and children over 16 years of age:** 500 mg as a single dose on day 1 followed by 250 mg once daily on days 2–5 for a total dose of 1.5 g.
*Nongonococcal urethritis and cervicitis due to C. trachomatis or genital ulcer disease due to H. ducreyi.*
1 g given as a single dose.
*Gonococcal urethritis/cervicitis due to N. gonnorheae.*
2 g given as a single dose.
*Prophylaxis of bacterial endocarditis.*
**Adults:** 500 mg 1 hour before procedure. **Children:** 50 mg/kg PO 1 hour before procedure.

• **Tablets**
*Prophylaxis of M. avium complex in advanced HIV infections.*
1,200 mg once a week (two 600-mg tablets).

• **Oral Suspension**
*Pediatric: otitis media or community-acquired pneumonia.*
10 mg/kg (not to exceed 500 mg) on day 1, followed by 5 mg/kg (not to exceed 250 mg/day) on days 2–5.
*Pediatric: pharyngitis/tonsillitis.*
12 mg/kg/day for 5 days, not to exceed 500 mg/day.

• **IV**
*Community-acquired pneumonia.*

500 mg IV as a single daily dose for at least 2 days followed by a single daily dose of 500 mg PO to complete a 7- to 10-day course of therapy.

*Pelvic inflammatory disease.*
500 mg IV as a single daily dose for 1 or 2 days followed by a single daily dose of 250 mg PO to complete a 7-day course of therapy.

### DENTAL CONCERNS

See also *Dental Concerns* for *Erythromycins.*
**Client/Family Teaching**
1. Do not administer capsules with meals because food decreases absorption.
2. Avoid ingesting aluminum- or magnesium-containing antacids simultaneously with azithromycin.
3. Notify provider if N&V or diarrhea is excessive.
4. Avoid sun exposure and use protection when necessary.
5. Report if no symptom improvement after 48–72 hr.
6. Use an additional nonhormonal form of birth control if taking oral contraceptives because their effectiveness may be diminished.

**B**

# Beclomethasone dipropionate

(be-kloh-**METH**-ah-zohn)
**Pregnancy Category:** C
**Aerosol Inhaler:** Alti-Beclomethasone Dipropionate ✦, Beclodisk Diskhaler ✦, Becloforte Inhaler ✦, Beclovent, Beclovent Rotacaps or Rotahaler ✦, Vanceril, Vanceril DS **(Rx)**, **Intranasal:** Beclodisk for Oral Inhalation ✦, Beconase AQ Nasal, Beconase Inhalation, Gen-Beclo Aq. ✦, Vancenase AQ 84 mcg Double Strength, Vancenase AQ Forte, Vancenase AQ Nasal, Vancenase Nasal Inhaler **(Rx)**, **Topical:** Propaderm ✦
**Classification:** Glucocorticoid

See also *Corticosteroids.*
**Action/Kinetics:** t½: 15 hr. Rapidly inactivated, thereby resulting in few systemic effects.

*NOTE:* If a client is on systemic steroids, transfer to beclomethasone may be difficult because recovery from impaired renal function may be slow.
**Uses:** Relief of symptoms of seasonal or perennial rhinitis in clients not responsive to more conventional therapy, to prevent recurrence of nasal polyps following surgical removal, and to treat allergic or nonallergic (vasomotor) rhinitis (spray formulations). Inhalation therapy for chronic use in bronchial asthma. In glucocorticoid-dependent clients, beclomethasone often permits a decrease in the dosage of the systemic agent. Withdrawal of systemic corticosteroids must be carried out gradually.
**Contraindications:** Status asthmaticus, acute episodes of asthma, hypersensitivity to drug or aerosol ingredients.
**Special Concerns:** Safe use during lactation and in children under 6 years of age not established.
**Side Effects:** *Intranasal:* Headache, pharyngitis, coughing, epistaxis, nasal burning, pain, conjunctivitis, myalgia, tinnitus. Rarely, ulceration of the nasal mucosa and nasal septum perforation. *Oral:* Dry mouth, candidiasis.
**How Supplied:** *Metered dose inhaler:* 0.042 mg/inh; *Nasal Spray:* 0.042 mg/inh, 0.084 mg/inh

**Dosage**

• **Metered Dose Inhaler**

---

✦ = Available in Canada    ***bold italic*** = life-threatening side effect

*Asthma.*
*Beclovent.* **Adults:** 2 inhalations (total of 84 mcg beclomethasone) t.i.d.–q.i.d. In some clients, 4 inhalations (168 mcg) b.i.d. have been effective. Do not exceed 20 inhalations (840 mcg) daily. **Pediatric, 6–12 years:** 1–2 inhalations (42–84 mcg) t.i.d.–q.i.d. In some, 4 inhalations (168 mcg) b.i.d. have been effective. Do not to exceed 10 inhalations (420 mcg) daily. Dosage has not been determined in children less than 6 years of age.

*Vanceril.* **Adults:** 2 inhalations (total of 168 mcg) b.i.d. In those with severe asthma, start with 6–8 inhalations/day and adjust dose downward as determined by client response. Do not exceed 10 inhalations (840 mcg) daily. **Children, 6–12 years:** 2 inhalations (168 mcg) b.i.d. Do not exceed 5 inhalations (420 mcg) daily. Dosage has not been determined in children less than 6 years of age.

*NOTE:* Vanceril DS can be used once daily for treatment of asthma.

In clients also receiving systemic glucocorticosteroids, beclomethasone should be started when client's condition is relatively stable.
* **Nasal Aerosol or Spray**
*Allergic or nonallergic rhinitis, Prophylaxis of nasal polyps.*
**Adults and children over 12 years:** 1 inhalation (42 mcg) in each nostril b.i.d.–q.i.d. (i.e., total daily dose: 168–336 mcg). If no response after 3 weeks, discontinue therapy. **Maintenance, usual:** 1 inhalation in each nostril t.i.d. (252 mcg/day). For nasal polyps, treatment may be required for several weeks or more before a therapeutic effect can be assessed fully. Two sprays of the double-strength product (Vancenase AQ 84 mcg Double Strength) are administered once daily.

Vancenase AQ Forte may be used once daily for treatment of rhinitis.

## DENTAL CONCERNS
### General
1. Monitor vital signs at every appointment because of cardiovascular and respiratory side effects.
2. The patient may require a semi-supine position for the dental chair to help with breathing.
3. Dental procedures may cause the patient anxiety which could result in an asthma attack. Make sure that the patient has his or her sympathomimetic inhaler present or have the inhaler from the office emergency kit present.
4. Morning and shorter appointments, as well as methods for addressing anxiety levels in the patient, can help to reduce the amount of stress that the patient is experiencing.
5. Sulfites present in vasoconstrictors can precipitate an asthma attack.
6. Decreased saliva flow can put the patient at risk for dental caries, periodontal disease, and candidiasis.
### Consultation with Primary Care Provider
1. Consultation may be necessary in order to evaluate the patient's level of disease control.
2. Consultation may be necessary in order to determine the patient's ability to tolerate stress.
### Client/Family Teaching
1. Daily home fluoride treatments for persistent dry mouth.
2. Avoid alcohol-containing mouth rinses and beverages.
3. Avoid caffeine-containing beverages.
4. Dry mouth can be treated with tart, sugarless gum or candy, water, sugar-free beverages, or with saliva substitutes if dry mouth persists.
5. Review use, care, and storage of inhaler. Rinse out mouth and wash the mouth piece, spacer, sprayer and dry after each use.
6. Review technique for use and care of prescribed inhalers and respiratory equipment. Rinsing of equipment and of mouth after use is imperative in preventing oral fungal infections.

# Benazepril hydrochloride

(beh-**NAYZ**-eh-prill)
**Pregnancy Category:** D
Lotensin **(Rx)**
**Classification:** Antihypertensive, ACE inhibitor

See also *Angiotensin-Converting Enzyme Inhibitors*

**Action/Kinetics:** Both supine and standing BPs are reduced with mild-to-moderate hypertension and no compensatory tachycardia. Also an antihypertensive effect in clients with low-renin hypertension. Food does not affect the extent of absorption. Almost completely converted to the active benazeprilat, which has greater ACE inhibitor activity. **Onset:** 1 hr. **Duration:** 24 hr. **Peak plasma levels, benazepril:** 30–60 min. **Peak plasma levels, benazeprilat:** 1–2 hr if fasting and 2–4 hr if not fasting. **t½, benazeprilat:** 10–11 hr. **Peak reduction in BP:** 2–4 hr after dosing. **Peak effect with chronic therapy:** 1–2 weeks. Highly bound to plasma protein and excreted through the urine with about 20% of a dose excreted as benazeprilat.

**Uses:** Alone or in combination with thiazide diuretics to treat hypertension.

**Contraindications:** Hypersensitivity to benazepril or any other ACE inhibitor.

**Special Concerns:** Use with caution during lactation. Safety and effectiveness have not been determined in children.

**Side Effects:** *CNS:* Headache, dizziness, fatigue, anxiety, insomnia, nervousness. *GI:* N&V, constipation, abdominal pain, melena. *CV:* Symptomatic hypotension, postural hypotension, syncope, angina pectoris, palpitations, peripheral edema, ECG changes. *Dermatologic:* Dermatitis, pruritus, rash, flushing, diaphoresis. *GU:* Decreased libido, impotence, UTI. *Respiratory:* Cough, asthma, bronchitis, dyspnea, sinusitis, bronchospasm. *Neuromuscular:* Paresthesias, arthralgia, arthritis, as-

thenia, myalgia. *Hematologic:* Occasionally, eosinophilia, leukopenia, neutropenia, decreased hemoglobin. *Miscellaneous:* Angioedema, which may be associated with involvement of the tongue, glottis, or larynx; hypertonia; proteinuria; hyponatremia; infection.

**Drug Interactions:** See also *Angiotensin-Converting Enzyme Inhibitors*

**How Supplied:** *Tablet:* 5 mg, 10 mg, 20 mg, 40 mg

## Dosage

• **Tablets**
*Clients not receiving a diuretic.*
**Initial:** 10 mg once daily; **maintenance:** 20–40 mg/day given as a single dose or in two equally divided doses. Total daily doses greater than 80 mg have not been evaluated.
*Clients receiving a diuretic.*
**Initial:** 5 mg/day.
*Ccr < 30 mL/min/1.73 m².* The recommended starting dose is 5 mg/day; **maintenance:** titrate dose upward until BP is controlled or to a maximum total daily dose of 40 mg.

### DENTAL CONCERNS

See also *Dental Concerns* for *Angiotensin-Converting Enzyme Inhibitors* and *Antihypertensive Agents.*

# Benztropine mesylate

(**BENS**-troh-peen)
**Pregnancy Category:** C
Apo-Benztropine ✝, Cogentin, PMS-Benztropine ✝ **(Rx)**
**Classification:** Synthetic anticholinergic, antiparkinson agent

See also *Cholinergic Blocking Agents.*

**Action/Kinetics:** Synthetic anticholinergic possessing antihistamine and local anesthetic properties. **Onset, PO:** 1–2 hr; **IM, IV:** Within a few minutes. Effects are cumulative; is long-acting (24 hr). Full effects are manifested in 2–3 days. Low incidence of side effects.

---

*bold italic* = life-threatening side effect

**B**

**Uses:** Adjunct in the treatment of parkinsonism (all types). To reduce severity of extrapyramidal effects in phenothiazine or other antipsychotic drug therapy (not effective in tardive dyskinesia).

**Special Concerns:** Not recommended for children under 3 years of age. Geriatric and emaciated clients cannot tolerate large doses. Certain drug-induced extrapyramidal symptoms may not respond to benztropine.

**How Supplied:** *Injection:* 1 mg/mL; *Tablet:* 0.5 mg, 1 mg, 2 mg

**Dosage** ————————————
• **Tablets**
  *Parkinsonism.*
  **Adults:** 1–2 mg/day (range: 0.5–6 mg/day).
  *Idiopathic parkinsonism.*
  **Adults, initial:** 0.5–1 mg/day, increased gradually to 4–6 mg/day, if necessary.
  *Postencephalitic parkinsonism.*
  **Adults:** 2 mg/day in one or more doses.
  *Drug-induced extrapyramidal effects.*
  **Adults:** 1–4 mg 1–2 times/day.
• **IM, IV (Rarely)**
  *Acute dystonic reactions.*
  **Adults, initial:** 1–2 mg; **then,** 1–2 mg PO b.i.d. usually prevents recurrence. Clients can rarely tolerate full dosage.

————————————

## DENTAL CONCERNS

See also *Dental Concerns* for *Cholinergic Blocking Agents*.
1. Avoid using ingestible sodium bicarbonate products within 1 hour of taking benztropine mesylate.

# Betaxolol hydrochloride
(beh-**TAX**-oh-lohl)
**Pregnancy Category:** C
Betoptic, Betoptic S, Kerlone **(Rx)**
**Classification:** Beta-adrenergic blocking agent
————————————
See also *Beta-Adrenergic Blocking Agents*.

**Action/Kinetics:** Inhibits beta-1-adrenergic receptors although beta-2 receptors will be inhibited at high doses. Has some membrane stabilizing activity but no intrinsic sympathomimetic activity. Low lipid solubility. When used in the eye, betaxolol reduces the production of aqueous humor, thus, reducing intraocular pressure. It has no effect on pupil size or accommodation. **t½:** 14–22 hr. Metabolized in the liver with most excreted through the urine; about 15% is excreted unchanged.

**Uses: PO:** Hypertension, alone or with other antihypertensive agents (especially diuretics). **Ophthalmic:** Ocular hypertension and chronic open-angle glaucoma (used alone or in combination with other antiglaucoma drugs).

**Contraindications:** Oral Tablets: Hypersensitivity to betaxolol, cardiogenic shock, 2nd or 3rd degree heart block, sinus bradycardia, congestive heart failure, cardiac failure. Ophthalmic Drops: Hypersensitivity to beta-blockers, cardiogenic shock, 2nd or 3rd degree heart block, sinus bradycardia, congestive heart failure, right ventricular failure, congenital glaucoma (infants), COPD.

**Special Concerns:** Use with caution during lactation. Geriatric clients are at greater risk of developing bradycardia. Aortic or mitral valve disease, asthma, COPD, diabetes mellitus, major surgery, renal disease, thyroid disease, well-compensated heart failure.

**Side Effects:** *Oral:* Dry mouth. *CV:* Bradycardia, dysrhythmias, hypotension. *CNS:* Depression, dizziness, fatigue, insomnia, lethargy. *GI:* Diarrhea, dyspepsia, vomiting. *Hematologic:* **Aranulocytosis**, thrombocytopenia. *Skin:* Pruritus, rash, increased skin pigmentation, sweating, dry skin, alopecia, skin irritation, psoriasis. *Ophthalmic:* Dry, burning eyes, conjunctivitis, keratitis. *GU:* Impotence. *Respiratory:* **Bronchospasm**, dyspnea, pharyngitis.

**Drug Interactions:** See also Drug Interactions of concern to the dental practitioner for *Beta-Adrenergic Blocking Agents* and *Antihypertensive Agents*.

**How Supplied:** *Ophthalmic Solution:* 0.5%; *Ophthalmic Suspension:* 0.25%; *Tablet:* 10 mg, 20 mg

**Dosage**
• **Tablets**
*Hypertension.*
**Initial:** 10 mg once daily either alone or with a diuretic. If the desired effect is not reached, the dose can be increased to 20 mg although doses higher than 20 mg will not increase the therapeutic effect. In geriatric clients the initial dose should be 5 mg/day.
• **Ophthalmic Solution, Suspension**
**Adults:** 1–2 gtt b.i.d. If used to replace another drug, continue the drug being used and add 1 gtt of betaxolol b.i.d. The previous drug should be discontinued the following day. If transferring from several antiglaucoma drugs being used together, adjust one drug at a time at intervals of not less than 1 week. The agents being used can be continued and add 1 gtt betaxolol b.i.d. The next day, another agent should be discontinued. The remaining antiglaucoma drug dosage can be decreased or discontinued depending on the response of the client.

**DENTAL CONCERNS**

See also *Dental Concerns* for *Beta-Adrenergic Blocking Agents* and *Antihypertensive Agents*.
**Client/Family Teaching**
1. Review the importance of good oral hygiene in order to prevent soft tissue inflammation.
2. Review the proper use of oral hygiene aids to prevent injury.
3. Daily home fluoride treatments for persistent dry mouth.
4. Avoid alcohol-containing mouth rinses and beverages.
5. Avoid caffeine-containing beverages.
6. Dry mouth can be treated with tart, sugarless gum or candy, water, sugar-free beverages, or with saliva substitutes if dry mouth persists.
7. You may want to wear dark glasses to avoid photophobia, which can occur with the dental light.

# Bethanechol chloride
(beh-**THAN**-eh-kohl)
**Pregnancy Category:** C
Duvoid, Myotonachol, PMS-Bethanechol Chloride ✦, Urecholine **(Rx)**
**Classification:** Cholinergic (parasympathomimetic), direct-acting

**Action/Kinetics:** Directly stimulates cholinergic receptors, primarily muscarinic type. This results in stimulation of gastric motility, increases gastric tone, and stimulates the detrusor muscle of the urinary bladder. Produces a slight transient fall of DBP, accompanied by minor reflex tachycardia. The drug is resistant to hydrolysis by acetylcholinesterase, which increases its duration of action. **PO: Onset,** 30–90 min; **maximum:** 60–90 min; **duration:** up to 6 hr. **SC: Onset,** 5–15 min; **maximum:** 15–30 min; **duration:** 2 hr.
**Uses:** Postpartum or postoperative urinary retention, neurogenic atony of the bladder with urinary retention. *Non-FDA Approved Uses:* Reflux esophagitis in adults and gastroesophageal reflux in infants and children.
**Contraindications:** Hypotension, hypertension, CAD, coronary occlusion, AV conduction defects, vasomotor instability, pronounced bradycardia, peptic ulcer, asthma (latent or active), hyperthyroidism, parkinsonism, epilepsy, obstruction of the bladder, if the strength or integrity of the GI or bladder wall is questionable, peritonitis, GI spastic disease, inflammatory lesions of the GI tract, marked vagotonia. Not to be used IM or IV.
**Special Concerns:** Use with caution during lactation. Safety and effectiveness have not been determined in children.

**Side Effects:** Serious side effects are uncommon with PO dosage but more common following SC use. *Oral:* Salivation. *GI:* Nausea, diarrhea, GI upset, involuntary defecation, cramps, colic, belching, rumbling/gurgling of stomach. *CV:* Hypotension with reflex tachycardia, vasomotor response. *CNS:* Headache, malaise. *Other:* Flushing, sensation of heat about the face, sweating, urinary urgency, attacks of asthma, bronchial constriction, miosis, lacrimation.

**Drug Interactions**
*Cholinergic inhibitors* / Additive cholinergic effects

**How Supplied:** *Injection:* 5 mg/mL; *Tablet:* 5 mg, 10 mg, 25 mg, 50 mg

**Dosage** ⎯⎯⎯⎯⎯⎯⎯⎯⎯
• **Tablets**
*Urinary retention.*
**Adults, usual:** 10–50 mg t.i.d.–q.i.d. The minimum effective dose can be determined by giving 5–10 mg initially and repeating this dose q 1–2 hr until a satisfactory response is observed or a maximum of 50 mg has been given.
*Treat reflux esophagitis in adults.*
25 mg q.i.d.
*Gastroesophageal reflex in infants and children.*
3 mg/m²/dose t.i.d.
• **SC**
*Urinary retention.*
**Adults, usual:** 5 mg t.i.d.–q.i.d. The minimum effective dose is determined by giving 2.5 mg initially and repeating this dose at 15–30-min intervals to a maximum of four doses or until a satisfactory response is obtained.
*Diagnosis of reflux esophagitis in adults.*
Two 50-mcg/kg doses 15 min apart.

## DENTAL CONCERNS
**General**
1. Monitor vital signs at every appointment because of cardiovascular side effects.
2. Have the patient sit up slowly and remain seated for at least two minutes after being supine in order to minimize the risk of orthostatic hypotension.

**Consultation with Primary Care Provider**
1. Excessive salivation is usually limited to treatment duration. If it persists, the patient should consult with the appropriate health care provider.

# Biperiden hydrochloride
(bye-**PER**-ih-den)
**Pregnancy Category:** C
Akineton Hydrochloride **(Rx)**
**Classification:** Synthetic anticholinergic, antiparkinson agent

See also *Antiparkinson Drugs* and *Cholinergic Blocking Agents.*
**Action/Kinetics:** Tolerance may develop to this synthetic anticholinergic. Tremor may increase as spasticity is relieved. Slight respiratory and CV effects. **Time to peak levels:** 60–90 min. **Peak levels:** 4–5 mcg/L. **t½:** About 18–24 hr.
**Uses:** Parkinsonism, especially of the postencephalitic, arteriosclerotic, and idiopathic types. Drug-induced (e.g., phenothiazines) extrapyramidal manifestations.
**Additional Contraindications:** Children under the age of 3 years.
**Special Concerns:** Use with caution in older children.
**Additional Side Effects:** Muscle weakness, inability to move certain muscles.
**How Supplied:** *Tablet:* 2 mg.

**Dosage** ⎯⎯⎯⎯⎯⎯⎯⎯⎯
• **Tablets**
*Parkinsonism.*
**Adults:** 2 mg t.i.d.–q.i.d., to a maximum of 16 mg/day.
*Drug-induced extrapyramidal effects.*
**Adults:** 2 mg 1–3 times/day. Maximum daily dose: 16 mg.
**Adults:** 2 mg; repeat q 30 min until symptoms improve, but not more than four doses daily. **Pediatric:** 0.04 mg/kg (1.2 mg/m²); repeat q 30 min until symptoms improve, but not more than four doses daily.

## DENTAL CONCERNS

See also *Dental Concerns* for *Antiparkinson Drugs* and *Cholinergic Blocking Agents.*

---

# Bitolterol mesylate

(bye-**TOHL**-ter-ohl)
**Pregnancy Category:** C
Tornalate Aerosol **(Rx)**
**Classification:** Bronchodilator

---

See also *Sympathomimetic Drugs.*
**Action/Kinetics:** Bitolterol is a pro-drug in that it is converted by esterases in the body to the active colterol. Colterol combines with beta-2-adrenergic receptors, producing dilation of bronchioles. Minimal beta-1-adrenergic activity. **Onset following inhalation:** 3–4 min. **Time to peak effect:** 30–60 min. **Duration:** 5–8 hr.
**Uses:** Prophylaxis and treatment of bronchial asthma and bronchospasms. Treatment of bronchitis, emphysema, bronchiectasis, and COPD. May be used with theophylline and/or steroids.
**Special Concerns:** Safety has not been established for use during lactation and in children less than 12 years of age. Use with caution in ischemic heart disease, hypertension, hyperthyroidism, diabetes mellitus, cardiac arrhythmias, seizure disorders, or in those who respond unusually to beta-adrenergic agonists. There may be decreased effectiveness in steroid-dependent asthmatic clients. Hypersensitivity reactions may occur.
**Additional Side Effects:** *CNS:* Hyperactivity, hyperkinesia, lightheadedness. *CV:* Premature ventricular contractions. *Other:* Throat irritation.
**Drug Interactions:** Additive effects with other beta-adrenergic bronchodilators.
**How Supplied:** *Metered dose inhaler:* 0.37 mg/inh; *Solution:* 0.2%

**Dosage** ————————
• **Metered Dose Inhaler**
  *Bronchodilation.*

**Adults and children over 12 years:** 2 inhalations at an interval of 1–3 min q 8 hr (if necessary, a third inhalation may be taken). The dose should not exceed 3 inhalations q 6 hr or 2 inhalations q 4 hr.
  *Prophylaxis of bronchospasm.*
**Adults and children over 12 years:** 2 inhalations q 8 hr.

---

## DENTAL CONCERNS

See also *Dental Concerns* for *Sympathomimetic Drugs.*

---

# Bretylium tosylate

(breh-**TILL**-ee-um **TOZ**-ill-ayt)
**Pregnancy Category:** C
Bretylate Parenteral ✶, Bretylol **(Rx)**
**Classification:** Antiarrhythmic, class III

**Action/Kinetics:** Bretylium inhibits catecholamine release at nerve endings by decreasing excitability of the nerve terminal. Initially there is a release of norepinephrine, which may cause tachycardia and a rise in BP; this is followed by a blockade of release of catecholamines. The drug also increases the duration of the action potential and the effective refractory period, which may assist in reversing arrhythmias. **Peak plasma concentration and effect:** 1 hr after IM injection. Antifibrillatory effect within a few minutes after IV use. Suppression of ventricular tachycardia and ventricular arrhythmias takes 20–120 min, whereas suppression of PVCs does not occur for 6–9 hr. **Therapeutic serum levels:** 0.5–1.5 mcg/mL. **t½:** Approximately 5–10 hr. **Duration:** 6–8 hr. From 0% to 8% is protein bound. Up to 90% of drug is excreted unchanged in the urine over 24 hr.
**Uses:** Life-threatening ventricular arrhythmias that have failed to respond to other antiarrhythmics. Prophylaxis and treatment of ventricular fibrillation. For short-term use only. *Non-FDA Approved Uses:* Second-line drug (after lidocaine) for advanced cardiac life support during CPR.

---

***bold italic*** = life-threatening side effect

**Contraindications:** Severe aortic stenosis, severe pulmonary hypertension.

**Special Concerns:** Safety and efficacy in children have not been established. Dosage adjustment is required in clients with impaired renal function.

**Side Effects:** *CV:* Hypotension (including postural hypotension), transient hypertension, increased frequency of PVCs, bradycardia, precipitation of anginal attacks, initial increase in arrhythmias, sensation of substernal pressure. *GI:* N&V (especially after rapid IV administration), diarrhea, abdominal pain, hiccoughs. *CNS:* Vertigo, dizziness, lightheadedness, syncope, anxiety, paranoid psychosis, confusion, mood swings. *Miscellaneous:* Renal dysfunction, flushing, hyperthermia, SOB, nasal stuffiness, diaphoresis, conjunctivitis, erythematous macular rash, lethargy, generalized tenderness.

**Drug Interactions**
*Digitoxin, Digoxin* / Bretylium may aggravate digitalis toxicity due to initial release of norepinephrine
*Procainamide, Quinidine* / Concomitant use with bretylium ↓ inotropic effect of bretylium and ↑ hypotension

**How Supplied:** *Injection:* 50 mg/mL

**Dosage** ────────────
• **IV**
*Ventricular fibrillation, hemodynamically unstable ventricular tachycardia.*
**Adults:** 5 mg/kg of undiluted solution given rapidly. Can increase to 10 mg/kg if ventricular fibrillation persists; repeat as needed. **Maintenance, IV infusion:** 1–2 mg/min; or, 5–10 mg/kg q 6 hr of diluted drug infused over more than 8 min. **Children:** 5 mg/kg/dose IV followed by 10 mg/kg at 15–30-min intervals for a maximum total dose of 30 mg/kg; **maintenance:** 5–10 mg/kg q 6 hr.
*Other ventricular arrhythmias.*
• **IV Infusion**
5–10 mg/kg of diluted solution over more than 8 min. **Maintenance:** 5–10 mg/kg q 6 hr over a period of 8 min or more or 1–2 mg/min by continuous IV infusion. **Children:** 5–10 mg/kg/dose q 6 hr.
• **IM**
*Other ventricular arrhythmias.*
**Adults:** 5–10 mg/kg of undiluted solution followed, if necessary, by the same dose at 1–2-hr intervals; **then,** give same dosage q 6–8 hr.

## DENTAL CONCERNS

See also *Dental Concerns* for *Antiarrhythmic Agents.*

# Bromocriptine mesylate
(broh-moh-**KRIP**-teen)
**Pregnancy Category:** B
Alti-Bromocriptine ✱, Apo-Bromocriptine ✱, Parlodel **(Rx)**
**Classification:** Prolactin secretion inhibitor; antiparkinson agent

**Action/Kinetics:** Bromocriptine is a nonhormonal agent that inhibits the release of the hormone prolactin by the pituitary. Should be used only when prolactin production by pituitary tumors has been ruled out. Its effect in parkinsonism is due to a direct stimulating effect on dopamine type 2 receptors in the corpus striatum. Use for parkinsonism may allow the dose of levodopa to be decreased, thus decreasing the incidence of severe side effects following long-term levodopa therapy. Less than 30% of the drug is absorbed from the GI tract. **Onset, lower prolactin:** 2 hr; **antiparkinson:** 30–90 min; **decrease growth hormone:** 1–2 hr. **Peak plasma concentration:** 1–3 hr. **t½, plasma:** 6–8 hr; **terminal:** 15 hr. **Duration, lower prolactin:** 24 hr (after a single dose); **decrease growth hormone:** 4–8 hr. Significant first-pass effect. Metabolized in liver, excreted mainly through bile and thus the feces.

**Uses:** Short-term treatment of amenorrhea with or without galactorrhea, infertilitiy, or hypogonadism. Alone or as an adjunct in the treatment of acromegaly. As adjunctive therapy with levodopa in the treatment of idiopathic or postencephalitic Parkinson's disease. May provide additional benefit in clients who are taking optimal doses of levodopa, in those who are developing tolerance to levodopa therapy, or in those who are manifesting levodopa "end of dose failure." Clients unresponsive to levodopa are not good candidates for bromocriptine therapy. No longer recommended to suppress postpartum lactation. *Non-FDA Approved Uses:* Hyperprolactinemia due to pituitary adenoma, neuroleptic malignant syndrome, cocaine dependence, cyclical mastalgia.

**Contraindications:** Sensitivity to ergot alkaloids. Pregnancy, lactation, children under 15 years of age. Peripheral vascular disease, ischemic heart disease.

**Special Concerns:** Geriatric clients may manifest more CNS effects. Use with caution in liver or kidney disease.

**Side Effects:** The type and incidence of side effects depend on the use of the drug. *When used for hyperprolactinemia. Oral:* Dry mouth. *GI:* N&V, abdominal cramps, diarrhea, constipation. *CNS:* Headache, dizziness, fatigue, drowsiness, lightheadedness, psychoses. *Other:* Nasal congestion, hypotension, CSF rhinorrhea.

*When used for acromegaly. Oral:* Dry mouth. *GI:* N&V, anorexia, dyspepsia, indigestion, GI bleeding. *CNS:* Dizziness, syncope, drowsiness, tiredness, headache, lightheadedness, lassitude, vertigo, sluggishness, paranoia, insomnia, heavy headedness, decreased sleep requirement, delusional psychosis, visual hallucinations. *CV:* Orthostatic hypotension, digital vasospasm, Raynaud's syndrome; rarely, arrhythmias, ventricular tachycardia, bradycardia, vasovagal attack. *Respiratory:* Nasal stuffiness, SOB. *Other:* Potentiation of effects of alcohol, hair loss, paresthesia, tingling of ears, muscle cramps, facial pallor, reduced tolerance to cold.

*When used for parkinsonism. Oral:* Dry mouth. *GI:* N&V, abdominal discomfort, constipation, anorexia, dysphagia. *CNS:* Confusion, hallucinations, fainting, drowsiness, dizziness, insomnia, depression, vertigo, anxiety, fatigue, headache, lethargy, nightmares. *GU:* Urinary incontinence, urinary retention, urinary frequency. *Other:* Abnormal involuntary movements, asthenia, visual disturbances, ataxia, hypotension, SOB, edema of feet and ankles, blepharospasm, erythromelalgia, skin mottling, nasal stuffiness, paresthesia, skin rash.

**Drug Interactions**
*Alcohol* / ↑ Chance of GI toxicity; alcohol intolerance
*Butyrophenones* / ↓ Effect of bromocriptine because butyrophenones are dopamine antagonists
*Erythromycins* / ↑ Levels of bromocriptine → ↑ pharmacologic and toxic effects
*Phenothiazines* / ↓ Effect of bromocriptine because phenothiazines are dopamine antagonists
*Sympathomimetics* / ↑ Side effects of bromocriptine, including ventricular tachycardia and cardiac dysfunction

**How Supplied:** *Capsule:* 5 mg; *Tablet:* 2.5 mg

**Dosage** ─────────
• **Capsules, Tablets**
*For hyperprolactinemic conditions.*
**Adults, initial:** 0.5–2.5 mg/day with meals; **then,** increase dose by 2.5 mg q 3–7 days until optimum response observed (usual: 5–7.5 mg/day; range: 2.5–15 mg/day). For amenorrhea/galactorrhea, do not use for more than 6 months. Side effects may be reduced by temporarily decreasing the dose to ½ tablet 2–3 times/day.
*Parkinsonism.*
**Initial:** 1.25 mg (½ tablet) b.i.d. with meals while maintaining dose of levodopa, if possible. Dosage may be increased q 14–28 days by 2.5 mg/day

with meals. The usual dosage range is 10–40 mg/day. Any decrease in dosage should be done gradually in 2.5-mg decrements.

*Acromegaly.*
**Initial:** 1.25–2.5 mg for 3 days with food and on retiring; **then,** increased by 1.25–2.5 mg q 3–7 days until optimum response observed. Usual optimum therapeutic range: 20–30 mg/day, not to exceed 100 mg/day. Clients should be reevaluated monthly and dosage adjusted accordingly.

*Hyperprolactinemia associated with pituitary adenomas.*
**Maintenance:** 0.625–10 mg/day for 6 to 52 months.

## DENTAL CONCERNS
### General
1. Monitor vital signs at every appointment because of cardiovascular side effects.
2. Have the patient sit up slowly and remain seated for at least two minutes after being supine in order to minimize the risk of orthostatic hypotension.
3. Decreased saliva flow can put the patient at risk for dental caries, periodontal disease, and candidiasis.
4. Shorter appointments may be necessary because of the effects of Parkinson's disease on muscle.
### Consultation with Primary Care Provider
1. Consultation may be required in order to assess extent of disease control.
### Client/Family Teaching
1. Daily home fluoride treatments for persistent dry mouth.
2. Avoid alcohol-containing mouth rinses and beverages.
3. Avoid caffeine-containing beverages.
4. Dry mouth can be treated with tart, sugarless gum or candy, water, sugar-free beverages, or with saliva substitutes if dry mouth persists.

# Brompheniramine maleate
(brohm-fen-**EAR**-ah-meen)
**Pregnancy Category:** B

Brombay, Chlorphed, Conjec-B, Cophene-B, Diamine T.D., Dimetane Extentabs, Dimetane-Ten, Histaject Modified, Nasahist B, ND Stat Revised, Oraminic II, Sinusol-B, Veltane (Rx; Dimetane and Dimetane Extentabs are OTC)
**Classification:** Antihistamine, alkylamine type

See also *Antihistamines.*
**Action/Kinetics:** Fewer sedative effects. **t½:** 25 hr. **Time to peak effect:** 3–9 hr. **Duration:** 4–25 hr.
**Uses:** Allergic rhinitis (oral). Parenterally to treat allergic reactions to blood or plasma; adjunct to treat anaphylaxis; uncomplicated allergic conditions when PO therapy is not possible or is contraindicated.
**Contraindications:** Use in neonates.
**Special Concerns:** Geriatric clients may be more sensitive to the usual adult dose.
**How Supplied:** *Capsule:* 4 mg; *Elixir:* 2 mg/5 mL; *Injection:* 10 mg/mL; *Tablet:* 4 mg; *Tablet, Extended Release:* 12 mg

## Dosage
- **Liqui-Gels**
  *Allergic rhinitis.*
**Adults and children over 12 years:** 4 mg q 4–6 hr, not to exceed 24 mg/day.
- **IM, IV, SC**
**Adults: usual,** 10 mg (range: 5–20 mg) b.i.d. (maximum daily dose: 40 mg); **pediatric, under 12 years:** 0.5 mg/kg/day (15 mg/m² /day) divided into three or four doses.

## DENTAL CONCERNS

See also *Dental Concerns* for *Antihistamines.*

# Bupivacaine hydrochloride
(Byou-**piv**-a-kane)
**Pregnancy Category:** C
Marcaine, Sensorcaine, Sensorcaine-MPF

# Bupivacaine hydrochloride with epinephrine

Marcaine Hydrochloride with Epinephrine, Sensorcaine with Epinephrine, Sensorcaine-MPF with Epinephrine

Classification: Amide local anesthetic agents

See also *Amide Local Anesthetic Agents.*

**Action/Kinetics:** Blocks nerve action potential by inhibiting ion fluxes across the cell membrane. **Onset:** 4-17 mins, **Duration:** 4-12 hr, Renally excreted, metabolized by the liver.

**Uses:** Local dental anesthesia, caudal anesthesia, epidural anesthesia, peripheral nerve anesthesia.

**Contraindications:** Hypersensitivity, 0.75% solution in dentistry.

**Special Concerns:** See also *Amide Local Anesthetic Agents.*

**Side Effects:** See also *Amide Local Anesthetic Agents.*

**Drug Interactions:** See also *Amide Local Anesthetic Agents.*

**How Supplied:** *Injection:* 0.25%, 0.5%, 0.75%; *Injection with Epinephrine:* 1:200,000 in 0.25%, 0.5%, 0.75%

## Dosage

• **0.5% Injection with 200,000 Epinephrine**

*Infiltration or conduction block.*

**Adults:** 9-90 mg. Dose should be adjusted down for medically compromised, debilitated, or elderly patients. (See also *Appendix 9.*)

## DENTAL CONCERNS

See also *Dental Concerns* for *Amide Local Anesthetic Agents.*

# Bupropion hydrochloride

(byou-**PROH**-pee-on)

**Pregnancy Category:** B
Wellbutrin, Wellbutrin SR, Zyban **(Rx)**
Classification: Antidepressant, miscellaneous

**Action/Kinetics:** Bupropion is an antidepressant whose mechanism of action is not known; the drug does not inhibit MAO and it only weakly blocks neuronal uptake of epinephrine, serotonin, and dopamine. The drug exerts moderate anticholinergic and sedative effects, but only slight orthostatic hypotension. **Peak plasma levels:** 2-3 hr. t½: 8-24 hr. **Time to steady state:** 1.5-5 days. Significantly metabolized by a first-pass effect through the liver to both active and inactive metabolites. During chronic use the plasma levels of two active metabolites may be higher than bupropion. Excreted through both the urine (87%) and the feces (10%). Zyban is a sustained-release formulation.

**Uses:** Short-term (6 weeks or less) treatment of depression. Aid to stop smoking (may be combined with a nicotine transdermal system).

**Contraindications:** Seizure disorders; presence or history of bulimia or anorexia nervosa due to the higher incidence of seizures in such clients. Concomitant use of an MAO inhibitor. Wellbutrin, Wellbutrin SR, and Zyban all contain bupropion; do not use together.

**Special Concerns:** Use with caution in clients with a history of seizures, cranial trauma, with drugs that lower the seizure threshold, and other situations that might cause seizures (e.g., abrupt cessation of a benzodiazepine). Use with caution and in lower doses in clients with liver or kidney disease and in those with a recent history of MI or unstable heart disease. Assess benefits versus risks during lactation. Safety and efficacy have not been established in clients less than 18 years of age.

**Side Effects:** Listed are side effects with an incidence of 0.1% or greater. *CNS:* Insomnia, abnormal dreams, dizziness, disturbed concentration, nervousness, tremor, dysphoria, somnolence, agitation, abnormal thinking, depression, irritability, CNS stimulation, confusion, decreased libido, decreased memory, depersonalization, emotional lability, hostility, hyperkinesia, hypertonia, hypesthesia, paresthesia, suicidal ideation, vertigo. *Oral:* Dry mouth, gingivitis, glossitis, stomatitis, mouth ulcer. *GI:* Nausea, constipation, diarrhea, anorexia, thirst, increased appetite, dyspepsia, flatulence, vomiting, abnormal liver function, bruxism, dysphagia, gastric reflux, jaundice. *CV:* Palpitations, hypertension, flushing, migraine, postural hypotension, hot flashes, **stroke,** tachycardia, vasodilation. *Body as a whole:* Abdominal pain, accidental injury, neck pain, chest pain, facial edema, asthenia, fever, headache, back pain, chills, inguinal hernia, musculoskeletal chest pain, pain, photosensitivity. *Dermatologic:* Rash, pruritus, urticaria, dry skin, sweating, acne, dry skin. *Musculoskeletal:* Arthralgia, myalgia, leg cramps. *Respiratory:* Rhinitis, bronchitis, increased cough, pharyngitis, sinusitis, epistaxis, dyspnea. *GU:* Urinary frequency, impotence, polyuria, urinary urgency. *Ophthalmic:* Amblyopia, abnormal accommodation, dry eye. *Miscellaneous:* Taste perversion, tinnitus, ecchymosis, edema, increased weight, peripheral edema.

**Drug Interactions**

*Alcohol* / Alcohol ↓ seizure threshold; use with bupropion may precipitate seizures

*Carbamazepine* / ↑ Bupropion metabolism → ↓ plasma levels

*Cimetidine* / Cimetidine inhibits the metabolism of bupropion

*Fluoxetine* / Panic symptoms and psychotic reactions

*Levodopa* / ↑ Risk of side effects

*MAO inhibitors* / Acute toxicity to bupropion may ↑, especially if used with phenelzine

*Phenobarbital* / ↑ Bupropion metabolism → ↓ plasma levels

*Phenytoin* / ↑ Bupropion metabolism → ↓ plasma levels

**How Supplied:** *Tablet:* 75 mg, 100 mg; *Tablet Extended Release:* 100 mg, 150 mg

**Dosage** ————————
• **Tablets**
*Antidepressant.*

**Adults, initial:** 100 mg in the morning and evening for the first 3 days; **then,** 100 mg t.i.d., given in the morning, midday, and in the evening (6 hr should elapse between doses). If no response is observed after 4 weeks or longer, the dose may be increased to 450 mg/day with individual doses not to exceed 150 mg. Doses higher than 450 mg should not be administered. The sustained-release dosage form may be used for twice-daily dosing. **Maintenance:** Lowest dose to control depression.

*Smoking deterrent.*

Begin dosing at 150 mg/day for the first 3 days followed by 150 mg b.i.d. Eight hours or more should elapse between successive doses.

## DENTAL CONCERNS

See also *Dental Concerns* for *Antidepressants, Tricyclic.*

**General**

1. Decreased saliva flow can put the patient at risk for dental caries, periodontal disease, and candidiasis.

2. Consider shorter appointments and different methods of reducing stress in very anxious patients.

3. Review other smoking cessation techniques with the patient (see section on nicotine transdermal systems).

**Consultation with Primary Care Provider**

1. Consultation may be required in order to assess extent of disease control.

2. Health care provider should be informed of the oral adverse effects of these drugs.

# Buspirone hydrochloride

(byou-**SPYE**-rohn)
**Pregnancy Category:** B
Apo-Buspirone ✱, BuSpar, Linbuspirone ✱, Nu-Buspirone ✱ **(Rx)**
**Classification:** Nonbenzodiazepine antianxiety agent

**Action/Kinetics:** The mechanism of action is unknown. Not chemically related to the benzodiazepines; no anticonvulsant or muscle relaxant properties. Significant sedation has not been observed. The drug binds to serotonin (5-HT$_{1A}$) and dopamine (D$_2$) receptors in the CNS; it is thus possible that dopamine-mediated neurologic disorders may occur. These include dystonia, Parkinson-like symptoms, akathisia, and tardive dyskinesia. **Peak plasma levels:** 1–6 ng/mL 40–90 min after a single PO dose of 20 mg. **t½:** 2–3 hr. Extensive first-pass metabolism; active and inactive metabolites excreted in the urine and through the feces.

**Uses:** Anxiety disorders, short-term use to relieve symptoms of anxiety due to motor tension, apprehension, autonomic hyperactivity, or hyperattentiveness. Not usually indicated for treatment of anxiety and tension due to stress of everyday living.

**Contraindications:** Psychoses, severe liver or kidney impairment, lactation.

**Special Concerns:** Safety and efficacy in children less than 18 years of age not established. A decrease in dose may be necessary in geriatric clients due to age-related impairment of renal function.

**Side Effects:** *CNS:* Dizziness, drowsiness, insomnia, fatigue, nervousness, excitement, dream disturbances, dysphoria, noise intolerance, euphoria, depersonalization, akathisia, hallucinations, suicidal ideation, seizures, decreased concentration, confusion, anger or hostility, depression. *CV:* Nonspecific chest pain, hypotension, palpitations, tachycardia, syncope, hypertension. *Oral:* Dry mouth, altered taste. *GI:* N&V, diarrhea, constipation, abdominal distress, increased appetite, irritable colon. *Ophthalmologic:* Redness and itching of eyes, conjunctivitis, photophobia, eye pain. *Dermatologic:* Skin rash, pruritus, dry skin, edema of face, acne, easy bruising, flushing. *Neurologic:*

Paresthesia, tremor, numbness, incoordination. *GU:* Urinary hesitancy or frequency, enuresis, amenorrhea, pelvic inflammatory disease. *Miscellaneous:* Tinnitus, sore throat, nasal congestion, altered smell, muscle aches or pains, skin rash, headache, sweating, hyperventilation, SOB, hair loss, galactorrhea, decreased or increased libido, delayed ejaculation.

**Drug Interactions:** Use with MAO inhibitors may cause an increase in BP.

**How Supplied:** *Tablet:* 5 mg, 10 mg, 15 mg

**Dosage** ————————
• **Tablets**
**Adults:** 5 mg t.i.d. Dosage may be increased in increments of 5 mg/day q 2–3 days to achieve optimum effects; the total daily dose should not exceed 60 mg. BuSpar is available in a 15-mg tablet that is scored in 5-mg increments and notched in 7.5-mg increments so clients can take the drug b.i.d. rather than t.i.d.

## DENTAL CONCERNS

See also *Dental Concerns* for *Sedative-Hypnotics (Anti-anxiety)/Antimanic Drugs.*

# Busulfan
(byou-**SUL**-fan)
**Pregnancy Category:** D
Myleran (Abbreviation: Bus) **(Rx)**
**Classification:** Antineoplastic, alkylating agent

See also *Antineoplastic Agents.*

**Action/Kinetics:** Busulfan is cell cycle-phase nonspecific and acts predominately against cells of the granulocyte type and is thought to act by alkylating cellular thiol groups. Cross-linking of nucleoproteins occurs. May cause severe bone marrow depression. Leukocyte count drops during the second or third week. Thus, close medical supervision, including weekly laboratory tests, is mandatory. Resistance may develop and is thought to be due to the altered transport into the cell and/or increased intracellular inactivation. Rapidly absorbed from the GI tract; appears in serum 0.5–2 hr after PO administration. **t½:** 2.5 hr. Extensively metabolized and excreted in the urine.

Increased appetite and sense of well-being may occur a few days after therapy is started. Sometimes administered with allopurinol to prevent symptoms of clinical gout.

**Uses:** Chronic myelogenous leukemia (granulocytic, myelocytic, myeloid). Less effective in individuals with chronic myelogenous leukemia who lack the Philadelphia (Ph1) chromosome. Not effective in individuals where the disease is in the "blastic" phase.

**Contraindications:** Use during lactation only if benefits outweigh risks.

**Side Effects:** *Hematologic: **Pancytopenia, severe bone marrow hypoplasia,*** anemia, leukopenia, thrombocytopenia. *Pulmonary: **Bronchopulmonary dysplasia with interstitial pulmonary fibrosis.*** *Ophthalmologic:* Cataracts after prolonged use. *Dermatologic:* Hyperpigmentation, especially in clients with a dark complexion; also, urticaria, erythema multiforme, erythema nodosum, alopecia, porphyria cutanea tarda, excessive dryness and fragility of the skin with anhidrosis, dryness of the oral mucous membranes, cheilosis. *Metabolic:* Syndrome resembling adrenal insufficiency, including symptoms of weakness, severe fatigue, weight loss, anorexia, N&V, and melanoderma (especially after prolonged use). Also, hyperuricemia and hyperuricosuria in clients with chronic myelogenous leukemia. *Oral:* Dry mouth, stomatitis, cheilosis. *Miscellaneous:* Cellular dysplasia in various organs, including lymph nodes, pancreas, thyroid, adrenal glands, bone marrow, and liver. Also, gynecomastia, seizures after high doses, cataracts after prolonged use, ***hepatotoxicity,*** cholestatic jaundice, myasthenia gravis, sterility, ***en-docardial fibrosis,*** and suppression of ovarian function.

**Drug Interactions**
*Aspirin* / ↑ Increased risk of bleeding
**How Supplied:** *Tablet:* 2 mg

**Dosage** ————————————————
• **Tablets**
Individualized according to leukocyte count.
  *Chronic myelocytic leukemia.*
**Adults, remission, induction, usual dose:** 4–8 mg/day until leukocyte count falls below 15,000/mm3; **maintenance:** 1–3 mg/day. Discontinue therapy if there is a precipitous fall in leukocyte count. **Children, induction:** 0.06–0.12 mg/kg or 1.8 mg/m2 daily; **maintenance:** dosage is titrated to maintain a leukocyte count of 20,000/mm3.

## DENTAL CONCERNS

See also *Dental Concerns* for *Antineoplastic Agents.*

# Butenafine hydrochloride
(byou-**TEN**-ah-feen)
**Pregnancy Category:** B
Mentax **(Rx)**
**Classification:** Antifungal drug

See also *Anti-Infectives.*
**Action/Kinetics:** Acts by inhibiting epoxidation of squalene, thus blocking the synthesis of ergosterol, an essential component of fungal cell membranes. Depending on the concentration and the fungal species, the drug may be fungicidal. Although applied topically, some of the drug is absorbed into the general circulation.
**Uses:** Treatment of interdigital tinea pedia (athlete's foot) due to *Epidermophyton floccosum, Trichophyton mentagrophytes,* or *T. rubrum.*
**Special Concerns:** Use with caution in clients sensitive to allylamine antifungal drugs as the drugs may be cross-reactive. Use with caution during lactation. Safety and efficacy have not been determined in children less than 12 years of age.

**Side Effects:** *Dermatologic:* Contact dermatitis, burning or stinging, worsening of the condition, erythema, irritation, itching.
**How Supplied:** *Cream:* 1%

**Dosage**
- **Cream, 1%**
  *Athlete's foot.*
Apply the cream to cover the affected area and immediate surrounding skin once daily for 4 weeks. Review the diagnosis if no beneficial effects are noted after the treatment period.

## DENTAL CONCERNS

See also *Dental Concerns* for *All Anti-Infectives.*

# Butorphanol tartrate
(byou-**TOR**-fah-nohl)
**Pregnancy Category:** C
Stadol, Stadol NS **(C-IV) (Rx)**
**Classification:** Opioid agonist/antagonist

See also *Opioid Analgesics.*
**Action/Kinetics:** Has both opioid agonist and antagonist properties. Analgesic potency is said to be up to 7 times that of morphine and 30–40 times that of meperidine. Overdosage responds to naloxone. **Onset, IM:** 10–15 min; **IV:** rapid; **nasal:** within 15 min. **Duration, IM, IV:** 3–4 hr; **nasal:** 4–5 hr. **Peak analgesia, IM, IV:** 30–60 min; **nasal:** 1–2 hr. **t½, IM:** 2.1–8.8 hr; **nasal:** 2.9–9.2 hr. The t½ is increased up to 25% in clients over 65 years of age. Metabolized in the liver and excreted by the kidney. The drug has about 1/40 the narcotic antagonist activity as naloxone. A metered-dose nasal spray is now available.
**Uses: Parenteral and nasal:** Moderate to severe pain, especially after surgery. **Parenteral:** Preoperative medication (as part of balanced anesthesia). Pain during labor. **Nasal:** Treatment of migraine headaches.

**Contraindications:** Use of the nasal form during labor or delivery.
**Special Concerns:** Safe use during pregnancy, during labor for premature infants, or in children under 18 years not established. Use with extreme caution in clients with AMI, ventricular dysfunction, and coronary insufficiency (morphine or meperidine are preferred). Use in clients physically dependent on narcotics will result in precipitation of a withdrawal syndrome. Geriatric clients may be more sensitive to side effects, especially dizziness.
**Additional Side Effects:** The most common side effects are somnolence, dizziness, N&V. The nasal product commonly causes nasal congestion and insomnia.
**Drug Interactions:** Barbiturate anesthetics may increase respiratory and CNS depression of butorphanol.
**How Supplied:** *Injection:* 1 mg/mL, 2 mg/mL; *Spray:* 10 mg/mL

**Dosage**
- **IM**
  *Analgesia.*
**Adults, usual:** 2 mg q 3–4 hr, as necessary; **range:** 1–4 mg q 3–4 hr. Single doses should not exceed 4 mg.
  *Preoperative/preanesthetic.*
**Adults:** 2 mg 60–90 min before surgery. Individualize dosage.
  *Labor.*
**Adults:** 1–2 mg if at full term and during early labor. May be repeated after 4 hr.
- **IV**
  *Analgesia.*
**Adults, usual:** 1 mg q 3–4 hr; **range:** 0.5–2 mg q 3–4 hr. **Not recommended for use in children.**
  *Balanced anesthesia.*
**Adults:** 2 mg just before induction or 0.5–1 mg in increments during anesthesia. The increment may be up to 0.06 mg/kg, depending on drugs previously given. Total dose range: less than 4 mg to less than 12.5 mg.

*Labor.*
**Adults:** 1–2 mg if at full term and during early labor. May be repeated after 4 hr.

• **Nasal Spray**
*Analgesia.*
**Adults:** 1 spray (1 mg) in one nostril. If pain relief is not reached within 60–90 min, an additional 1 mg may be given. The two-dose sequence may be repeated in 3–4 hr if necessary. In severe pain, 2 mg (1 spray in each nostril) may be given initially followed in 3–4 hr by additional 2-mg doses if needed. **Geriatric clients, initial:** 1 mg; wait 90–120 min before determining if a second 1-mg dose is required.

## DENTAL CONCERNS

See also *Dental Concerns* for *Opioid Analgesics.*

# Cabergoline
(cah-**BER**-goh-leen)
**Pregnancy Category:** B
Dostinex **(Rx)**
**Classification:** Drug to treat hyperprolactinemia

**Action/Kinetics:** Secretion of prolactin occurs through the release of dopamine from tuberofundibular neurons. Cabergoline is a synthetic ergot derivative that is a dopamine receptor agonist at $D_2$ receptors. Inhibits basal and metoclopramide-induced prolactin secretion. **Peak plasma levels:** 2–3 hr. Undergoes a significant first-pass effect. Extensively metabolized in the liver and excreted in both the urine and feces. **t½, elimination:** 63–69 hr.

**Uses:** Treatment of hyperprolactinemia, either idiopathic or due to pituitary adenomas. *Non-FDA Approved Uses:* Shrink tumors in clients with microprolactinoma or macroprolactinoma. Parkinson's disease. Normalize androgen levels and improve menstrual cyclicity in polycystic ovary syndrome.

**Contraindications:** Uncontrolled hypertension or in pregnancy-induced hypertension (i.e., pre-eclampsia, eclampsia). Hypersensitivity to ergot alkaloids. Lactation. Not to be used to inhibit or suppress physiologic lactation.

**Special Concerns:** Use with caution in those with impaired hepatic function or with other drugs that lower BP. Safety and efficacy have not been determined in children.

**Side Effects:** *Oral:* Dry mouth, toothache. *GI:* N&V, constipation, abdominal pain, dyspepsia, diarrhea, flatulence, throat irritation, anorexia, weight loss or gain. *CNS:* Headache, dizziness, somnolence, vertigo, paresthesia, depression, nervousness, anxiety, insomnia. *CV:* Postural hypotension, hypotension, palpitations. *GU:* Breast pain, dysmenorrhea, increased libido. *Body as a whole:* Asthenia, fatigue, syncope, flu-like symptoms, malaise, periorbital edema, peripheral edema, hot flashes. *Miscellaneous:* Nasal stuffiness, abnormal vision, acne, epistaxis, pruritus.

**Drug Interactions**
*Antihypertensive drugs* / Additive hypotension
*Butyrophenones* / ↓ Effects of cabergoline
*Metoclopramide* / Effects of cabergoline
*Phenothiazines* / Effects of cabergoline
*Thioxanthenes* / Effects of cabergoline
**How Supplied:** *Tablets:* 0.5 mg

## Dosage

• **Tablets**
*Hyperprolactinemia.*
**Adults, initial:** 0.5 mg twice a week. Dose may be increased by

0.25 mg twice weekly to less than or equal to 1 mg twice a week, depending on the serum prolactin level. Dosage increases should not occur more often than every 4 weeks.

*Parkinson's disease.*
**Adults:** 7.5 mg/day.
*Improve menstrual cyclicity in polycystic ovary syndrome.*
**Adults:** 0.5 mg/week.

## DENTAL CONCERNS

None reported.

**Client/Family Teaching**
1. Review the importance of good oral hygiene in order to prevent soft tissue inflammation.
2. Review the proper use of oral hygiene aids in order to prevent injury.
3. Instruct patient to continually update the health/medication record at each visit.

# Calcium carbonate

(**KAL**-see-um **KAR**-bon-ayt)
Alka-Mints, Amitone, Antacid Tablets, Apo-Cal ✦, Cal Carb-HD, Calci-Chew, Calciday-667, Calci-Mix, Calcite 500, Calcium 600, Cal-Plus, Calsan ✦, Caltrate ✦, Caltrate 600, Caltrate Jr., Children's Mylanta Upset Stomatch Relief, Chooz, Dicarbosil, Equilet, Extra Strength Antacid, Extra Strength Tums, Florical, Gencalc 600, Maalox Antacid Caplets, Mallamint, Mylanta Lozenges, Nephro-Calci, Os-Cal 500, Os-Cal 500 Chewable, Oysco 500 Chewable, Oyst-Cal 500, Oystercal 500, Oyster Shell Calcium-500, Tums, Tums Ultra, Webber Calcium Carbonate ✦ **(OTC)**
**Classification:** Calcium salt

See also *Calcium Salts* and *Antacids.*
**Uses:** Mild hypocalcemia, antacid, antihyperphosphatemic.
**Special Concerns:** Dosage has not been established in children.
**Drug Interactions:** May interfere with the absorption of anticholinergics, ketoconazole, tetracyclines, and sodium fluoride.
**How Supplied:** *Capsule:* 500 mg, 600 mg, 900 mg, 1250 mg; *Chew Tablet:* 300 mg, 420 mg, 500 mg, 600 mg, 650 mg, 1,250 mg, 1,500 mg; *Lozenge/Troche:* 240 mg; *Suspension:* 500 mg/5 mL; *Tablet* 10 mg, 250 mg, 375 mg, 420 mg, 500 mg, 600 mg, 625 mg, 650 mg, 750 mg, 1,000 mg, 1,250 mg; *Tablet, Extended Release:* 500 mg; *Wafer:* 1,250 mg

## Dosage

• **Chewable Tablets, Tablets, Suspension, Gum, Lozenges, Wafers**
**Adults:** 0.5–1.5 g, as needed.
• **Capsules, Suspension, Tablets, Chewable Tablets**
*Hypocalcemia, nutritional supplement.*
**Adults:** 1.25–1.5 g 1–3 times/day with or after meals.
*Antihyperphosphatemic.*
**Adults:** 5–13 g/day in divided doses with meals.
*NOTE:* The preparation contains 40% elemental calcium and 400 mg elemental calcium/g (20 mEq/g).
• **Florical**
1 capsule or tablet daily (also contains 8.3 mg sodium fluoride per capsule or tablet).
• **Children's Mylanta Upset Stomach Relief Chewable Tablets or Liquid**
*Upset stomach in children.*
1 tablet or 5 mL for children weighing 24–47 pounds (or those aged 2–5 years) and 2 tablets or 10 mL for children weighing 48–95 pounds (or those aged 6–11).

## DENTAL CONCERNS
**General**
1. Monitor vital signs at every appointment because of cardiovascular side effects.
2. A semisupine position for the dental chair may be necessary to help minimize or avoid GI adverse effects.

# Captopril

(**KAP**-toe-prill)
**Pregnancy Category:** C (first trimester); D (second and third trimesters)
Alti-Captopril ✦, Apo-Capto ✦, Capoten, Gen-Captopril ✦, Med-Capto-

pril ✱, Novo-Captoril ✱, Nu-Capto ✱
**(Rx)**
**Classification:** Antihypertensive, inhibitor of angiotensin synthesis

See also *Angiotensin-Converting Enzyme Inhibitors.*

**Action/Kinetics: Onset:** 15 min. **Peak serum levels:** 30–90 min; presence of food decreases absorption by 30%–40%. **Plasma protein binding:** 25%–30%. **Time to peak effect:** 60–90 min. **Duration:** 6–12 hr. $t\frac{1}{2}$, **normal renal function:** 2 hr; $t\frac{1}{2}$, **impaired renal function:** 3.5–32 hr. More than 95% of absorbed dose excreted in urine (40%–50% unchanged). Food decreases bioavailability of captopril by 30%–40%.

**Uses:** Antihypertensive, step I therapy in clients with normal renal function. Concomitant use with diuretic therapy may, however, cause precipitous hypotension. In combination with diuretics and digitalis in treatment of CHF not responding to conventional therapy. To improve survival following MI in clinically stable clients with LV dysfunction manifested as an ejection fraction of 40% or less. Treatment of diabetic nephropathy (proteinuria > 500 mg/day) in those with type I insulin-dependent diabetes and retinopathy. *Non-FDA Approved Uses:* Rheumatoid arthritis, hypertensive crisis, neonatal and childhood hypertension, hypertension related to scleroderma renal crisis, diagnosis of anatomic renal artery stenosis, diagnosis of primary aldosteronism, Raynaud's syndrome, hypertension of Takayasu's disease, idiopathic edema, and Bartter's syndrome.

**Contraindications:** Use with a history of angioedema related to previous use of ACE inhibitors.

**Special Concerns:** Use with caution in cases of impaired renal function and during lactation. Use in children only if other antihypertensive therapy has proven ineffective in controlling BP. May cause a profound drop in BP following the first dose.

**Side Effects:** *Dermatologic:* Rash (usually maculopapular) with pruritus and occasionally fever, eosinophilia, and arthralgia. Alopecia, erythema multiforme, photosensitivity, exfoliative dermatitis, **Stevens-Johnson syndrome,** reversible pemphigoid-like lesions, bullous pemphigus, onycholysis, flushing, pallor, scalded mouth sensation. *Oral:* Dysgeusia, aphthous ulcers, dry mouth, glossitis. *GI:* N&V, anorexia, constipation or diarrhea, gastric irritation, abdominal pain, peptic ulcers, dyspepsia, pancreatitis. *Hepatic:* Jaundice, cholestasis, hepatitis. *CNS:* Headache, dizziness, insomnia, malaise, fatigue, paresthesias, confusion, depression, nervousness, ataxia, somnolence. *CV:* Hypotension, angina, **MI,** Raynaud's phenomenon, chest pain, palpitations, tachycardia, **CVA, CHF, cardiac arrest,** orthostatic hypotension, rhythm disturbances. *Renal:* Renal insufficiency or failure, proteinuria, urinary frequency, oliguria, polyuria, nephrotic syndrome, interstitial nephritis. *Respiratory:* **Bronchospasm,** cough, dyspnea, asthma, **pulmonary embolism, pulmonary infarction.** *Hematologic:* Agranulocytosis, neutropenia, thrombocytopenia, pancytopenia, **aplastic or hemolytic anemia.** *Other:* Decrease or loss of taste perception with weight loss (reversible), angioedema, asthenia, syncope, fever, myalgia, arthralgia, vasculitis, blurred vision, impotence, hyperkalemia, hyponatremia, myasthenia, gynecomastia, rhinitis, eosinophilic pneumonitis.

**Drug Interactions:** See also *Angiotensin-Converting Enzyme Inhibitors.*

**How Supplied:** *Tablet:* 12.5 mg, 25 mg, 50 mg, 100 mg

**Dosage** ——————
• **Tablets**
*Hypertension.*
**Adults, initial:** 25 mg b.i.d.–t.i.d. If unsatisfactory response after 1–2 weeks, increase to 50 mg b.i.d.–t.i.d.; if still unsatisfactory after another 1–2 weeks, thiazide diuretic should be added (e.g., hydrochloro-

thiazide, 25 mg/day). Dosage may be increased to 100–150 mg b.i.d.–t.i.d., not to exceed 450 mg/day.

*Accelerated or malignant hypertension.*

Stop current medication (except for the diuretic) and initiate captopril at a dose of 25 mg b.i.d.–t.i.d. The dose may be increased q 24 hr until a satisfactory response is obtained or the maximum dose reached. Furosemide may be indicated.

*Heart failure.*

**Initial:** 25 mg t.i.d.; **then,** if necessary, increase dose to 50 mg t.i.d. and evaluate response; **maintenance:** 50–100 mg t.i.d., not to exceed 450 mg/day.

*NOTE:* For adults, an initial dose of 6.25–12.5 mg (0.15 mg/kg t.i.d. in children) should be given b.i.d.–t.i.d. to clients who are sodium- and water-depleted due to diuretics, who will continue to be on diuretic therapy, and who have renal impairment.

*Left ventricular dysfunction after MI.*

Therapy may be started as early as 3 days after the MI. **Initial dose:** 6.25 mg; **then,** begin 12.5 mg t.i.d. and increase to 25 mg t.i.d. over the next several days. The target dose is 50 mg t.i.d. over the next several weeks. Other treatments for MI may be used concomitantly (e.g., aspirin, beta blockers, thrombolytic drugs).

*Diabetic nephropathy.*

25 mg t.i.d. for chronic use. Other antihypertensive drugs (e.g., beta blockers, centrally-acting drugs, diuretics, vasodilators) may be used with captopril if additional drug therapy is needed to reduce BP.

*Hypertensive crisis.*

**Initial:** 25 mg; **then,** 100 mg 90–120 min later, 200–300 mg/day for 2–5 days (then adjust dose). Sublingual captopril, 25 mg, has also been used successfully.

*Rheumatoid arthritis.*

75–150 mg/day in divided doses.

*NOTE:* For all uses, doses should be reduced in clients with renal impairment.

## DENTAL CONCERNS

See also *Dental Concerns* for *Angiotensin-Converting Enzyme Inhibitors* and *Antihypertensive Agents.*

# Carbamazepine
(kar-bah-**MAYZ**-eh-peen)
**Pregnancy Category:** C
Apo-Carbamazepine ✦, Atretol, Depitol, Epitol, Mazepine ✦, Novo–Carbamaz ✦, Nu–Carbamazepine ✦, PMS-Carbamazepine ✦, Taro-Carbamazepine ✦, Tegretol, Tegretol Chewtabs ✦, Tegretol CR ✦, Tegretol XR **(Rx)**
**Classification:** Anticonvulsant, miscellaneous

See also *Anticonvulsants.*

**Action/Kinetics:** The anticonvulsant action is not known but may involve depressing activity in the nucleus ventralis anterior of the thalamus, resulting in a reduction of polysynaptic responses and blocking posttetanic potentiation. Due to the potentially serious blood dyscrasias, a benefit-to-risk evaluation should be undertaken before the drug is instituted. **Peak serum levels:** 4–5 hr. **t½** (serum): 12–17 hr with repeated doses. **Therapeutic serum levels:** 4–12 mcg/mL. Metabolized in the liver to an active metabolite (epoxide derivative) with a half-life of 5–8 hr. Metabolites are excreted through the feces and urine.

**Uses:** Partial seizures with complex symptoms (psychomotor, temporal lobe). Tonic-clonic seizures, diseases with mixed seizure patterns or other partial or generalized seizures. Carbamazepine is often a drug of choice due to its low incidence of side effects. For children with epilepsy who are less than 6 years of age for the treatment of partial seizures, generalized tonic-clonic seizures, and mixed seizure patterns and for treating trigeminal neuralgia. To treat pain associated with tic douloureux (trigeminal neuralgia) and glossopharyngeal neuralgia. *Non-FDA Approved Uses:* Bipolar disorders, unipolar depression, schizoaffective illness, resistant schizophrenia, dyscontrol syndrome associated with limbic system dysfunction, intermittent explosive disorder, PTSD, atypical psychosis. Management of alcohol, cocaine, and benzodiazepine withdrawal symptoms. Restless leg syndrome, nonhereditary chorea in children.

**Contraindications:** History of bone marrow depression. Hypersensitivity to drug or tricyclic antidepressants. Lactation. In clients taking MAO inhibitors. Use for relief of general aches and pains.

**Special Concerns:** Safety and effectiveness have not been established in children less than 6 years of age. Use with caution in glaucoma and in hepatic, renal, CV disease, and a history of hematologic reaction. Use with caution in clients with mixed seizure disorder that includes atypical absence seizures (carbamazepine is not effective and may be associated with an increased frequency of generalized convulsions). Use in geriatric clients may cause an increased incidence of confusion, agitation, AV heart block, syndrome of inappropriate antidiuretic hormone, and bradycardia.

**Side Effects:** *Oral:* Dry mouth, glossitis, stomatitis. *GI:* N&V (common), diarrhea, constipation, gastric distress, abdominal pain, anorexia. *Hematologic:* **Aplastic anemia,** leukopenia, eosinophilia, thrombocytopenia, **agranulocytosis,** leukocytosis, pancytopenia, **bone marrow depression.** *CNS:* Dizziness, drowsiness, disturbances of coordination, headache, fatigue, confusion, speech disturbances, visual hallucinations, depression with agitation, talkativeness, hyperacusis, abnormal involuntary movements, behavioral changes in children. *CV:* CHF, aggravation of hypertension, hypotension, syncope and collapse, edema, recurrence of or primary thrombophlebitis, aggravation of

CAD, paralysis and other symptoms of cerebral arterial insufficiency, ***arrhythmias (including AV block).*** *GU:* Urinary frequency, acute urinary retention, oliguria with hypertension, impotence, renal failure, azotemia, albuminuria, glycosuria, increased BUN, microscopic deposits in urine. *Pulmonary:* Pulmonary hypersensitivity characterized by fever, dyspnea, pneumonitis, or pneumonia. *Dermatologic:* Pruritus, urticaria, photosensitivity, exfoliative dermatitis, erythematous rashes, alterations in pigmentation, alopecia, sweating, purpura, toxic epidermal necrolysis (Lyell's syndrome), ***Stevens-Johnson syndrome,*** aggravation of disseminated lupus erythematosus, alopecia, erythema nodosum or multiforme. *Ophthalmologic:* Nystagmus, double vision, blurred vision, oculomotor disturbances, conjunctivitis; scattered, punctate lens opacities. *Hepatic:* Abnormal liver function tests, cholestatic or hepatocellular jaundice, hepatitis, acute intermittent porphyria. *Other:* Peripheral neuritis, paresthesias, tinnitus, fever, chills, joint and muscle aches and leg cramps, adenopathy or lymphadenopathy, inappropriate ADH secretion syndrome.

**Drug Interactions**

*Acetaminophen* / ↑ Breakdown of acetaminophen → ↓ effect and ↑ risk of hepatotoxicity

*Contraceptives, oral* / ↓ Effect of contraceptives due to ↑ breakdown by liver

*Doxycycline* / ↓ Effect of doxycycline due to ↑ breakdown by liver

*Erythromycin* / ↑ Effect of carbamazepine due to ↓ breakdown by liver

*Fluoxetine* / ↑ Carbamazepine levels → possible toxicity

*Fluvoxamine* / ↑ Carbamazepine levels → possible toxicity

*Haloperidol* / ↓ Effect of haloperidol due to ↑ breakdown by liver

*Macrolide antibiotics* / Effect of carbamazepine due to breakdown by liver

*MAO inhibitors* / Exaggerated side effects of carbamazepine

*Muscle relaxants, nondepolarizing /* Resistance to or reversal of the neuromuscular blocking effects of these drugs

*Phenobarbital /* ↓ Effect of carbamazepine due to ↑ breakdown by liver

*Phenytoin /* ↓ Effect of carbamazepine due to ↑ breakdown by liver; also, phenytoin levels may ↑ or ↓

*Propoxyphene /* ↑ Effect of carbamazepine due to ↓ breakdown by liver

*Succinimides /* ↓ Effect of succinimides due to ↑ breakdown by the liver

*Terfenadine /* May ↑ carbamazepine levels

*Tricyclic antidepressants /* ↓ Effect of tricyclic antidepressants due to ↑ breakdown by liver; also, ↓ levels of tricyclic antidepressants

*Troleandomycin /* ↑ Effect of carbamazepine due to ↓ breakdown by liver

**How Supplied:** *Chew Tablet:* 100 mg; *Suspension:* 100 mg/5 mL; *Tablet:* 200 mg; *Tablet, Extended Release:* 100 mg, 200 mg, 400 mg

**Dosage** ─────────────
• **Oral Suspension, Tablets, Chewable Tablets, Extended-Release Tablets**

*Anticonvulsant.*

**Adults and children over 12 years, initial:** 200 mg b.i.d. on day 1 (100 mg q.i.d. of suspension). Increase by 200 mg/day at weekly intervals until best response is attained. Divide total dose and administer q 6–8 hr; the extended-release tablets may be used for twice-daily dosing instead of dosing 3 or 4 times a day. **Maximum dose, children 12–15 years:** 1,000 mg/day; **adults and children over 15 years:** 1,200 mg/day. **Maintenance:** decrease dose gradually to minimum effective level, usually 800–1,200 mg/day. **Children, 6–12 years: initial,** 100 mg b.i.d. on day 1 (50 mg q.i.d. of suspension); **then,** increase slowly, at weekly intervals, by 100 mg/day;

dose is divided and given q 6–8 hr. Daily dose should not exceed 1,000 mg. **Maintenance:** 400–800 mg/day. **Children, less than 6 years:** 10–20 mg/kg/day in two to three divided doses; dose can be increased slowly in weekly increments to maintenance levels of 250–300 mg/day (not to exceed 400 mg/day).

*Trigeminal neuralgia.*

**Initial:** 100 mg b.i.d. on day 1 (50 mg q.i.d. of suspension); increase by no more than 200 mg/day, using increments of 100 mg q 12 hr as needed, up to maximum of 1,200 mg/day. **Maintenance: Usual:** 400–800 mg/day (range: 200–1,200 mg/day). Attempt discontinuation of drug at least 1 time q 3 months.

*Restless legs syndrome.*

100–300 mg at bedtime.

*Nonhereditary chorea in children.*

15–25 mg/kg/day.

## DENTAL CONCERNS

See also *Dental Concerns* for *Anticonvulsants.*

# Carbidopa

(**KAR**-bih-doh-pah)
Lodosyn **(Rx)**

─────COMBINATION DRUG─────

# Carbidopa/Levodopa

(**KAR**-bih-doh-pah/**LEE**-voh-doh-pah)
Sinemet-10/100, -25/100, or -25/250, Sinemet CR **(Rx)**
**Classification:** Antiparkinson agent

See also *Levodopa.*

**Content:    Carbidopa/Levodopa:** Each 10/100 tablet contains: carbidopa, 10 mg, and levodopa, 100 mg. Each 25/100 tablets contains: carbidopa, 25 mg, and levodopa, 100 mg. Each 25/250 tablet contains: carbidopa, 25 mg, and levodopa, 250 mg. Each sustained-release tablet contains: carbidopa, 50 mg, and levodopa, 200 mg.

**Action/Kinetics:** Carbidopa inhibits peripheral decarboxylation (breakdown) of levodopa. Since peripheral decarboxylation is inhibited, this allows more levodopa to be available for transport to the brain, where it will be converted to dopamine, thus relieving the symptoms of parkinsonism. It is recommended that both carbidopa and levodopa be given together (e.g., Sinemet). However, *the dosage of levodopa must be reduced by up to 80% when combined with carbidopa.* This decreases the incidence of levodopa-induced side effects. *NOTE:* Pyridoxine will not reverse the action of carbidopa/levodopa. **t½, carbidopa:** 1–2 hr; when given with levodopa, the t½ of levodopa increases from 1 hr to 2 hr (may be as high as 15 hr in some clients). About 30% carbidopa is excreted unchanged in the urine.

**Uses:** All types of parkinsonism (idiopathic, postencephalitic, following injury to the nervous system due to carbon monoxide and manganese intoxication). Carbidopa alone is used in clients who require individual titration of carbidopa and levodopa. *Non-FDA Approved Uses:* Postanoxic intention myoclonus. **Warning:** Levodopa must be discontinued at least 8 hr before carbidopa/levodopa therapy is initiated. Also, clients taking carbidopa/levodopa must not take levodopa concomitantly, because the former is a combination of carbidopa and levodopa.

**Contraindications:** History of melanoma. MAO inhibitors should be stopped 2 weeks before therapy. Lactation.

**Special Concerns:** Use during pregnancy only if benefits outweigh risks. Safety and efficacy in children less than 18 years of age have not been determined. Lower doses may be necessary in geriatric clients due to aged-related decreases in peripheral dopa decarboxylase.

**Side Effects:** Because more levodopa reaches the brain, dyskinesias may occur at lower doses with carbidopa/levodopa than with levodopa alone. Clients abruptly withdrawn from levodopa may experience neuroleptic malignant-like syndrome in-

cluding symptoms of muscular rigidity, hyperthermia, increased serum phosphokinase, and changes in mental status.

**Drug Interactions:** Use with tricyclic antidepressants may cause hypertension and dyskinesia.

**How Supplied:** Carbodopa: *Tablet:* 25 mg. Carbidopa/Levodopa: See Content

## Dosage

- **Tablets**
  *Parkinsonism, clients not receiving levodopa.*
**Initial:** 1 tablet of 10 mg carbidopa/100 mg levodopa t.i.d.–q.i.d. or 25 mg carbidopa/100 mg levodopa t.i.d.; **then,** increase by 1 tablet q 1–2 days until a total of 8 tablets/day is taken. If additional levodopa is required, substitute 1 tablet of 25 mg carbidopa/250 mg levodopa t.i.d.–q.i.d.
  *Parkinsonism, clients receiving levodopa.*
**Initial:** Carbidopa/levodopa dosage should be about 25% of prior levodopa dosage (levodopa dosage is discontinued 8 hr before carbidopa/levodopa is initiated); **then,** adjust dosage as required. Suggested starting dose is 1 tablet of 25 mg carbidopa/250 mg levodopa t.i.d.–q.i.d. for clients taking more than 1500 mg levodopa or 25 mg carbidopa/100 mg levodopa for clients taking less than 1500 mg levodopa.

- **Sustained-Release Tablets**
  *Parkinsonism, clients not receiving levodopa.*
1 tablet b.i.d. at intervals of not less than 6 hr. Depending on the response, dosage may be increased or decreased. Usual dose is 2–8 tablets/day in divided doses at intervals of 4–8 hr during waking hours (if divided doses are not equal, the smaller dose should be given at the end of the day).
  *Parkinsonism, clients receiving levodopa.*
1 tablet b.i.d. Carbidopa is available alone for clients requiring additional carbidopa (i.e., inadequate reduction in N&V); in such clients, carbido-

pa may be given at a dose of 25 mg with the first daily dose of carbidopa/levodopa. If necessary, additional carbidopa, at doses of 12.5 or 25 mg, may be given with each dose of carbidopa/levodopa.

*Clients receiving carbidopa/levodopa who require additional carbidopa.*
In clients taking 10 mg carbidopa/100 mg levodopa, 25 mg carbidopa may be given with the first dose each day. Additional doses of 12.5 or 25 mg may be given during the day with each dose. If the client is taking 25 mg carbidopa/250 mg levodopa, a dose of 25 mg carbidopa may be given with any dose, as needed. The maximum daily dose of carbidopa is 200 mg.

## DENTAL CONCERNS

See also *Dental Concerns* for *Levodopa.*

## Carteolol hydrochloride

(kar-**TEE**-oh-lohl)
**Pregnancy Category:** C
Cartrol, Ocupress **(Rx)**
**Classification:** Beta-adrenergic blocking agent

See also *Beta-Adrenergic Blocking Agents.*
**Action/Kinetics:** Has both beta-1 and beta-2 receptor blocking activity. It has no membrane-stabilizing activity but does have moderate intrinsic sympathomimetic effects. Low lipid solubility. **t½:** 6 hr. **Duration, ophthalmic use:** 12 hr. Approximately 50%–70% excreted unchanged in the urine.
**Uses: PO.** Hypertension. *Non-FDA Approved Uses:* Reduce frequency of anginal attacks. **Ophthalmic:** Chronic open-angle glaucoma and intraocular hypertension alone or in combination with other drugs.
**Contraindications:** Hypersensitivity to carteolol, cardiogenic shock, 2nd or 3rd degree heart block, sinus bradycardia, congestive heart failure, cardiac failure, right ventricular failure. Severe, persistent bradycardia. Bronchial asthma or bronchospasm, including severe COPD. Congenital glaucoma (infants).
**Special Concerns:** Use with caution during lactation. Geriatric clients are at greater risk of developing bradycardia. Coronary artery disease, COPD, diabetes mellitus, major surgery, non-allergic bronchospams, renal disease, thyroid disease, well-compensated heart failure. Dosage has not been established in children.
**Side Effects:** *Oral:* Dry mouth. *CV:* ***AV block, bradycardia, CHF, chest pain,*** dysrhythmias, hypotension, orthostatic hypotension, palpitations, ***peripheral vascular insufficiency, ventricular dysrhythmias.*** *CNS:* Anxiety, ataxia, catatonia, decreased concentration, depression, dizziness, drowsiness, fatigue, headache, insomnia, lethargy, mental changes, nightmares, paresthesia. *GI:* Anorexia, constipation, diarrhea, flatulence, vomiting. *Hematologic:* ***Agranulocytosis,*** thrombocytopenia. *Skin:* Pruritus, rash, increased skin pigmentation, alopecia. *GU:* Impotence, ejaculation failure, urinary retention. *Respiratory:* ***Bronchospasm,*** dyspnea, nasal stuffiness, pharyngitis, wheezing.
**Additional Side Effects: Ophthalmic use.** Transient irritation, burning, tearing, conjunctival hyperemia, edema, blurred or cloudy vision, photophobia, decreased night vision, ptosis, blepharoconjunctivitis, abnormal corneal staining, corneal sensitivity.
**Drug Interactions:** See also *Drug Interactions* for *Beta-Adrenergic Blocking Agents* and *Antihypertensive Agents.*
**How Supplied:** *Ophthalmic solution:* 1%; *Tablet:* 2.5 mg, 5 mg

## Dosage
• **Tablets**
*Hypertension.*
**Initial:** 2.5 mg once daily either alone or with a diuretic. If response is inadequate, the dose may be in-

creased gradually to 5 mg and then 10 mg/day as a single dose. **Maintenance:** 2.5–5 mg once daily. Doses greater than 10 mg/day are not likely to increase the beneficial effect and may decrease the response. Increase the dosage interval in clients with renal impairment.

*Reduce frequency of anginal attacks.*
10 mg/day.

• **Ophthalmic Solution**
**Usual:** 1 gtt in affected eye b.i.d. If the response is unsatisfactory, concomitant therapy may be initiated.

## DENTAL CONCERNS

See also *Dental Concerns* for *Beta-Adrenergic Blocking Agents* and *Antihypertensive Agents.*
**Client/Family Teaching**
1. Review the importance of good oral hygiene in order to prevent soft tissue inflammation.
2. Review the proper use of oral hygiene aids in order to prevent injury.
3. Daily home fluoride treatments for persistent dry mouth.
4. Avoid alcohol-containing mouth rinses and beverages.
5. Avoid caffeine-containing beverages.
6. Dry mouth can be treated with tart, sugarless gum or candy, water, sugar-free beverages, or with saliva substitutes if dry mouth persists.
7. You may want to wear dark glasses to avoid photophobia, which can occur with the examination light.

---

# Carvedilol

(kar-**VAY**-dih-lol)
**Pregnancy Category:** C
Coreg **(Rx)**
**Classification:** Alpha/beta-adrenergic blocking agent

---

See also *Adrenergic Blocking Agents.*
**Action/Kinetics:** Has both alpha- and beta-adrenergic blocking activity. Thus, the drug decreases cardiac output, reduces exercise- or isoproterenol-induced tachycardia, reduces reflex orthostatic hypotension, causes vasodilation, and reduces peripheral vascular resistance. Significant beta-blocking activity occurs within 60 min while alpha-blocking action is observed within 30 min. BP is lowered more in the standing than in the supine position. Significantly lowers plasma renin activity when given for at least 4 weeks. Rapidly absorbed after PO administration, but there is a significant first-pass effect. **Terminal t½:** 7–10 hr. Food delays the rate of absorption. Over 98% is bound to plasma protein. Plasma levels average 50% higher in geriatric compared with younger clients. Extensively metabolized in the liver, with metabolites excreted primarily via the bile into the feces.

**Uses:** Essential hypertension used either alone or in combination with other antihypertensive drugs, especially thiazide diuretics. Used with digitalis, diuretics, and ACE inhibitors to reduce the progression of mild to moderate CHF of ischemic or cardiomyopathic origin. *Non-FDA Approved Uses:* Angina pectoris, idiopathic cardiomyopathy.

**Contraindications:** Clients with New York Heart Association Class IV decompensated cardiac failure, bronchial asthma, or related bronchospastic conditions, second- or third-degree AV block, sick sinus syndrome (unless a permanent pacemaker is in place), cardiogenic shock, severe bradycardia, drug hypersensitivity. Hepatic impairment. Lactation.

**Special Concerns:** Use with caution in hypertensive clients with CHF controlled with digitalis, diuretics, or an ACE inhibitor. Use with caution in peripheral vascular disease, in surgical procedures using anesthetic agents that depress myocardial function, in diabetics receiving insulin or oral hypoglycemic drugs, in those subject to spontaneous hypoglycemia, or in thyrotoxicosis. Clients with a history of severe anaphylactic reaction to a variety of allergens may be more reactive to repeated challenge while taking beta blockers. Safety and efficacy have not been established in children less than 18 years of age.

**Side Effects:** *CV:* Bradycardia, postural hypotension, dependent or peripheral edema, AV block, extrasystoles, hypertension, hypotension, palpitations, peripheral ischemia, syncope, angina, *cardiac failure,* myocardial ischemia, tachycardia, CV disorder. *CNS:* Dizziness, headache, somnolence, insomnia, ataxia, hypesthesia, paresthesia, vertigo, depression, nervousness, migraine, neuralgia, paresis, amnesia, confusion, sleep disorder, impaired concentration, abnormal thinking, paranoia, emotional lability. *Body as a whole:* Fatigue, viral infection, rash, allergy, asthenia, malaise, pain, injury, fever, infection, somnolence, sweating, *sudden death. Oral:* Dry mouth. *GI:* Diarrhea, abdominal pain, bilirubinemia, N&V, flatulence, anorexia, dyspepsia, melena, periodontitis, increased hepatic enzymes, *GI hemorrhage. Respiratory:* Rhinitis, pharyngitis, sinusitis, bronchitis, dyspnea, *asthma, bronchospasm,* pulmonary edema, respiratory alkalosis, dyspnea, respiratory disorder, URTI, coughing. *GU:* UTI, albuminuria, hematuria, frequency of micturition, abnormal renal function, impotence. *Dermatologic:* Pruritus; erythematous, maculopapular, and psoriaform rashes, photosensitivity reaction, exfoliative dermatitis. *Metabolic:* Hypertriglyceridemia, hypercholesterolemia, hyperglycemia, hypovolemia, hyperuricemia, increased weight, gout, dehydration, hypervolemia, glycosuria, hyponatremia, hypokalemia, hyperkalemia, diabetes mellitus. *Hematologic:* Thrombocytopenia, anemia, leukopenia, pancytopenia, purpura, atypical lymphocytes. *Musculoskeletal:* Back pain, arthralgia, myalgia, arthritis. *Otic:* Decreased hearing, tinnitus. *Miscellaneous:* Hot flushes, leg cramps, abnormal vision, *anaphylactoid reaction.*

**Drug Interactions**
*Epinephrine* / ↑ Chance for hypertension, bradycardia
*Halothane* / ↑ Risk of severe myocardial depression → hypotension
*Indomethacin* / ↓ Hypotensive effects of labetolol
*Lidocaine* / ↓ Metabolism of labetol
*NSAIDs* / ↓ Hypotensive effects of labetolol
*Sympathomimetics* / ↓ Effects of labetolol / ↑ Chance of hypertension, bradycardia

**How Supplied:** *Tablet:* 6.25 mg, 12.5 mg, 25 mg

**Dosage**
• **Tablets**
*Essential hypertension.*
**Initial:** 6.25 mg b.i.d. If this is tolerated, using standing systolic pressure measured about 1 hr after dosing, maintain the dose for 7–14 days. **Then,** increase to 12.5 mg b.i.d., if necessary, based on trough BP, using standing systolic pressure 2 hr after dosing. This dose should be maintained for 7–14 days and can then be adjusted upward to 25 mg b.i.d. if necessary and tolerated. The total daily dose should not exceed 50 mg.
*Congestive heart failure.*
**Initial:** 3.125 mg b.i.d. for 2 weeks. If this is tolerated, increase to 6.25 mg b.i.d. Dosing is doubled every 2 weeks to the highest tolerated level, up to a maximum of 25 mg b.i.d. in those weighing less than 85 kg and 50 mg b.i.d. in those weighing over 85 kg.
*Angina pectoris.*
25–50 mg b.i.d.
*Idiopathic cardiomyopathy.*
6.25–25 mg b.i.d.

## DENTAL CONCERNS

See also *Dental Concerns* for *Antihypertensive Agents* and *Alpha-1-* and *Beta Adrenergic Blocking Agents.*

# Cefaclor
**(SEF**-ah-klor**)**
**Pregnancy Category:** B

Ceclor, Ceclor CD **(Rx)**
**Classification:** Cephalosporin, second-generation

See also *Anti-Infectives* and *Cephalosporins.*
**Action/Kinetics: Peak serum levels:** 5–15 mcg/mL after 1 hr. **t½: PO,** 36–54 min. Well absorbed from GI tract. From 60% to 85% excreted in urine within 8 hr.

**Uses:** Otitis media due to *Streptococcus pneumoniae, Hemophilus influenzae, Streptococcus pyogenes,* and staphylococci. Upper respiratory tract infections (including pharyngitis and tonsillitis) caused by *S. pyogenes.* Lower respiratory tract infections (including pneumonia) due to *S. pneumoniae, H. influenzae,* and *S. pyogenes.* Skin and skin structure infections due to *Staphylococcus aureus* and *S. pyogenes.* UTIs (including pyelonephritis and cystitis) caused by *Escherichia coli, Proteus mirabilis, Klebsiella,* and coagulase-negative staphylococci. *Extended-release tablets:* Acute bacterial exacerbations of chronic bronchitis due to non-β-lactamase-producing strains of *H. influenzae, Moraxella catarrhalis* (including β-lactamase-producing strains), or *S. pneumoniae.* Secondary bacterial infections of acute bronchitis due to *H. influenzae* (non-β-lactamase-producing strains only), *M. catarrhalis* (including β-lactamase-producing strains), or *S. pneumoniae.* Pharyngitis or tonsillitis due to *S. pyogenes.* Uncomplicated skin and skin structure infections due to *S. aureus* (methicillin-susceptible). *Non-FDA Approved Uses:* Acute uncomplicated UTIs in select populations using a single dose of 2 g.

**Contraindications:** Hypersensitivity to cephalosporins or related penicillin antibiotics.

**Special Concerns:** Safety for use in infants less than 1 month of age has not been established.

**Side Effects:** See also *Cephalosporins.*
**Additional Side Effects:** Cholestatic jaundice, lymphocytosis.

**Drug Interactions:** See also *Cephalosporins.*

**How Supplied:** *Capsule:* 250 mg, 500 mg; *Powder for reconstitution:* 125 mg/5 mL, 187 mg/5 mL, 250 mg/5 mL, 375 mg/5 mL; *Tablet, Extended Release:* 375 mg, 500 mg

**Dosage** ———————————
• **Capsules, Oral Suspension**
*All uses.*
**Adults:** 250 mg q 8 hr. Dose may be doubled in more severe infections or those caused by less susceptible organisms. Total daily dose should not exceed 4 g. **Children:** 20 mg/kg/day in divided doses q 8 hr. Dose may be doubled in more serious infections, otitis media, or for infections caused by less susceptible organisms. For otitis media and pharyngitis, the total daily dose may be divided and given q 12 hr. Total daily dose should not exceed 1 g.
• **Tablets, Extended Release**
*Acute bacterial exacerbations, chronic bronchitis, secondary bacterial infections of acute bronchitis.*
500 mg q 12 hr for 7 days.
*Pharyngitis, tonsillitis.*
375 mg q 12 hr for 10 days.
*Uncomplicated skin and skin structure infections.*
375 mg q 12 hr for 7–10 days.

## DENTAL CONCERNS

See also *General Dental Concerns for All Anti-Infectives* and *Cephalosporins.*
**Client/Family Teaching**
1. Take entire prescription as directed; do not stop when feeling better.
2. Report any adverse response or lack of improvement after 48–72 hr.

# Cefadroxil monohydrate
(sef-ah-**DROX**-ill)
**Pregnancy Category:** B
Duricef **(Rx)**
**Classification:** Cephalosporin, first-generation

See also *Anti-Infectives* and *Cephalosporins.*

**Action/Kinetics: Peak serum levels: PO,** 15–33 mcg/mL after 90 min. t½: **PO,** 70–80 min. Ninety percent of drug is excreted unchanged in urine within 24 hr.

**Uses:** UTIs caused by *Escherichia coli, Proteus mirabilis,* and *Klebsiella.* Skin and skin structure infections due to staphylococci or streptococci. Pharyngitis and tonsillitis due to group A beta-hemolytic streptococci. Prevention of bacterial endocarditis in patients who cannot tolerate or are allergic to penicillin. *Note:* Cephalosporins should not be used in individuals with immediate-type hypersensitivity reactions to penicillins.

**Contraindications:** See also *Cephalosporins.*

**Special Concerns:** Safe use in children not established. $C_{CR}$ determinations must be carried out in clients with renal impairment.

**Side Effects:** See also *Cephalosporins.*

**Drug Interactions:** See also *Cephalosporins.*

**How Supplied:** *Capsule:* 500 mg; *Powder for Reconstitution:* 125 mg/5 mL, 250 mg/5 mL, 500 mg/5 mL; *Tablet:* 1 g

**Dosage** ——————————
• **Capsules, Oral Suspension, Tablets**
*Pharyngitis, tonsillitis.*
**Adults:** 1 g/day in single or two divided doses for 10 days. **Children:** 30 mg/kg/day in single or two divided doses (for beta-hemolytic streptococcoal infection, dose should be given for 10 days).

*Skin and skin structure infections.*
**Adults:** 1 g/day in single or two divided doses. **Children:** 30 mg/kg/day in divided doses q 12 hr.

*UTIs.*
**Adults:** 1–2 g/day in single or two divided doses for uncomplicated lower UTI (e.g., cystitis). For all other UTIs, the usual dose is 2 g/day in two divided doses. **Children:** 30 mg/kg/day in divided doses q 12 hr.

*Bacterial endocarditis prophylaxis.*

**Adults:** 2 g 1 hr before dental procedure. **Children:** 50 mg/kg of body weight, not to exceed adult dose, 1 hr before dental procedure.

*For clients with $C_{CR}$ rates below 50 mL/min.*
**Initial:** 1 g; **maintenance,** 500 mg at following dosage intervals: q 36 hr for $C_{CR}$ rates of 0–10 mL/min; q 24 hr for $C_{CR}$ rates of 10–25 mL/min; q 12 hr for $C_{CR}$ rates of 25–50 mL/min.

## DENTAL CONCERNS

See also *General Dental Concerns for All Anti-Infectives* and *Cephalosporins.*
**Client/Family Teaching**
1. Take prescription as directed.
2. Report adverse side effects or lack of response.

## Cefazolin sodium
(sef-**AYZ**-oh-lin)
**Pregnancy Category:** B
Ancef, Kefzol, Zolicef **(Rx)**
**Classification:** Cephalosporin, first-generation

See also *Anti-Infectives* and *Cephalosporins.*

**Action/Kinetics: Peak serum concentration: IM** 17–76 mcg/mL after 1 hr. **t½: IM, IV:** 90–130 min. From 80% to 100% excreted unchanged in urine.

**Uses:** Infections of the urinary tract, biliary tract, respiratory tract, bones, joints, soft tissue, and skin. Endocarditis, septicemia, prophylaxis in surgery.

**Contraindications:** See also *Cephalosporins.*

**Special Concerns:** Safety in infants under 1 month of age has not been determined.

**Side Effects:** See also *Cephalosporins.*
**Additional Side Effects:** When high doses are used in renal failure clients: extreme confusion, *tonic-clonic seizures,* mild hemiparesis.

**Drug Interactions:** See also *Cephalosporins.*

---

**How Supplied:** *Injection:* 1 g/50 mL, 500 mg/50 mL; *Powder for injection:* 500 mg, 1 g, 5 g, 10 g

**Dosage**

- **IM, IV Only**
  *Mild infections due to gram-positive cocci.*
  **Adults:** 250–500 mg q 8 hr.
  *Mild to moderate infections.*
  **Children over 1 month:** 25–50 mg/kg/day in three to four doses.
  *Moderate to severe infections.*
  **Adults:** 0.5–1 g q 6–8 hr.
  *Acute, uncomplicated UTIs.*
  **Adults:** 1 g q 12 hr. *For severe infections,* up to 100 mg/kg/day may be used.
  *Endocarditis, septicemia.*
  **Adults:** 1–1.5 g q 6 hr (rarely, up to 12 g/day).
  *Pneumococcal pneumonia.*
  **Adults:** 0.5 g q 12 hr.
  *Preoperative.*
  **Adults:** 1 g 30–60 min prior to surgery.
  *During surgery.*
  **Adults:** 0.5–1 g.
  *Postoperative.*
  **Adults:** 0.5–1 g q 6–8 hr for 24 hr (may be given up to 5 days, especially in open heart surgery or prosthetic arthroplasty).
  *Bacterial endocarditis prophylaxis*
  **Adults:** 1 g IM or IV within 30 minutes of starting the procedure. **Children:** 25 mg/kg of body weight not to exceed adult dose, IM or IV within 30 minutes of starting the procedure. *Note:* Not to be used in patients with immediate-type hypersensitivity reactions to penicillins.
  *Impaired renal function.*
  **Initial:** 0.5 g; **then,** maintenance doses are given, depending on C$_{CR}$, according to schedule provided by manufacturer.

## DENTAL CONCERNS

See also *General Dental Concerns for All Anti-Infectives* and *Cephalosporins.*
**Client/Family Teaching**
1. Take prescription as directed.
2. Report adverse side effects or lack of response.

# Cefepime hydrochloride
(**SEF**-eh-pim)
**Pregnancy Category:** B
Maxipime **(Rx)**
**Classification:** Cephalosporin

See also *Cephalosporins.*
**Action/Kinetics:** Antibacterial activity against both gram-negative and gram-positive pathogens, including those resistant to other β-lactam antibiotics. High affinity for the multiple penicillin-binding proteins that are essential for cell wall synthesis. **Peak serum levels, after IV:** 78 mcg/mL. **t½, terminal:** 2 hr. About 85% of the drug is excreted unchanged in the urine.
**Uses:** Uncomplicated and complicated UTIs (including pyelonephritis) caused by *Escherichia coli* or *Klebsiella pneumoniae;* when the infection is severe or caused by *E. coli, K. pneumoniae,* or *Proteus mirabilis;* when the infection is mild to moderate, including infections associated with concurrent bacteremia with these microorganisms. Uncomplicated skin and skin structure infections caused by *Staphylococcus aureus* (methicillin-susceptible strains only) or *Streptococcus pyogenes.* Moderate to severe pneumonia due to *Streptococcus pneumoniae,* including cases associated with concurrent bacteremia, *Pseudomonas aeruginosa, K. pneumoniae,* or *Enterobacter* species. Monotherapy for empiric treatment of febrile neutropenia.
**Contraindications:** Use in those who have had an immediate hypersensitivity reaction to cefepime, cephalosporins, pencillins, or any other β-lactam antibiotics.
**Special Concerns:** Use with caution during lactation. Safety and efficacy have not been determined in children less than 12 years of age.
**Side Effects:** See *Cephalosporins.* The most common side effects include rash, phlebitis, pain, and/or inflammation.
**Drug Interactions**
*Aminoglycosides /* ↑ Risk of nephrotoxicity and ototoxicity

*Furosemide* / ↑ Risk of nephrotoxicity

**How Supplied:** *Powder for injection:* 500 mg, 1 g, 2 g

**Dosage**
- **IM, IV**

*Mild to moderate uncomplicated or complicated UTIs, including pyelonephritis, due to* E. coli, K. pneumoniae, *or* P. mirabilis.

**Adults and children over 12 years:** 0.5–1 g IV or IM (for *E. coli* infections) q 12 hr for 7–10 days.

*Severe uncomplicated or complicated UTIs, including pyelonephritis, due to* E. coli *or* K. pneumoniae.

**Adults and children over 12 years:** 2 g IV q 12 hr for 10 days.

*Moderate to severe pneumonia due to* S. pneumoniae, P. aeruginosa, K. pneumoniae, *or* Enterobacter *species.*

**Adults and children over 12 years:** 1–2 g IV q 12 hr for 10 days.

*Moderate to severe uncomplicated skin and skin structure infections due to* S. aureus *or* S. pyogenes.

**Adults and children over 12 years:** 2 g IV q 12 hr for 10 days.

*Febrile neutropenia.*

2 g IV q 8 hr for 7 days, or until resolution of neutropenia.

## DENTAL CONCERNS

See also *Dental Concerns* for *Cephalosporins.*

# Cefixime oral

(seh-**FIX**-eem)
**Pregnancy Category:** B
Suprax **(Rx)**
**Classification:** Cephalosporin, third-generation

See also *Anti-Infectives* and *Cephalosporins.*

**Action/Kinetics:** Stable in the presence of beta-lactamase enzymes. **Peak serum levels:** 2–6 hr. **t½:** averages 3–4 hr. About 50% excreted unchanged in the urine and approximately 10% in the bile.

**Uses:** Uncomplicated UTIs caused by *E. coli* and *P. mirabilis.* Otitis media due to *H. influenzae* (beta-lactamase positive and negative strains), *Moraxella catarrhalis,* and *S. pyogenes.* Pharyngitis and tonsillitis caused by *S. pyogenes.* Acute bronchitis and acute exacerbations of chronic bronchitis caused by *S. pneumoniae* and *H. influenzae* (beta-lactamase positive and negative strains). Uncomplicated cervical or urethral gonorrhea due to *N. gonorrhoeae* (both penicillinase- and non-penicillinase-producing strains).

**Contraindications:** See also *Cephalosporins.*

**Special Concerns:** Safe use in infants less than 6 months old has not been established.

**Side Effects:** See also *Cephalosporins.*

**Additional Side Effects:** *GI:* Flatulence. *Hepatic:* Elevated alkaline phosphatase levels. *Renal:* Transient increases in BUN or creatinine.

**Drug Interactions:** See also *Cephalosporins.*

**How Supplied:** *Powder for reconstitution:* 100 mg/5 mL; *Tablet:* 200 mg, 400 mg

**Dosage**
- **Oral Suspension, Tablets**

**Adults:** Either 400 mg once daily or 200 mg q 12 hr. **Children:** Either 8 mg/kg once daily or 4 mg/kg q 12 hr. Clients on renal dialysis or in whom $C_{CR}$ is 21–60 mL/min, the dose should be 75% of the standard dose (i.e., 300 mg/day). If the $C_{CR}$ is less than 20 mL/min, the dose should be 50% of the standard dose (i.e., 200 mg/day).

*Uncomplicated gonorrhea.*
One 400-mg tablet.

## DENTAL CONCERNS

See also *General Dental Concerns for All Anti-Infectives* and for *Cephalosporins.*

# Cefpodoxime proxetil
(sef-poh-**DOX**-eem)

**Pregnancy Category:** B
Vantin **(Rx)**
**Classification:** Cephalosporin, second-generation

See also *Anti-Infectives* and *Cephalosporins*.
**Action/Kinetics:** From 29% to 33% is excreted unchanged in the urine.
**Uses:** Acute, community-acquired pneumonia due to *Streptococcus pneumoniae* or *Hemophilus influenzae* (only non-β-lactamase-producing strains). Acute bacterial exacerbation of chronic bronchitis caused by *S. pneumoniae,* non-beta-lactamase-producing *H. influenzae,* or *Moraxella catarrhalis.* Acute otitis media caused by *S. pneumoniae, H. influenzae* (including beta-lactamase-producing strains), and *M. catarrhalis.* Pharyngitis or tonsillitis due to *Streptococcus pyogenes.* Acute, uncomplicated urethral and cervical gonorrhea caused by *Neisseria gonorrhoeae* (including penicillinase-producing strains). Acute, uncomplicated anorectal infections in women due to *N. gonorrhoeae* (including penicillinase-producing strains). Uncomplicated skin and skin structure infections due to *Staphylococcus aureus* (including penicillinase-producing strains) or *S. pyogenes.* Uncomplicated UTIs (cystitis) due to *Escherichia coli, Klebsiella pneumoniae, Proteus mirabilis,* or *Staphyloccus saprophyticus.*
**Contraindications:** Hypersensitivity to cephalosporins. Use in infants < 1 month of age.
**Special Concerns:** Hypersensitivity to penicillin antibiotics. Renal disease.
**Side Effects:** See also *Anti-Infectives* and *Cephalosporins.*
**Drug Interactions:** See also *Anti-Infectives* and *Cephalosporins.*
**How Supplied:** *Granule for reconstitution:* 50 mg/5 mL, 100 mg/5 mL; *Tablet:* 100 mg, 200 mg

**Dosage**
• **Tablets, Suspension**
*Acute community-acquired pneumonia.*
**Adults and children over 13 years:** 200 mg q 12 hr for 14 days.

*Acute bacterial exacerbations of chronic bronchitis.*
**Adults and children over 13 years:** 200 mg q 12 hr for 10 days.
*Uncomplicated gonorrhea (men and women) and rectal gonococcal infections (women).*
**Adults and children over 13 years:** Single dose of 200 mg.
*Skin and skin structure infections.*
**Adults and children over 13 years:** 400 mg q 12 hr for 7–14 days.
*Pharyngitis, tonsillitis.*
**Adults and children over 13 years:** 100 mg q 12 hr for 5–10 days.
**Children, 6 months–12 years:** 5 mg/kg (maximum of 100 mg/dose) q 12 hr (maximum daily dose: 200 mg) for 5–10 days.
*Uncomplicated UTIs.*
**Adults and children over 13 years:** 100 mg q 12 hr for 7 days.
*Acute otitis media.*
**Children, 6 months–12 years:** 5 mg/kg (maximum of 200 mg/dose) q 12 hr or 10 mg/kg q 24 hr for 10 days. The maximum daily dose should not exceed 400 mg.

## DENTAL CONCERNS

See also *General Dental Concerrns for All Anti-Infectives* and *Cephalosporins.*
**Client/Family Teaching**
1. Avoid mouth rinses with alcohol because of drying effects and possible drug-drug interactions

# Cefprozil
(**SEF**-proh-zill)
**Pregnancy Category:** B
Cefzil **(Rx)**
**Classification:** Cephalosporin, second-generation

See also *Anti-Infectives* and *Cephalosporins.*
**Action/Kinetics:** Sixty percent is recovered in the urine unchanged.
**Uses:** Pharyngitis and tonsillitis due to *Streptococcus pyogenes.* Acute bacterial sinusitis due to *Streptococcus pneumoniae, Staphylococcus aureus, Haemophilus influenzae,* and *Moraxella catarrhalis.* Otitis media

caused by *S. pneumoniae, H. influenzae,* and *M. catarrhalis.* Uncomplicated skin and skin structure infections due to *S. aureus* (including penicillinase-producing strains) and *S. pyogenes.* Secondary bacterial infection of acute bronchitis and acute bacterial exacerbation of chronic bronchitis due to *S. pneumoniae, H. influenzae* (beta-lactamase positive and negative strains), and *M. catarrhalis.*

**Contraindications:** Hypersensitivity to cephalosporins.

**Special Concerns:** Hypersensitivity to penicillins. Use caution in the elderly and those with renal disease.

**Side Effects:** See also *Cephalosporins.*

**Drug Interactions:** See also *Cephalosporins* .

**How Supplied:** *Powder for reconstitution:* 125 mg/5 mL, 250 mg/5 mL; *Tablet:* 250 mg, 500 mg

**Dosage** ————————————
• **Suspension, Tablets**
*Pharyngitis, tonsillitis, acute sinusitis.*
**Adults and children over 13 years of age:** 500 mg q 24 hr for at least 10 days (especially for *S. pyogenes* infections). **Children, 2–12 years of age:** 7.5 mg/kg q 12 hr for at least 10 days (especially for *S. pyogenes* infections).
*Secondary bacterial infections of acute bronchitis and acute bacterial exacerbation of chronic bronchitis.*
**Adults and children over 13 years of age:** 500 mg q 12 hr for 10 days.
*Uncomplicated skin and skin structure infections.*
**Adults and children over 13 years of age:** Either 250 mg q 12 hr, 500 mg q 24 hr, or 500 mg q 12 hr (all for a duration of 10 days).
*Otitis media.*
**Infants     and     children     6 months–12 years:** 15 mg/kg q 12 hr for 10 days.

## DENTAL CONCERNS

See also *General Dental Concerns*

*for All Anti-Infectives* and *Cephalosporins.*

**Client/Family Teaching**
1. Avoid mouth rinses with alcohol because of drying effects and possible drug-drug interactions

# Ceftibuten
(sef-**TYE**-byou-ten)
**Pregnancy Category:** B
Cedax **(Rx)**
**Classification:** Cephalosporin

See also *Cephalosporins.*

**Action/Kinetics:** Resistant to beta-lactamase. Has the broadest gram-negative spectrum of any of the current PO cephalosporins. Is well absorbed from the GI tract. Food delays the time to peak serum concentration, lowers the peak concentration, and decreases the total amount of drug absorbed. **Peak serum levels:** 2 to 3 hr. **t½:** 2 hr. Excreted in the urine.

**Uses:** Acute bacterial exacerbations of chronic bronchitis due to *Haemophilus influenzae* (including beta-lactamase-producing strains), *Moraxella catarrhalis* (including beta-lactamase-producing strains), and penicillin-susceptible strains of *Streptococcus pneumoniae.* Acute bacterial otitis media due to *H. influenzae, M. catarrhalis,* and *Staphylococcus pyogenes.* Pharyngitis and tonsillitis due to *S. pyogenes.*

**Contraindications:** Hypersensitivity to cephalosporins.

**Special Concerns:** Although ceftibuten has been approved for pharyngitis or tonsillitis, only penicillin has been shown to be effective in preventing rheumatic fever. Not approved to treat urinary infections. Hypersensitivity to penicillins. Use with caution in patients with renal impairement, infants < 6 months, and in patients with pseudomembraneous colitis. Oral suspension contains 1 g sucrose per 5 mL.

**Side Effects:** See *Cephalosporins.* Ceftibuten is usually well tolerated.

The most common side effect is diarrhea.

**Drug Interactions:** See also *Cephalosporins,*

*Aminoglycosides /* ↑ Nephrotoxic potential of cefibuten

**How Supplied:** *Capsules:* 400 mg; *Oral suspension:* 90 mg/5mL, 180 mg/5 mL.

**Dosage** ─────────────

• **Capsules, Oral Suspension**
  *All uses.*

**Adults and children over 12 years of age:** 400 mg once daily for 10 days. The maximum daily dose is 400 mg. Adjust the dose in clients with a creatinine clearance ($C_{CR}$) less than 50 mL/min as follows. If the $C_{CR}$ is between 30 and 49 mL/min, the recommended dose is 4.5 mg/kg or 200 mg once daily. If the $C_{CR}$ is between 5 and 29 mL/min, the recommended dose is 2.25 mg/kg or 100 mg once daily. In clients undergoing hemodialysis 2 or 3 times/week, a single 400-mg dose of ceftibuten capsules or a single dose of 9 mg/kg (maximum of 400 mg) of PO suspension can be given at the end of each hemodialysis session.

*Children: pharyngitis, tonsillitis, acute bacterial otitis media.*
9 mg/kg, up to a maximum of 400 mg daily, for a total of 10 days. Give children over 45 kg the maximum daily dose of 400 mg.

---

## DENTAL CONCERNS

See also *Dental Concerns* for *Anti-Infectives* and *Cephalosporins.*
**General**
1. Oral suspension contains sucrose. Instruct the patient to rinse and spit following each dose.
**Consultation with Primary Care Provider**
1. Consultation with the appropriate health care provider may be necessary to assess disease control.

---

# Cefuroxime axetil
(sef-your-**OX**-eem)
**Pregnancy Category:** B

Ceftin **(Rx)**
Classification: Cephalosporin, second-generation
─────────────

See also *Anti-Infectives* and *Cephalosporins.*

**Action/Kinetics:** Cefuroxime axetil is used PO, whereas cefuroxime sodium is used either IM or IV.

**Uses: PO (axetil).** Pharyngitis, tonsillitis, otitis media, sinusitis, acute bacterial exacerbations of chronic bronchitis and secondary bacterial infections of acute bronchitis, uncomplicated UTIs, uncomplicated skin and skin structure infections, uncomplicated gonorrhea (urethral and endocervical) caused by non-penicillinase-producing strains of *Neisseria gonorrhoeae.* Early Lyme disease due to *Borrelia burgdorferi.* The suspension is indicated for children from 3 months to 12 years to treat pharyngitis, tonsillitis, acute bacterial otitis media, and impetigo.

**Contraindications:** Hypersensitivity to cephalosporins. Use in infants < 1 month.

**Special Concerns:** Hypersensitivity to penicillin antibiotics. Those with renal disease.

**Side Effects:** See also *Cephalosporins.*
**Additional Side Effects:** Decrease in H&H.

**Drug Interactions:** See also *Cephalosporins.*

**How Supplied:** *Powder for reconstitution:* 125 mg/5 mL; *Tablet:* 125 mg, 250 mg, 500 mg.

**Dosage** ─────────────

• **Tablets**
  *Pharyngitis, tonsillits.*

**Adults and children over 13 years:** 250 mg q 12 hr for 10 days.
**Children:** 125 mg q 12 hr for 10 days.

*Acute bacterial exacerbations of chronic bronchitis and secondary bacterial infections of acute bronchitis, uncomplicated skin and skin structure infections.*

**Adults and children over 13 years:** 250 or 500 mg q 12 hr for 10 days (5 days for secondary bacterial infections of acute bronchitis).

*Uncomplicated UTIs.*

**Adults and children over 13 years:** 125 or 250 mg q 12 hr for 7–10 days. **Infants and children less than 12 years:** 125 mg b.i.d.

*Acute otitis media.*

**Children:** 250 mg b.i.d. for 10 days.

*Uncomplicated gonorrhea.*

**Adults and children over 13 years:** 1,000 mg as a single dose.

*Early Lyme disease.*

500 mg/day for 20 days.

• **Suspension**

*Pharyngitis, tonsillitis.*

**Children, 3 months to 12 years:** 20 mg/kg/day in 2 divided doses, not to exceed 500 mg total dose/day, for 10 days.

*Acute otitis media, impetigo.*

**Children, 3 months to 12 years:** 30 mg/kg/day in 2 divided doses, not to exceed 1,000 mg total dose/day, for 10 days.

## DENTAL CONCERNS

See also *General Dental Concerns for All Anti-Infectives* and *Cephalosporins.*

**Client/Family Teaching**

1. Avoid mouth rinses with alcohol because of drying effects and possible drug-drug interactions

# Celecoxib

(**sell**-ah-**KOX**-ihb)

**Pregnancy Category:** C (D after 34 weeks gestation or close to delivery)

Celebrex

**Classification:** Selective cyclooxygenase-2 Inhibitor

**Action/Kinetics:** Inhibits prostaglandin synthesis by decreasing the activity of cyclo-oxygenase-2 (COX-2). This results in a reduction of the formation of prostaglandin precursors. **Serum half-life:** 11 hr. **Time to peak:** 3 hr.

**Uses:** Treatment of osteoarthritis and rheumatoid arthritis in adults.

**Contraindications:** Hypersensitivity

**Special Concerns:** Patients with a history of GI bleeding, decreased re-

nal function, liver dysfunction, CHF, hypertension, asthma, aspirin sensitivity.

**Side Effects:** *Oral:* Dry mouth, taste changes, tooth disorder. *The following side effects occurred in greater than 2% of the population studied: GI:* Dyspepsia, diarrhea, abdominal pain, nausea, flatulence. *CNS:* Headache, insomnia, dizziness. *CV:* Peripheral edema. *Pulmonary:* URTI, sinusitis, pharyngitis, rhinitis. *Dermatologic:* skin rash. *Neuromuscular:* Back pain. *Miscellaneous:* Accidental injury.

**Drug Interactions**

*Aspirin* / ↑ Risk of GI bleeding

*Fluconazole* / ↑ Celecoxib levels

**How Supplied:** *Capsules:* 100 mg, 200 mg

## Dosage

• **Capsule**

*Osteoarthritis.*

**Adults:** 200 mg q.d. or 100 mg b.i.d.

*Rheumatiod arthritis.*

**Adults:** 100–200 mg b.i.d.

## DENTAL CONCERNS

**General**

1. Decreased saliva flow can put the patient at risk for dental caries, periodontal disease, and candidiasis.

2. A semisupine position for the dental chair may be necessary to help minimize or avoid GI adverse effects or be tolerable for patients with rheumatoid arthritis.

3. The patient should avoid prescription and over-the-counter aspirin-containing drug products.

**Consultation with Primary Care Provider**

1. Consultation may be required in order to assess extent of disease control.

**Client/Family Teaching**

1. Take with a full glass of water or milk, with meals, or with a prescribed antacid and remain upright 30 min following administration to reduce gastric irritation or ulcer formation.

2. Avoid alcohol or aspirin because of increased risk for GI bleeding.

---

3. Daily home fluoride treatments for persistent dry mouth.
4. Avoid alcohol-containing mouth rinses or beverages.
5. Avoid caffeine-containing beverages.
6. Dry mouth can be treated with tart, sugarless gum or candy, water, sugarless beverages, or with saliva substitutes if dry mouth persists.

# Cephalexin hydrochloride monohydrate
(sef-ah-**LEX**-in)
**Pregnancy Category:** B
Keftab **(Rx)**

# Cephalexin monohydrate
(sef-ah-**LEX**-in)
**Pregnancy Category:** B
Apo-Cephalex ✤, Biocef, Dom-Cephalexin ✤, Keflex, Novo-Lexin ✤, Nu-Cephalex ✤, PMS-Cephalexin ✤, STCC-Cephalexin ✤ **(Rx)**
**Classification:** Cephalosporin, first-generation

See also *Anti-Infectives* and *Cephalosporins.*
**Action/Kinetics:** Peak serum levels: **PO,** 9–39 mcg/mL after 1 hr. t½, **PO:** 30–72 min. Absorption delayed in children. The HCl monohydrate does not require conversion in the stomach before absorption. Ninety percent of drug excreted unchanged in urine within 8 hr.
**Uses:** Respiratory tract infections caused by *Streptococcus pneumoniae* and group A β-hemolytic streptococci. Otitis media due to *S. pneumoniae, Hemophilus influenzae, Moraxella catarrhalis* (use monohydrate only), staphylococci, and streptococci. Genitourinary tract infections (including acute prostatitis) due to *Escherichia coli, Proteus mirabilis,* and *Klebsiella.* Bone infections caused by *P. mirabilis* and staphylococci. Skin and skin structure infections due to staphylococci and streptococci. Bacterial endocarditis prophylaxis.
**Contraindications:** Hypersensitivity to cephalosporins.

**Special Concerns:** Safety and effectiveness of the HCl monohydrate have not been determined in children. Hypersensitivity to penicillins. Use in patients with renal impairment.
**Side Effects:** See also *Cephalosporins.*
**Additional Side Effects:** Nephrotoxicity, cholestatic jaundice.
**Drug Interactions:** See also *Cephalosporins.*
**How Supplied:** Cephalexin hydrochloride monohydrate: *Tablet:* 500 mg. Cephalexin monohydrate: *Capsule:* 250 mg, 500 mg; *Powder for reconstitution:* 125 mg/5 mL, 250 mg/5 mL; *Tablet:* 250 mg, 500 mg

## Dosage
• **Capsules, Oral Suspension, Tablets**
*General infections.*
**Adults, usual:** 250 mg q 6 hr up to 4 g/day. **Pediatric:** *Monohydrate,* 25–50 mg/kg/day in four equally divided doses.
*Infections of skin and skin structures, streptococcal pharyngitis, uncomplicated cystitis, over 15 years.*
**Adults:** 500 mg q 12 hr. Large doses may be needed for severe infections or for less susceptible organisms. For streptococcal pharyngitis in children over 1 year and for skin and skin structure infections, the total daily dose should be divided and given q 12 hr. In severe infections, the dose should be doubled.
*Otitis media.*
**Pediatric:** 75–100 mg/kg/day in four divided doses.
*Bacterial endocarditis prophylaxis.*
**Adults:** 2 g 1 hr before procedure for patients unable to take amoxicillin. **Pediatric:** 20 mg/kg of body weight 1 hr before procedure. *Note:* Should not be used in patients with immediate-type hypersensitivity reactions to penicillins.

## DENTAL CONCERNS

See also *General Dental Concerns for All Anti-Infectives* and *Cephalosporins.*
**Client/Family Teaching**
1. Avoid mouth rinses with alcohol

because of drying effects and possible drug-drug interactions

# Cephradine

(**SEF**-rah-deen)
**Pregnancy Category:** B
Anspor, Velosef **(Rx)**
**Classification:** Cephalosporin, first-generation

See also *Anti-Infectives* and *Cephalosporins*.
**Action/Kinetics:** Similar to cephalexin. Rapidly absorbed PO or IM (30 min–2 hr); 60%–90% excreted after 6 hr. **Peak serum levels: PO,** 8–24 mcg/mL after 30–60 min; **IM,** 5.6–13.6 mcg/mL after 1–2 hr. **t½:** 42–120 min; 80%–95% excreted in urine unchanged.
**Uses:** Infections of the respiratory tract (including lobar pneumonia, tonsillitis, pharyngitis), urinary tract (including prostatitis and enterococcal infections), skin, skin structures, and bone. Otitis media, septicemia, prophylaxis in surgery, following cesarean section to prevent infection. In severe infections, therapy is usually initiated parenterally.
**Contraindications:** Hypersensitivity to cephalosporins.
**Special Concerns:** Safe use during pregnancy, of the parenteral form in infants under 1 month of age, and of the PO form in children less than 9 months of age have not been established. Hypersensitivity to penicillins. Use in renal impairment.
**Side Effects:** See also *Cephalosporins*.
**Drug Interactions:** See also *Cephalosporins*.
**How Supplied:** *Capsule:* 250 mg, 500 mg; *Powder for reconstitution:* 125 mg/5 mL, 250 mg/5 mL

## Dosage

• **Capsules, Oral Suspension**
*Skin and skin structures, respiratory tract infections.*
**Adults, usual:** 250 mg q 6 hr or 500 mg q 12 hr.
*Lobar pneumonia.*
**Adults:** 500 mg q 6 hr or 1 g q 12 hr.

*Uncomplicated UTIs.*
**Adults, usual:** 500 mg q 12 hr.
*More serious infections and prostatitis.*
500 mg q 6 hr or 1 g q 12 hr (severe, chronic infections may require up to 1 g q 6 hr).
**Pediatric, over 9 months:** 25–50 mg/kg/day in equally divided doses q 6–12 hr (75–100 mg/kg/day for otitis media).
• **Deep IM, IV**
*General infections.*
**Adults:** 2–4 g/day in equally divided doses q.i.d.
*Surgical prophylaxis.*
**Adults:** 1 g 30–90 min before surgery; **then,** 1 g q 4–6 hr for one to two doses (or up to 24 hr postoperatively).
*Cesarean section, prophylaxis.*
**IV:** 1 g when the umbilical cord is clamped; **then,** give two additional 1-g doses **IV or IM** 6 and 12 hr after the initial dose. **Pediatric, over 1 year:** 50–100 mg/kg/day in equally divided doses q.i.d.

## DENTAL CONCERNS

See also *General Dental Concerns for All Anti-Infectives* and *Cephalosporins*.
**Client/Family Teaching**
1. Avoid mouth rinses with alcohol because of drying effects and possible drug-drug interactions.

# Cerivastatin sodium

(seh-**RIHV**-ah-stat-in)
**Pregnancy Category:** X
Baycol **(Rx)**
**Classification:** Antihyperlipidemic agent—HMG-CoA reductase inhibitors

See also *Antihyperlipidemic Agents—HMG-CoA Reductase Inhibitors*.
**Action/Kinetics:** Competitive inhibitor of HMG-CoA reductase leading to inhibition of cholesterol synthesis and decrease in plasma cholesterol levels. **Peak plasma levels:** 2.5 hr.

---

✦ = Available in Canada          ***bold italic*** = life-threatening side effect

**t½, terminal:** 2–3 hr. Food does not affect blood levels. Metabolized in liver and excreted through urine and feces.

**Uses:** Adjunct to diet to reduce elevated total and LDL cholesterol in clients with primary hypercholesterolemia and mixed dyslipidemia when response to diet or other non-pharmacologic approaches have not been adequate.

**Contraindications:** Use in active liver disease or unexplained elevation of serum transaminases. Pregnancy, lactation.

**Special Concerns:** Use in women of child-bearing age only when pregnancy is unlikely and they have been informed of potential risks. Drug has not been evaluated in rare homozygous familial hypercholesterolemia. Due to interference with cholesterol synthesis and lower cholesterol levels, may be blunting of adrenal or gonadal steroid hormone production. Use with caution in renal or hepatic insufficiency. Safety and efficacy have not been determined in children.

**Side Effects:** See also *HMG-CoA Reductase Inhibitors. Musculoskeletal:* Rarely, rhabdomyolysis with acute renal failure secondary to myoglobinemia.

**Drug Interactions:** ↑ Risk of myopathy when used with azole antifungals, cyclosporine, and erythromycin.

**How Supplied:** *Tablets:* 0.2 mg, 0.3 mg

**Dosage** ————————
• **Tablets**
  *Hypercholesterolemia.*
**Adults:** 0.3 mg once daily in evening. Recommended starting dose in those with significant renal impairment ($C_{CR}$ less than 60 mL/min/1.73 m$^2$) is 0.2 mg once daily in evening.

## DENTAL CONCERNS

See also *Dental Concerns* for *Antibyperlipidemic Agents—HMG-CoA Reductase Inhibitors.*

# Cetirizine hydrochloride
(seh-**TIH**-rah-zeen)
**Pregnancy Category:** B
Reactine ✱, Zyrtec **(Rx)**
**Classification:** Antihistamine

See also *Antihistamines.*

**Action/Kinetics:** A potent H$_1$-receptor antagonist. A mild bronchodilator that protects against histmine-induced bronchospasm; negligible anticholinergic and sedative activity. Rapidly absorbed after PO administration; however, food delays the time to peak serum levels but does not decrease the total amount of drug absorbed. Poorly penetrates the CNS, but high levels are distributed to the skin. **t½:** 8.3 hr (longer in elderly clients and in those with impaired liver or renal function). Excreted mostly unchanged (70%) in the urine; 10% is excreted in the feces.

**Uses:** Relief of symptoms associated with seasonal allergic rhinitis due to ragweed, grass, and tree pollens; perennial allergic rhinitis due to allergens such as dust mites, animal dander, and molds. Chronic idiopathic urticaria.

**Contraindications:** Lactation. In those hypersensitive to hydroxyzine.

**Special Concerns:** Due to the possibility of sedation, use with caution in situations requiring mental alertness. Safety and efficacy have not been determined in children less than 12 years of age.

**Side Effects:** See *Antihistamines.* The most common side effects are somnolence, dry mouth, fatigue, pharyngitis, and dizziness.

**How Supplied:** *Tablets:* 5 mg, 10 mg

**Dosage** ————————
• **Tablets**
  *Seasonal or perennial allergic rhinitis, chronic urticaria.*
**Adults and children over 6 years of age, initial:** Depending on the severity of the symptoms, 5 or 10 mg (most common initial dose) once daily. In clients with decreased renal function ($C_{CR}$: 11–31 mL/min), in hemodialysis clients ($C_{CR}$ less than 7

mL/min), and in those with impaired hepatic function, the dose is 5 mg once daily.

## DENTAL CONCERNS
**General**
1. Decreased saliva flow can put the patient at risk for dental caries, periodontal disease, and candidiasis.
**Client/Family Teaching**
1. Daily home fluoride treatments for persistent dry mouth.
2. Avoid alcohol-containing mouth rinses and beverages.
3. Avoid caffeine-containing beverages.
4. Dry mouth can be treated with tart, sugarless gum or candy, water, sugar-free beverages, or with saliva substitutes if dry mouth persists.

# Chloral hydrate
(**KLOH**-ral **HY**-drayt)
**Pregnancy Category:** C
Aquachloral Supprettes, Novo-Chlorhydrate ✿, PMS-Chloral Hydrate ✿ **(C-IV) (Rx)**
**Classification:** Nonbenzodiazepine, nonbarbiturate sedative-hypnotic

**Action/Kinetics:** Chloral hydrate is metabolized to trichloroethanol, which is the active metabolite causing CNS depression. Produces only slight hangover effects and is said not to affect REM sleep. High doses lead to severe CNS depression, as well as depression of respiratory and vasomotor centers (hypotension). Both psychologic and physical dependence develop. **Onset:** Within 30 min. **Duration:** 4–8 hr. **t½, trichloroethanol:** 7–10 hr. Readily absorbed from the GI tract and distributed to all tissues; passes the placental barrier and appears in breast milk. Metabolites excreted by kidney.

**Uses:** Short-term hypnotic. Daytime sedative and sedation prior to EEG procedures. Preoperative sedative and postoperative as adjunct to analgesics. Prevent or reduce symptoms of alcohol withdrawal.

**Contraindications:** Marked hepatic or renal impairment, severe cardiac disease, lactation. PO use in clients with esophagitis, gastritis, or gastric or duodenal ulcer.

**Special Concerns:** Use by nursing mothers may cause sedation in the infant. A decrease in dose may be necessary in geriatric clients due to age-related decrease in both hepatic and renal function.

**Side Effects:** *CNS:* Paradoxical paranoid reactions. Sudden withdrawal in dependent clients may result in "chloral delirium." *Sudden intolerance to the drug following prolonged use may result in respiratory depression, hypotension, cardiac effects, and possibly death.* *Oral:* Bad taste in mouth, mucosal irritation. *GI:* N&V, diarrhea, gastritis, increased peristalsis. *GU:* Renal damage, decreased urine flow and uric acid excretion. *Miscellaneous:* Skin reactions, hepatic damage, allergic reactions, leukopenia, eosinophilia.

Chronic toxicity is treated by gradual withdrawal and rehabilitative measures such as those used in treatment of the chronic alcoholic. Poisoning by chloral hydrate resembles acute barbiturate intoxication; the same supportive treatment is indicated (see *Barbiturates*).

**Drug Interactions**
*CNS depressants* / Additive CNS depression; concomitant use may lead to drowsiness, lethargy, stupor, respiratory collapse, coma, or death

**How Supplied:** *Capsule:* 500 mg; *Suppository:* 325 mg, 500 mg, 650 mg; *Syrup:* 250 mg/5 mL, 500 mg/5 mL

## Dosage
• **Capsules, Syrup**
*Daytime sedative.*
**Adults:** 250 mg t.i.d. after meals.
*Preoperative sedative.*
**Adults:** 0.5–1.0 g 30 min before surgery.
*Hypnotic.*
**Adults:** 0.5–1 g 15–30 min before bedtime. **Pediatric:** 50 mg/kg (1.5

g/m²) at bedtime (up to 1 g may be given as a single dose).
*Daytime sedative.*
**Pediatric:** 8.3 mg/kg (250 mg/m²) up to a maximum of 500 mg t.i.d. after meals.
*Premedication prior to EEG procedures.*
**Pediatric:** 20–25 mg/kg.
- **Suppositories, Rectal**
*Daytime sedative.*
**Adults:** 325 mg t.i.d. **Pediatric:** 8.3 mg/kg (250 mg/m²) t.i.d.
*Hypnotic.*
**Adults:** 0.5–1 g at bedtime. **Pediatric:** 50 mg/kg (1.5 g/m²) at bedtime (up to 1 g as a single dose).

## DENTAL CONCERNS
### General
1. A semisupine position for the dental chair may be necessary to help minimize or avoid adverse GI effects.
2. Mix the liquid in fruit juice or punch in order to mask the unpleasant taste and minimize adverse GI effects.
3. This drug is contraindicated in patients with peptic ulcer disease.
4. There is a risk for physical and psychological dependence with chronic use.
### Client/Family Teaching
1. Avoid activities that require mental alertness. Have someone drive you to and from your appointment.

# Chlorhexidine gluconate
(klor-**HEX** i-deen)
**Pregnancy Category: B**
PerioGard
**Classification:** Anti-infective oral rinse

**Action/Kinetics:** Chorhexidine is absorbed onto the tooth surface, dental plaque, and oral mucosa allowing for a sustained reduction of plaque organisms. Poorly absorbed orally, 30% retained in the oral cavity and slowly released.
**Uses:** Treatment of gingivitis between dental visits. *Non-FDA Approved Uses:* Acute aphthous ulcers, denture stomatitis.

**Contraindications:** Hypersensitivity.
**Special Concerns:** Efficacy not established in children < 18 years of age, lactation, not intended for periodontitis.
**Side Effects:** *Oral:* Altered sense of taste, increased calculus formation, staining of teeth, tongue, and restorations, mucosal desquamation and irritation, transient parotitis.
**Drug Interactions**
*Alcohol* / ↑ Chance of disulfiram-like reaction
*Disfulfiram* / ↑ Chance of disulfiram-like reaction
*Metronidazole* / ↑ Chance of disulfiram-like reaction
**How Supplied:** *Oral rinse:* 0.12%

## Dosage
- **Oral rinse**
*Gingivitis.*
**Adults:** Rinse with 15 mL for 30 seconds b.i.d. after brushing and flossing teeth, then expectorate.
*Denture stomatitis.*
Soak dentures for 1 to 2 min b.i.d. Have the patient follow the oral rinse instructions.

## DENTAL CONCERNS
### General
1. Patients require dental examination and prophylaxis/scaling/root planing prior to the rinse.
2. Patients require frequent visits due to oral side effects.
3. The medication may not be appropriate for patients with anterior facial restorations with rough surfaces or margins.
### Client/Family Teaching
1. Patients should be instructed to eat, brush, and floss prior to using the rinse.
2. Do not rinse with water after using the rinse.
3. Inform patients of the oral side effects of this drug.

# Chlorpheniramine maleate
(klor-fen-**EAR**-ah-meen)
**Pregnancy Category: B**
**Syrup, Tablets, Chewable Tablets:**
Aller-Chlor, Allergy, Chlo-Amine,

Chlor-Trimeton Allergy 4 Hour, Chlor-Tripolon ✚ **(OTC), Extended-release Tablets:** Chlor-Trimeton 8 Hour and 12 Hour **(OTC), Injectable:** Chlorpheniramine maleate **(Rx)**
**Classification:** Antihistamine, alkylamine type

See also *Antihistamines.*
**Action/Kinetics:** Moderate anticholinergic and low sedative activity. **Onset:** 15–30 min. **t½:** 21–27 hr. **Time to peak effect:** 6 hr. **Duration:** 3–6 hr.
**Uses:** *PO:* Allergic rhinitis. *IM, SC:* Allergic reactions to blood and plasma and adjunct to anaphylaxis therapy.
**Contraindications:** IV or intradermal use. Not recommended for children under 6 years of age.
**Special Concerns:** Geriatric clients may be more sensitive to the adult dose. Parenteral route not recommended for neonates.
**How Supplied:** *Capsule, Extended Release:* 8 mg, 12 mg; *Chew Tablet:* 2 mg; *Injection:* 10 mg/mL; *Syrup:* 2 mg/5 mL; *Tablet:* 4 mg; *Tablet, Extended Release:* 8 mg, 12 mg, 16 mg

**Dosage**
• **Syrup, Tablets, Chewable Tablets**
**Adults and children over 12 years:** 4 mg q 6 hr, not to exceed 24 mg in 24 hr. **Pediatric, 6–12 years:** 2 mg (break 4-mg tablets in half) q 4–6 hr, not to exceed 12 mg in 24 hr. **2–6 years:** 1 mg (¼ of a 4-mg tablet) q 4–6 hr.
• **Extended-Release Tablets**
**Adults and children over 12 years:** 8 mg q 8–12 hr or 12 mg q 12 hr, not to exceed 24 mg in 24 hr.
• **IM, SC**
**Adults and children over 12 years:** 5–40 mg for uncomplicated allergic reactions; 10–20 mg for amelioration of allergic reactions to blood or plasma or to treat anaphylaxis. Maximum dose per 24 hr: 40 mg.

**DENTAL CONCERNS**

See also *Dental Concerns* for *Antihistamines.*

# Chlorpromazine
(klor-**PROH**-mah-zeen)
Thorazine **(Rx)**

# Chlorpromazine hydrochloride
(klor-**PROH**-mah-zeen)
Apo-Chlorpromazine ✚, Chlorprom ✚, Chlorpromanyl ✚, Largactil ✚, Novo–Chlorpromazine ✚, Ormazine, Thorazine, Thor-Prom **(Rx)**
**Classification:** Antipsychotic, dimethylamino-type phenothiazine

See also *Antipsychotic Agents, Phenothiazines.*
**Action/Kinetics:** Has significant antiemetic, hypotensive, and sedative effects; moderate to strong anticholinergic effects and weak to moderate extrapyramidal effects. **Peak plasma levels:** 2–3 hr after both PO and IM administration. **t½** (after IV, IM): **Initial,** 4–5 hr; **final,** 3–40 hr. Extensively metabolized in the intestinal wall and liver; certain of the metabolites are active. **Steady-state plasma levels** (in psychotics): 10–1,300 ng/mL. After 2–3 weeks of therapy, plasma levels decline, possibly because of reduction in drug absorption and/or increase in drug metabolism.
**Uses:** Acute and chronic psychoses, including schizophrenia; manic phase of manic-depressive illness. Acute intermittent porphyria. Preanesthetic, adjunct to treat tetanus, intractable hiccoughs, severe behavioral problems in children, neuroses, and N&V. Treatment of choreiform movements in Huntington's disease.
**Special Concerns:** Use during pregnancy only if benefits outweigh risks. PO dosage for psychoses and N&V has not been established in children less than 6 months of age.
**Additional Drug Interactions**
*Epinephrine* / Chlorpromazine ↓ peripheral vasoconstriction and may reverse action of epinephrine
*Norepinephrine* / Chlorpromazine ↓ pressor effect and eliminates bradycardia due to norepinephrine

---

✚ = Available in Canada                    ***bold italic*** = life-threatening side effect

**How Supplied:** Chlorpromazine: *Suppository:* 25 mg. Chlorpromazine hydrochloride: *Capsule, Extended Release:* 30 mg, 75 mg, 150 mg; *Concentrate:* 30 mg/mL, 100 mg/mL; *Injection:* 25 mg/mL; *Syrup:* 10 mg/5 mL; *Tablet:* 10 mg, 25 mg, 50 mg, 100 mg, 200 mg

## Dosage

• **Tablets, Extended-Release Capsules, Oral Concentrate, Syrup**
*Psychotic disorders.*
**Adults and adolescents:** 10–25 mg (of the base) b.i.d.–q.i.d.; dosage may be increased by 20–50 mg/day q 3–4 days as needed. Or, 30–300 mg (of the base) using the extended-release capsules 1–3 times/day (the 300-mg extended-release capsules are used only in severe neuropsychiatric situations). **Pediatric:** 0.55 mg/kg (15 mg/m²) q 4–6 hr.
*N&V.*
**Adults and adolescents:** 10–25 mg (of the base) q 4 hr; dosage may be increased as needed. **Pediatric:** 0.55 mg/kg (15 mg/m²) q 4–6 hr.
*Preoperative sedation.*
**Adults and adolescents:** 25–50 mg (of the base) 2–3 hr before surgery. **Pediatric:** 0.55 mg/kg (15 mg/m²) 2–3 hr before surgery.
*Hiccoughs or porphyria.*
**Adults and adolescents:** 25–50 mg (of the base) t.i.d.–q.i.d.
• **IM**
*Severe psychoses.*
**Adults:** 25–50 mg (of the base) repeated in 1 hr if needed; **then,** repeat the dose q 3–4 hr as needed and tolerated (the dose may be increased gradually over several days). **Pediatric, over 6 months:** 0.55 mg/kg (15 mg/m²) q 6–8 hr as needed.
*N&V.*
**Adults:** 25 mg (base) as a single dose; **then,** increase to 25–50 mg q 3–4 hr as needed until vomiting ceases. **Pediatric:** 0.55 mg/kg q 6–8 hr as needed.
*N&V during surgery.*
**Adults:** 12.5 mg (base) as a single dose; repeat in 30 min if needed. **Pediatric,** 0.275 mg/kg; repeat in 30 min if needed.

*Preoperative sedative.*
**Adults:** 12.5–25 mg (base) 1–2 hr before surgery. **Pediatric:** 0.55 mg/kg 1–2 hr before surgery.
*Hiccoughs.*
**Adults:** 25–50 mg (base) t.i.d.–q.i.d.
*Porphyria.*
**Adults:** 25 mg (base) q 6–8 hr until client can take PO therapy.
*Tetanus.*
**Adults:** 25–50 mg (base) t.i.d.–q.i.d. (dose can be increased as needed and tolerated).
• **IV**
*N&V during surgery.*
**Adults:** 25 mg (base) diluted to 1 mg/mL with 0.9% NaCl injection given at a rate of no more than 2 mg/2 min. **Pediatric:** 0.275 mg/kg diluted to 1 mg/mL with 0.9% NaCl injection given at a rate of no more than 1 mg q 2 min.
*Tetanus.*
**Adults:** 25–50 mg (base) diluted to 1 mg/mL with 0.9% NaCl injection and given at a rate of 1 mg/min. **Pediatric:** 0.55 mg/kg diluted to 1 mg/mL with 0.9% NaCl injection and given at a rate of 1 mg/2 min.
• **Suppositories**
*N&V.*
**Adults and adolescents:** 50–100 mg q 6–8 hr as needed up to a maximum of 400 mg/day. **Pediatric:** 1 mg/kg q 6–8 hr as needed (do not use the 100-mg suppository in children).

## DENTAL CONCERNS

See also *Dental Concerns* for *Antipsychotic Agents, Phenothiazines.*

# Chlorpropamide
(klor-**PROH**-pah-myd)
**Pregnancy Category:** C
Apo-Chlorpropamide ✸, Diabinese, Novo–Propamide ✸ **(Rx)**
**Classification:** Sulfonylurea, first-generation

See also *Antidiabetic Agents: Hypoglycemic Agents and Insulin.*
**Action/Kinetics:** May be effective in clients who do not respond well to other antidiabetic agents. **Onset:** 1 hr. **t½:** 35 hr. **Time to peak levels:**

2–4 hr. **Duration:** Up to 60 hr (due to slow excretion). Eighty percent metabolized in liver; 80%–90% excreted in the urine.

**Additional Uses:** *Non-FDA Approved Uses:* Neurogenic diabetes insipidus.

**Special Concerns:** If the client is susceptible to fluid retention or has impaired cardiac function, frequent monitoring is necessary.

**Additional Side Effects:** Side effects are frequent. Severe diarrhea, occasionally accompanied by bleeding in the lower bowel. Relieve severe GI distress by dividing total daily dose in half. In older clients, hypoglycemia may be severe. Inappropriate ADH secretion, leading to hyponatremia, water retention, low serum osmolality, and high urine osmolality.

**Additional Drug Interactions**

*Disulfiram* / More likely to interact with chlorpropamide than other oral antidiabetics

*Probenecid* / ↑ Effect of chlorpropamide

*Sodium bicarbonate* / ↓ Effect of chlorpropamide due to ↑ excretion by kidney

**How Supplied:** *Tablet:* 100 mg, 250 mg

**Dosage**

- **Tablets**

    *Diabetes.*

**Adults, middle-aged clients, mild to moderate diabetes, initial:** 250 mg/day as a single or divided dose; **geriatric, initial:** 100–125 mg/day. **All clients, maintenance:** 100–250 mg/day as single or divided doses. Severe diabetics may require 500 mg/day; doses greater than 750 mg/day are not recommended.

    *Neurogenic diabetes insipidus.*
**Adults:** 200–500 mg/day.

## DENTAL CONCERNS

See also *Dental Concerns* for *Antidiabetic Agents: Hypoglycemic Agents (Including Sulfonylureas).*

# Cholestyramine resin

(koh-less-**TEER**-ah-meen)
Alti-Cholestyramine Light ✼, Lo-Cholest, Novo-Cholaine Light ✼, PMS-Cholestyramine ✼, Prevalite, Questran, Questran Light **(Rx)**
**Classification:** Hypocholesterolemic agent, bile acid sequestrant

**Action/Kinetics:** Binds sodium cholate (bile salts) in the intestine; thus, the principal precursor of cholesterol is not absorbed due to formation of an insoluble complex, which is excreted in the feces. Decreases cholesterol and LDL and either has no effect or increases triglycerides, VLDL, and HDL. Also, itching is relieved as a result of removing irritating bile salts. The antidiarrheal effect results from the binding and removal of bile acids. **Onset, to reduce plasma cholesterol:** Within 24–48 hr, but levels may continue to fall for 1 yr; **to relieve pruritus:** 1–3 weeks; **relief of diarrhea associated with bile acids:** 24 hr. Cholesterol levels return to pretreatment levels 2–4 weeks after discontinuance. Fat-soluble vitamins (A, D, K) and possibly folic acid may have to be administered IM during long-term therapy because cholestyramine binds these vitamins in the intestine.

**Uses:** Adjunct to reduce elevated serum cholesterol in primary hypercholesterolemia in those who do not respond adequately to diet. Pruritus associated with partial biliary obstruction. Diarrhea due to bile acids. *Non-FDA Approved Uses:* Antibiotic-induced pseudomembranous colitis (i.e., due to toxin produced by *Clostridium difficile*), digitalis toxicity, treatment of chlordecone (Kepone) poisoning, treatment of thyroid hormone overdose.

**Contraindications:** Complete obstruction or atresia of bile duct, hypersensitivity.

**Special Concerns:** Use during pregnancy only if benefits outweigh risks. Use with caution during lactation and in children. Long-term effects and efficacy in decreasing cholesterol levels in pediatric clients are not known. Geriatric clients may be more likely to manifest GI side effects as well as adverse nutritional effects. Caution should be exercised by phenylketonurics as Prevalite contains 14.1 mg phenylalanine per 5.5-g dose.

**Side Effects:** *Oral:* Dental bleeding, sour taste. *GI:* Constipation (may be severe), N&V, diarrhea, heartburn, GI bleeding, anorexia, flatulence, belching, abdominal distention, abdominal pain or cramping, loose stools, indigestion, aggravation of hemorrhoids, rectal bleeding or pain, black stools, bleeding duodenal ulcer, peptic ulceration, GI irritation, dysphagia, dental bleeding, hiccoughs, sour taste, pancreatitis, diverticulitis, cholescystitis, cholelithiasis. Fecal impaction in elderly clients. Large doses may cause steatorrhea. *CNS:* Migraine or sinus headaches, dizziness, anxiety, vertigo, insomnia, fatigue, lightheadedness, syncope, drowsiness, femoral nerve pain, paresthesia. *Hypersensitivity:* Urticaria, dermatitis, asthma, wheezing, rash. *Hematologic:* Increased PT, ecchymosis, anemia. *Musculoskeletal:* Muscle or joint pain, backache, arthritis, osteoporosis. *GU:* Hematuria, dysuria, burnt odor to urine, diuresis. *Other:* Bleeding tendencies (due to hypoprothrombinemia). Deficiencies of vitamins A and D. Uveitis, weight loss or gain, osteoporosis, swollen glands, increased libido, weakness, SOB, edema, swelling of hands/feet; hyperchloremic acidosis in children, rash and irritation of the skin, tongue, and perianal area.

**Drug Interactions**
*Aspirin* / ↓ Absorption of aspirin from GI tract
*Cephalexin* / ↓ Absorption of cephalexin from GI tract
*Clindamycin* / ↓ Absorption of clindamycin from GI tract
*Corticosteroids* / ↓ Absorption of corticosteroids from GI tract
*Hydrocortisone* / ↓ Effect of hydrocortisone due to ↓ absorption from GI tract

*Penicillin G* / ↓ Effect of penicillin G due to ↓ absorption from GI tract
*Phenobarbital* / ↓ Absorption of phenobarbital from GI tract
*Piroxicam* / ↑ Elimination
*Tetracyclines* / ↓ Effect of tetracyclines due to ↓ absorption from GI tract

*NOTE:* These drug interactions may also be observed with colestipol.

**How Supplied:** *Powder for reconstitution:* 4 g/5 g, 4 g/5.5 g, 4 g/5.7 g, 4 g/9 g

**Dosage**
• **Powder**
**Adults, initial:** 1 g 1–2 times/day. Dose is individualized. **Maintenance:** 2–4 packets or scoopfuls/day (8–16 g anhydrous cholestyramine resin) mixed with 60–180 mL water or noncarbonated beverage. The recommended dosing schedule is b.i.d. but it can be given in one to six doses/day. Maximum daily dose: 6 packets or scoopsful.

## DENTAL CONCERNS
**General**
1. Review life-style, duration of illness, and attempts made to control with diet, exercise, and weight reduction.
2. Consider repositioning dental chair to semisupine condition for patient discomfort because of GI side effects.

## Cidofovir
(sih-**DOF**-oh-veer)
**Pregnancy Category:** C
Vistide **(Rx)**
**Classification:** Antiviral drug

See also *Antiviral Drugs.*

**Action/Kinetics:** A nucleotide analog that suppresses CMV replication by selective inhibition of viral DNA synthesis. Must be administered with probenecid.

**Uses:** Treatment of CMV retinitis in clients with AIDS.

**Contraindications:** History of severe hypersensitivity to probenecid or other sulfa-containing drugs. Use by direct intraocular injection.

**Special Concerns:** Safety and efficacy have not been determined for children or for treatment of other CMV infections, including pneumonitis, gastroenteritis, congenital or neonatal CMV disease, or CMV disease in non-HIV-infected clients. Increased risk of ocular hypotony in those with preexisting diabetes. Use in clients with a baseline serum creatinine greater than 1.5 mg/dL or creatinine clearances of 55 mL/min or less only when potential benefits outweigh potential risks.

**Side Effects:** *Renal/GU:* Nephrotoxicity, Fanconi's syndrome and decreases in serum bicarbonate associated with renal tubular damage, proteinuria, elevated serum creatinine, glycosuria, hematuria, urinary incontinence, UTI. *Oral:* Tongue discoloration, oral candidiasis, stomatitis, apththous stomatitis, mouth ulceration, dry mouth. *GI:* N&V, diarrhea, anorexia, abdominal pain, colitis, constipation, dyspepsia, dysphagia, flatulence, gastritis, hepatomegaly, abnormal liver function tests, melena, rectal disorder. *CNS:* Headache, asthenia, amnesia, anxiety, confusion, ***convulsions,*** depression, dizziness, abnormal gait, hallucinations, insomnia, neuropathy, paresthesia, somnolence. *CV:* Hypotension, postural hypotension, pallor, syncope, tachycardia, vasodilation. *Hematologic:* Neutropenia, granulocytopenia, thrombocytopenia, anemia. *Respiratory:* Asthma, bronchitis, coughing, dyspnea, hiccup, increased sputum, lung disorder, pharyngitis, pneumonia, rhinitis, sinusitis. *Dermatologic:* Alopecia, rash, acne, skin discoloration, dry skin, herpes simplex, pruritus, rash, sweating, urticaria. *Musculoskeletal:* Arthralgia, myasthenia, myalgia. *Metabolic:* Edema, dehydration, weight loss. *Ophthalmic:* Ocular hypotony, amblyopia, conjunctivitis, eye disorder, iritis, retinal detachment, uveitis, abnormal vision. *Miscellaneous:* Allergic reactions, facial edema, malaise, back pain, chest pain, neck pain, ***sarcoma, sepsis,*** fever, infections, chills.

**Drug Interactions**
*Amphotericin B* / ↑ Risk of nephrotoxicity
*Aminoglycosides* / ↑ Risk of nephrotoxicity
*Foscarnet* / Risk of nephrotoxicity
*Pentamidine, IV* / ↑ Risk of nephrotoxicity
*Zidovudine* / ↓ Clearance of zidovudine

**How Supplied:** *Injection:* 75 mg/mL

## Dosage
- **IV Infusion**
  *CMV retinitis.*

**Induction:** 5 mg/kg given once weekly for 2 consecutive weeks as an IV infusion at a constant rate over 1 hr. **Maintenance:** 5 mg/kg given once q 2 weeks as an IV infusion at a constant rate over 1 hr. With each dose of cidofovir, probenecid, 2 g PO, must be given 3 hr prior to the cidofovir dose and 1 g PO given at 2 hr and again at 8 hr after completion of the 1-hr cidofovir infusion. Also, with each dose of cidofovir, the client should receive a total of 1 L of 0.9% NaCl solution IV over a 1- to 2-hr period just before the cidofovir infusion. If the client can tolerate it, give a second liter of 0.9% NaCl solution either at the start of the cidofovir infusion or immediately afterward and infuse over a 1- to 3-hr period. If serum creatinine increases by 0.3 to 0.4 mg/dL, reduce the dose of cidofovir from 5 to 3 mg/kg. Discontinue cidofovir if the serum creatinine increases by 0.5 mg/dL or more or if there is development of 3+ or more proteinuria.

## DENTAL CONCERNS

See also *Dental Concerns* for *Antiviral Drugs.*
**Client/Family Teaching**
1. Review the importance of good oral hygiene in order to prevent soft tissue inflammation.

C

2. Review the proper use of oral hygiene aids in order to prevent injury.
3. Daily home fluoride treatments for persistent dry mouth.
4. Avoid alcohol-containing mouth rinses or beverages.
5. Avoid caffeine-containing beverages.
6. Dry mouth can be treated with tart, sugarless gum or candy, water, sugar-free beverages, or with saliva substitutes if dry mouth persists.

# Cimetidine
(sye-MET-ih-deen)
**Pregnancy Category:** B
Apo-Cimetidine ✳, Novo–Cimetine ✳, Nu-Cimet ✳, Peptol ✳, Tagamet **(Rx)**, Tagamet HB **(OTC)**
**Classification:** Histamine $H_2$ receptor blocking agent

See also *Histamine $H_2$ Antagonists.*
**Action/Kinetics:** Reduces postprandial daytime and nighttime gastric acid secretion by about 50%–80%. It also inhibits cytochrome P-450 and P-448, which will affect metabolism of drugs. Well absorbed from GI tract. **Peak plasma level, PO:** 45–90 min. **Time to peak effect, after PO:** 1–2 hr. **Peak plasma levels, after PO use:** 0.7–3.2 mcg/mL (after a 300 mg dose; **after IV:** 3.5–7.5 mcg/mL. **Protein binding:** 13%–25%. **Duration, nocturnal:** 6–8 hr; **basal:** 4–5 hr. **$t\frac{1}{2}$:** 2 hr, longer in presence of renal impairment. After PO use, most metabolized in liver; after parenteral use, about 75% of drug excreted unchanged in the urine.
**Uses: Rx.** Treatment and maintenance of active duodenal ulcers. Short-term (6 weeks) treatment of benign gastric ulcers (in rare cases, healing has occurred). As part of multidrug regimen to eradicate *Helicobacter pylori*. Management of gastric acid hypersecretory states (Zollinger-Ellison syndrome, systemic mastocytosis). Gastroesophageal reflux disease, including erosive esophagitis. Prophylaxis of upper GI bleeding in critically ill hospitalized clients. *Non-FDA Approved Uses:* Prior to surgery to prevent aspiration pneumo-

nitis, secondary hyperparathyroidism in chronic hemodialysis clients, prophylaxis of stress-induced ulcers, hyperparathyroidism, dyspepsia, herpes virus infections, tinea capitis, hirsute women, chronic idiopathic urticaria, dermatologic anaphylaxis, acetaminophen overdosage, warts, colorectal cancer.
**OTC:** Relief of symptoms of heartburn, acid indigestion, and sour stomach.
**Contraindications:** Children under 16, lactation. Cirrhosis, impaired liver and renal function.
**Special Concerns:** In geriatric clients with impaired renal or hepatic function, confusion is more likely to occur. Not recommended for children less than 16 years of age.
**Side Effects:** *GI:* Diarrhea, pancreatitis (rare), hepatitis, hepatic fibrosis. *CNS:* Dizziness, sleepiness, headache, confusion, delirium, hallucinations, double vision, dysarthria, ataxia. Severely ill clients may manifest agitation, anxiety, depression, disorientation, hallucinations, mental confusion, and psychosis. *CV:* Hypotension and arrhythmias following rapid IV administration. *Hematologic:* Agranulocytosis, thrombocytopenia, *hemolytic or aplastic anemia,* granulocytopenia. *GU:* Impotence (high doses for prolonged periods of time), gynecomastia (long-term treatment). *Dermatologic:* Exfoliative dermatitis, erythroderma, erythema multiforme. *Musculoskeletal:* Arthralgia, reversible worsening of joint symptoms with preexisting arthritis (including gouty arthritis). *Other:* Hypersensitivity reactions, pain at injection site, myalgia, rash, cutaneous vasculitis, peripheral neuropathy, galactorrhea, alopecia, bronchoconstriction.
**Drug Interactions**
*Antacids /* ↓ Effect of cimetidine due to ↓ absorption from GI tract
*Anticholinergics /* ↓ Effect of cimetidine due to ↓ absorption from GI tract
*Benzodiazepines /* ↑ Effect of benzodiazepines due to ↓ breakdown by liver

*Caffeine* / ↑ Effect of caffeine due to ↓ breakdown by liver

*Carbamazepine* / ↑ Effect of carbamazepine due to ↓ breakdown by liver

*Chlorpromazine* / ↓ Effect of chlorpromazine due to ↓ absorption from GI tract

*Fluconazole* / ↓ Effect of fluconazole due to ↓ absorption from GI tract

*Indomethacin* / ↓ Effect of indomethacin due to ↓ absorption from GI tract

*Ketoconazole* / ↓ Effect of ketoconazole due to ↓ absorption from GI tract

*Lidocaine* / ↑ Effect of lidocaine due to ↓ breakdown by liver

*Metronidazole* / ↑ Effect of metronidazole due to ↓ breakdown by liver

*Opioid Analgesics* / Possible ↑ toxic effects (respiratory depression) of narcotics

*Phenytoin* / ↑ Effect of phenytoin due to ↓ breakdown by liver

*Succinylcholine* / ↑ Neuromuscular blockade → respiratory depression and extended apnea

*Sulfonylureas* / ↑ Effect of sulfonylureas due to ↓ breakdown by liver

*Tetracyclines* / ↓ Effect of tetracyclines due to ↓ absorption from GI tract

*Tricyclic antidepressants* / ↑ Effect of tricyclic antidepressants due to ↓ breakdown by liver

**How Supplied:** *Injection:* 150 mg/mL, 300 mg/50 mL; *Solution:* 300 mg/5 mL; *Tablet:* 100 mg, 200 mg, 300 mg, 400 mg, 800 mg

## Dosage
- **Tablets, Oral Solution**
  *Duodenal ulcers, short-term.*
**Adults:** 800 mg at bedtime. Alternate dosage: 300 mg q.i.d. with meals and at bedtime for 4–6 weeks (administer with antacids, staggering the dose of antacids) or 400 mg b.i.d. (in the morning and evening). **Maintenance:** 400 mg at bedtime.

*Active benign gastric ulcers.*
**Adults:** 800 mg at bedtime (preferred regimen) or 300 mg q.i.d. with meals and at bedtime for no more than 8 weeks.

*Pathologic hypersecretory conditions.*
**Adults:** 300 mg q.i.d. with meals and at bedtime up to a maximum of 2,400 mg/day for as long as needed.

*Erosive gastroesophageal reflux disease.*
**Adults:** 800 mg b.i.d. or 400 mg q.i.d. for 12 weeks. Use beyond 12 weeks has not been determined.

*Heartburn, acid indigestion, sour stomach (OTC only).*
200 mg with water as symptoms present up to b.i.d.

*Dyspepsia.*
**Adults:** 400 mg b.i.d.

*Prophylaxis of aspiration pneumonitis.*
**Adults:** 400–600 mg 60–90 min before anesthesia.

*Primary hyperparathyroidism, secondary hyperparathyroidism in chronic hemodialysis clients.*
Up to 1 g/day.

- **IM, IV, IV Infusion**
  *Hospitalized clients with pathologic hypersecretory conditions or intractable ulcers or those unable to take PO medication.*
**Adults:** 300 mg IM or IV q 6–8 hr. If an increased dose is necessary, administer 300 mg more frequently than q 6–8 hr, not to exceed 2,400 mg/day.

*Prophylaxis of upper GI bleeding.*
**Adults:** 50 mg/hr by continuous IV infusion. If $C_{CR}$ is less than 30 mL/min, use one-half the recommended dose. Treatment beyond 7 days has not been studied.

*Prophylaxis of aspiration pneumonitis.*
**Adults:** 300 mg IV 60–90 min before induction of anesthetic.

## DENTAL CONCERNS

See also *Dental Concerns* for *Histamine $H_2$ Antagonists.*

# Cinoxacin

(sin-**OX**-ah-sin)
**Pregnancy Category:** B
Cinobac Pulvules **(Rx)**
**Classification:** Urinary anti-infective

See also *Anti-Infectives*.
**Action/Kinetics:** Related chemically to nalidixic acid. Acts by inhibiting DNA replication, resulting in a bactericidal action. Rapidly absorbed after PO administration; a 500-mg dose results in a urine concentration of 300 mcg/mL during the first 4-hr period and 100 mcg/mL during the second 4-hr period. Within 24 hr, 97% is excreted in the urine, 60% unchanged. **Mean serum t½:** 1.5 hr. Food decreases peak serum levels by approximately 30% but not the total amount absorbed.
**Uses:** Initial and recurrent UTIs caused by *Escherichia coli, Proteus mirabilis, P. vulgaris, Klebsiella,* and *Enterobacter* species. Prevents UTIs for up to 5 months in women with a history of UTIs. *NOTE:* Cinoxacin is ineffective against *Pseudomonas,* staphylococci, and enterococci infections. Prophylaxis of UTIs.
**Contraindications:** Hypersensitivity to cinoxacin or other quinolones. Infants and prepubertal children. Anuric clients. Lactation.
**Special Concerns:** Use with caution in clients with hepatic or kidney disease. Safety and efficacy in children less than 18 years of age have not been determined.
**Side Effects:** *GI:* N&V, anorexia, abdominal cramps and pain, diarrhea, altered sensation of taste. *CNS:* Headache, dizziness, insomnia, drowsiness, confusion, nervousness. *Hypersensitivity:* Rash, pruritus, urticaria, edema, angioedema, eosinophilia, **anaphylaxis (rare),** toxic epidermal necrolysis (rare), erythema multiforme, ***Stevens-Johnson syndrome***. *Other:* Tingling sensation, photophobia, perineal burning, tinnitus, thrombocytopenia.
**Drug Interactions:** *Probenecid / ↓* Excretion of cinoxacin → ↓ concentration in the urine.

**How Supplied:** *Capsule:* 250 mg, 500 mg

**Dosage** ―――――――
• **Capsules**
*UTIs.*
**Adults:** 1 g/day in two to four divided doses for 7–14 days. *In clients with impaired renal function:* **Initial,** 500 mg; **then,** dosage schedule based on creatinine clearance (see package insert).
*Prophylaxis of UTIs in women.*
250 mg at bedtime for up to 5 months.

## DENTAL CONCERNS

See also *General Dental Concerns for All Anti-Infectives.*

# Ciprofloxacin hydrochloride

(sip-row-**FLOX**-ah-sin)
**Pregnancy Category:** C
Ciloxan Ophthalmic, Cipro, Cipro Cystitis Pack, Cipro I.V. **(Rx)**
**Classification:** Fluoroquinolone anti-infective

See also *Fluoroquinolones*.
**Action/Kinetics:** Effective against both gram-positive and gram-negative organisms. Rapidly and well absorbed following PO administration. Food delays absorption of the drug. **Maximum serum levels:** 2–4 mcg/mL 1–2 hr after dosing. **t½:** 4 hr for PO use and 5–6 hr for IV use. Avoid peak serum levels above 5 mcg/mL. About 40%–50% of a PO dose and 50%–70% of an IV dose is excreted unchanged in the urine.
**Uses: Systemic.** UTIs caused by *Escherichia coli, Enterobacter cloacae, Citrobacter diversus, Citrobacter freundii, Klebsiella pneumoniae, Proteus mirabilis, Providencia rettgeri, Pseudomonas aeruginosa, Morganella morganii, Serratia marcescens, Serratia epidermidis,* and *Streptococcus faecalis.* Uncomplicated cervical and urethral gonorrhea due to *Neisseria gonorrhoeae.* Chancroid due to *Haemophilus ducreyi;* un-

complicated or disseminated gono-coccal infections.

Mild to moderate chronic bacterial prostatitis due to *E. coli* or *P. mirabilis.*

Mild to moderate sinusitis due to *S. pneumoniae, H. influenzae,* or *M. catarrhalis.*

Lower respiratory tract infections caused by *E. coli, E. cloacae, K. pneumoniae, P. mirabilis, P. aeruginosa, Haemophilus influenzae, H. parainfluenzae,* and *Streptococcus pneumoniae.*

Bone and joint infections due to *E. cloacae, P. aeruginosa,* and *S. marcescens.*

Skin and skin structure infections caused by *E. coli, E. cloacae, Citrobacter freundii, M. morganii, K. pneumoniae, P. aeruginosa, P. mirabilis, Proteus vulgaris, Providencia stuartii, Staphylococcus pyogenes, Staphylococcus epidermidis,* and penicillinase- and non-penicillinase-producing strains of *Staphylococcus aureus.*

Infectious diarrhea caused by enterotoxigenic strains of *E. coli.* Also, *Campylobacter jejuni, Shigella flexneri,* and *Shigella sonnei.*

Typhoid fever (enteric fever) due to *Salmonella typhi.* Efficacy in eradicating the chronic typhoid carrier state has not been shown.

IV as empirical therapy in febrile neutropenia.

*Non-FDA Approved Uses:* Clients, over 14 years of age, with cystic fibrosis who have pulmonary exacerbations due to susceptible microorganisms. Malignant external otitis. In combination with rifampin and other tuberculostatics for tuberculosis.

**Ophthalmic.** Superficial ocular infections due to *Staphylococcus* species (including *S. aureus*), *Streptococcus* species (including *S. pneumoniae, S. pyogenes*), *E. coli, H. ducreyi, H. influenzae, H. parainfluenzae, K. pneumoniae, N. gonorrhoeae, Proteus* species, *Klebsiella* species, *Acinetobacter calcoaceticus, Enterobacter aerogenes, P. ae-*

*ruginosa, S. marcescens, Chlamydia trachomatis, Vibrio* species, and *Providencia* species.

**Contraindications:** Hypersensitivity to quinolones. Use in children. Lactation. Ophthalmic use in the presence of dendritic keratitis, varicella, vaccinia, and mycobacterial and fungal eye infections and after removal of foreign bodies from the cornea.

**Special Concerns:** Safety and effectiveness of ophthalmic, PO, or IV use have not been determined in children.

**Additional Side Effects:** See also *Side Effects* for *Fluoroquinolones.*
*Oral:* Dry, painful mouth, oral candidiasis. *GI:* N&V, abdominal pain/discomfort, diarrhea, dry/painful mouth, dyspepsia, heartburn, constipation, flatulence, pseudomembranous colitis, oral candidiasis, *intestinal perforation,* anorexia, GI bleeding, bad taste in mouth. *CNS:* Headache, dizziness, fatigue, lethargy, malaise, drowsiness, restlessness, insomnia, nightmares, hallucinations, tremor, lightheadedness, irritability, confusion, ataxia, mania, weakness, psychotic reactions, depression, depersonalization, seizures. *GU:* Nephritis, hematuria, cylindruria, renal failure, urinary retention, polyuria, vaginitis, urethral bleeding, acidosis, renal calculi, interstitial nephritis, vaginal candidiasis. *Skin:* Urticaria, photosensitivity, hypersensitivity, flushing, erythema nodosum, cutaneous candidiasis, hyperpigmentation, rash, paresthesia, edema (of lips, neck, face, conjunctivae, hands), angioedema, toxic epidermal necrolysis, exfoliative dermatitis, *Stevens-Johnson syndrome. Ophthalmic:* Blurred or disturbed vision, double vision, eye pain, nystagmus. *CV:* Hypertension, syncope, angina pectoris, palpitations, atrial flutter, *MI, cerebral thrombosis,* ventricular ectopy, *cardiopulmonary arrest,* postural hypotension. *Respiratory:* Dyspnea, *bronchospasm, pulmonary embolism, edema of larynx or lungs,* hemoptysis, hic-

coughs, epistaxis. *Hematologic:* Eosinophilia, pancytopenia, leukopenia, anemia, leukocytosis, **agranulocytosis,** bleeding diathesis. *Miscellaneous:* Superinfections; fever; chills; tinnitus; joint pain or stiffness; back, neck, or chest pain; flare-up of gout; flushing; worsening of myasthenia gravis; **hepatic necrosis;** cholestatic jaundice; hearing loss, dysphasia.

*After ophthalmic use:* Irritation, burning, itching, angioneurotic edema, urticaria, maculopapular and vesicular dermatitis, crusting of lid margins, conjunctival hyperemia, bad taste in mouth, corneal staining, keratitis, keratopathy, allergic reactions, photophobia, decreased vision, tearing, lid edema. Also, a white, crystalline precipitate in the superficial part of corneal defect (onset within 1–7 days after initiating therapy; lasts about 2 weeks and does not affect continued use of the medication).

**How Supplied:** *Injection:* 10 mg/mL, 200 mg/100 mL, 400 mg/200 mL; *Ophthalmic solution:* 0.3%; *Tablet:* 100 mg, 250 mg, 500 mg, 750 mg

**Dosage** ———————————
• **Tablets**
*UTIs.*
250 mg (mild to moderate) to 500 mg (severe/complicated) q 12 hr for 7–14 days.
*Mild to moderate chronic bacterial prostatitis.*
**Adults:** 500 mg b.i.d. for 28 days.
*Mild to moderate sinusitis.*
**Adults:** 500 mg b.i.d. for 10 days.
*Urethral or cervical gonococcal infections, uncomplicated.*
250 mg in a single dose.
*Infectious diarrhea.*
500 mg q 12 hr for 5–7 days.
*Skin, skin structures, lower respiratory tract, bone and joint infections.*
500 mg (mild to moderate) to 750 mg (severe or complicated) q 12 hr for 7–14 days. Treatment may be required for 4–6 weeks in bone and joint infections.
*Typhoid fever.*

500 mg (mild to moderate) q 12 hr for 10 days.
*Chancroid (*H. ducreyi *infection).*
500 mg b.i.d. for 3 days.
*Disseminated gonococcal infections.*
500 mg b.i.d. to complete a full week of therapy after initial treatment with ceftriaxone, 1 g IM or IV q 24 hr for 24–48 hr after improvement begins.
*Uncomplicated gonococcal infections.*
500 mg in a single dose plus doxycycline.
*NOTE:* Dose must be reduced with a $C_{CR}$ less than 50 mL/min. The PO dose should be 250–500 mg q 12 hr if the $C_{CR}$ is 30–50 mL/min and 250–500 mg q 18 hr (IV: 200–400 mg q 18–24 hr) if the $C_{CR}$ is 5–29 mL/min. If the client is on hemodialysis or peritoneal dialysis, the PO dose should be 250–500 mg q 24 hr after dialysis.
• **Cipro Cystitis Pack**
*Uncomplicated UTI infections.*
100 mg b.i.d. for 3 days. The pack contains six 100-mg tablets of ciprofloxacin and is intended to increase compliance.
• **IV Infusion**
*UTIs.*
200 mg (mild to moderate) to 400 mg (severe or complicated) q 12 hr for 7–14 days.
*Skin, skin structures, respiratory tract, bone and joint infections.*
400 mg (for mild to moderate infections) q 12 hr for 7–14 days.
• **Ophthalmic Solution**
*Acute infections.*
**Initial,** 1–2 gtt q 15–30 min; **then,** reduce dosage as infection improves.
*Moderate infections.*
1–2 gtt 4–6 (or more) times/day.

## DENTAL CONCERNS

See also *Dental Concerns for All Anti-infectives* and *Fluoroquinolones.*

—————————————
# Cisapride
(**SISS**-ah-pryd)

**Pregnancy Category: C**
Prepulsid ✸, Propulsid **(Rx)**
Classification: GI drug

**Action/Kinetics:** Cisapride is a GI prokinetic agent. Acts by enhancing release of acetylcholine at the myenteric plexus, resulting in increased strength of esophageal peristalsis and an increase in lower esophageal sphincter pressure. Also increases gastric emptying time. Rapidly absorbed. **Onset:** 30–60 min. **Peak plasma levels:** 1–1.5 hr. **Terminal t½:** 6–12 hr (up to 20 hr following IV use). Metabolized in the liver with less than 10% excreted unchanged through the urine and feces.

**Uses:** Symptomatic treatment of clients with nocturnal heartburn due to gastroesophageal reflux disease (GERD).

**Contraindications:** Use when an increase in GI motility could be harmful (i.e., in the presence of GI hemorrhage, mechanical obstruction, perforation). Concomitant use with clarithromycin, erythromycin, fluconazole, itraconazole, ketoconazole, IV miconazole, or troleandomycin.

**Special Concerns:** Use with caution during lactation. Safety and efficacy have not been demonstrated in children. Steady-state plasma levels are generally higher in older clients as a result of increased elimination half-life although doses used are similar to those in younger adults. The increased rate of gastric emptying time due to cisapride could affect the rate of absorption of other drugs.

**Side Effects:** *Oral:* Dry mouth. *GI:* Diarrhea, abdominal pain, nausea, constipation, flatulence, dyspepsia, vomiting, dry mouth. *CNS:* Headache, insomnia, anxiety, nervousness, dizziness, depression, tremor, *seizures,* extrapyramidal effects, somnolence, migraine. *CV:* Palpitation, sinus tachycardia, tachycardia. ***Rarely, serious cardiac arrhythmias, including ventricular arrhythmias and torsades de pointes associated with QT prolongation*** (usually in those taking antifungal drugs and other multiple medications and who had preexisting cardiac disease or arrhythmia risk factors). *Respiratory:* Rhinitis, sinusitis, coughing, pharyngitis, URTI. *GU:* UTI, increased frequency of urination, vaginitis. *Hepatic:* Hepatitis, elevated liver enzymes. *Musculoskeletal:* Arthralgia, back pain, myalgia. *Hematologic:* Thrombocytopenia, leukopenia, ***aplastic anemia, pancytopenia,*** granulocytopenia (rare). *Miscellaneous:* Pain, fever, viral infection, rash, pruritus, abnormal vision, chest pain, fatigue, dehydration, edema.

**Drug Interactions**
*Alcohol* / Possible ↑ sedative effect
*Anticholinergics* / ↓ Effect of cisapride
*Benzodiazepines* / Possible ↑ sedative effect
*Cimetidine* / ↑ Peak plasma levels of cisapride; also ↑ GI absorption of cimetidine
*Clarithromycin* / ↑ Cisapride plasma levels due to ↓ metabolism, resulting in prolonged QT intervals and possibility of ventricular arrhythmias and torsades de pointes
*Erythromycin* / ↑ Cisapride plasma levels due to ↓ metabolism, resulting in prolonged QT intervals and possibility of ventricular arrhythmias and torsades de pointes
*Fluconazole* / ↑ Cisapride plasma levels due to ↓ metabolism, resulting in prolonged QT intervals and possibility of ventricular arrhythmias and torsades de pointes
*Itraconazole* / ↑ Cisapride plasma levels due to ↓ metabolism, resulting in prolonged QT intervals and possibility of ventricular arrhythmias and torsades de pointes
*Ketoconazole* / ↑ Cisapride plasma levels due to ↓ metabolism, resulting in prolonged QT intervals and possibility of ventricular arrhythmias and torsades de pointes
*Miconazole (IV)* / ↑ Cisapride plasma levels due to ↓ metabolism, resulting in prolonged QT intervals and possibility of ventricular arrhythmias and torsades de pointes

*Ranitidine* / ↑ GI absorption of ranitidine

*Troleandomycin* / ↑ Cisapride plasma levels due to ↓ metabolism, resulting in prolonged QT intervals and possibility of ventricular arrhythmias and torsades de pointes

**How Supplied:** *Suspension:* 1 mg/mL; *Tablet:* 10 mg, 20 mg

## Dosage
- **Suspension, Tablets**
  *GERD.*

**Adults, initial:** 10 mg q.i.d. at least 15 min before meals and at bedtime. May need to increase in some clients to 20 mg q.i.d. 15 min before meals and at bedtime.

## DENTAL CONCERNS
### General
1. Decreased saliva flow can put the patient at risk for dental caries, periodontal disease, and candidiasis.
2. A semisupine position for the dental chair may be necessary to help minimize or avoid GI effect of the disease.
3. Patients on chronic drug therapy may develop blood dyscrasias. Symptoms include fever, sore throat, bleeding, and poor wound healing.

### Consultation with Primary Care Provider
1. Patients with symptoms of blood dyscrasias should be referred to their primary care provider for complete blood counts. Treatment should be postponed until the results are known.
2. Consultation may be required in order to assess extent of disease control.

### Client/Family Teaching
1. Review the importance of good oral hygiene in order to prevent soft tissue inflammation.
2. Review the proper use of oral hygiene aids in order to prevent injury.
3. Daily home fluoride treatments for persistent dry mouth.
4. Avoid alcohol-containing mouth rinses and beverages.
5. Avoid caffeine-containing beverages.
6. Dry mouth can be treated with tart, sugarless gum or candy, water, sugar-free beverages, or with saliva substitutes if dry mouth persists.

# Citalopram hydrobromide
(sigh-**TAL**-oh-pram)
**Pregnancy Category:** C
Celexa
**Classification:** Selective serotonin reuptake inhibitor

See also *Selective Serotonin Reuptake Inhibitors.*

**Action/Kinetics:** Inhibits the reuptake of serotonin in the central nervous system. **Absolute bioavailabity:** 80% and not affected by food. Metabolized in the liver and excreted by the kidneys to a small extent.

**Uses:** Major depression. *Non-FDA Approved Uses*: Obsessive-compulsive disorder, panic disorder, schizophrenia, alcoholism, diabetic peripheral neuropathy.

**Contraindications:** Should not be used within 14 days before or after use of an MAOI.

**Side Effects:** *Oral:* Dry mouth. *GI:* Nausea, diarrhea. *CNS:* Somnolence, mania, hypomania, seizures, tremor. *GU:* Delayed ejaculation. *Miscellaneous:* Increased sweating, hyponatremia, syndrome of inappropriate anitdiuretic hormone secretion.

**Drug Interactions:** No drug interactions reported.

**How Supplied:** *Tablets:* 20 mg, 40 mg

## Dosage
- **Tablets**
  *Depression.*

**Adults:** 20 mg q.d. (either morning or evening) which can be increased to 40 mg q.d.

## DENTAL CONCERNS

See *Dental Concerns* for *Selective Serotonin Reuptake Inhibitors.*

# Clarithromycin
(klah-**rith**-roh-**MY**-sin)
**Pregnancy Category:** C
Biaxin **(Rx)**
**Classification:** Antibiotic, macrolide

See also *Anti-Infectives.*

**Action/Kinetics:** Clarithromycin is a macrolide antibiotic that acts by binding to the 50S ribosomal subunit of susceptible organisms, thus interfering with or inhibiting microbial protein synthesis. Rapidly absorbed from the GI tract although food slightly delays the onset of absorption and the formation of the active metabolite but does not affect the extent of the bioavailability. **Peak serum levels:** When fasting, 2 hr for the tablet and 3 hr for the suspension. **Steady-state peak serum levels:** 1 mcg/mL within 2–3 days after 250 mg q 12 hr and 2–3 mcg/mL after 500 mg q 12 hr. Clarithromycin and 14-OH clarithromycin (active metabolite) are readily distributed to body tissues and fluids. **t½, elimination:** 3–7 hr (depending on the dose) for clarithromycin and 5–6 hr for 14-OH clarithromycin. Up to 30% of a dose is excreted unchanged in the urine.

**Uses:** Mild to moderate infections caused by susceptible strains of the following. **Adults.** Pharyngitis/tonsillitis due to *Streptococcus pyogenes*. Acute maxillary sinusitis or acute bacterial exacerbaton of chronic bronchitis due to *Sreptococcus pneumoniae, Haemophilus influenzae,* and *Moraxella catarrhalis*. The active metabolite, 14-OH clarithromycin, has significant activity (twice the parent compound) against *H. influenzae*. Pneumonia due to *Mycoplasma pneumoniae, S. pneumoniae,* or *Chlamydia pneumoniae*. Uncomplicated skin and skin structure infections due to *Staphylococcus aureus* or *S. pyogenes*. Treatment of disseminated mycobacterial infections due to *Mycobacterium avium* (commonly seen in AIDS clients) and *M. intracellulare*. Prevention of disseminated *M. avium* complex in individuals with advanced HIV.

Used with omeprazole or ranitidine bismuth citrate (Tritec) for the eradication of *Helicobacter pylori* infection in clients with active duodenal ulcers associated with *H. pylori* infection also with amoxicillin and lansoprazole for the same purpose.

**Children.** Pharyngitis or tonsillitis due to *S. pyogenes*. Acute maxillary sinusitis or acute otitis media due to *S. pneumoniae, H. influenzae,* and *M. catarrhalis*. Uncomplicated skin and skin structure infections due to *S. aureus* or *S. pyogenes*. Disseminated mycobacterial infections due to *M. avium* or *M. intracellulare*. Prevention of disseminated *M. avium* complex disease in clients with advanced HIV infection. Community-acquired pneumonia caused by *M. pneumoniae, Chlamydia pneumoniae,* and *S. pneumoniae.*

**Contraindications:** Hypersensitivity to clarithromycin, other macrolide antibiotics, or erythromycin. Clients taking astemizole, terfenadine, cisapride, or pimozide.

**Special Concerns:** Use with caution in severe renal impairment with or without concomitant hepatic impairment and during lactation. Safety and effectiveness in children less than 6 months of age have not been determined. Safety has not been determined in MAC clients less than 20 months of age.

**Side Effects:** *Oral:* Abnormal taste, glossitis, stomatitis, oral candidiasis. *GI:* Diarrhea, nausea, dyspepsia, abdominal discomfort or pain, pseudomembranous colitis, vomiting. *CNS:* Headache, dizziness, behavioral changes, confusion, depersonalization, disorientation, hallucinations, insomnia, nightmares, vertigo. *Allergic:* Urticaria, mild skin eruptions and, rarely, ***anaphylaxis and Stevens-Johnson syndrome.*** *Hepatic:* Hepatocellular cholestatic hepatitis with or without jaundice, increased liver enzymes, ***hepatic failure.*** *Miscellaneous:* Hearing loss (usually reversible), alteration of sense of smell (usually with taste perversion).

In children, the most common side effects are diarrhea, vomiting, abdominal pain, rash, and headache.

---

**Drug Interactions**
See also Drug Interactions for Eryth-romycins.
Anticholinergic drugs / ↓ Effects of anticholinergic drugs
Astemizole / Combination not to be used in clients who have preexisting cardiac abnormalities or electrolyte disturbances
Carbamazepine / ↑ Blood levels of carbamazepine
Cisapride / Possibility of serious cardiac arrhythmias, including ventricular tachycardia, ventricular fibrillation, torsade de pointes, and QT prolongation
Oral contraceptives / ↓ Effectiveness of oral contraceptives
Pimozide / ↑ Risk of sudden death; do not use together
Terfenadine / ↑ Plasma levels of the active acid metabolite of terfenadine; ↑ risk of cardiac arrhythmias, including QT interval prolongation
Triazolam / ↑ Risk of somnolence and confusion
**How Supplied:** Granule for reconstitution: 125 mg/5 mL, 250 mg/5 mL; Tablet: 250 mg, 500 mg

**Dosage** —————————
• **Tablets, Oral Suspension**
Pharyngitis, tonsillitis.
250 mg q 12 hr for 10 days.
Acute exacerbation of chronic bronchitis due to S. pneumoniae or M. catarrhalis; pneumonia due to S. pneumoniae or M. pneumoniae; skin and skin structure infections.
250 mg q 12 hr for 7–14 days.
Acute maxillary sinusitis, acute exacerbation of chronic bronchitis due to H. influenzae.
500 mg q 12 hr for 7–14 days.
Disseminated M. avium complex or prophylaxis of M. avium complex.
**Adults:** 500 mg b.i.d.; **children:** 7.5 mg/kg b.i.d. up to 500 mg b.i.d.
NOTE: The usual daily dose for children is 15 mg/kg q 12 hr for 10 days.
Community-acquired pneumonia in children.
15 mg/kg/day of the suspension, divided and given q 12 hr for 10 days.

Active duodenal ulcers associated with H. pylori infection.
Clarithromycin, 500 mg t.i.d., with omeprazole, 40 mg, each morning for 2 weeks. **Then,** omeprazole is given alone at a dose of 20 mg/day for 2 more weeks. Or, clarithromycin, 500 mg t.i.d., with ranitidine bismuth citrate, 400 mg b.i.d., for 2 weeks. **Then,** ranitidine bismuth citrate is given alone at a dose of 400 mg b.i.d. for 2 more weeks or, clarithromycin 500 mg, plus lansoprazole, 30 mg, and amoxicillin, 1 g b.i.d. for 2 weeks.

## DENTAL CONCERNS

See also Dental Concerns for Anti-Infectives and Erythromycins.
**Client/Family Teaching**
1. May take with or without meals; food delays onset of absorption. Drug may cause a bitter taste.
2. Report any persistent diarrhea; an antibiotic-associated colitis may be precipitated by C. difficile and require alternative management.
3. Report if no symptom improvement after 48–72 hr.
4. Use an additional nonhormonal form of birth control if taking oral contraceptives because their effectiveness may be diminished.
5. Review the importance of good oral hygiene in order to prevent soft tissue inflammation.

# Clindamycin hydrochloride hydrate
(klin-dah-**MY**-sin)
Cleocin Hydrochloride, Dalacin C ✸ **(Rx)**

# Clindamycin palmitate hydrochloride
(klin-dah-**MY**-sin)
Cleocin Pediatric, Dalacin C Palmitate ✸ **(Rx)**

# Clindamycin phosphate
(klin-dah-**MY**-sin)
**Pregnancy Category:** B (vaginal cream, topical gel, lotion, solution)

Cleocin Vaginal Cream, Cleocin Phosphate, Cleocin T, Clinda-Derm, C/T/S, Dalacin C Phosphate ✹, Dalacin T Topical ✹, Dalacin Vaginal Cream ✹ **(Rx)**
**Classification:** Antibiotic, clindamycin and lincomycin

See also *Anti-Infectives.*

**Action/Kinetics:** A semisynthetic antibiotic that suppresses protein synthesis by microorganism by binding to ribosomes (50S subunit) and preventing peptide bond formation. Is both bacteriostatic and bactericidal. **Peak serum concentration: PO,** 4 mcg/mL after 300 mg; **IM,** 4.9 mcg/mL after 300 mg; **IV,** 14.7 mcg/mL after 300 mg. **t½:** 2.4–3 hr. In serious infections the rate of IV administration is adjusted to maintain appropriate serum drug concentrations: 4–6 mcg/mL.

**Uses:** Should not be used for trivial infections. **Systemic.** Serious respiratory tract infections (e.g., empyema, lung abscess, pneumonia) caused by staphylococci, streptococci, and pneumococci. Serious skin and soft tissue infections, septicemia, intraabdominal infections, pelvic inflammatory disease, female genital tract infections. May be the drug of choice for *Bacteroides fragilis.* In combination with aminoglycosides for mixed aerobic and anaerobic bacterial infections. Staphylococci-induced acute hematogenous osteomyelitis. Adjunct to surgery for chronic bone/joint infections. Bacterial endocarditis prophylaxis. *Non-FDA Approved Uses:* Alternative to sulfonamides in combination with pyrimethamine in the acute treatment of CNS toxoplasmosis in AIDS clients. In combination with primaquine to treat *Pneumocystis carinii* pneumonia. Chlamydial infections in women. Bacterial vaginosis due to *Gardnerella vaginalis.* **Topical Use.** Used topically for inflammatory acne vulgaris. Vaginally to treat bacterial vaginosis. *Non-FDA Approved Uses:* Treatment of rosacea (lotion used).

**Contraindications:** Hypersensitivity to either clindamycin or lincomycin. Use in treating viral and minor bacterial infections or in clients with a history of regional enteritis, ulcerative colitis, or antibiotic-associated colitis. Lactation.

**Special Concerns:** Use with caution in infants up to 1 month of age, in clients with GI disease, liver or renal disease, or a history of allergy or asthma. Safety and efficacy of topical products have not been established in children less than 12 years of age.

**Side Effects:** *Oral:* Candidiasis. *GI:* N&V, diarrhea, bloody diarrhea, abdominal pain, GI disturbances, tenesmus, flatulence, bloating, anorexia, weight loss, esophagitis. Nonspecific colitis, pseudomembranous colitis (may be severe). *Allergic:* Morbilliform rash (most common). Also, maculopapular rash, urticaria, pruritus, fever, hypotension. Rarely, polyarteritis, anaphylaxis, erythema multiforme. *Hematologic:* Leukopenia, neutropenia, eosinophilia, thrombocytopenia, ***agranulocytosis.*** *Miscellaneous:* Superinfection. Also sore throat, fatigue, urinary frequency, headache.

*Following IV use:* Thrombophlebitis, erythema, pain, swelling. *Following IM use:* Pain, induration, sterile abscesses.

*Following topical use:* Erythema, irritation, dryness, peeling, itching, burning, oiliness of skin.

*Following vaginal use:* Cervicitis, vaginitis, vulvar irritation, urticaria, rash.

*NOTE:* The injection contains benzyl alcohol, which has been associated with ***a fatal "gasping syndrome"*** in infants.
**Drug Interactions**
*Antiperistaltic antidiarrheals (opiates, Lomotil)* / ↑ Diarrhea due to ↓ removal of toxins from colon
*Ciprofloxacin HCl* / Additive antibacterial activity
*Erythromycin* / Cross-interference → ↓ effect of both drugs

---

*Inhaled hydrocarbon anesthetics* / ↑
Effect of inhaled hydrocarbon anesthetics
*Kaolin (e.g., Kaopectate)* / ↓ Effect due to ↓ absorption from GI tract
*Neuromuscular blocking agents* / ↑ Effect of blocking agents

**How Supplied:** Clindamycin hydrochloride hydrate: *Capsule:* 75 mg, 150 mg, 300 mg. Clindamycin palmitate hydrochloride: *Granule for reconstitution:* 75 mg/5 mL. Clindamycin phosphate: *Vaginal cream:* 2%; *Gel:* 1%; *Injection:* 150 mg/mL, 300 mg/50 mL, 600 mg/50 mL, 900 mg/50 mL; *Lotion:* 1%; *Solution:* 1%; *Swab:* 1%

**Dosage** ———————————
• **PO only: Capsules, Oral Solution**
**Adults: Clindamycin HCl, Clindamycin palmitate HCl:** 150–450 mg q 6 hr, depending on severity of infection. **Pediatric: Clindamycin HCl hydrate:** 8–20 mg/kg/day divided into three to four equal doses; clindamycin palmitate HCl: 8–25 mg/kg/day divided into three to four equal doses. **Children less than 10 kg:** Minimum recommended dose is 37.5 mg t.i.d.
• **IV**
**Clindamycin phosphate. Adults:** 0.6–2.7 g/day in two to four equal doses depending on severity of infection.
*Life-threatening infections.*
4.8 g. **Pediatric over 1 month:** 15–40 mg/kg/day in three to four equal doses depending on severity of infections.
*Severe infections.*
No less than 300 mg/day, regardless of body weight.
*Acute pelvic inflammatory disease.*
**IV:** 600 mg q.i.d. plus gentamicin, 2 mg/kg IV; **then,** gentamicin, 1.5 mg/kg t.i.d. IV. IV therapy should be continued for 2 days after client improves. The 10–14-day treatment cycle should be completed using clindamycin, **PO:** 450 mg q.i.d.
• **Topical Gel, Lotion, or Solution**

Apply thin film b.i.d. to affected areas. One or more pledgets may also be used.
• **Vaginal Cream (2%)**
One applicatorful (containing about 100 mg clindamycin phosphate), preferably at bedtime, for 7 consecutive days.
*Bacterial endocarditis prophylaxis.*
**Adult:** 600 mg 1 hr prior to procedure. **Children:** 20 mg/kg of body weight 1 hr prior to procedure not to exceed adult dose. IV dose form for patients who cannot take oral medications.

## DENTAL CONCERNS

See also *General Dental Concerns for All Anti-Infectives.*

# Clofibrate
(kloh-**FYE**-brayt)
**Pregnancy Category:** C
Atromid-S, Claripex ✹, Novo-Fibrate ✹ **(Rx)**
**Classification:** Antihyperlipidemic agent

**Action/Kinetics:** Clofibrate decreases triglycerides and VLDL; cholesterol and LDL are decreased less predictably and less effectively. The mechanism is not known with certainty but may be due to increased catabolism of VLDL to LDL and decreased synthesis of VLDL by the liver. Cholesterol formation is inhibited early in the biosynthetic chain; excretion of neutral streoids is increased. **Peak plasma levels:** 3–6 hr. **t½, plasma:** 15 hr. **Therapeutic effect: Onset,** 2–5 days; **maximum effect:** 3 weeks. Triglycerides return to pretreatment levels 2–3 weeks after therapy is terminated. Clofibrate is hydrolyzed to the active *p*-chlorophenoxyisobutyric acid which is further metabolized and excreted in the urine. The drug may concentrate in fetal blood. LFTs should be performed during therapy.
**Uses:** Dysbetalipoproteinemia (type III hyperlipidemia) not responding to diet. Hyperlipidemia (types IV and V) with a risk of abdominal pain

and pancreatitis not responding to diet.

**Contraindications:** Impaired hepatic or renal function, primary biliary cirrhosis, lactation, pregnancy, children.

**Special Concerns:** Use with caution in clients with gout and peptic ulcer. Reduced dosage may be required in geriatric clients due to age-related decreases in renal function.

**Side Effects:** *Oral:* Stomatitis. *GI:* Nausea, dyspepsia, weight gain, gastritis, vomiting, bloating, flatulence, abdominal distress, loose stools, diarrhea, hepatomegaly, cholelithiasis, gallstones. *CNS:* Headaches, dizziness, fatigue, weakness, drowsiness. *CV:* Changes in blood-clotting time, arrhythmias, increased or decreased angina, intermittent claudication, thromboembolic events, thrombophlebitis, swelling and phlebitis at xanthoma site, pulmonary embolism. *Skeletal muscle:* Asthenia, arthralgia, myalgia, weakness, muscle cramps, aches. *GU:* Impotence, dysuria, hematuria, decreased urine output, decreased libido, proteinuria. *Hematologic:* Anemia, leukopenia, eosinophilia. *Dermatologic:* Allergic reactions, including urticaria, skin rash, dry skin, pruritus, dry brittle hair, alopecia. *Other:* Dyspnea, polyphagia, flu-like symptoms, ***noncardiovascular death.***

**Drug Interactions:** No significant drug interactions that affect oral health or with medications commonly used in dentistry.

**How Supplied:** *Capsule:* 500 mg

**Dosage** ————————
• **Capsules**
*Antihyperlipidemic.*
**Adults:** 500 mg q.i.d. Therapeutic response may take several weeks to become apparent. Drug must be administered on a continuous basis because lowered levels of cholesterol and other lipids will return to elevated state within several weeks after administration is stopped. Discontinue after 3 months if response is poor.

## DENTAL CONCERNS

None reported.
**Client/Family Teaching**
1. Stress the importance of good oral hygiene in order to prevent soft tissue damage.

# Clomipramine hydrochloride
(kloh-**MIP**-rah-meen)
**Pregnancy Category:** C
Anafranil, Apo–Clomipramine ✽, Gen-Clomipramine ✽, Novo-Clopamine ✽ **(Rx)**
**Classification:** Antidepressant, tricyclic

————————

See also *Antidepressants, Tricyclic.*
**Action/Kinetics:** Significant anticholinergic and sedative effects as well as moderate orthostatic hypotension. Significant serotonin uptake blocking activity and moderate blocking activity for norepinephrine. $t\frac{1}{2}$: 19–37 hr. **Effective plasma levels:** 80–100 ng/mL. **Time to reach steady state:** 7–14 days. Metabolized to the active desmethylclomipramine.

**Uses:** Obsessive-compulsive disorder in which the obsessions or compulsions cause marked distress, significantly interfere with social or occupational activities, or are time-consuming. Panic attacks and cataplexy associated with narcolepsy.

**Contraindications:** To relieve symptoms of depression.

**Special Concerns:** Safety has not been established for use during lactation or in children less than 10 years of age.

**Additional Side Effects:** Hyperthermia, especially when used with other drugs. Increased risk of ***seizures.*** Aggressive reactions, asthenia, anemia, eructation, failure to ejaculate, laryngitis, vestibular disorders, muscle weakness.

**How Supplied:** *Capsule:* 25 mg, 50 mg, 75 mg

## Dosage

- **Capsules**

**Adult, initial:** 25 mg/day; **then,** increase gradually to approximately 100 mg during the first 2 weeks (depending on client tolerance). The dose may then be increased slowly to a maximum of 250 mg/day over the next several weeks. **Adolescents, children, initial:** 25 mg/day; **then,** increase gradually during the first 2 weeks to a maximum of 100 mg or 3 mg/kg, whichever is less. The dose may then be increased to a maximum daily dose of 3 mg/kg or 200 mg, whichever is less. **Maintenance, adults and children:** Adjust the dose to the lowest effective dose with periodic reassessment to determine need for continued therapy.

## DENTAL CONCERNS

See also *Dental Concerns* for *Antidepressants, Tricyclic.*

# Clonazepam

(kloh-**NAY**-zeh-pam)

Alti-Clonazepam ✽, Apo-Clonazepam ✽, Dom-Clonazepam ✽, Klonopin, Nu-Clonazepam ✽, PMS–Clonazepam ✽, Rivotril ✽ **(C-IV) (Rx)**

**Classification:** Anticonvulsant, miscellaneous

See also *Anticonvulsants.*

**Action/Kinetics:** Benzodiazepine derivative which increases presynaptic inhibition and suppresses the spread of seizure activity. **Peak plasma levels:** 1–2 hr. **t½:** 18–60 hr. **Therapeutic serum levels:** 20–80 ng/mL. More than 80% bound to plasma protein; metabolized almost completely in the liver to inactive metabolites, which are excreted in the urine.

Even though a benzodiazepine, clonazepam, is used only as an anticonvulsant. However, contraindications, side effects, and so forth are similar to those for diazepam.

**Uses:** Absence seizures (petit mal) including Lennox-Gastaut syndrome, akinetic and myoclonic seizures. Some effectiveness in clients resistant to succinimide therapy. *Non-FDA Approved Uses:* Parkinsonian dysarthria, acute manic episodes of bipolar affective disorder, leg movements (periodic) during sleep, adjunct in treating schizophrenia, neuralgias, multifocal tic disorders.

**Contraindications:** Sensitivity to benzodiazepines. Severe liver disease, acute narrow-angle glaucoma. Pregnancy.

**Special Concerns:** Effects on lactation not known.

**Side Effects:** *Oral:* Dry mouth, increased salivation, increased bleeding. See also *Sedative Hypnotics (Antianxiety), Antimanic Drugs,* .

**Additional Side Effects:** In clients in whom different types of seizure disorders exist, clonazepam may elicit or precipitate **grand mal seizures.**

**Drug Interactions**

*CNS depressants* / Potentiation of CNS depressant effect of clonazepam

*Phenobarbital* / ↓ Effect of clonazepam due to ↑ breakdown by liver

*Phenytoin* / ↓ Effect of clonazepam due to ↑ breakdown by liver

**How Supplied:** *Tablet:* 0.5 mg, 1 mg, 2 mg

## Dosage

- **Tablets**

*Seizure disorders.*

**Adults, initial:** 0.5 mg t.i.d. Increase by 0.5–1 mg/day q 3 days until seizures are under control or side effects become excessive; **maximum:** 20 mg/day. **Pediatric up to 10 years or 30 kg:** 0.01–0.03 mg/kg/day in two to three divided doses up to a maximum of 0.05 mg/kg/day. Increase by increments of 0.25–0.5 mg q 3 days until seizures are under control or maintenance of 0.1–0.2 mg/kg is attained.

*Parkinsonian dysarthria.*

**Adults:** 0.25–0.5 mg/day.

*Acute manic episodes of bipolar affective disorder.*

**Adults:** 0.75–16 mg/day.
*Periodic leg movements during sleep.*
**Adults:** 0.5–2 mg nightly.
*Adjunct to treat schizophrenia.*
**Adults:** 0.5–2 mg/day.
*Neuralgias.*
**Adults:** 2–4 mg/day.
*Multifocal tic disorders.*
**Adults:** 1.5–12 mg/day.

## DENTAL CONCERNS

See also *Dental Concerns* for *Sedative-Hypnotics (Anti-anxiety)/Antimanic Drugs* and *Anticonvulsants*.

## Clonidine hydrochloride

(**KLOH**-nih-deen)
**Pregnancy Category:** C
Apo-Clonidine ✸; Catapres; Catapres-TTS-1, -2, and -3; Dixarit ✸; Duraclon, Novo-Clonidine ✸, Nu-Clonidine ✸ **(Rx)**
**Classification:** Antihypertensive, centrally acting antiadrenergic

See also *Antihypertensive Agents*.

**Action/Kinetics:** Stimulates alpha-adrenergic receptors of the CNS, which results in inhibition of the sympathetic vasomotor centers and decreased nerve impulses. Thus, bradycardia and a fall in both SBP and DBP occur. Plasma renin levels are decreased, while peripheral venous pressure remains unchanged. Few orthostatic effects. Although NaCl excretion is markedly decreased, potassium excretion remains unchanged. Tolerance to the drug may develop. **Onset, PO:** 30–60 min; **transdermal:** 2–3 days. **Peak plasma levels, PO:** 3–5 hr; **transdermal:** 2–3 days. **Maximum effect, PO:** 2–4 hr. **Duration, PO:** 12–24 hr; **transdermal:** 7 days (with system in place). **t½:** 12–16 hr. Approximately 50% excreted unchanged in the urine; 20% excreted through the feces.

The transdermal dosage form contains the following levels of drug: Catapres-TTS-1 contains 2.5 mg clonidine (surface area 3.5 cm²), with 0.1 mg released daily; Catapres-TTS-2 contains 5 mg clonidine (surface area 7 cm²), with 0.2 mg released daily; and Catapres-TTS-3 contains 7.5 mg clonidine (surface area 10.5 cm²), with 0.3 mg released daily.

Epidural use causes analgesia at presynaptic and postjunctional alpha-2-adrenergic receptors in the spinal cord due to prevention of pain signal transmission to the brain. **t½, distribution, epidural:** 19 min; **elimination:** 22 hr.

**Uses: Oral, Transdermal:** Mild to moderate hypertension. A diuretic or other antihypertensive drugs, or both, are often used concomitantly. *Non-FDA Approved Uses:* Alcohol withdrawal, atrial fibrillation, attention deficit hyperactivity disorder, constitutional growth delay in children, cyclosporine-associated nephrotoxicity, diabetic diarrhea, Gilles de la Tourette's syndrome, hyperhidrosis, hypertensive emergencies, mania, menopausal flushing, opiate detoxification, diagnosis of pheochromocytoma, postherpetic neuralgia, psychosis in schizophrenia, reduce allergen-induced inflammatory reactions in extrinsic asthma, restless leg syndrome, facilitate smoking cessation, ulcerative colitis.

**Epidural:** With opiates for severe pain in cancer clients not relieved by opiate analgesics alone. Most effective for neuropathic pain.

**Contraindications:** Hypersensitivity to the drug or its components.

**Special Concerns:** Use with caution in presence of severe coronary insufficiency, recent MI, cerebrovascular disease, or chronic renal failure. Use with caution during lactation. Safe use in children not established. Geriatric clients may be more sensitive to the hypotensive effects; a decreased dosage may also be necessary in these clients due to age-related decreases in renal function. For children, restrict epidural use to severe intractable pain from malignancy that is not responsive to epidural or spinal opiates or other analgesic approaches.

**Side Effects:** *CNS:* Drowsiness (common), sedation, confusion, dizziness, headache, fatigue, malaise, nightmares, nervousness, restlessness, anxiety, mental depression, increased dreaming, insomnia, hallucinations, delirium, agitation. *Oral:* Dry mouth (common), taste changes. *GI:* Constipation, anorexia, N&V, parotid pain, weight gain, hepatitis, parotitis, ileus, pseudo-obstruction, abdominal pain. *CV:* CHF, severe hypotension, Raynaud's phenomenon, abnormalities in ECG, palpitations, tachycardia and bradycardia, postural hypotension, conduction disturbances, sinus bradycardia, *CVA. Dermatologic:* Urticaria, skin rashes, sweating, *angioneurotic edema,* pruritus, thinning of hair, alopecia, skin ulcer. *GU:* Impotence, urinary retention, decreased sexual activity, loss of libido, nocturia, difficulty in urination, UTI. *Respiratory:* Hypoventilation, dyspnea. *Musculoskeletal:* Muscle or joint pain, leg cramps, weakness. *Other:* Gynecomastia, increase in blood glucose (transient), increased sensitivity to alcohol, chest pain, tinnitus, hyperaesthesia, pain, infection, thrombocytopenia, syncope, blurred vision, withdrawal syndrome, dryness of mucous membranes of nose; itching, burning, dryness of eyes; skin pallor, fever.

*Transdermal products:* Localized skin reactions, pruritus, erythema, allergic contact sensitization and contact dermatitis, localized vesiculation, hyperpigmentation, edema, excoriation, burning, papules, throbbing, blanching, generalized macular rash.

*NOTE:* Rebound hypertension may be manifested if clonidine is withdrawn abruptly.

**Drug Interactions**
*Alcohol* / ↑ Depressant effects
*CNS depressants* / ↑ Depressant effect
*Levodopa* / ↓ Effect of levodopa
*Local anesthetics* / Epidural clonidine → prolonged duration of epidural local anesthetics

*Opioid analgesics* / Potentiation of hypotensive effect of clonidine
*NSAIDs, especially indomethacin* / ↓ Hypotensive effects
*Sympathomimetics* / ↓ Hypotensive effects
*Tricyclic antidepressants* / Blocks antihypertensive effect

**How Supplied:** *Film, extended release:* 0.1 mg/24 hr, 0.2 mg/24 hr, 0.3 mg/24 hr; *Tablet:* 0.1 mg, 0.2 mg, 0.3 mg

## Dosage

• **Tablets**
  *Hypertension.*
**Initial:** 100 mcg b.i.d.; **then,** increase by 100–200 mcg/day until desired response is attained; **maintenance:** 200–600 mcg/day in divided doses (maximum: 2400 mcg/day). Tolerance necessitates increased dosage or concomitant administration of a diuretic. Gradual increase of dosage after initiation minimizes side effects. **Pediatric:** 50–400 mcg b.i.d.

*NOTE:* In hypertensive clients unable to take PO medication, clonidine may be administered sublingually at doses of 200–400 mcg/day.

  *Alcohol withdrawal.*
300–600 mcg q 6 hr.

  *Atrial fibrillation.*
75 mcg 1–2 times/day with or without digoxin.

  *Attention deficit hyperactivity disorder.*
5 mcg/kg/day for 8 weeks.

  *Constitutional growth delay in children.*
37.5–150 mcg/m²/day.

  *Diabetic diarrhea.*
100–600 mcg q 12 hr.

  *Gilles de la Tourette syndrome.*
150–200 mcg/day.

  *Hyperhidrosis.*
250 mcg 3–5 times/day.

  *Hypertensive urgency (diastolic > 120 mm Hg).*
**Initial:** 100–200 mcg; **then,** 50–100 mcg q hr to a maximum of 800 mcg.

  *Menopausal flushing.*
100–400 mcg/day.

  *Withdrawal from opiate dependence.*

15–16 mcg/kg/day.
*Diagnosis of pheochromocytoma.*
300 mcg.
*Postherpetic neuralgia.*
200 mcg/day.
*Psychosis in schizophrenia.*
Less than 900 mcg/day.
*Reduce allergen-induced inflammation in extrinsic asthma.*
150 mcg for 3 days or 75 mcg/1.5 mL saline by inhalation.
*Restless leg syndrome.*
100–300 mcg/day, up to 900 mcg/day.
*Facilitate cessation of smoking.*
150–400 mcg/day.
*Ulcerative colitis.*
300 mcg t.i.d.
• **Transdermal**
*Hypertension.*
**Initial:** Use 0.1-mg system; **then,** if after 1–2 weeks adequate control has not been achieved, can use another 0.1-mg system or a larger system. The antihypertensive effect may not be seen for 2–3 days. The system should be changed q 7 days.
*Cyclosporine-associated nephrotoxicity.*
100–200 mcg/day.
*Diabetic diarrhea.*
0.3 mg/24 hr patch (1 or 2 patches/week).
*Menopausal flushing.*
100 mcg/24-hr patch.
*Facilitate cessation of smoking.*
200 mcg/24-hr patch.
• **Epidural infusion**
*Analgesia.*
**Initial:** 30 mcg/hr. Dose may then be titrated up or down, depending on pain relief and side effects.

## DENTAL CONCERNS

See also *Dental Concerns* for *Antihypertensive Agents.*
**General**
1. If patient is experiencing changes in taste, consider clonidine as the causative agent.

# Clopidogrel bisulfate
(kloh-**PID**-oh-grel)

**Pregnancy Category:** B
Plavix **(Rx)**
**Classification:** Antiplatelet drug

**Action/Kinetics:** Inhibits platelet aggregation by inhibiting binding of adenosine diphosphate (ADP) to its platelet receptor and subsequent ADP-mediative activation of glycoprotein GPIIb/IIIa complex. Drug modifies receptor irreversibly; thus, platelets are affected for remainder of their lifespan. Also inhibits platelet aggregation caused by agonists other than ADP by blocking amplification of platelet activation by released ADP. Rapidly absorbed from GI tract; food does not affect bioavailability. **Peak plasma levels:** About 1 hr. Extensively metabolized in liver; about 50% excreted in urine and 46% in feces. **t½, elimination:** 8 hr.

**Uses:** Reduction of MI, stroke, and vascular death in clients with atherosclerosis documented by recent stroke, MI, or established peripheral arterial disease.

**Contraindications:** Lactation. Active pathological bleeding such as peptic ulcer or intracranial hemorrhage.

**Special Concerns:** Use with caution in those at risk of increased bleeding from trauma, surgery, or other pathological conditions. Safety and efficacy have not been determined in children.

**Side Effects:** *CV:* Edema, hypertension, ***intracranial hemorrhage***. *GI:* Abdominal pain, dyspepsia, diarrhea, nausea, hemorrhage, ulcers (peptic, gastric, duodenal). *CNS:* Headache, dizziness, depression. *Body as a whole:* Chest pain, accidental injury, flu-like symptoms, pain, fatigue. *Respiratory:* Upper respiratory tract infection, dyspnea, rhinitis, bronchitis, coughing. *Hematologic:* Purpura, epistaxis. *Musculoskeletal:* Arthralgia, back pain. *Dermatologic:* Disorders of skin/appendages, rash, pruritus. *Miscellaneous:* Urinary tract infection.

**Drug Interactions**

*Aspirin* / ↑ Risk of bleeding and occult blood loss

*NSAIDs* / ↑ Risk of bleeding and occult blood loss

**How Supplied:** *Tablets:* 75 mg

**Dosage** ⸺⸺⸺

• **Tablets**

*Reduction of atherosclerotic events.*

**Adults:** 75 mg once daily with or without food.

## DENTAL CONCERNS
**General**

Patients taking this drug require PT test prior to their dental visit because of the increased risk for prolonged bleeding.

1. Local hemostatic measures may be necessary to prevent excessive bleeding.

2. Platelet aggregation returns to normal within 5–7 days of discontinuing therapy.

**Consultation with Primary Care Provider**

1. Consultation with primary care provider may be necessary to assess patient status (disease control and ability to tolerate stress). Include patient's most current PT time.

**Client/Family Teaching**

1. Use caution when using oral hygiene aids.

2. Brush teeth with a soft-bristle tooth brush.

3. Avoid OTC agents especially aspirin and NSAIDs.

4. Report any unusual bruising or bleeding; advise others esp. dentist of prescribed therapy, before surgery or new meds added.

5. Drug should be discontinued 7 days prior to elective surgery (including oral surgery).

⸺⸺⸺⸺⸺⸺

# Clotrimazole
(kloh-**TRY**-mah-zohl)

**Pregnancy Category:** C (systemic use); B (topical/vaginal use)

Canesten ✤, Canestin 1 ✤, Canestin 3 ✤, Clotrimaderm ✤, FemCare, Gyne-Lotrimin, Lotrimin, Lotrimin AF, Mycelex, Mycelex-7, Mycelex-G, My-celex OTC, Myclo-Derm ✤, Myclo-Gyne ✤, Neo-Zol **(OTC) (Rx)**

**Classification:** Antifungal

⸺⸺⸺⸺⸺⸺

See also *Anti-Infectives.*

**Action/Kinetics:** Depending on concentration, may be fungistatic or fungicidal. Acts by inhibiting the biosynthesis of sterols, resulting in damage to the cell wall and subsequent loss of essential intracellular elements due to altered permeability. May also inhibit oxidative and peroxidative enzyme activity and inhibit the biosynthesis of triglycerides and phospholipids by fungi. When used for *Candida albicans,* the drug inhibits transformation of blastophores into the invasive mycelial form. Poorly absorbed from the GI tract and metabolized in the liver to inactive compounds that are excreted through the feces. **Duration:** up to 3 hr.

**Uses:** Broad-spectrum antifungal effective against *Malassezia furfur, Trichophyton rubrum, Trichophyton mentagrophytes, Epidermophyton floccosum, Microsporum canis, C. albicans.* *Oral troche:* Oropharyngeal candidiasis. Reduce incidence of oropharyngeal candidiasis in clients who are immunocompromised due to chemotherapy, radiotherapy, or steroid therapy used for leukemia, solid tumors, or kidney transplant. *Topical OTC products:* Topically to treat tinea pedis, tinea cruris, and tinea corporis. *Topical prescription products:* Same as OTC plus candidiasis and tinea versicolor. *Vaginal products:* Vulvovaginal candidiasis.

**Contraindications:** Hypersensitivity. First trimester of pregnancy.

**Special Concerns:** Use with caution during lactation. Safety and effectiveness for PO use in children less than 3 years of age has not been determined.

**Side Effects:** *Skin:* Irritation including rash, stinging, pruritus, urticaria, erythema, peeling, blistering, edema. *Vaginal:* Lower abdominal cramps; urinary frequency; bloating; vaginal irritation, itching or burning; dyspareunia. *Hepatic:* Abnormal liver function tests. *GI:* N&V following use of troche.

**Drug Interactions**
*Astemizole* / Serious CV side effects, including torsades de pointes and other ventricular arrhythmias (including QT interval prolongation), cardiac arrest, and death
*Terfenadine* / Serious CV side effects, including torsades de pointes and other ventricular arrhythmias (including QT interval prolongation), cardiac arrest, and death

**How Supplied:** *Kit; Lotion:* 1%; *Lozenge/Troche:* 10 mg; *Solution:* 1%; *Topical cream:* 1%; *Vaginal cream:* 1%; *Vaginal tablet:* 100 mg, 500 mg

**Dosage**
• **Troche**
*Treatment of oropharyngeal candidiasis.*
One troche (10 mg) 5 times/day for 14 consecutive days.
*Prophylaxis of oropharyngeal candidiasis.*
One troche t.i.d. for duration of chemotherapy or until maintenance doses of steroids are instituted.
• **Topical Cream, Lotion, Solution (each 1%)**
Massage into affected skin and surrounding areas b.i.d. in morning and evening for 7 consecutive days. Diagnosis should be reevaluated if no improvement occurs in 4 weeks.
• **Vaginal Tablets**
One 100-mg tablet/day at bedtime for 7 days. One 500-mg tablet can be inserted once at bedtime.
• **Vaginal Cream (1%)**
5 g (one full applicator)/day at bedtime for 7 consecutive days.
• **Vaginal Inserts and Clotrimazole, 1%**
*Vaginal yeast infections.*
Insert daily for 3 consecutive days.

---

## DENTAL CONCERNS

See also *General Dental Concerns for All Anti-Infectives.*
**Client/Family Teaching**
1. Soak full or partial dentures in an antifungal solution overnight until oral infection heals. Prolonged infection may require new dentures.
2. Replace toothbrush used during treatment of oral infection in order to prevent reinfection.
3. Long-term therapy may be necessary. Complete the full course of antifungal therapy.

---

# Cloxacillin sodium
(klox-ah-**SILL**-in)
**Pregnancy Category:** B
Apo-Cloxi ✱, Cloxapen, Novo-Cloxin ✱, Nu-CLoxi ✱, Orbenin ✱, Taro-Cloxacillin ✱, Tegopen **(Rx)**
**Classification:** Antibiotic, penicillin

See also *Anti-Infectives* and *Penicillins.*
**Action/Kinetics:** Resistant to penicillinase and is acid stable. **Peak plasma levels:** 7–15 mcg/mL after 30–60 min. **t½:** 30 min. Protein binding: 88%–96%. Well absorbed from GI tract. Mostly excreted in urine, but some excreted in bile.
**Uses:** Infections caused by penicillinase-producing staphylococci, including pneumococci, group A beta-hemolytic streptococci, and penicillin G-sensitive staphylococci.
**Contraindications:** Hypersensitivity to penicillins.
**Special Concerns:** Hypersensitivity to cephalosporins.
**Side Effects:** See also *Anti-Infectives* and *Penicillins.*
**Drug Interactions**
*Probenecid* / ↑ Cloxacillin concentrations

See also *Anti-Infectives* and *Penicillins.*
**How Supplied:** *Capsule:* 250 mg, 500 mg; *Powder for reconstitution:* 125 mg/5 mL

**Dosage**
• **Capsules, Oral Solution**
*Skin and soft tissue infections, mild to moderate URTIs.*
**Adults and children over 20 kg:** 250 mg q 6 hr; **pediatric, less than 20 kg:** 50 mg/kg/day in divided doses q 6 hr.

---

*Lower respiratory tract infections or disseminated infections.*
**Adults and children over 20 kg:** 0.5 g q 6 hr; **pediatric, less than 20 kg:** 100 (or more) mg/kg/day in divided doses q 6 hr. Alternatively, a dose of 50–100 mg/kg/day (up to a maximum of 4 g/day) divided q 6 hr may be used for infants and children.

## DENTAL CONCERNS

See also *Dental Concerns* for *Anti-Infectives* and *Penicillins.*
**Client/Family Teaching**
1. Review appropriate guidelines for administration; include frequency and amount. Shake well before using; refrigerate; discard any left after 14 days.
2. Take as directed, 1 hr before or 2 hr after meals; food interferes with absorption of drug.
3. Complete prescription even feeling better.

# Clozapine
(**KLOH**-zah-peen)
**Pregnancy Category:** B
Clozaril **(Rx)**
**Classification:** Antipsychotic

**Action/Kinetics:** Interferes with the binding of dopamine to both D-1 and D-2 receptors; more active at limbic than at striatal dopamine receptors. Thus, is relatively free from extrapyramidal side effects and does not induce catalepsy. Also acts as an antagonist at adrenergic, cholinergic, histaminergic, and serotonergic receptors. Increases the amount of time spent in REM sleep. Food does not affect the bioavailability of clozapine. **Peak plasma levels:** 2.5 hr. **Average maximum concentration at steady state:** 122 ng/mL plasma after 100 mg b.i.d. Highly bound to plasma proteins. **t½:** 12 hr. Metabolized in the liver to inactive compounds and excreted through the urine (50%) and feces (30%).

**Uses:** Severely ill schizophrenic clients who do not respond adequately to conventional antipsychotic therapy, either because of ineffectiveness or intolerable side effects from other drugs. Due to the possibility of development of agranulocytosis and seizures, avoid continued use in clients failing to respond.

**Contraindications:** Myeloproliferative disorders. Use with other agents known to suppress bone marrow function. Severe CNS depression or coma due to any cause. Lactation.

**Special Concerns:** Use with caution in clients with known CV disease, prostatic hypertrophy, narrow angle glaucoma, hepatic or renal disease.

**Side Effects:** *Hematologic: **Agranulocytosis,*** leukopenia, neutropenia, eosinophilia. *CNS: **Seizures*** (appear to be dose dependent), drowsiness or sedation, dizziness, vertigo, headache, tremor, restlessness, nightmares, hypokinesia, akinesia, agitation, akathisia, confusion, rigidity, fatigue, insomnia, hyperkinesia, weakness, lethargy, slurred speech, ataxia, depression, anxiety, epileptiform movements. *CV:* Orthostatic hypotension (especially initially), tachycardia, syncope, hypertension, angina, chest pain, ***cardiac abnormalities,*** changes in ECG. *Neuroleptic malignant syndrome: **Hyperpyrexia,*** muscle rigidity, altered mental status, irregular pulse or BP, tachycardia, diaphoresis, cardiac dysrhythmias. *Oral:* Dry mouth, excessive salivation, glossitis, numb or sore tongue. *GI:* Constipation, nausea, heartburn, abdominal discomfort, vomiting, diarrhea, anorexia. *GU:* Urinary abnormalities, incontinence, abnormal ejaculation, urinary frequency or urgency, urinary retention. *Musculoskeletal:* Muscle weakness, pain (back, legs, neck), muscle spasm, muscle ache. *Respiratory:* Dyspnea, SOB, throat discomfort, nasal congestion. *Miscellaneous:* Sweating, visual disturbances, fever (transient), rash, weight gain.

**Drug Interactions**
*Anticholinergic drugs* / Additive anticholinergic effects
*Benzodiazepines* / Possible respiratory depression and collapse

*Epinephrine* / Clozapine may reverse effects if epinephrine is given for hypotension

**How Supplied:** *Tablet:* 25 mg, 100 mg

**Dosage** ————————
• **Tablets**
*Schizophrenia.*
**Adults, initial:** 25 mg 1–2 times/day; **then,** if drug is tolerated, the dose can be increased by 25–50 mg/day to a dose of 300–450 mg/day at the end of 2 weeks. Subsequent dosage increments should occur no more often than once or twice a week in increments not to exceed 100 mg. **Usual maintenance dose:** 300–600 mg/day (although doses up to 900 mg/day may be required in some clients). Total daily dose should not exceed 900 mg.

**DENTAL CONCERNS**

See also *Dental Concerns* for *Antipsychotic Agents, Phenothiazines.*

# Codeine phosphate
(**KOH**-deen)
Pregnancy Category: C
Paveral ✳ (C-II) (Rx)

# Codeine sulfate
(**KOH**-deen )
Pregnancy Category: C
(C-II) (Rx)
Classification: Opioid analgesic, morphine type

See also *Opioid Analgesics.*
**Action/Kinetics:** Resembles morphine pharmacologically but produces less respiratory depression and N&V. Moderately habit-forming and constipating. Dosages over 60 mg often cause restlessness and excitement and irritate the cough center. However, in lower doses, it is a potent antitussive and is an ingredient in many cough syrups. **Onset:** 10–30 min. **Peak effect:** 30–60 min. **Duration:** 4–6 hr. **t½:** 3–4 hr. Codeine is

two-thirds as effective PO as parenterally.
**Uses:** Relief of mild to moderate pain. Antitussive to relieve chemical or mechanical respiratory tract irritation. In combination with aspirin or acetaminophen to enhance analgesia.
**Contraindications:** Premature infants or during labor when delivery of a premature infant is expected.
**Special Concerns:** May increase the duration of labor. Use with caution and reduce the initial dose in clients with seizure disorders, acute abdominal conditions, renal or hepatic disease, fever, Addison's disease, hypothyroidism, prostatic hypertrophy, ulcerative colitis, urethral stricture, following recent GI or GU tract surgery, and in the young, geriatric, or debilitated clients.
**Additional Drug Interactions:** Combination with chlordiazepoxide may induce coma.
**How Supplied:** Codeine Phosphate: *Injection:* 15 mg/mL, 30 mg/mL, 60 mg/mL; *Solution:* 15 mg/5 mL; *Tablet:* 30 mg, 60 mg. Codeine Sulfate: *Tablet:* 15 mg, 30 mg, 60 mg

**Dosage** ————————
• **Solution, Tablets, IM, IV, SC**
*Analgesia.*
**Adults:** 15–60 mg q 4–6 hr, not to exceed 360 mg/day. **Pediatric, over 1 year:** 0.5 mg/kg q 4–6 hr. IV should not be used in children.
*Antitussive.*
**Adults:** 10–20 mg q 4–6 hr, up to maximum of 120 mg/day. **Pediatric, 2–6 years:** 2.5–5 mg PO q 4–6 hr, not to exceed 30 mg/day; **6–12 years:** 5–10 mg q 4–6 hr, not to exceed 60 mg/day.

**DENTAL CONCERNS**

See also *Dental Concerns* for *Opioid Analgesics.*
**Client/Family Teaching**
1. Take only as directed. Acetaminophen or aspirin act synergistically with codeine and are usually given together.

# Colestipol hydrochloride

(koh-**LESS**-tih-poll)
Colestid **(Rx)**
Classification: Hypocholesterolemic, bile acid sequestrant

**Action/Kinetics:** Colestipol, an anion exchange resin, binds bile acids in the intestine, forming an insoluble complex excreted in the feces. The loss of bile acids results in increased oxidation of cholesterol to bile acids and a decrease in LDL and serum cholesterol. Does not affect (or may increase) triglycerides or HDL and may increase VLDL. Not absorbed from the GI tract. **Onset:** 1–2 days; **maximum effect:** 1 month. Return to pretreatment cholesterol levels after discontinuance of therapy: 1 month.

**Uses:** As adjunctive therapy in hyperlipoproteinemia (types IIA and IIB) to reduce serum cholesterol in clients who do not respond adequately to diet. *Non-FDA Approved Uses:* Digitalis toxicity.

**Contraindications:** Complete obstruction or atresia of bile duct.

**Special Concerns:** Use during pregnancy only if benefits outweigh risks. Use with caution during lactation and in children. Children may be more likely to develop hyperchloremic acidosis although dosage has not been established. Clients over 60 years of age may be at greater risk of GI side effects and adverse nutritional effects.

**Side Effects:** *Oral:* Tongue irritation. *GI:* Constipation (may be severe and accompanied by fecal impaction), N&V, diarrhea, heartburn, GI bleeding, anorexia, flatulence, steatorrhea, abdominal distention/cramping, bloating, loose stools, indigestion, rectal bleeding/pain, black stools, hemorrhoidal bleeding, *bleeding duodenal ulcer, peptic ulceration,* ulcer attack, GI irritation, dysphagia, dental bleeding/caries, hiccoughs, sour taste, pancreatitis, diverticulitis, cholecystitis, cholelithiasis. *CV:* Chest pain, angina, tachycardia (rare). *CNS:* Migraine or sinus headache, anxiety, vertigo, dizziness, lightheadedness, insomnia, fatigue, tinnitus, syncope, drowsiness, femoral nerve pain, paresthesia. *Hematologic:* Ecchymosis, anemia, bleeding tendencies due to hypoprothrombinemia. *Allergic:* Urticaria, dermatitis, asthma, wheezing, rash. *Musculoskeletal:* Backache, muscle/joint pain, arthritis. *Renal:* Hematuria, burnt odor to urine, dysuria, diuresis. *Miscellaneous:* Uveitis, fatigue, weight loss or gain, increased libido, swollen glands, SOB, edema, weakness, swelling of hands/feet, osteoporosis, calcified material in biliary tree and gall bladder, hyperchloremic acidosis in children.

**Drug Interactions:** See *Cholestyramine.*

**How Supplied:** *Granule for reconstitution:* 5 g/7.5 g, 5 g/packet, 5 g/scoopful; *Tablet:* 1 g

## Dosage ───────────────

• **Oral Granules**
*Antihyperlipidemic.*
**Adults, initial:** 5 g 1–2 times/day; **then,** can increase 5 g/day at 1–2-month intervals. **Total dose:** 5–30 g/day given once or in two to three divided doses.

• **Tablets**
**Adults, initial:** 2 g 1–2 times/day. Dose can be increased by 2 g, once or twice daily, at 1–2-month intervals. **Total dose:** 2–16 g/day given once or in divided doses.
*Digitalis toxicity.*
10 g followed by 5 g q 6–8 hr.

## DENTAL CONCERNS

See also *Dental Concerns* for *Cholestyramine.*

# Cromolyn sodium (Sodium cromoglycate)

(**CROH**-moh-lin)
**Pregnancy Category:** B
Crolom, Gastrocrom, Intal, Nalcrom ✦, Nasalcrom, Novo–Cromolyn ✦, Opticrom ✦, PMS–Sodium Chromoglycate ✦, Rynacrom ✦, Vistacrom ✦ **(OTC) (Rx)**
**Classification:** Antiasthmatic, antiallergic drug

**Action/Kinetics:** Acts locally to inhibit the degranulation of sensitized mast cells that occurs after exposure to certain antigens. Prevents the release of histamine, slow-reacting substance of anaphylaxis, and other endogenous substances causing hypersensitivity reactions. When effective, reduces the number and intensity of asthmatic attacks as well as decreasing allergic reactions in the eye. The drug has no antihistaminic, antiinflammatory, or bronchodilator effects and has no role in terminating an acute attack of asthma. After inhalation, some of the drug is absorbed systemically. **t½:** 81 min; from lungs: 60 min. About 50% excreted unchanged through the urine and 50% through the bile. When used in the eye, approximately 0.03% is absorbed. **Onset, ophthalmic:** Several days. **Onset, nasal:** Less than 1 week. **Time to peak effect, nasal:** Up to 4 weeks.

**Uses: Inhalation:** Prophylactic and adjunct in the management of severe bronchial asthma in selected clients. Prophylaxis of exercise-induced bronchospasms and bronchospasms due to allergens, cold dry air, or environmental pollutants. **Ophthalmologic:** Conjunctivitis, including vernal keratoconjunctivitis, vernal conjunctivitis, and vernal keratitis. **Nasal, OTC:** Prophylaxis and treatment of allergic rhinitis. **PO:** Mastocytosis (improves symptoms including diarrhea, flushing, headaches, vomiting, urticaria, nausea, abdominal pain, and itching). *Non-FDA Approved Uses:* PO to treat food allergies.

**Contraindications:** Hypersensitivity. Acute attacks and status asthmaticus. Due to the presence of benzalkonium chloride in the product, soft contact lenses should not be worn if the drug is used in the eye. For mastocytosis in premature infants.

**Special Concerns:** Dosage of the ophthalmic product has not been established in children less than 4 years of age; dosage of the nasal product has not been established in children less than 6 years of age. Use with caution for long periods of time, in the presence of renal or hepatic disease, and during lactation.

**Side Effects:** *Respiratory:* **Bronchospasm, laryngeal edema (rare),** cough, eosinophilic pneumonia. *CNS:* Dizziness, drowsiness, headache. *Allergic:* Urticaria, rash, angioedema, serum sickness, **anaphylaxis.** *Other:* Nausea, urinary frequency, dysuria, joint swelling and pain, lacrimation, swollen parotid gland.

**Following nebulization:** Sneezing, wheezing, itching, nose bleeds, burning, nasal congestion. **Following nasal solution:** Burning, stinging, irritation of nose; sneezing, nose bleeds, headache, bad taste in mouth, postnasal drip. **Following ophthalmic use:** Stinging and burning after use. Also, conjunctival injection, watery or itchy eyes, dryness around the eye, puffy eyes, eye irritation, styes.

**Following PO use:** *Oral:* Taste perversion, burning of mouth and throat, dry mouth. *GI:* Diarrhea, taste perversion, spasm of esophagus, flatulence, dysphagia, burning of mouth and throat. *CNS:* Headache, dizziness, fatigue, migraine, paresthesia, anxiety, depression, psychosis, behavior changes, insomnia, hallucinations, lethargy, lightheadedness after eating. *Dermatologic:* Flushing, angioedema, urticaria, skin burning, skin erythema. *Musculoskeletal:* Arthralgia, stiffness and weakness in legs. *Miscellaneous:* Altered liver function test, dyspnea, dysuria, polycythemia, neutropenia.

**How Supplied:** *Concentrate:* 100 mg/5 mL; *Metered dose inhaler:* 0.8 mg/inh; *Ophthalmic solution:* 4%; *Solution:* 10 mg/mL; *Nasal spray:* 5.2 mg/inh

**Dosage**
• **Capsules or Metered Dose Inhaler**

---

*Prophylaxis of bronchial asthma.*
**Adults:** 20 mg q.i.d. at regular intervals. Adjust dosage as required.
*Prophylaxis of bronchospasm.*
**Adults:** 20 mg as a single dose just prior to exposure to the precipitating factor. If used chronically, 20 mg q.i.d, up to a maximum of 160 mg/day.

- **Ophthalmic Solution**
  *Allergic ocular disorders.*
**Adults and children over 4 years:** 1–2 gtt of the 4% solution in each eye 4–6 times/day at regular intervals.

- **Nasal Spray (OTC)**
  *Allergic rhinitis.*
**Adults and children over 6 years:** 5.2 mg in each nostril 3–4 times/day at regular intervals (e.g., q 4–6 hr). May be used up to 6 times/day.

- **Oral Capsules**
  *Mastocytosis.*
**Adults:** 200 mg q.i.d. 30 min before meals and at bedtime. **Pediatric, term to 2 years:** 20 mg/kg/day in four divided doses; should be used in this age group only in severe incapacitating disease where benefits outweigh risks. **Pediatric, 2–12 years:** 100 mg q.i.d. 30 min before meals and at bedtime. If relief is not seen within 2–3 weeks, dose may be increased, but should not exceed 40 mg/kg/day for adults and children over 2 years of age and 30 mg/kg/day for children 6 months–2 years.

## DENTAL CONCERNS
### General
1. The patient may require a semisupine position for the dental chair to help with breathing.
2. Dental procedures may cause the patient anxiety which could result in an asthma attack. Make sure that the patient has his or her sympathomimetic inhaler present or have the inhaler from the office emergency kit present.
3. Morning and shorter appointments, as well as methods for addressing anxiety levels in the patient, can help to reduce the amount of stress that the patient is experiencing.
4. Sulfites present in vasoconstrictors can precipitate an asthma attack.
5. Decreased saliva flow can put the patient at risk for dental caries, periodontal disease, and candidiasis.
### Consultation with Primary Care Provider
1. Consultation may be necessary in order to evaluate the patient's level of disease control.
2. Consultation may be necessary in order to determine the patient's ability to tolerate stress.
### Client/Family Teaching
1. Daily home fluoride treatments for persistent dry mouth.
2. Avoid alcohol-containing mouth rinses and beverages.
3. Avoid caffeine-containing beverages.
4. Dry mouth can be treated with tart, sugarless gum or candy, water, sugar-free gum, or with saliva substitutes if dry mouth persists.
5. Review technique for use and care of prescribed inhalers and respiratory equipment. Rinsing of equipment and of mouth after use is imperative in preventing oral fungal infections.

# Cyclophosphamide
(sye-kloh-**FOS**-fah-myd)
**Pregnancy Category:** D
Cytoxan, Cytoxan Lyophilized, Neosar, Procytox ✣ (Abbreviation: CYC)
**(Rx)**
**Classification:** Antineoplastic, alkylating agent

See also *Antineoplastic Agents.*
**Action/Kinetics:** Metabolized in the liver to both active antineoplastic alkylating agents and inactive metabolites. The active metabolites alkylate nucleic acids, thus interfering with the growth of neoplastic and normal tissues. The cytotoxic action is due to cross-linking of strands of DNA and RNA and inhibition of protein synthesis. Also possesses immunosuppressive activity. $t\frac{1}{2}$: 3–12 hr, but remnants of drug and/or metab-

olites detectable in serum after 72 hr; in children, the t½ averages 4.1 hr. Metabolites are excreted through the urine with up to 25% of cyclophosphamide excreted unchanged. Cyclophosphamide is also excreted in milk.

**Uses:** Often used in combination with other antineoplastic drugs. *Malignancies:* Malignant lymphomas (Stages III and IV, Ann Arbor Staging System), Hodgkin's disease, lymphocytic lymphoma (nodular or diffuse), mixed-cell-type lymphoma, histiocytic lymphoma, Burkitt's lymphoma, multiple myeloma, neuroblastoma (disseminated), adenocarcinoma of the ovary, retinoblastoma, carcinoma of the breast. *Leukemias:* Chronic lymphocytic and granulocytic leukemia, acute myelogenous and monocytic leukemia, acute lymphoblastic leukemia in children. *Other:* Mycosis fungoides, nephrotic syndrome in children. *Non-FDA Approved Uses:* Rheumatic diseases including rheumatoid arthritis and lupus erythematosus, Wegemer's granulomatosis, multiple sclerosis, polyarteritis nodosa, polymyositis (use with corticosteroids), severe neuropsychiatric lupus erythematosus.

**Contraindications:** Lactation. Severe bone marrow depression.

**Special Concerns:** Use with caution in clients with thrombocytopenia, leukopenia, previous radiation therapy, bone marrow infiltration of tumor cells, previous therapy causing cytotoxicity, and impaired liver and kidney function. May interfere with wound healing.

**Side Effects:** *Oral:* Swelling of lips and tongue, stomatitis. *GI:* Nausea, vomiting, diarrhea, weight loss, *hepatoxicity*, colitis. *CNS:* Headache, dizziness. *CV: Cardiotoxicity (high doses).* *Pulmonary: Fibrosis.* Hematolog-

*ic: Thrombocytopenia, leukopenia, pancytopenia, myelosuppression.* *GU: Hemorrhagic cystitis, hematuria, neoplasms, amenorrhea, azoospermia, impotence, sterility, ovarian fibrosis.* *Skin:* Alopecia, dermatitis.

**Drug Interactions**
*Allopurinol* / ↑ Chance of bone marrow toxicity
*Anticoagulants* / ↑ Effect of anticoagulants
*Chloramphenicol* / ↓ Metabolism of cyclophosphamide to active metabolites → ↓ pharmacologic effect
*Digoxin* / ↓ Serum digoxin levels
*Insulin* / ↑ Hypoglycemia
*Phenobarbital* / ↑ Rate of metabolism of cyclophosphamide in liver
*Quinolone antibiotics* / ↓ Antimicrobial effect of quinolones
*Succinylcholine* / ↑ Neuromuscular blockade due to ↓ cholinesterase activity

**How Supplied:** *Powder for injection:* 100 mg, 200 mg, 500 mg, 1 g, 2 g; *Tablet:* 25 mg, 50 mg

**Dosage** ————————————
• **IV**
*Malignancies.*
**Initial, with no hematologic deficiency:** 40–50 mg/kg in divided doses over 2–5 days. *Alternative therapy:* 10–15 mg/kg q 7–10 days or 3–5 mg/kg twice weekly.
• **Tablets**
*Malignancies.*
**Initial and maintenance:** 1–5 mg/kg depending on client tolerance. Attempt to maintain leukocyte count at 3,000–4,000/mm³. Adjust dosage for kidney or liver disease.
*Nephrotic syndrome in children.*
2.5–3 mg/kg/day for 60–90 days.

## DENTAL CONCERNS

See also *Dental Concerns* for *Antineoplastic Agents.*

# Daclizumab

(dah-**KLIZ**-you-mab)
**Pregnancy Category:** C
Zenapax **(Rx)**
**Classification:** Immunosuppressive drug

**Action/Kinetics:** Daclizumab is a humanized IgG1 monoclonal antibody produced by recombinant DNA technology. As an antagonist, it binds to the alpha subunit (Tac subunit) of the human high affinity interleukin-2 (IL-2) receptor found on the surface of activated lymphocytes. This results in inhibition of IL-2 mediated activation of lymphocytes, a critical pathway in the cellular immune response involved in allograft rejection. **t½, terminal:** Estimated to be 20 days.

**Uses:** Prophylaxis of acute organ rejection in renal transplants. Used with cyclosporine and corticosteroids.

**Contraindications:** Lactation.

**Special Concerns:** Increased risk for developing lymphoproliferative disorders and opportunistic infections. Use with caution in geriatric clients. Adequate studies have not been performed in children.

**Side Effects:** Incidence of 2% or more is reported. *GI:* Constipation, N&V, abdominal pain, pyrosis, dyspepsia, abdominal distention, epigastric pain, flatulence, gastritis, hemorrhoids. *CNS:* Tremor, headache, dizziness, prickly sensation, depression, anxiety. *CV:* Hypertension, hypotension, aggravated hypertension, tachycardia, thrombosis, bleeding. *Respiratory:* Dyspnea, pulmonary edema, coughing atelectasis, congestion, pharyngitis, rhinitis, hypoxia, rales, abnormal breathing sounds, pleural effusion. *GU:* Oliguria, dysuria, renal tubular necrosis, renal damage, hydronephrosis, urinary tract bleeding, urinary tract disorder, renal insufficiency, urinary retention. *Dermatologic:* Impaired wound healing without infection, acne, pruritus, hirsutism, rash, night sweats, increased sweating. *Musculoskeletal:* Musculoskeletal pain, back pain, arthralgia, leg cramps, myalgia. *Body as a whole:* Post-traumatic pain, chest pain, fever, pain, fatigue, insomnia, lymphocele, shivering, general weakness, injection site reaction, infections. *Metabolic:* Peripheral edema, edema, fluid overload, diabetes mellitus, hyperglycemia. *Miscellaneous:* Blurred vision.

**Drug Interactions:** None reported.

**How Supplied:** *Injection concentrate:* 25 mg/5mL

## Dosage

- **IV**

    *Prevent kidney transplant rejection.*

1 mg/kg q 14 days for total of five doses. Regimen also includes cyclosporine and corticosteroids.

## DENTAL CONCERNS

### General

1. Though most patients receive this drug in the hospital, some patients may continue therapy at home. These patients may come in for dental treatment while receiving this drug.

2. Transplant patients may be receiving other medications which could suppress the immune system.

3. Shorter appointments and stress reduction may be necessary for anxious patients.

### Consultation with Primary Care Provider

1. Antibiotic prophylaxis may be necessary for patients with organ transplants or for those who are otherwise immunocompromised.

### Client/Family Teaching

1. Review the importance of good oral hygiene in order to prevent soft tissue inflammation.

2. Review the proper use of oral hygiene aids in order to prevent injury.

3. Instruct patient to continually up-

date the health/medication record at each visit.

# Danaparoid sodium
(dah-**NAP**-ah-royd)
**Pregnancy Category:** B
Orgaran **(Rx)**
**Classification:** Anticoagulant, glyco-saminoglycan

See also *Anticoagulants*.
**Action/Kinetics:** A low molecular weight sulfated glycosaminoglycans obtained from porcine mucosa. Prevents fibrin formation in the coagulation pathway via thrombin generation inhibition by anti-Xa and anti-IIa effects. Minimal effect on clotting assays, fibrinolytic activity, or bleeding time. 100% bioavailable with SC use. **t½:** About 24 hr. Excreted primarily through the kidneys.
**Uses:** Prophylaxis of postoperative deep vein thrombosis (DVT) in clients undergoing elective hip replacement surgery. *Non-FDA Approved Uses*: Thromboembolism, anticoagulation during hemodialysis, hemofiltration during CV operation, and increased risk of thrombosis during pregnancy.
**Contraindications:** Use in hemophilia, idiopathic thrombocytopenic purpura, active major bleeding state (including hemorrhagic stroke in the acute phase), and type II thrombocytopenia associated with a positive in vitro test for antiplatelet antibody in the presence of danaparoid. Hypersensitivity to pork products. IM use.
**Special Concerns:** Cannot be dosed interchangeably (unit for unit) with either heparin or low molecular weight heparins. Use with extreme caution in disease states where there is an increased risk of hemorrhage, including severe uncontrolled hypertension, acute bacterial endocarditis, congenital or acquired bleeding disorders, active ulcerative and angiodysplastic GI disease, nonhemorrhagic stroke, postoperative indwelling epidural catheter use, and shortly after brain, spinal, or ophthalmologic surgery. Use with caution during lactation and in those with severely impaired renal function. Use with caution in clients receiving oral anticoagulants or platelet inhibitors. Safety and efficacy have not been determined in children.
**Side Effects:** *CV:* Intraoperative blood loss, postoperative blood loss. *GI:* N&V, constipation. *CNS:* Insomnia, headache, dizziness. *Dermatologic:* Rash, pruritus. *GU:* UTI, urinary retention. *Miscellaneous:* Fever, pain at injection site, peripheral edema, joint disorder, edema, asthenia, anemia, pain, infection.
**How Supplied:** *Injection:* 750 anti-Xa units/0.6 mL.

## Dosage
- **SC only**
  *Prophylaxis of DVT in hip replacement surgery.*
**Adults:** 750 anti-Xa units b.i.d. SC, beginning 1 to 4 hr preoperatively and then not sooner than 2 hr postoperatively. Continue treatment throughout the postoperative period until the risk of deep vein thrombosis has decreased. Average duration of treatment is 7 to 10 days, up to 14 days.

## DENTAL CONCERNS

See also *Dental Concerns* for *Anticoagulants*.

# Delavirdine mesylate
(deh-lah-**VIR**-deen)
**Pregnancy Category:** C
Rescriptor **(Rx)**
**Classification:** Antiviral drug, reverse transcriptase inhibitor

See also *Antiviral Drugs*.
**Action/Kinetics:** Non-nucleoside reverse transcriptase inhibitor that binds directly to reverse transcriptase and blocks RNA-dependent and DNA-dependent DNA polymerase activities. Effect is additive if used with other antiviral drugs. Delavirdine may confer cross-resistance to other non-nucleoside reverse tran-

scriptase inhibitors when used alone or in combination. Rapidly absorbed. **Peak plasma levels:** About 1 hr. Extensively bound to plasma albumin. Converted to inactive metabolites which are excreted in urine and feces. It inhibits its own metabolism.

**Uses:** Treatment of HIV-1 infections in combination with appropriate antiretroviral agents.

**Contraindications:** Hypersensitivity; cisipride.

**Special Concerns:** Use with caution in impaired hepatic function. Safety and efficacy in combination with other antiretroviral drugs have not been determined in HIV-1-infected clients less than 16 years of age.

**Side Effects:** *Body as a whole:* Headache, fatigue, asthenia, allergic reaction, chest pain, chills, general or local edema, fever, flu syndrome, lethargy, malaise, neck rigidity, general or local pain, trauma. *CV:* Bradycardia, migraine, pallor, palpitation, postural hypotension, syncope, tachycardia, vasodilation. *CNS:* Abnormal coordination, agitation, amnesia, anxiety, change in dreams, cognitive impairment, confusion, decreased libido, depression, disorientation, dizziness, emotional lability, hallucinations, hyperesthesia, hyperreflexia, hypesthesia, impaired coordination, insomnia, mania, nervousness, neuropathy, nightmares, paralysis, paranoia, paresthesia, restlessness, somnolence, tingling, tremor, vertigo, weakness. *Oral:* Aphthous stomatitis, dry mouth, mouth ulcers, taste perversion, gingivitis, gum hemorrhage, increased saliva, lipedema, sialadenitis, stomatitis, tongue edema. *GI:* N&V, diarrhea, anorexia, bloody stool, colitis, constipation, appetite decreased or increased, diarrhea, duodenitis, diverticulitis, dyspepsia, dysphagia, fecal incontinence, flatulence, enteritis, esophagitis, gastritis, gagging, gastroesophageal reflux, GI bleeding or disorder, increased thirst, abdominal cramps/distention/pain, hepatitis (nonspecified), pancreatitis, rectal disorder, ulceration. *Dermatologic:* Skin rashes, maculopapular rash, pruritus, angioedema, dermal leukocytoblastic vasculitis, dermatitis, desquamation, diaphoresis, dry skin, erythema, erythema multiforme, folliculitis, fungal dermatitis, alopecia, nail disorder, petechial rash, seborrhea, skin disorder, skin nodule, *Stevens-Johnson syndrome,* vesiculobullous rash, sebaceous cyst. *GU:* Breast enlargement, kidney calculi, epididymitis, hematuria, hemospermia, impotence, kidney pain, metrorrhagia, nocturia, polyuria, proteinuria, vaginal moniliasis. *Musculoskeletal:* Back pain, neck rigidity, arthritis or arthralgia of single or multiple joints, bone disorder or pain, leg cramps, muscle weakness, myalgia, tendon disorder, tenosynovitis, tetany, muscle cramps. *Respiratory:* Upper respiratory infection, bronchitis, chest congestion, cough, dyspnea, epistaxis, laryngismus, pharyngitis, rhinitis, sinusitis. *Hematologic:* Anemia, bruises, ecchymosis, eosinophilia, granulocytosis, neutropenia, pancytopenia, petechiae, purpura, spleen disorder, thrombocytopenia. *Ophthalmic:* Nystagmus, blepharitis, conjunctivitis, diplopia, dry eyes, photophobia. *Miscellaneous:* Alcohol intolerance, peripheral edema, weight increase or decrease, tinnitus, ear pain.

**Drug Interactions**

*Antacids* / ↓ Absorption of delavirdine; separate doses by 1 hr

*Astemizole* / Possible serious or life-threatening side effects of astemizole due to ↓ metabolism

*Benzodiazpines* / Possible serious or life-threatening side effects of benzodiazepines due to ↓ metabolism

*Carbamazepine* / Possible serious or life-threatening side effects of carbamazepine due to ↓ metabolism

*Cisapride* / Possible serious or life-threatening side effects of cisapride due to ↓ metabolism

*Clarithromycin* / Significant ↑ in amount absorbed of both drugs; possible serious side effects
*Ketoconazole* / Possible serious or life-threatening side effects of ketoconazole due to ↓ metabolism
*Terfenadine* / Possible serious or life-threatening side effects of terfenadine due to ↓ metabolism

**Dosage** ─────────────
• **Tablets**
*HIV-1 infection.*
400 mg (4–100 mg tablets) t.i.d. in combination with other antiretroviral therapy.

## DENTAL CONCERNS

See also *General Dental Concerns for All Anti-Infectives* and *Antiviral Drugs.*
**General**
1. Examine patients for oral signs and symptoms of opportunistic infection.
2. Patients on chronic drug therapy may develop blood dyscrasias. Symptoms include fever, sore throat, bleeding, and poor wound healing.
3. Decreased saliva flow can put the patient at risk for dental caries, periodontal disease, and candidiasis.
4. Have the patient sit up slowly and remain seated for at least two minutes after being supine in order to minimize the risk of orthostatic hypotension.
5. Do not use ingestible sodium bicarbonate products within 2 hours of taking delavirdine (i.e., air polishing system).
**Consultation with Primary Care Provider**
1. Patients with symptoms of blood dyscrasias should be referred to their primary care provider for complete blood counts. Treatment should be postponed until the results are known.
2. Medical consultation may be necessary in order to assess patient's ability to tolerate stress.
3. Medical consultation may be nec

essary in order to assess patient's level of disease control.
**Client/Family Teaching**
1. Review the importance of good oral hygiene in order to prevent soft tissue inflammation.
2. Review the proper use of oral hygiene aids in order to prevent injury.
3. Daily home fluoride treatments for persistent dry mouth.
4. Avoid alcohol-containing mouth rinses and beverages.
5. Avoid caffeine-containing beverages.
6. Dry mouth can be treated with tart, sugarless gum or candy, water, sugar-free beverages, or with saliva substitutes if dry mouth persists.
7. Report oral sores, lesions, or bleeding to the dentist.
8. Update patient's dental record (medication/health history) as needed.

# Desipramine hydrochloride
(dess-**IP**-rah-meen)
Alti-Desipramine ✤, Apo-Desipramine ✤, Dom-Desipramine ✤, Norpramin, Novo-Desipramine ✤, Nu-Desipramine ✤, Pertofrane ✤, PMS-Desipramine ✤ **(Rx)**
**Classification:** Antidepressant, tricyclic

See also *Antidepressants, Tricyclic.*
**Action/Kinetics:** Slight anticholinergic and sedative effects and slight ability to cause orthostatic hypotension. **Effective plasma levels:** 125–300 ng/mL. **t½:** 12–24 hr. **Time to reach steady state:** 2–11 days. Response usually seen within the first week.
**Uses:** Symptoms of depression. Bulimia nervosa. To decrease craving and depression during cocaine withdrawal. To treat severe neurogenic pain. Cataplexy associated with narcolepsy. Attention deficit disorders with or without hyperactivity in children over 6 years of age.

**Contraindications:** Use in children less than 12 years of age.

**Special Concerns:** Safe use during pregnancy has not been established. Safety and efficacy have not been established in children.

**Additional Side Effects:** Bad taste in mouth, hypertension during surgery.

**How Supplied:** *Tablet:* 10 mg, 25 mg, 50 mg, 75 mg, 100 mg, 150 mg

**Dosage** ————————————
• **Tablets**
   *Antidepressant.*
**Initial:** 100–200 mg/day in single or divided doses. **Maximum daily dose:** 300 mg in severely ill clients. **Maintenance:** 50–100 mg/day. **Geriatric clients:** 25–50 mg/day in divided doses up to a maximum of 150 mg/day. **Adolescents and geriatric clients:** 25–50 mg/day in divided doses up to a maximum of 150 mg.
   *Cocaine withdrawal.*
50–200 mg/day.

## DENTAL CONCERNS

See also *Dental Concerns* for *Antidepressants, Tricyclic.*

# Dextroamphetamine sulfate

(dex-troh-am-**FET**-ah-meen)
**Pregnancy Category:** C
Dexedrine, Oxydess II, Spancap No. 1 **(C-II) (Rx)**
**Classification:** Central nervous system stimulant, amphetamine type

See also *Amphetamines and Derivatives.*

**Action/Kinetics:** Has stronger CNS effects and weaker peripheral action than does amphetamine; thus, dextroamphetamine manifests fewer undesirable CV effects. After PO administration, completely absorbed in 3 hr. **Duration: PO,** 4–24 hr; **t½, adults:** 10–12 hr; **children:** 6–8 hr. Excreted in urine. Acidification will increase excretion, while alkalinization will decrease it.

**Uses:** Attention deficit disorders in children, narcolepsy.

**Contraindications:** See also *Amphetamines and Derivatives.*

**Additional Contraindications:** Lactation. Use for obesity.

**Special Concerns:** Use of extended-release capsules for attention deficit disorders in children less than 6 years of age and the elixir or tablets for attention deficit disorders in children less than 3 years of age is not recommended. Dosage for narcolepsy has not been determined in children less than 6 years of age.

**Side Effects:** See also *Amphetamines and Derivatives.*

**Drug Interactions:** See also *Amphetamines and Derivatives.*

**How Supplied:** *Capsule, Extended Release:* 5 mg, 10 mg, 15 mg; *Tablet:* 5 mg, 10 mg

**Dosage** ————————————
• **Tablets**
   *Attention deficit disorders in children.*
**3–5 years, initial:** 2.5 mg/day; increase by 2.5 mg/day at weekly intervals until optimum dose is achieved (usual range 0.1–0.5 mg/kg/dose each morning). **6 years and older, initial:** 5 mg 1–2 times/day; increase in increments of 5 mg/week until optimum dose is achieved (rarely over 40 mg/day).
   *Narcolepsy.*
**Adults:** 5–60 mg in divided doses daily. **Children over 12 years, initial:** 10 mg/day; increase in increments of 10 mg/day at weekly intervals until optimum dose is reached. **Children, 6–12 years, initial:** 5 mg/day; increase in increments of 5 mg/week until optimum dose is reached (maximum is 60 mg/day).
• **Extended-Release Capsule**
   *Attention deficit disorders.*
**Children, 6 years and older:** 5–15 mg/day.
   *Narcolepsy.*
**Adults:** 5–30 mg/day. **Children, 6–12 years:** 5–15 mg/day; **12 years and older:** 10–15 mg/day.

## DENTAL CONCERNS

See also *Dental Concerns* for *Amphetamines and Derivatives.*

# Diazepam

(dye-**AYZ**-eh-pam)
**Pregnancy Category:** D
Apo-Diazepam ✹, Diastat, Diazemuls ✹, Diazepam Intensol, Dizac, E Pam ✹, Meval ✹, Novo-Dipam ✹, PMS-Diazepam ✹, Valium, Valium Roche ✹, Vivol ✹ **(C-IV) (Rx)**
**Classification:** Antianxiety agent, anticonvulsant, skeletal muscle relaxant

---

See also *Sedative Hynotics*.

**Action/Kinetics:** The skeletal muscle relaxant effect of diazepam may be due to enhancement of GABA-mediated presynaptic inhibition at the spinal level as well as in the brain stem reticular formation. **Onset: PO,** 30–60 min; **IM,** 15–30 min; **IV,** more rapid. **Peak plasma levels: PO,** 0.5–2 hr; **IM,** 0.5–1.5; **IV,** 0.25 hr. **Duration:** 3 hr. **t½:** 20–50 hr. Metabolized in the liver to the active metabolites desmethyldiazepam, oxazepam, and temazepam. Diazepam and metabolites are excreted through the urine. Diazepam is 97%–99% bound to plasma protein.

**Uses:** Anxiety, tension (more effective than chlordiazepoxide), alcohol withdrawal, muscle relaxant, adjunct to treat seizure disorders, antipanic drug. Used prior to gastroscopy and esophagoscopy, preoperatively and prior to cardioversion. In dentistry to induce sedation. Treatment of status epilepticus. Relief of skeletal muscle spasm due to inflammation of muscles or joints or trauma; spasticity caused by upper motor neuron disorders such as cerebral palsy and paraplegia; athetotis; and stiff-man syndrome. Relieve spasms of facial muscles in occlusion and temporomandibular joint disorders. IV: Status epilepticus, severe recurrent seizures, and tetanus. Rectal gel: Treat epilepsy in those with stable regimens of anticonvulsant drugs who require intermittent diazepam to control increased seizure activity.

**Additional          Contraindications:** Narrow-angle glaucoma, children under 6 months, lactation, and parenterally in children under 12 years.

**Special Concerns:** When used as an adjunct for seizure disorders, diazepam may increase the frequency or severity of clonic-tonic seizures, for which an increase in the dose of anticonvulsant medication is necessary. Safety and efficacy of parenteral diazepam have not been determined in neonates less than 30 days of age. Prolonged CNS depression has been observed in neonates, probably due to inability to biotransform diazepam into inactive metabolites.

**Additional Drug Interactions:** Diazepam potentiates antihypertensive effects of thiazides and other diuretics.

Diazepam potentiates muscle relaxant effects of *d*-tubocurarine and gallamine.

*Fluoxetine* / ↑ Half-life of diazepam.
*Isoniazid* / ↑ Half-life of diazepam.
*Ranitidine* / ↓ GI absorption of diazepam.

**How Supplied:** *Concentrate:* 5 mg/mL; *Injection:* 5 mg/mL; *Solution:* 5 mg/5 mL; *Tablet* 2 mg, 5 mg, 10 mg

## Dosage

- **Tablets, Oral Solution**
  *Antianxiety, anticonvulsant, adjunct to skeletal muscle relaxants.*
  **Adults:** 2–10 mg b.i.d.–q.i.d. **Elderly, debilitated clients:** 2–2.5 mg 1–2 times/day. May be gradually increased to adult level. **Pediatric, over 6 months, initial:** 1–2.5 mg (0.04–0.2 mg/kg or 1.17–6 mg/m²) b.i.d.–t.i.d.
  *Alcohol withdrawal.*
  **Adults:** 10 mg t.i.d.–q.i.d. during the first 24 hr; **then,** decrease to 5 mg t.i.d.–q.i.d. as required.
  *Anticonvulsant.*
  **Adults:** 15–30 mg once daily.
- **Rectal Gel**
  *Anticonvulsant.*
  **Over 12 years:** 0.2 mg/kg. **Children, 6–11 years:** 0.3 mg/kg; **2–5**

---

**D**

**years:** 0.5 mg/kg. If required, a second dose can be given 4 to 12 hr after the first dose. Do not treat more than five episodes per month or more than one episode every 5 days. Adjust dose downward in elderly or debilitated clients to reduce ataxia or oversedation.

- **IM, IV**

  *Preoperative or diagnostic use.*
  **Adults:** 10 mg IM 5–30 min before procedure.

  *Adjunct to treat skeletal muscle spasm.*
  **Adults, initial:** 5–10 mg IM or IV; **then,** repeat in 3–4 hr if needed (larger doses may be required for tetanus).

  *Moderate anxiety.*
  **Adults:** 2–5 mg IM or IV q 3–4 hr if necessary.

  *Severe anxiety, muscle spasm.*
  **Adults:** 5–10 mg IM or IV q 3–4 hr, if necessary.

  *Acute alcohol withdrawal.*
  **Initial:** 10 mg IM or IV; **then,** 5–10 mg q 3–4 hr.

  *Preoperatively.*
  **Adults:** 10 mg IM prior to surgery.

  *Endoscopy.*
  **IV:** 10 mg or less although doses up to 20 mg can be used; **IM:** 5–10 mg 30 min prior to procedure.

  *Cardioversion.*
  **IV:** 5–15 mg 5–10 min prior to procedure.

  *Tetanus in children.*
  **IM, IV, over 1 month:** 1–2 mg, repeated q 3–4 hr as necessary; **5 years and over:** 5–10 mg q 3–4 hr.

- **IV**

  *Status epilepticus.*
  **Adults, initial:** 5–10 mg; **then,** dose may be repeated at 10–15-min intervals up to a maximum dose of 30 mg. Dosage may be repeated after 2–4 hr. **Children, 1 month–5 years:** 0.2–0.5 mg q 2–5 min, up to maximum of 5 mg. Can be repeated in 2–4 hr. **5 years and older:** 1 mg q 2–5 min up to a maximum of 10 mg; dose can be repeated in 2–4 hr, if needed.

  *NOTE:* Elderly or debilitated clients should not receive more than 5 mg parenterally at any one time.

## DENTAL CONCERNS

See also *Dental Concerns* for *Sedative-Hypnotic (Anti-anxiety)/Antimanic Drugs.*
1. Review anxiety level and identify any contributing factors.
2. Elderly clients may experience adverse reactions more quickly than younger clients; use a lower dose in this group.
3. Have someone drive the patient to and from the dental appointment if this drug is used for conscious sedation.
4. Assist the patient to and from the dental chair because of the possibility of dizziness.

# Diclofenac potassium
(dye-**KLOH**-fen-ack)
**Pregnancy Category:** B
Cataflam **(Rx)**

# Diclofenac sodium
(dye-**KLOH**-fen-ack)
**Pregnancy Category:** B
Apo-Diclo ✦, Apo-Diclo SR ✦, Novo–Difenac ✦, Novo–Difenac SR ✦, Nu-Diclo ✦, Taro-Diclofenac ✦, Voltaren, Voltaren Ophtha ✦, Voltaren Ophthalmic, Voltaren SR ✦, Voltaren-XR **(Rx)**
**Classification:** Nonsteroidal anti-inflammatory analgesic

See also *Nonsteroidal Anti-Inflammatory Drugs.*
**Action/Kinetics:** Available as both the potassium (immediate-release) and sodium (delayed-release) salts. *Immediate-release product.* **Onset:** 30 min. **Peak plasma levels:** 1 hr. **Duration:** 8 hr. *Delayed-release product.* **Peak plasma levels:** 2–3 hr. **t½:** 1–2 hr. For all dosage forms, food will affect the rate, but not the amount, absorbed from the GI tract. Metabolized in the liver and excreted by the kidneys.
**Uses: PO, Immediate-release:** Analgesic, primary dysmenorrhea. **PO, Immediate- or Delayed-release:** Rheumatoid arthritis, osteoarthritis, ankylosing spondylitis. **PO, Delayed-release:** Osteoarthritis, rheu-

matoid arthritis. *Non-FDA Approved Uses:* Mild to moderate pain, juvenile rheumatoid arthritis, acute painful shoulder, sunburn. **Ophthalmic:** Postoperative inflammation following cataract extraction.

**Contraindications:** Wearers of soft contact lenses.

**Special Concerns:** Use with caution during lactation. Safety and effectiveness has not been determined in children. When used ophthalmically, may cause increased bleeding of ocular tissues in conjunction with ocular surgery. Healing may be slowed or delayed.

**Side Effects:** *Following ophthalmic use:* Keratitis, increased intraocular pressure, ocular allergy, N&V, anterior chamber reaction, viral infections, transient burning and stinging on administration. When used with soft contact lenses, may cause ocular irritation, including redness and burning.

**How Supplied:** Diclofenac potassium: *Tablet:* 50 mg. Diclofenac sodium: *Enteric coated tablet:* 25 mg, 50 mg, 75 mg; *Ophthalmic solution:* 0.1%; *Tablet, extended release:* 100 mg

**Dosage** ⎯⎯⎯⎯⎯⎯⎯⎯⎯⎯
• **Immediate-Release      Tablets, Delayed-Release Tablets**
*Analgesia, primary dysmenorrhea.*
**Adults:** 50 mg t.i.d. of immediate-release tablets. In some, an initial dose of 100 mg followed by 50-mg doses may achieve better results. After the first day, the total daily dose should not exceed 150 mg.
*Rheumatoid arthritis.*
**Adults:** 100–200 mg/day in divided doses (e.g., 50 mg t.i.d. or q.i.d.; 75 mg b.i.d. of the sodium salt). For chronic therapy, use extended-release tablets, 100 mg once or twice daily, not to exceed 225 mg/day.
*Osteoarthritis.*
**Adults:** 100–150 mg/day in divided doses (e.g., 50 mg b.i.d. or t.i.d.; 75 mg b.i.d. of the sodium salt). For chronic therapy, use extended-re-

lease tablets, 100 mg/day. Doses greater than 200 mg/day have not been evaluated.
*Ankylosing spondylitis.*
**Adults:** 25 mg q.i.d. with an extra 25-mg dose at bedtime, if necessary. Doses greater than 125 mg/day have not been evaluated.
• **Ophthalmic Solution**
1 gtt of the 0.1% solution in the affected eye q.i.d. beginning 24 hr after cataract surgery and for 2 weeks thereafter.

### DENTAL CONCERNS

See also *Dental Concerns* for *Nonsteroidal Anti-Inflammatory Drugs.*

# Dicyclomine hydrochloride
(dye-**SYE**-kloh-meen)
**Pregnancy Category:** C
Antispas, A-Spas, Bentyl, Bentylol ✦, Byclomine, Dibent, Di-Cyclonex, Di-lomine, Di-Spaz, Formulex ✦, Or-Tyl **(Rx)**
**Classification:** Cholinergic blocking agent

See also *Cholinergic Blocking Agents.*
**Action/Kinetics: t½, initial:** 1.8 hr; **secondary:** 9–10 hr.
**Uses:** Hypermotility and spasms of GI tract associated with irritable colon and spastic colitis, mucous colitis.
**Additional      Contraindications:** Use for peptic ulcer.
**Special Concerns:** Lower doses may be needed in elderly clients due to confusion, agitation, excitement, or drowsiness.
**Additional Side Effects:** Brief euphoria, slight dizziness, feeling of abdominal distention. **Use of the syrup in infants less than 3 months of age:** *Seizures,* syncope, respiratory symptoms, fluctuations in pulse rate, *asphyxia,* muscular hypotonia, *coma.*
**How Supplied:** *Capsules:* 10 mg; *Injection:* 10 mg/mL; *Syrup:* 10 mg 1.5 mL; *Tablets:* 20 mg

**Dosage**

• **Capsules, Syrup, Tablets**
*Hypermotility and spasms of GI tract.*

**Adults:** 10–20 mg t.i.d.–q.i.d.; **then,** may increase to total daily dose of 160 mg if side effects do not limit this dosage. **Pediatric, 6 years and older, capsules or tablets:** 10 mg t.i.d.–q.i.d.; adjust dosage to need and incidence of side effects. **Pediatric, 6 months–2 years, syrup:** 5–10 mg t.i.d.–q.i.d.; **2 years and older:** 10 mg t.i.d.–q.i.d. The dose should be adjusted to need and incidence of side effects.

• **IM**
*Hypermotility and spasms of GI tract.*

**Adults:** 20 mg q 4–6 hr. **Not for IV use.**

## DENTAL CONCERNS

See also *Dental Concerns* for *Cholinergic Blocking Agents.*

---

# Didanosine (ddl, dideoxyinosine)
(die-**DAN**-oh-seen)
**Pregnancy Category:** B
Videx **(Rx)**
**Classification:** Antiviral

See also *Antiviral Agents.*

**Action/Kinetics:** Didanosine is a nucleoside analog of deoxyadenosine. After entering the cell, it is converted to the active dideoxyadenosine triphosphate (ddATP) by cellular enzymes. Due to the chemical structure of ddATP, its incorporation into viral DNA leads to chain termination and therefore inhibition of viral replication. ddATP also inhibits viral replication by interfering with the HIV–RNA-dependent DNA polymerase by competing with the natural nucleoside triphosphate for binding to the active site of the enzyme. Didanosine has shown in vitro antiviral activity in a variety of HIV-infected T cell and monocyte/macrophage cell cultures. Is broken down quickly at acidic pH; therefore, PO products contain buffering agents to increase the pH of the stomach. Food decreases the rate of absorption. t½, **elimination:** 1.6 hr for adults and 0.8 hr for children. Metabolized in the liver and excreted mainly through the urine.

**Uses:** Advanced HIV infection in adult and pediatric (over 6 months of age) clients who are intolerant of AZT therapy or who have demonstrated decreased effectiveness of AZT therapy. Use in adults with HIV infection who have received prolonged AZT therapy. Treatment of HIV infection when antiretroviral therapy is indicated. AZT should be considered as initial therapy for the treatment of advanced HIV infection, unless contraindicated, since this drug prolongs survival and decreases the incidence of opportunistic infections. May be used as monotherapy for the treatment of AIDS.

**Contraindications:** Lactation.

**Special Concerns:** Use with caution in renal and hepatic impairment and in those on sodium-restricted diets. Opportunistic infections and other complications of HIV infection may continue to develop; thus, keep clients under close observation.

**Side Effects:** Commonly pancreatitis and peripheral neuropathy (manifested by distal numbness, tingling, or pain in the feet or hands). Neuropathy occurs more frequently in clients with a history of neuropathy or neurotoxic drug therapy.

**In adults.** *Oral:* Dry mouth, stomatitis, mouth sores, oral moniliasis, sialadenitis, oral thrush. *GI:* Diarrhea, abdominal pain, N&V, anorexia, ileus, colitis, constipation, eructation, flatulence, gastroenteritis, *GI hemorrhage, stomach ulcer hemorrhage,* melena, liver abnormalities. *CNS:* Headache, *tonic-clonic seizures,* abnormal thinking, anxiety, nervousness, twitching, confusion, depression, acute brain syndrome, amnesia, aphasia, ataxia, dizziness, hyperesthesia, hypertonia, incoordination, *intracranial hemorrhage,* paralysis, paranoid reaction, psychosis, insomnia, sleep disorders, speech disorders, tremor. *Hematologic:* Leukopenia, granulocytopenia, thrombocytopenia, microcytic anemia, **hemorrhage,** ecchymosis, petechiae. *Dermatologic:* Rash, pruritus, herpes simplex, skin disorder, sweating, eczema, impetigo, excoriation, erythema. *Musculoskeletal:* Asthenia, myopathy, arthralgia, arthritis, myalgia, muscle atrophy, decreased strength, hemiparesis, neck rigidity, joint disorder, leg cramps. *CV:* Chest pain, hypertension, hypotension, migraine, palpitation, peripheral vascular disorder, syncope, vasodilation, arrhythmias. *Body as a whole:* Chills, fever, infection, allergic reaction, pain, abscess, cellulitis, cyst, dehydration, malaise, flu syndrome, numbness of hands and feet, weight loss, alopecia. *Respiratory:* Pneumonia, dyspnea, asthma, bronchitis, increased cough, rhinitis, rhinorrhea, epistaxis, laryngitis, decreased lung function, pharyngitis, hypoventilation, sinusitis, rhonchi, rales, congestion, interstitial pneumonia, respiratory disorders. *Ophthalmic:* Blurred vision, conjunctivitis, diplopia, dry eye, glaucoma, retinitis, photophobia, strabismus. *Otic:* Ear disorder, otitis (externa and media), ear pain. *GU:* Impotency, kidney calculus, kidney failure, abnormal kidney function, nocturia, urinary frequency, vaginal hemorrhage. *Miscellaneous:* Peripheral edema, sarcoma, hernia, hypokalemia, lymphoma-like reaction.

**In children.** *Oral:* Stomatitis, mouth sores, oral thrush, dry mouth. *GI:* Diarrhea, N&V, liver abnormalities, abdominal pain, pancreatitis, anorexia, increase in appetite, constipation, melena. *CNS:* Headache, nervousness, insomnia, dizziness, poor coordination, lethargy, neurologic symptoms, **seizures.** *Hematologic:* Ecchymosis, **hemorrhage,** petechiae, leukopenia, granulocytopenia, thrombocytopenia, anemia. *Dermatologic:* Rash, pruritus, skin disorder, eczema, sweating, impetigo, excoriation, erythema. *Musculoskeletal:* Ar-

thritis, myalgia, muscle atrophy, decreased strength. *Body as a whole:* Chills, fever, asthenia, pain, malaise, failure to thrive, weight loss, flu syndrome, alopecia, dehydration. *CV:* Vasodilation, arrhythmia. *Respiratory:* Cough, rhinitis, dyspnea, asthma, rhinorrhea, epistaxis, pharyngitis, hypoventilation, sinusitis, rhonchi, rales, congestion, pneumonia. *Ophthalmic:* Photophobia, strabismus, visual impairment. *Otic:* Ear pain, otitis. *Miscellaneous:* Urinary frequency, diabetes mellitus, diabetes insipidus, liver abnormalities.

**Drug Interactions**

*Itraconazole* / ↓ Absorption of itraconazole due to gastric pH change caused by buffering agents in didanosine

*Ketoconazole* / ↓ Absorption of ketoconazole due to gastric pH change caused by buffering agents in didanosine

*Metronidazole* / ↑ Risk of pancreatitis and ↑ risk of peripheral neuropathy

*Nitrous oxide* / ↑ Risk of peripheral neuropathy

*Quinolone antibiotics* / ↓ Plasma levels of quinolone antibiotics

*Ranitidine* / ↓ Absorption of ranitidine due to gastric pH change caused by buffering agents in didanosine

*Sulfonamides* / ↑ Risk of pancreatitis

*Sulindac* / ↑ Risk of pancreatitis

*Tetracyclines* / ↓ Absorption of tetracyclines from the stomach due to the buffering agents in didanosine and ↑ risk of pancreatitis

**How Supplied:** *Chew Tablet:* 25 mg, 50 mg, 100 mg, 150 mg; *Powder for reconstitution:* 100 mg, 167 mg, 250 mg, 2 g, 4 g

## Dosage

- **Chewable/Dispersible Buffered Tablets, Buffered Powder for Oral Solution, Powder for Pediatric Oral Solution**

**Adults, initial, weight over 60 kg:** 200 mg q 12 hr (with 250 mg buffered powder q 12 hr). **Weight less than 60 kg:** 125 mg q 12 hr (with 167 mg buffered powder q 12 hr). **Pediatric, BSA 1.1–1.4 m²:** Two 50-mg tablets q 12 hr or 125 mg of the pediatric powder q 12 hr; **BSA 0.8–1.0 m²:** One 50- and one 25-mg tablet q 12 hr or 94 mg of the pediatric powder q 12 hr. **BSA 0.5–0.7 m²:** Two 25-mg tablets q 12 hr or 62 mg of the pediatric powder q 12 hr. **BSA less than 0.4 m²:** One 25-mg tablet q 12 hr or 31 mg of the pediatric powder q 12 hr.

## DENTAL CONCERNS

See also *Dental Concerns* for *Antiviral Agents.*

### General

1. Monitor vital signs at every appointment because of cardiovascular and respiratory side effects.
2. Patients on chronic drug therapy may develop blood dyscrasias. Symptoms include fever, sore throat, bleeding, and poor wound healing.
3. Avoid direct dental light in the patient's eyes. Keep dark glasses available for patient comfort.

### Consultation with Primary Care Provider

1. Patients with symptoms of blood dyscrasias should be referred to their primary care provider for complete blood counts. Treatment should be postponed until the results are known.
2. Medical consultation may be necessary in order to assess patient's cardiovascular status and ability to tolerate stress.

### Client/Family Teaching

1. Review the importance of good oral hygiene in order to prevent soft tissue inflammation.
2. Review the proper use of oral hygiene aids in order to prevent injury.
3. Daily home fluoride treatments for persistent dry mouth.
4. Avoid alcohol-containing mouth rinses and beverages.
5. Avoid caffeine-containing beverages.
6. Dry mouth can be treated with tart, sugarless gum or candy, water,

sugar-free beverages, or with saliva substitutes if dry mouth persists.

# Diflunisal
(dye-FLEW-nih-sal)
**Pregnancy Category:** C
Apo-Diflunisal ✦, Dolobid, Novo-Diflunisal ✦, Nu-Diflunisal ✦ **(Rx)**
**Classification:** Nonsteroidal analgesic, anti-inflammatory, antipyretic

**Action/Kinetics:** Diflunisal is a salicylic acid derivative although it is not metabolized to salicylic acid. Mechanism not known; may be an inhibitor of prostaglandin synthetase. **Onset:** 20 min (analgesic, antipyretic). **Peak plasma levels:** 2–3 hr. **Peak effect:** 2–3 hr. **Duration:** 4–6 hr **t½:** 8–12 hr. Ninety-nine percent protein bound. Metabolites excreted in urine.

**Uses:** Analgesic, rheumatoid arthritis, osteoarthritis, ankylosing spondylitis, psoriatic arthritis, musculoskeletal pain. Prophylaxis and treatment of vascular headaches.

**Contraindications:** Hypersensitivity to diflunisal, aspirin, or other anti-inflammatory drugs. Acute asthmatic attacks, urticaria, or rhinitis precipitated by aspirin. During lactation and in children less than 12 years of age.

**Special Concerns:** Use with caution in presence of ulcers or in clients with a history thereof, in clients with hypertension, compromised cardiac function, or in conditions leading to fluid retention. Use with caution in only first two trimesters of pregnancy. Geriatric clients may be at greater risk of GI toxicity.

**Side Effects:** *GI:* Nausea, dyspepsia, GI pain and bleeding, diarrhea, vomiting, constipation, flatulence, peptic ulcer, eructation, anorexia. *CNS:* Headache, fatigue, fever, malaise, dizziness, somnolence, insomnia, nervousness, vertigo, depression, paresthesias. *Dermatologic:* Rashes, pruritus, sweating, ***Stevens-Johnson syndrome,*** dry mucous membranes, erythema multiforme. *CV:* Palpitations, syncope, edema. *Other:* Tinnitus, asthenia, chest pain, hypersensitivity reactions, **anaphylaxis,** dyspnea, dysuria, muscle cramps, thrombocytopenia.

**Drug Interactions**

*Acetaminophen* / ↑ Plasma levels of acetaminophen

*Antacids* / ↓ Plasma levels of diflunisal

*Anticoagulants* / ↑ PT

*Furosemide* / ↓ Hyperuricemic effect of furosemide

*Hydrochlorothiazide* / ↑ Plasma levels and ↓ hyperuricemic effect of hydrochlorothiazide

*Indomethacin* / ↓ Renal clearance of indomethacin → ↑ plasma levels

*Naproxen* / ↓ Urinary excretion of naproxen and metabolite

**How Supplied:** *Tablet:* 250 mg, 500 mg

**Dosage** ────────────

• **Tablets**

*Mild to moderate pain.*

**Adults, initial:** 1,000 mg; **then,** 250–500 mg q 8–12 hr.

*Rheumatoid arthritis, osteoarthritis.*

**Adults:** 250–500 mg b.i.d. Doses in excess of 1,500 mg/day are not recommended. For some, an initial dose of 500 mg followed by 250 mg q 8–12 hr may be effective. Reduce dosage with impaired renal function.

─────────────────

**DENTAL CONCERNS**

See also *Dental Concerns* for *Nonsteroidal Anti-Inflammatory Drugs.*

─────────────────

# Digitoxin

(dih-jih-**TOX**-in)

**Pregnancy Category:** C

Crystodigin, Digitaline ✿ **(Rx)**

**Classification:** Cardiac glycoside

─────────────────

See also *Cardiac Glycosides.*

**Action/Kinetics:** Most potent of the digitalis glycosides. Slow onset makes it unsuitable for emergency use. Almost completely absorbed from GI tract. **Onset: PO,** 1–4 hr; maximum effect: 8–12 hr. **t½:** 5–9 days; **Duration:** 2 weeks. Significant protein binding (over 90%). Metabolized by the liver and excreted as in-

active metabolites through the urine. **Therapeutic serum levels:** 14–26 ng/mL. Withhold drug and check with provider if serum level exceeds 35 ng/mL, indicating toxicity.

**Uses:** Maintenance in CHF.

**Contraindications:** See also *Cardiac Glycosides.*

**Special Concerns:** Digitalis tablets may not be suitable for small children; thus, other digitalis products should be considered.

**Side Effects:** See also *Cardiac Glycosides.*

**Drug Interactions:** See also *Cardiac Glycosides.*

**Additional Drug Interactions**

*Barbiturates* / ↓ Effect of digitoxin due to ↑ breakdown by liver

*Phenylbutazone* / ↓ Effect of digitoxin due to ↑ breakdown by liver

**How Supplied:** *Tablet:* 0.1 mg

**Dosage** ────────────

• **Tablets**

*Digitalizing (loading) dose: Rapid.*

**Adults:** 0.6 mg followed by 0.4 mg in 4–6 hr; **then,** 0.2 mg q 4–6 hr until therapeutic effect achieved.

*Digitalizing (loading) dose: Slow.*

**Adults:** 0.2 mg b.i.d. for 4 days.

*Digitalizing (loading) dose: children.*

After the neonatal period, the doses are as follows: **Under one year:** 0.045 mg/kg/day divided into three, four, or more doses with 6 hr between doses; **one to two years:** 0.04 mg/kg/day divided into three, four, or more doses with 6 hr between doses; **over two years:** 0.03 mg/kg/day (0.75 mg/m²) divided into three, four, or more doses with 6 hr between doses.

*Maintenance dose: PO.*

**Adults:** 0.05–0.3 mg/day (**usual:** 0.15 mg/day). **Children:** Give one-tenth of the digitalizing dose.

─────────────────

**DENTAL CONCERNS**

See also *Dental Concerns* for *Cardiac Glycosides.*

# Digoxin
(dih-**JOX**-in)
Pregnancy Category: A
Lanoxicaps, Lanoxin, Novo–Digoxin
✦ **(Rx)**
Classification: Cardiac glycoside

See also *Cardiac Glycosides.*
**Action/Kinetics:** Action prompter and shorter than that of digitoxin. **Onset: PO,** 0.5–2 hr; **time to peak effect:** 2–6 hr. **Duration:** Over 24 hr. **Onset, IV:** 5–30 min; **time to peak effect:** 1–4 hr. **Duration:** 6 days. t½: 30–40 hr. **Therapeutic serum level:** 0.5–2.0 ng/mL. From 20% to 25% is protein bound. Serum levels above 2.5 ng/mL indicate toxicity. Fifty percent to 70% is excreted unchanged by the kidneys. Bioavailability depends on the dosage form: tablets (60%–80%), capsules (90%–100%), and elixir (70%–85%). Thus, changing dosage forms may require dosage adjustments.
**Uses:** May be drug of choice for CHF because of rapid onset, relatively short duration, and ability to be administered PO or IV.
**Contraindications:** See also *Cardiac Glycosides.*
**Side Effects:** See also *Cardiac Glycosides.*
**Drug Interactions:** See also *Cardiac Glycosides.*
**Additional Drug Interactions**
The following drugs increase serum digoxin levels, leading to possible toxicity: anticholinergics, benzodiazepines, erythromycin, ibuprofen, indomethacin, tetracyclines.
**How Supplied:** *Capsule:* 0.05 mg, 0.1 mg, 0.2 mg; *Elixir:* 0.05 mg/mL; *Injection:* 0.1 mg/mL, 0.25 mg/mL; *Tablet:* 0.125 mg, 0.25 mg, 0.5 mg

## Dosage
• **Capsules**
*Digitalization: Rapid.*
**Adults:** 0.4–0.6 mg initially followed by 0.1–0.3 mg q 6–8 hr until desired effect achieved.
*Digitalization: Slow.*
**Adults:** A total of 0.05–0.35 mg/day divided in two doses for a period of 7–22 days to reach steady-state serum levels. **Pediatric.** Digitalizing dosage is divided into three or more doses with the initial dose being about one-half the total dose; doses are given q 4–8 hr. **Children, 10 years and older:** 0.008–0.012 mg/kg. **5–10 years:** 0.015–0.03 mg/kg. **2–5 years:** 0.025–0.035 mg/kg. **1 month–2 years:** 0.03–0.05 mg/kg. **Neonates, full-term:** 0.02–0.03 mg/kg. **Neonates, premature:** 0.015–0.025 mg/kg.
*Maintenance.*
**Adults:** 0.05–0.35 mg once or twice daily. **Premature neonates:** 20%–30% of total digitalizing dose divided and given in two to three daily doses. **Neonates to 10 years:** 25%–35% of the total digitalizing dose divided and given in two to three daily doses.
• **Elixir, Tablets**
*Digitalization: Rapid.*
**Adults:** A total of 0.75–1.25 mg divided into two or more doses each given at 6–8-hr intervals.
*Digitalization: Slow.*
**Adults:** 0.125–0.5 mg/day for 7 days. **Pediatric.** (Digitalizing dose is divided into two or more doses and given at 6–8-hr intervals.) **Children, 10 years and older, rapid or slow:** Same as adult dose. **5–10 years:** 0.02–0.035 mg/kg. **2–5 years:** 0.03–0.05 mg/kg. **1 month–2 years:** 0.035–0.06 mg/kg. **Premature and newborn infants to 1 month:** 0.02–0.035 mg/kg.
*Maintenance.*
**Adults:** 0.125–0.5 mg/day. **Pediatric:** One-fifth to one-third the total digitalizing dose daily. *NOTE:* An alternate regimen (referred to as the "small-dose" method) is 0.017 mg/kg/day. This dose causes less toxicity.
• **IV**
*Digitalization.*
**Adults:** Same as tablets. **Maintenance:** 0.125–0.5 mg/day in divided doses or as a single dose. **Pediatric:** Same as tablets.

## DENTAL CONCERNS

See also *Dental Concerns* for *Cardiac Glycosides.*

# Diltiazem hydrochloride
(dill-**TIE**-ah-zem)

**Pregnancy Category:** C

Alti-Diltiazem ✹, Apo-Diltiaz ✹, Cardizem, Cardizem CD, Cardizem Injectable, Cardizem Lyo-Ject, Cardizem-SR, Dilacor XR, Diltiazem HCl Extended Release, Gen-Diltiazem ✹, Novo-Diltiazem ✹, Nu-Diltiaz ✹, Tiazac **(Rx)**

**Classification:** Calcium channel blocking agent (antianginal, antihypertensive)

---

See also *Calcium Channel Blocking Agents.*

**Action/Kinetics:** Decreases SA and AV conduction and prolongs AV node effective and functional refractory periods. The drug also decreases myocardial contractility and peripheral vascular resistance. **Tablets: Onset,** 30–60 min; **time to peak plasma levels:** 2–3 hr; t½, **first phase:** 20–30 min; **second phase:** about 3–4.5 hr (5–8 hr with high and repetitive doses); **duration:** 4–8 hr. **Extended-Release Capsules: Onset,** 2–3 hr; **time to peak plasma levels:** 6–11 hr; t½: 5–7 hr; **duration:** 12 hr. **Therapeutic serum levels:** 0.05–0.2 mcg/mL. Metabolized to desacetyldiltiazem, which manifests 25%–50% of the activity of diltiazem. Excreted through both the bile and urine.

**Uses: Tablets:** Vasospastic angina (Prinzmetal's variant). Chronic stable angina (classic effort-associated angina), especially in clients who cannot use beta-adrenergic blockers or nitrates or who remain symptomatic after clinical doses of these agents. **Sustained-Release Capsules:** Essential hypertension, angina. **Parenteral:** Atrial fibrillation or flutter. Paroxysmal SVT. Cardizem Lyo-Ject is used on an emergency basis for atrial fibrillation or atrial flutter. *Non-FDA Approved Uses:* Prophylaxis of reinfarction of nonQ wave MI; tardive dyskinesia, Raynaud's syndrome.

**Contraindications:** Hypotension. Second- or third-degree AV block and sick sinus syndrome except in presence of a functioning ventricular pacemaker. Acute MI, pulmonary congestion. Lactation.

**Special Concerns:** Safety and effectiveness in children have not been determined. The half-life may be increased in geriatric clients. Use with caution in hepatic disease and in CHF. Abrupt withdrawal may cause an increase in the frequency and duration of chest pain. Use with beta blockers or digitalis is usually well tolerated, although the effects of co-administration cannot be predicted (especially in clients with left ventricular dysfunction or cardiac conduction abnormalities).

**Side Effects:** *CV:* AV block, bradycardia, CHF, hypotension, syncope, palpitations, peripheral edema, *arrhythmias,* angina, tachycardia, *abnormal ECG, ventricular extrasystoles.* *GI:* N&V, diarrhea, constipation, anorexia, abdominal discomfort, cramps, dry mouth, dysgeusia. *CNS:* Weakness, nervousness, dizziness, lightheadedness, headache, depression, psychoses, hallucinations, disturbances in sleep, somnolence, insomnia, amnesia, abnormal dreams. *Dermatologic:* Rashes, dermatitis, pruritus, urticaria, erythema multiforme, *Stevens-Johnson syndrome.* *Other:* Photosensitivity, joint pain or stiffness, flushing, nasal or chest congestion, dyspnea, SOB, nocturia/polyuria, sexual difficulties, weight gain, paresthesia, tinnitus, tremor, asthenia, gynecomastia, gingival hyperplasia, petechiae, ecchymosis, purpura, bruising, hematoma, leukopenia, double vision, epistaxis, eye irritation, thirst, alopecia, *bundle branch block,* abnormal gait, hyperglycemia.

**Drug Interactions**

*Anesthetics* / ↑ Risk of depression of cardiac contractility, conductivity, and automaticity as well as vascular dilation

*Barbiturates* / ↓ Effect of ditiazem

*Carbamazepine* / ↑ Effect of diltiazem due to ↓ breakdown by liver

---

*Cimetidine* / ↑ Bioavailability of diltiazem

*Cyclosporine* / ↑ Effect of cyclosporine possibly leading to renal toxicity

*Digoxin* / ↑ Serum digoxin levels are possible

*Indomethacin* / ↓ Effect of diltiazem

*Lithium* / ↑ Risk of neurotoxicity

*NSAIDs* / ↓ Possible effect of diltiazem

*Phenobarbital* / ↓ Effect of diltiazem

*Ranitidine* / ↑ Bioavailability of diltiazem

*Theophyllines* / ↑ Risk of pharmacologic and toxicologic effects of theophyllines

*Other drugs with hypotensive effects* / ↑ Effect of diltiazem

**How Supplied:** *Capsule, Extended Release:* 60 mg, 90 mg, 120 mg, 180 mg, 240 mg, 300 mg, 360 mg; *Injection:* 5 mg/mL; *Powder for injection:* 25 mg *Tablet:* 30 mg, 60 mg, 90 mg, 120 mg

## Dosage

- **Tablets**

  *Angina.*

  **Adults, initial:** 30 mg q.i.d. before meals and at bedtime; **then,** increase gradually to total daily dose of 180–360 mg (given in three to four divided doses). Increments may be made q 1–2 days until the optimum response is attained.

- **Capsules, Sustained-Release**

  *Angina.*

  **Cardizem CD: Adults, initial:** 120 or 180 mg once daily. Up to 480 mg/day may be required. Dosage adjustments should be carried out over a 7–14-day period.

  **Dilacor XR: Adults, initial:** 120 mg once daily; **then,** dose may be titrated, depending on the needs of the client, up to 480 mg once daily. Titration may be carried out over a 7–14-day period.

  *Hypertension.*

  **Cardizem CD: Adults, initial:** 180–240 mg once daily. Maximum antihypertensive effect usually reached within 14 days. Usual range is 240–360 mg once daily.

**Cardizem SR: Adults, initial:** 60–120 mg b.i.d.; **then,** when maximum antihypertensive effect is reached (approximately 14 days), adjust dosage to a range of 240–360 mg/day.

**Dilacor XR: Adults, initial:** 180–240 mg once daily. Usual range is 180–480 mg once daily. The dose may be increased to 540 mg/day with little or no increased risk of side effects.

**Tiazac: Adults, initial:** 120–240 mg once daily. Usual range is 120–360 mg once daily, although doses up to 540 mg once daily have been used.

- **IV Bolus**

  *Atrial fibrillation/flutter; paroxysmal SVT.*

  **Adults, initial:** 0.25 mg/kg (average 20 mg) given over 2 min; **then,** if response is inadequate, a second dose may be given after 15 min. The second bolus dose is 0.35 mg/kg (average 25 mg) given over 2 min. Subsequent doses should be individualized. Some clients may respond to an initial dose of 0.15 mg/kg (duration of action may be shorter).

- **IV Infusion**

  *Atrial fibrillation/flutter.*

  **Adults:** 10 mg/hr following IV bolus dose(s) of 0.25 mg/kg or 0.35 mg/kg. Some clients may require 5 mg/hr while others may require 15 mg/hr. Infusion may be maintained for 24 hr.

- **Cardizem Lyo-Ject**

  *Atrial fibrillation/atrial flutter.*

  Delivery system consists of a dual-chamber, prefilled, calibrated syringe containing 25 mg of diltiazem hydrochloride in one chamber and 5 mL of diluent in the other chamber.

## DENTAL CONCERNS

See also *Dental Concerns* for *Calcium Channel Blocking Agents.*

**General**

1. Quarterly visits to assess for gingival hyperplasia.

2. In cases of taste alteration, consider diltiazem as the causative agent.

# Dimenhydrinate
(dye-men-**HY**-drih-nayt)
**Pregnancy Category:** B
**Oral Liquid, Syrup, Tablets, Chewable Tablets:** Apo-Dimenhydrinate ✦, Calm-X, Dimentabs, Dramamine, Gravol ✦, Marmine, Motion-Aid, PMS-Dimenhydrinate ✦, Travamine, Travel Tabs ✦, Traveltabs ✦, Triptone **(OTC). Injection:** Dimenhydrinate Injection ✦, Dinate, Dramanate, Dramilin, Dymenate, Gravol ✦, Hydrate, Marmine, Reidamine **(Rx)**
**Classification:** Antihistamine, antiemetic

See also *Antihistamines* and *Antiemetics.*
**Action/Kinetics:** Contains both diphenhydramine and chlorotheophylline. Antiemetic mechanism not known, but it does depress labyrinthine and vestibular function. May mask ototoxicity due to aminoglycosides. Possesses anticholinergic activity. **Duration:** 3–6 hr.
**Uses:** Motion sickness, especially to relieve nausea, vomiting, or dizziness. Treat vertigo.
**Special Concerns:** Use of the injectable form is not recommended in neonates. Geriatric clients may be more sensitive to the usual adult dose.
**How Supplied:** *Chew Tablet:* 50 mg; *Injection:* 50 mg/mL; *Liquid:* 12.5 mg/4 mL, 12.5 mg/5 mL; *Tablet:* 25 mg, 50 mg

**Dosage** —————————
• **Elixir, Syrup, Tablets, Chewable Tablets**
*Motion sickness.*
**Adults:** 50–100 mg q 4 hr, not to exceed 400 mg/day. **Pediatric, 6–12 years:** 25–50 mg q 6–8 hr, not to exceed 150 mg/day; **2–6 years:** 12.5–25 mg q 6–8 hr, not to exceed 75 mg/day.
• **IM, IV**
**Adults:** 50 mg as required. **Pediatric, over 2 years:** 1.25 mg/kg (37.5 mg/m²) q.i.d., not to exceed 300 mg/day.
• **IV**

**Adults:** 50 mg in 10 mL sodium chloride injection given over 2 min; may be repeated q 4 hr as needed.
**Pediatric:** 1.25 mg/kg (37.5 mg/m²) in 10 mL of 0.9% sodium chloride injection given slowly over 2 min; may be repeated q 6 hr, not to exceed 300 mg/day.

## DENTAL CONCERNS

See also *Dental Concerns* for *Antihistamines* and *Antiemetics.*

# Diphenhydramine hydrochloride
(dye-fen-**HY**-drah-meen)
**Pregnancy Category:** B
Allerdryl ✦, AllerMax, AllerMax Allergy & Cough Formula, Banophen Caplets, Benadryl, Benadryl Allergy, Benadryl Allergy Ultratabs, Benadryl Dye-Free Allergy, Benadryl Dye-Free Allergy Liqui Gels, Diphen AF, Diphen Cough, Diphenhist, Genahist, Hyrexin-50, Nytol ✦, Nytol Extra Strength ✦, PMS-Diphenhydramine ✦, Scheinpharm Diphenhydramine ✦, Scot-Tussin DM, Siladryl, Tusstat **(OTC and Rx). Sleep-Aids:** Dormin, Miles Nervine, Nighttime Sleep Aid, Nytol, Sleepeze 3, Sleep-Eze D ✦, Sleepwell 2-nite, Sominex **(OTC)**
**Classification:** Antihistamine, ethanolamine-type; antiemetic

See also *Antihistamines, Antiemetics,* and *Antiparkinson Drugs.*
**Action/Kinetics:** High sedative, anticholinergic, and antiemetic effects.
**Uses:** Hypersensitivity reactions, motion sickness (PO only), parkinsonism, nighttime sleep aid (PO only), antitussive (syrup only).
**Contraindications:** Topically to treat chickenpox, poison ivy, or sunburn. Topically on large areas of the body or on blistered or oozing skin.
**How Supplied:** *Balm:* 2%; *Capsule:* 25 mg, 50 mg; *Chew Tablet:* 12.5 mg; *Cream:* 1%, 2%; *Elixir:* 12.5 mg/5 mL; *Injection:* 10 mg/mL, 50 mg/mL; *Liquid:* 6.25 mg/5 mL, 12.5 mg/5 mL, 50 mg/15 mL; *Lotion:* 0.5%;

**D**

*Spray:* 1%, 2%; *Syrup:* 12.5 mg/5 mL; *Tablet:* 25 mg, 50 mg

**Dosage**
• **Capsules, Chewable Tablets, Elixir, Liquid, Syrup, Tablets**
*Antihistamine, antiemetic, anti-motion sickness, parkinsonism.*
**Adults:** 25–50 mg t.i.d.–q.i.d.; **pediatric, over 10 kg:** 12.5–25 mg t.i.d.–q.i.d. (or 5 mg/kg/day not to exceed 300 mg/day or 150 mg/m²/day).
*Sleep aid.*
**Adults and children over 12 years:** 50 mg at bedtime.
*Antitussive (Syrup only).*
**Adults:** 25 mg q 4 hr, not to exceed 100 mg/day; **pediatric, 6–12 years:** 12.5–25 mg q 4 hr, not to exceed 50 mg/day; **pediatric, 2–6 years:** 6.25 mg q 4 hr, not to exceed 25 mg/day.
• **IV, Deep IM**
*Parkinsonism.*
**Adults:** 10–50 mg up to 100 mg if needed (not to exceed 400 mg/day); **pediatric:** 1.25 mg/kg (or 37.5 mg/m²) q.i.d., not to exceed a total of 300 mg/day.

## DENTAL CONCERNS

See also *Dental Concerns* for *Antihistamines, Antiemetics,* and *Antiparkinson Drugs.*
**General**
1. Patients on chronic drug therapy may develop blood dyscrasias. Symptoms include fever, sore throat, bleeding, and poor wound healing.
**Consultation with Primary Care Provider**
1. Patients with symptoms of blood dyscrasias should be referred to their primary care provider for complete blood counts. Treatment should be postponed until the results are known.

# Disulfiram
(dye-**SUL**-fih-ram)
**Pregnancy Category:** C
Antabuse **(Rx)**
**Classification:** Treatment of alcoholism

**Action/Kinetics:** Produces severe hypersensitivity to alcohol. A single dose of disulfiram may be effective for 1–2 weeks. **Onset:** May be delayed up to 12 hr because disulfiram is initially localized in fat stores.
**Uses:** To prevent further ingestion of alcohol in chronic alcoholics. Should be given only to cooperating clients fully aware of the consequences of alcohol ingestion.
**Contraindications:** Alcohol intoxication. Severe myocardial or occlusive coronary disease. Use of paraldehyde or alcohol-containing products such as cough syrups. If client is exposed to ethylene dibromide.
**Special Concerns:** Use in pregnancy only if benefits outweigh risks. Use with caution in narcotic addicts or clients with diabetes, goiter, epilepsy, psychosis, hypothyroidism, hepatic cirrhosis, or nephritis.
**Side Effects: In the absence of alcohol,** the following symptoms have been reported: Drowsiness (most common), headache, restlessness, fatigue, psychoses, peripheral neuropathy, dermatoses, hepatotoxicity, metallic or garlic taste, arthropathy, impotence. **In the presence of alcohol,** the following symptoms may be manifested. *CV:* Flushing, chest pain, palpitations, tachycardia, hypotension, syncope, arrhythmias, *CV collapse, MI, acute CHF. CNS:* Throbbing headaches, vertigo, weakness, uneasiness, confusion, unconsciousness, *seizures, death. Oral:* Metallic taste. *GI:* Nausea, severe vomiting, thirst. *Respiratory:* Respiratory difficulties, dyspnea, hyperventilation, *respiratory depression. Other:* Throbbing in head and neck, sweating. In the event of an Antabuse-alcohol interaction, measures should be undertaken to maintain BP and treat shock. Oxygen, antihistamines, ephedrine, and/or vitamin C may also be used.
**Drug Interactions**
*Barbiturates* / ↑ Effect of barbiturates due to ↓ breakdown by liver
*Chlordiazepoxide, diazepam* / ↑ Effect of chlordiazepoxide or diazepam due to ↓ plasma clearance

Metronidazole / Acute toxic psychosis or confusional state
Phenytoin / ↑ Effect of phenytoin due to ↓ breakdown by liver
Tricyclic antidepressants / Acute organic brain syndrome
**How Supplied:** *Tablet:* 250 mg, 500 mg

**Dosage**
• **Tablets**
  *Alcoholism.*
**Adults, initial (after alcohol-free interval of 12–48 hr):** 500 mg/day for 1–2 weeks; **maintenance: usual,** 250 mg/day (range: 120–500 mg/day). Dose should not exceed 500 mg/day.

**DENTAL CONCERNS**
**Consultation with Primary Care Provider**
1. Consultation with appropriate health care provider may be necessary in order to assess the extent of disease control.
**Client/Family Teaching**
1. Avoid alcohol-containing mouth rinses.

# Dolasetron mesylate
(dohl-**AH**-seh-tron)
Pregnancy Category: B
Anzemet **(Rx)**
Classification: Antinauseant/antiemetic, serotonin 5-HT₃ antagonist

**Action/Kinetics:** Selective serotonin 5-HT₃ antagonist that prevents N&V by inhibiting released serotonin from combining with receptors on vagal efferents that initiate vomiting reflex. May also cause acute, usually reversible, PR and QT$_c$ prolongation and QRS widening, perhaps due to blockade of sodium channels by active metabolite of dolasetron. Well absorbed from GI tract. Metabolized to active hydrodolasetron: **peak plasma levels:** 1 hr; t½: 8.1 hr. Food does not affect bioavailability. Hydrodolasetron is excreted through urine and feces. Is eliminated more quickly in children than in adults.

**Uses:** Prevention of N&V associated with moderately-emetogenic cancer chemotherapy (initially and repeat courses). Prevention of postoperative N&V.
**Contraindications:** Hypersensitivity.
**Special Concerns:** Use with caution during lactation and in those who have or may develop prolongation of cardiac conduction intervals, including QT$_c$. These include clients with hypokalemia or hypomagnesemia, those taking diuretics with potential for electrolyte abnormalities, in congenital QT syndrome, those taking anti-arrhythmic drugs or other drugs which lead to QT prolongation, and cumulative high dose anthracycline therapy. Safety and efficacy in children less than 2 years of age have not been determined.
**Side Effects: Chemotherapy clients.** Headache, fatigue, diarrhea, bradycardia, dizziness, pain, tachycardia, dyspepsia, chills, shivering.
**Postoperative clients.** Headache, hypotension, dizziness, fever, pruritus, oliguria, hypertension, tachycardia.
**Chemotherapy or postoperative clients.** C*V:* Hypotension, edema, peripheral edema, peripheral ischemia, thrombophlebitis, phlebitis. *Oral:* Taste perversion. *GI:* Constipation, dyspepsia, abdominal pain, anorexia, pancreatitis. *CNS:* Flushing, vertigo, paresthesia, tremor, ataxia, twitching, agitation, sleep disorder, depersonalization, confusion, anxiety, abnormal dreaming. *Dermatologic:* Rash, increased sweating. *Hematologic:* Hematuria, epistaxis, anemia, purpura, hematoma, thrombocytopenia. *Hypersensitivity:* Rarely, ***anaphylaxis,*** facial edema, urticaria. *Musculoskeletal:* Myalgia, arthralgia. *Respiratory:* Dyspnea, bronchospasm. *GU:* Dysuria, polyuria, acute renal failure. *Ophthalmic:* Abnormal vision, photophobia. *Miscellaneous:* Tinnitus.
**Drug Interactions:** There is the potential for dolasetron to interact with

other drugs that prolong the $QT_c$ interval.

## Dosage

• **Tablets**

*Prevention of N&V during chemotherapy.*

**Adults:** 100 mg within 1 hr before chemotherapy. **Children, 2 to 16 years:** 1.8 mg/kg within 1 hr before chemotherapy, up to a maximum of 100 mg.

*Prevention of postoperative N&V.*

**Adults:** 100 mg within 2 hr before surgery. **Children, 2 to 16 years:** 1.2 mg/kg within 2 hr before surgery, up to a maximum of 100 mg.

• **IV**

*Prevention of N&V during chemotherapy.*

**Adults:** 1.8 mg/kg as a single dose about 30 min before chemotherapy. Alternatively, a fixed dose of 100 mg can be given over 30 seconds. **Children, 2 to 16 years:** 1.8 mg/kg as a single dose about 30 min before chemotherapy, up to a maximum of 100 mg.

*Prevention of postoperative N&V.*

**Adults:** 12.5 mg given as a single dose. **Children, 2 to 16 years:** 0.35 mg/kg, up to a maximum of 12.5 mg. For adults and children, give about 15 min before cessation of anesthesia or as soon as nausea and vomiting presents.

**Note:** For children, injection may be mixed with apple or apple-grape juice and used for oral dosing. When injection is used PO, recommended dose for prevention of cancer chemotherapy N&V is 1.8 mg/kg (up to a maximum of 100 mg) and dose for prevention of postoperative N&V is 1.2 mg/kg (up to a maximum of 100 mg). Diluted injection may be kept up to 2 hr at room temperature before use.

## DENTAL CONCERNS

### General

1. Patients should be monitored for untoward effects.

2. Alternative analgesics for dental pain should be considered for patients with acute or chronic pain

who are already taking opioid analgesics.

3. Patients may require chlorhexidine mouth rinse prior to and during chemotherapy in order to help reduce the severity of mucositis.

4. Other medications may be required to treat the oral side effects of cancer chemotherapy.

### Client/Family Teaching

1. Patients should be aware of the oral side effects of this drug and cancer chemotherapy.

2. Patients recovering from anesthesia after dental treatment should report any excessive nausea and vomiting.

# Donepezil hydrochloride
(dohn-**EP**-eh-zil)
**Pregnancy Category:** C
Aricept **(Rx)**
**Classification:** Psychotherapeutic drug for Alzheimer's disease

**Action/Kinetics:** A decrease in cholinergic function may be the cause of Alzheimer's disease. Donepezil is a cholinesterase inhibitor and exerts its effect by enhancing cholinergic function by increasing levels of acetylcholine. There is no evidence that the drug alters the course of the underlying dementing process. Well absorbed from the GI tract. **Peak plasma levels:** 3–4 hr. Food does not affect the rate or extent of absorption. Metabolized in the liver, and both unchanged drug and metabolites are excreted in the urine and feces.

**Uses:** Treatment of mild to moderate dementia of the Alzheimer's type.

**Contraindications:** Hypersensitivity to piperidine derivatives.

**Special Concerns:** Use with caution in clients with a history of asthma or obstructive pulmonary disease. Safety and efficacy have not been determined for use in children.

**Side Effects:** *NOTE:* Side effects with an incidence of 1% or greater are listed. *Oral:* Dry mouth, toothache, bad taste, gingivitis, tongue edema, coated tongue. *GI:* N&V, diarrhea, anorexia, fecal incontinence, GI bleeding, bloating, epigastric pain.

*CNS:* Insomnia, dizziness, depression, abnormal dreams, somnolence. *CV:* Hypertension, vasodilation, atrial fibrillation, hot flashes, hypotension, bradycardia. *Body as a whole:* Headache, pain (in various locations), accident, fatigue, influenza, chest pain. *Musculoskeletal:* Muscle cramps, arthritis, bone fracture. *Dermatologic:* Diaphoresis, urticaria, pruritus. *GU:* Urinary incontinence, nocturia, frequent urination. *Respiratory:* Dyspnea, sore throat, bronchitis. *Ophthalmic:* Cataract, eye irritation, blurred vision. *Miscellaneous:* Dehydration, syncope, ecchymosis, weight loss.

**Drug Interactions**
*Anticholinergic drugs* / The cholinesterase inhibitor activitiy of donepezil interferes with the activity of anticholinergics
*NSAIDs* / ↑ Gastric acid secretion → ↑ risk of active or occult GI bleeding
*Succinylcholine* / ↑ Muscle relaxant effect
**How Supplied:** *Tablet:* 5 mg, 10 mg

**Dosage** ─────────────
• **Tablets**
*Alzheimer's disease.*
**Initial:** 5 mg. Use of a 10-mg dose did not provide a clinical effect greater than the 5-mg dose; however, in some clients, 10 mg daily may be superior. Do not increase the dose to 10 mg until clients have been on a daily dose of 5 mg for 4 to 6 weeks.

**DENTAL CONCERNS**
**General**
1. Monitor vital signs at every appointment because of cardiovascular side effects.
2. Have the patient sit up slowly and remain seated for at least two minutes after being supine in order to minimize the risk of orthostatic hypotension.
3. Decreased saliva flow can put the patient at risk for dental caries, periodontal disease, and candidiasis.
4. Patients on chronic drug therapy

may develop blood dyscrasias. Symptoms include fever, sore throat, bleeding, and poor wound healing.
5. Place patient on frequent recall because of oral adverse effects.
6. A semisupine position for the dental chair may be necessary to help minimize or avoid GI adverse effects.
7. Use caution if dental surgery and anesthesia is required.
**Consultation with Primary Care Provider**
1. Patients with symptoms of blood dyscrasias should be referred to their primary care provider for complete blood counts. Treatment should be postponed until the results are known.
2. Consultation with the appropriate health care provider may be necessary in order to determine the extent of disease control and the patient's ability to tolerate stress.
**Client/Family Teaching**
1. Review the importance of good oral hygiene in order to prevent soft tissue inflammation.
2. Review the proper use of oral hygiene aids in order to prevent injury.
3. Daily home fluoride treatments for persistent dry mouth.
4. Avoid alcohol-containing mouth rinses and beverages.
5. Avoid caffeine-containing beverages.
6. Dry mouth can be treated with tart, sugarless gum or candy, water, sugar-free beverages, or with saliva substitutes if dry mouth persists.

# Doxazosin mesylate
(dox-**AYZ**-oh-sin)
**Pregnancy Category:** B
Cardura, Cardura-1, -2, -3 ✴ **(Rx)**
**Classification:** Antihypertensive

**Action/Kinetics:** Blocks the alpha-1 (postjunctional) adrenergic receptors resulting in a decrease in systemic vascular resistance and a corresponding decrease in BP. **Peak plasma levels:** 2–3 hr. **Peak effect:** 2–6 hr. Significantly bound (98%) to plasma proteins. Metabolized in the liver to active and inactive metabolites, which are excreted through the feces and urine. **t½:** 22 hr.

**Uses:** Alone or in combination with diuretics, calcium channel blockers, or beta blockers to treat hypertension. Treatment of BPH.

**Contraindications:** Clients allergic to prazosin or terazosin.

**Special Concerns:** Use with caution during lactation, in impaired hepatic function, or in those taking drugs known to influence hepatic metabolism. Safety and effectiveness have not been demonstrated in children. Due to the possibility of severe hypotension, do not use the 2-, 4-, and 8-mg tablets for initial therapy.

**Side Effects:** *Oral:* Dry mouth; *CV:* Dizziness (most frequent), syncope, vertigo, lightheadedness, edema, palpitation, arrhythmia, postural hypotension, tachycardia, peripheral ischemia. *CNS:* Fatigue, headache, paresthesia, kinetic disorders, ataxia, somnolence, nervousness, depression, insomnia. *Musculoskeletal:* Arthralgia, arthritis, muscle weakness, muscle cramps, myalgia, hypertonia. *GU:* Polyuria, sexual dysfunction, urinary incontinence, urinary frequency. *GI:* Nausea, diarrhea, constipation, dyspepsia, flatulence, abdominal pain, vomiting. *Respiratory:* Fatigue or malaise, rhinitis, epistaxis, dyspnea. *Miscellaneous:* Rash, pruritus, flushing, abnormal vision, conjunctivitis, eye pain, tinnitus, chest pain, asthenia, facial edema, generalized pain, slight weight gain.

**Drug Interactions**
*CNS Depressants* / ↑ Hypotensive effects
*Indomethacin* / ↓ Hypotensive effects
*NSAIDs* / ↓ Hypotensive effects
*Sympathomimetics* / ↓ Hypotensive Effects

**How Supplied:** *Tablet:* 1 mg, 2 mg, 4 mg, 8 mg

**Dosage** —————————
• **Tablets**
*Hypertension.*

**Adults: initial,** 1 mg once daily at bedtime; **then,** depending on the response (client's standing BP both 2–6 hr and 24 hr after a dose), the dose may be increased to 2 mg/day. A maximum of 16 mg/day may be required to control BP.
*Benign prostatic hyperplasia.*
**Initial:** 1 mg once daily. **Maintenance:** Depending on the urodynamics and symptoms, dose may be increased to 2 mg daily and then 4–8 mg once daily (maximum recommended dose). The recommended titration interval is 1–2 weeks.

---

## DENTAL CONCERNS

See also *Dental Concerns* for *Alpha-1 Adrenergic Blocking Agents* and *Antihypertensive Agents.*

---

# Doxepin hydrochloride
(**DOX**-eh-pin)
**Pregnancy Category:** C
Alti-Doxepin ✱, Apo-Doxepin ✱, Novo-Doxepin ✱, Rho-Doxepin ✱, Sinequan, Triadapin ✱, Zonalon ✱ **(Rx)**
**Classification:** Antidepressant, tricyclic

---

See also *Antidepressants, Tricyclic.*

**Action/Kinetics:** Metabolized to the active metabolite, desmethyldoxepin. Moderate anticholinergic effects and orthostatic hypotension; high sedative effects. **Minimum effective plasma level of both doxepin and desmethyldoxepin:** 100–200 ng/mL. **Time to reach steady state:** 2–8 days. **t½:** 8–24 hr.

**Uses:** Depression. Antianxiety agent, depression accompanied by anxiety and insomnia, depression in clients with manic-depressive illness. Depression or anxiety due to organic disease or alcoholism. Chronic, severe neurogenic pain. PUD. Dermatologic disorders including chronic urticaria, angioedema, and nocturnal pruritus due to atopic eczema.

**Additional Contraindications:** Glaucoma or a tendency for urinary retention.

**Special Concerns:** Safety has not been determined in pregnancy. Not recommended for use in children less than 12 years of age.

**Additional Side Effects:** Doxepin has a high incidence of side effects, including a high degree of sedation, decreased libido, extrapyramidal symptoms, dermatitis, pruritus, fatigue, weight gain, edema, paresthesia, breast engorgement, insomnia, tremor, chills, tinnitus, and photophobia.

**How Supplied:** *Capsule:* 10 mg, 25 mg, 50 mg, 75 mg, 100 mg, 150 mg; *Concentrate:* 10 mg/mL; *Cream:* 5%

**Dosage**
- **Capsules, Oral Concentrate**
  *Antidepressant, mild to moderate anxiety or depression.*
**Adults:** 25 mg t.i.d. (or up to 150 mg can be given at bedtime); **then,** adjust dosage to individual response (usual optimum dosage: 75–150 mg/day).
**Geriatric clients, initially:** 25–50 mg/day; dose can be increased as needed and tolerated.
  *Severe symptoms.*
**Initial:** 50 mg t.i.d.; **then,** gradually increase to 300 mg/day.
  *Emotional symptoms with organic disease.*
25–50 mg/day.
  *Antipruritic.*
10–30 mg at bedtime.
- **Cream 5%**
Apply a thin film q.i.d. with at least a 3–4 hr interval between applications.

**DENTAL CONCERNS**

See also *Dental Concerns* for *Antidepressants, Tricyclic.*

# Doxycycline calcium
(dox-ih-**SYE**-kleen)
**Pregnancy Category:** D
Vibramycin **(Rx)**

# Doxycycline hyclate
(dox-ih-**SYE**-kleen)
**Pregnancy Category:** D

Alti-Doxycycline ✦, Apo-Doxy ✦, Apo-Doxy-Tabs ✦, Atridox, Doryx, Doxy 100 and 200, Doxy-Caps, Doxycin ✦, Doxychel Hyclate, Doxytec ✦, Novo-Doxylin ✦, Nu-Doxycycline ✦, Rho-Doxycycline ✦, Vibramycin, Vibramycin IV, Vibra-Tabs, Vivox **(Rx)**

# Doxycycline monohydrate
(dox-ih-**SYE**-kleen)
**Pregnancy Category:** D
Monodox, Vibramycin **(Rx)**
**Classification:** Antibiotic, tetracycline

See also *Anti-Infectives* and *Tetracyclines.*

**Action/Kinetics:** More slowly absorbed, and thus more persistent, than other tetracyclines. Preferred for clients with impaired renal function for treating infections outside the urinary tract. From 80% to 95% is bound to serum proteins. **t½:** 14.5–22 hr; 30%–40% excreted unchanged in urine.

**Uses:** Syphilis, *Chylamydia trachomatis,* gonorrhea, lymphogranuloma venereum, uncommon gram negative and gram positive organisms, necrotizing ulcerative gingivostomatitis.

**Additional Uses:** Orally for uncomplicated gonococcal infections in adults (except anorectal infections in males); acute epididymo-orchitis caused by *Neisseria gonorrhoeae* and *C. trachomatis;* gonococcal arthritis-dermatitis syndrome; nongonococcal urethritis caused by *C. trachomatis* and *Ureaplasma urealyticum.* Prophylaxis of malaria due to *Plasmodium falciparum* in short-term travelers (< 4 months) to areas with chloroquine- or pyrimethamine-sulfadoxine-resistant strains.

**Contraindications:** Prophylaxis of malaria in pregnant individuals and in children less than 8 years old. Use during the last half of pregnancy and in children up to 8 years of age (tetracycline may cause permanent discoloration of the teeth). Lactation.

---

✦ = Available in Canada                    ***bold italic*** = life-threatening side effect

**Special Concerns:** Safety for IV use in children less than 8 years of age has not been established.

**Side Effects:** See also *Tetracyclines*.

**Drug Interactions**

*Antacids* / ↓ Absorption of antacids

*Anticoagulants* / ↑ Effectiveness of anticoagulants

*Barbiturates* / ↑ Metabolism of barbiturates

*Carbamazepine* / ↑ Metabolism of carbamazepines

*Cephalosporins* / ↓ Effects of cephalosporins

*Hydantoins* / ↑ Metabolism of hydantoins

*NaHCO₃* / ↓ Absorption of $NaHCO_3$

*Penicillins* / ↓ Effects of penicillins

**Additional Drug Interactions:** Carbamazepine, phenytoin, and barbiturates ↓ effect of doxycycline by ↑ breakdown of doxycycline by the liver.

**How Supplied:** Doxycycline calcium: *Syrup:* 50 mg/5 mL. Doxycyline hyclate: *Capsule:* 50 mg, 100 mg; *Enteric coated capsule:* 100 mg; *Powder for injection:* 100 mg, 200 mg; *Tablet:* 100 mg. Doxycycline monohydrate: *Capsule:* 50 mg, 100 mg; *Powder for reconstitution:* 25 mg/5 mL; *Gel:* Doxycycline 10%

**Dosage**

• **Capsules, Delayed-Release Capsules, Oral Suspension, Syrup, Tablets, IV**

*Infections.*

**Adult: First day,** 100 mg q 12 hr; **maintenance:** 100–200 mg/day, depending on severity of infection. **Children, over 8 years (45 kg or less): First day,** 4.4 mg/kg in 1–2 doses; **then,** 2.2–4.4 mg/kg/day in divided doses depending on severity of infection. Children over 45 kg should receive the adult dose.

*Acute gonorrhea.*

200 mg at once given PO; **then,** 100 mg at bedtime on first day, followed by 100 mg b.i.d. for 3 days. Alternatively, 300 mg immediately followed in 1 hr with 300 mg.

*Syphilis (primary/secondary).*

300 mg/day in divided PO doses for 10 days.

*C. trachomatis infections.*

100 mg b.i.d. PO for minimum of 7 days.

*Prophylaxis of "traveler's diarrhea."*

100 mg/day given PO.

*Prophylaxis of malaria.*

**Adults:** 100 mg PO once daily; **children, over 8 years of age:** 2 mg/kg/day up to 100 mg/day.

• **IV**

*Endometritis, parametritis, peritonitis, salpingitis.*

100 mg b.i.d. with 2 g cefoxitin, IV, q.i.d. continued for at least 4 days or 2 days after improvement observed. This is followed by doxycycline, PO, 100 mg b.i.d. for 10–14 days of total therapy.

*NOTE:* The Centers for Disease Control have established treatment schedules for STDs.

## DENTAL CONCERNS

See also *General Dental Concerns for All Anti-Infectives* and for *Tetracyclines*.

**Client/Family Teaching**

1. May take with food; take with a full glass of water to prevent esophageal ulceration.

# Dronabinol (Delta-9-tetrahydro-cannabinol)

(droh-**NAB**-ih-nohl)

**Pregnancy Category:** C

Marinol **(C-II) (Rx)**

**Classification:** Antinauseant

**Action/Kinetics:** As the active component in marijuana, significant psychoactive effects may occur. (See *Side Effects*.) Antiemetic effect may be due to inhibition of the vomiting center in the medulla. **Peak plasma levels:** 2–3 hr. Significant first-pass effect. The 11-hydroxytetrahydro-cannabinol metabolite is active. **t½, biphasic:** 4 hr and 25–36 hr. **t½, 11-hydroxy-THC:** 15–18 hr. Metabolized in the liver and mainly excreted in the feces. Cumulative toxicity using clinical doses may occur. Highly bound to plasma proteins and may thus displace other protein-bound drugs.

**Uses:** Nausea and vomiting associated with cancer chemotherapy, especially in clients who have not responded to other antiemetic treatment. To stimulate appetite and prevent weight loss in AIDS clients.

**Contraindications:** Nausea and vomiting from any cause other than cancer chemotherapy. Lactation. Hypersensitivity to sesame oil.

**Special Concerns:** Monitor pediatric and geriatric clients carefully due to an increased risk of psychoactive effects. Use with caution in clients with hypertension, occasional hypotension, syncope, tachycardia; those with a history of substance abuse, including alcohol abuse or dependence; clients with mania, depression, or schizophrenia (the drug may exacerbate these illnesses); clients receiving sedatives, hypnotics, or other psychoactive drugs (due to the potential for additive or synergistic CNS effects).

**Side Effects:** *CNS:* Side effects are due mainly to the psychoactive effects of the drug and, in addition to those listed in the preceding, include dizziness, muddled thinking, coordination difficulties, irritability, weakness, headache, ataxia, cannabinoid "high," paresthesia, hallucinations, visual distortions, depersonalization, confusion, nightmares, disorientation, and confusion. *CV:* Palpitations, tachycardia, vasodilation, facial flush, hypotension. *Oral:* Dry mouth. *GI:* Abdominal pain, N&V, diarrhea, fecal incontinence, anorexia. *Respiratory:* Cough, rhinitis, sinusitis. *Other:* Asthenia, conjunctivitis, myalgias, tinnitus, speech difficulty, vision difficulties, chills, headache, malaise, sweating, elevated hepatic enzymes.

*Symptoms of Abstinence Syndrome:* An abstinence syndrome has been reported following discontinuation of doses greater than 210 mg/day for 12–16 days. Symptoms include irritability, insomnia, and restlessness within 12 hr; within 24 hr, symptoms include "hot flashes," sweating, rhinorrhea, loose stools, hiccoughs, and anorexia. Disturbed sleep may occur for several weeks.

**Drug Interactions**

*Amphetamine* / Additive hypertension, tachycardia, possibly cardiotoxicity

*Anticholinergics* / Additive or super-additive tachycardia; drowsiness

*CNS depressants* / Additive CNS depressant effects

*Antidepressants, tricyclic* / Additive tachycardia, hypertension, drowsiness

*Ethanol* / During subchronic dronabinol use, lower and delayed peak alcohol blood levels

*Sympathomimetics* / See *Amphetamines and Derivatives*

**How Supplied:** *Capsule:* 2.5 mg, 5 mg, 10 mg

**Dosage**

• **Capsules**
*Antiemetic.*
**Adults and children, initial:** 5 mg/m$^2$ 1–3 hr before chemotherapy; **then,** 5 mg/m$^2$ q 2–4 hr for a total of four to six doses/day. If ineffective, this dose may be increased by 2.5 mg/m$^2$ to a maximum of 15 mg/m$^2$/dose. However, the incidence of serious psychoactive side effects increases dramatically at these higher dose levels.

*Appetite stimulation.*
**Initial:** 2.5 mg b.i.d. before lunch and dinner. If unable to tolerate 5 mg/day, reduce the dose to 2.5 mg/day as a single evening or bedtime dose. If side effects are absent or minimal and an increased effect is desired, the dose may be increased to 2.5 mg before lunch and 5 mg before dinner (or 5 mg at lunch and 5 mg after dinner). The dose may be increased to 20 mg/day in divided doses. The incidence of side effects increases at higher doses.

## DENTAL CONCERNS
**General**

1. Vasoconstrictors should be used with caution because of their CNS stimulating side effects.
2. Decreased saliva flow can put the patient at risk for dental caries, periodontal disease, and candidiasis.

**Consultation with Primary Care Provider**

1. It may be necessary to consult with the appropriate health care provider to determine the extent of disease control and the patient's ability to tolerate stress.

**Client/Family Teaching**

1. Daily home fluoride treatments for persistent dry mouth.
2. Avoid alcohol-containing mouth rinses and beverages.
3. Avoid caffeine-containing beverages.
4. Dry mouth can be treated with tart, sugarless gum or candy, water, sugar-free beverages, or with saliva substitutes if dry mouth persists.
5. Do not drive or perform hazardous tasks requiring mental acuity.

**E**

# Enalapril maleate

(en-**AL**-ah-prill)
**Pregnancy Category:** D
Apo-Enalapril ✹, Vasotec, Vasotec I.V., Vasotec Oral ✹ **(Rx)**
**Classification:** Angiotensin-converting enzyme inhibitor

See also *Angiotensin-Converting Enzyme Inhibitors.*

**Action/Kinetics:** Converted in the liver by hydrolysis to the active metabolite, enalaprilat. The parenteral product is enalaprilat injection. **Onset, PO:** 1 hr; **IV,** 15 min. **Time to peak action, PO:** 4–6 hr; **IV,** 1–4 hr. **Duration, PO:** 24 hr; **IV,** About 6 hr. Approximately 50%–60% is protein bound. **t½, enalapril, PO:** 1.3 hr; **IV,** 15 min. **t½, enalaprilat, PO:** 11 hr. Excreted through the urine (half unchanged) and feces; over 90% of enalaprilat is excreted through the urine.

**Uses:** Alone or in combination with a thiazide diuretic for the treatment of hypertension (step I therapy). As adjunct with digitalis and diuretic in acute and chronic CHF. *Non-FDA Approved Uses:* Hypertension in children, hypertension related to scleroderma renal crisis, diabetic nephropathy, asymptomatic left ventricular dysfunction following MI. Enalaprilat may be used for hypertensive emergencies (effect is variable).

**Contraindications:** See also *Angiotensin-Converting Enzyme Inhibitors.*

**Special Concerns:** Use with caution during lactation. Safety and effectiveness have not been determined in children.

**Side Effects:** *CV:* Palpitations, hypotension, chest pain, angina, ***CVA, MI,*** orthostatic hypotension, disturbances in rhythm, tachycardia, ***cardiac arrest,*** orthostatic effects, atrial fibrillation, bradycardia. *Oral:* Alterations in taste, dry mouth, glossitis, stomatitis. *GI:* N&V, diarrhea, abdominal pain, anorexia, constipation, dyspepsia, ileus, melena. *CNS:* Insomnia, headache, fatigue, dizziness, paresthesias, nervousness, sleepiness, ataxia, confusion, depression, vertigo. *Hepatic:* Hepatitis, hepatocellular or cholestatic jaundice, pancreatitis, elevated liver enzymes, hepatic failure. *Respiratory:* Bronchitis, cough, dyspnea, bronchospasm, upper respiratory infection, pneumonia, pulmonary infiltrates, asthma, ***pulmonary embolism and infarction, pulmonary edema.*** *Renal:* Renal dysfunction, oliguria, UTI, transient increases in creatinine and BUN. *Hematologic:* Rarely, neutropenia, thrombocytopenia, bone marrow depression, decreased H&H in hypertensive or CHF clients. Hemolytic anemia, including hemolysis, in clients with G6PD deficiency. *Dermatologic:* Rash, pruritus, alopecia, flushing, erythema multiforme, exfoliative dermatitis, photosensitivity, urticaria, increased sweating, pemphigus, *Stevens-Johnson syndrome,* herpes zoster, toxic epidermal necrolysis. *Other:* Angioedema, asthenia, impotence, blurred vision, fever, arthralgia, arthritis, vasculitis, eosinophilia, tinnitus, syncope, myalgia, rhinorrhea, sore throat, hoarseness, conjunctivitis, tearing, dry eyes, loss of sense of smell, hearing loss, peripheral neuropathy, anosmia, myositis, flank pain, gynecomastia.

**Drug Interactions:** See also *Angiotensin-Converting Enzyme Inhibitors.*

**How Supplied:** *Tablet:* 2.5 mg, 5 mg, 10 mg, 20 mg; *Injection:* 1.25 mg/mL

**Dosage** —————————
• **Tablets (Enalapril)**
*Antihypertensive in clients not taking diuretics.*
**Initial:** 5 mg/day; **then,** adjust dosage according to response (range: 10–40 mg/day in one to two doses).
*Antihypertensive in clients taking diuretics.*
**Initial:** 2.5 mg. Since hypotension may occur following the initiation of enalapril, the diuretic should be discontinued, if possible, for 2–3 days before initiating enalapril. If BP is not maintained with enalapril alone, diuretic therapy may be resumed.
*Adjunct with diuretics and digitalis in heart failure.*
**Initial:** 2.5 mg 1–2 times/day; **then,** depending on the response, 5–20 mg/day in two divided doses. Dose should not exceed 40 mg/day. Dosage must be adjusted in clients with renal impairment or hyponatremia.
*In clients with impaired renal function.*

**Initial:** 5 mg/day if $C_{CR}$ ranges between 30 and 80 mL/min and serum creatinine is less than 3 mg/dL; 2.5 mg/day if $C_{CR}$ is less than 30 mL/min and serum creatinine is more than 3 mg/dL and in dialysis clients on dialysis days.
*Renal impairment or hyponatremia.*
**Initial:** 2.5 mg/day if serum sodium is less than 130 mEq/L and serum creatinine is more than 1.6 mg/dL. The dose may be increased to 2.5 mg b.i.d. and then 5 mg b.i.d. or higher if required; dose is given at intervals of 4 or more days. Maximum daily dose is 40 mg.
*Asymptomatic LV dysfunction following MI.*
2.5–20 mg/day beginning 72 hr or longer after onset of MI. Therapy is continued for 1 year or longer.
*NOTE:* Dosage should be decreased in clients with a $C_{CR}$ less than 30 mL/min and a serum creatinine level greater than 3 mg/dL.
• **IV (Enalaprilat)**
*Hypertension.*
1.25 mg over a 5-min period; repeat q 6 hr.
*Antihypertensive in clients taking diuretics.*
**Initial:** 0.625 mg over 5 min; if an adequate response is seen after 1 hr, administer another 0.625-mg dose. Thereafter, 1.25 mg q 6 hr.
*Clients with impaired renal function.*
Give enalaprit, 1.25 mg q 6 hr for clients with a $C_{CR}$ more than 30 mL/min and an initial dose of 0.625 mg for clients with a $C_{CR}$ less than 30 mL/min. If there is an adequate response, an additional 0.625 mg may be given after 1 hr; thereafter, additional 1.25-mg doses can be given q 6 hr. For dialysis clients, the initial dose is 0.625 mg q 6 hr.

## DENTAL CONCERNS

See also *Dental Concerns* for *Angiotensin-Converting Enzyme Inhibitors* and *Antihypertensive Agents.*

# Enoxacin
(ee-**NOX**-ah-sin)
**Pregnancy Category:** C
Penetrex **(Rx)**
**Classification:** Antibacterial, fluoro-
quinolone derivative

See also *Fluoroquinolones.*

**Action/Kinetics:** The drug inhibits certain isozymes of the cytochrome P-450 hepatic microsomal enzyme system, resulting in alterations of metabolism of some drugs. **Peak plasma levels:** 0.83 mcg/mL 1–3 hr after a 200-mg dose and 2 mcg/mL 1–3 hr after a 400-mg dose. Mean peak plasma levels are 50% higher in geriatric clients than in young adults. Diffuses into the cervix, fallopian tubes, and myometrium at levels 1–2 times those seen in plasma and into kidney and prostate at levels 2–4 times those seen in plasma. **t½:** 3–6 hr. More than 40% excreted unchanged through the urine.

**Uses:** To treat uncomplicated urethral or cervical gonorrhea due to *Neisseria gonorrhoeae.* To treat uncomplicated UTIs due to *Escherichia coli, Staphylococcus epidermidis,* or *S. saprophyticus;* for complicated UTIs due to *E. coli, Klebsiella pneumoniae, Proteus mirabilis, Pseudomonas aeruginosa, S. epidermidis,* or *Enterobacter cloacae.* Not effective for syphilis.

**Contraindications:** Lactation.

**Special Concerns:** Safety and efficacy have not been determined in children less than 18 years of age. Dosage adjustment is not required in elderly clients with normal renal function. Not efficiently removed by hemodialysis or peritoneal dialysis.

**Additional Side Effects:** *Oral:* Candidiasis, dry mouth, stomatitis, unusual taste. *GI:* Anorexia, bloody stools, gastritis. *CNS:* Confusion, nervousness, anxiety, tremor, agitation, myoclonus, depersonalization, hypertonia. *Dermatologic:* Toxic epidermal necrolysis, ***Stevens-Johnson syndrome,*** urticaria, hyperhidrosis, mycotic infection, erythema multiforme. *CV:* Palpitations, tachycardia, vasodilation. *Respiratory:* Dyspnea, cough, epistaxis. *GU:* Vaginal moniliasis, urinary incontinence, renal failure. *Hematologic:* Eosinophilia, leukopenia, increased or decreased platelets, decreased hemoglobin, leukocytosis. *Miscellaneous:* Glucosuria, pyuria, increased or decreased potassium, asthenia, back or chest pain, myalgia, arthralgia, purpura, vertigo, tinnitus, conjunctivitis.

**Additional Drug Interactions**
*Bismuth subsalicylate* / Bioavailability of enoxacin is ↓ when bismuth subsalicylate is given within 1 hr; should not use together

**How Supplied:** *Tablet:* 200 mg, 400 mg

## Dosage
- **Tablets**
  *Uncomplicated gonorrhea.*
  **Adults:** 400 mg for one dose.
  *Uncomplicated UTIs, cystitis.*
  **Adults:** 200 mg q 12 hr for 7 days.
  *Complicated UTIs.*
  **Adults:** 400 mg q 12 hr for 14 days.

## DENTAL CONCERNS

See also *General Dental Concerns for All Anti-Infectives* and for *Fluoroquinolones.*

**General**
1. Ingestible sodium bicarbonate products (i.e., air polishing systems) can only be used 2 hours after taking enoxacin.
2. Use caution when prescribing caffeine-containing prescription and nonprescription drugs.
3. Determine why the patient is taking the medication.
4. Decreased saliva flow can put the patient at risk for dental caries, periodontal disease, and candidiasis.

**Consultation with Primary Care Provider**
1. Consult with the patient's health care provider if an acute dental infection occurs and the patient requires another anti-infective.

**Client/Family Teaching**
1. Review the importance of good oral hygiene in order to prevent soft tissue inflammation.
2. Daily home fluoride treatments for persistent dry mouth.

3. Avoid alcohol-containing mouth rinses and beverages.

4. Avoid caffeine-containing beverages.

5. Dry mouth can be treated with tart, sugarless gum or candy, water, sugar-free beverages, or with saliva substitutes if dry mouth persists.

6. You may want to wear dark glasses in order to avoid photophobia, which can occur with the dental light.

7. Discontinue treatment and inform dentist immediately if the patient experiences pain or inflammation in his or her tendons. Rest and avoid exercise.

# Ephedrine sulfate

(eh-**FED**-rin)

**Pregnancy Category:** C

**Nasal decongestants:** Kondon's Nasal, Pretz-D, Vatronol Nose Drops **(OTC). Systemic:** Ephed II (**Rx:** Injection; **OTC:** Oral dosage forms)

**Classification:** Adrenergic agent, direct- and indirect-acting

See also *Sympathomimetic Drugs* and *Nasal Decongestants*.

**Action/Kinetics:** Releases norepinephrine from synaptic storage sites. Has direct effects on alpha, beta-1, and beta-2 receptors, causing increased BP, bronchodilation, relaxation of GI tract smooth muscle, nasal decongestion, mydriasis, and increased tone of the bladder trigone and vesicle sphincter. It may also increase skeletal muscle strength, especially in myasthenia clients. Rapidly and completely absorbed following parenteral use. **Onset, IM:** 10–20 min; **PO:** 15–60 min; **SC:** < 20 min. **Duration, IM, SC:** 30–60 min; **PO:** 3–5 hr. **t½, elimination:** About 3 hr when urine is at a pH of 5 and about 6 hr when urinary pH is 6.3. Excreted mostly unchanged through the urine (rate dependent on urinary pH—increased in acid urine).

**Uses:** Bronchial asthma and reversible bronchospasms associated with obstructive pulmonary diseases. Nasal congestion in vasomotor rhinitis, acute sinusitis, hay fever, and acute coryza. Parenterally to treat narcolepsy and depression. Parenterally as a vasopressor to treat shock. In acute hypotension states, especially that associated with spinal anesthesia and Stokes-Adams syndrome with complete heart block.

**Additional Contraindications:** Angle closure glaucoma, anesthesia with cyclopropane or halothane, thyrotoxicosis, diabetes, obstetrics where maternal BP is greater than 130/80. Lactation.

**Special Concerns:** Geriatric clients may be at higher risk to develop prostatic hypertrophy. May cause hypertension resulting in intracranial hemorrhage; may also cause anginal pain in clients with coronary insufficiency or ischemic heart disease.

**Additional Side Effects:** *CNS:* Nervousness, shakiness, confusion, delirium, hallucinations. Anxiety and nervousness following prolonged use. *CV:* Precordial pain, *excessive doses may cause hypertension sufficient to result in cerebral hemorrhage*. *GU:* Difficult and painful urination, urinary retention in males with prostatism, decrease in urine formation. *Miscellaneous:* Pallor, respiratory difficulty, hypersensitivity reactions. *Abuse:* Prolonged abuse can cause an anxiety state, including symptoms of paranoid schizophrenia, tachycardia, poor nutrition and hygiene, dilated pupils, cold sweat, and fever.

**Additional Drug Interactions**

*Halothane* / Serious arrhythmias due to sensitization of the myocardium to sympathomimetics by halothane

*MAO Inhibitors* / ↑ Pressor effect → possible hypertensive crisis and intracranial hemorrhage

**How Supplied:** *Capsule:* 24.3 mg, 25 mg, 50 mg; *Injection:* 50 mg/mL; *Spray:* 0.25%

**Dosage**
• **Capsules**

---

*Bronchodilator, systemic nasal decongestant, CNS stimulant.*
**Adults:** 25–50 mg q 3–4 hr. **Pediatric:** 3 mg/kg (100 mg/m²) daily in four to six divided doses.

- **SC, IM, Slow IV**
  *Bronchodilator.*
**Adults:** 12.5–25 mg; subsequent doses determined by client response. **Pediatric:** 3 mg/kg (100 mg/m²) daily divided into four to six doses SC or IV.
  *Vasopressor.*
**Adults:** 25–50 mg (IM or SC) or 5–25 mg (by slow IV push) repeated at 5- to 10-min intervals, if necessary. Absorption following IM is more rapid than following SC use. **Pediatric (IM):** 16.7 mg/m² q 4–6 hr.
- **Topical (0.25% Spray)**
  *Nasal decongestant.*
**Adults and children over 6 years:** 2–3 gtt of solution or small amount of jelly in each nostril q 4 hr. Do not use topically for more than 3 or 4 consecutive days. Do not use in children under 6 years of age unless ordered by provider.

## DENTAL CONCERNS

See also *Dental Concerns* for *Sympathomimetic Drugs* and *Nasal Decongestants.*

# Epinephrine
(ep-ih-**NEF**-rin)
**Pregnancy Category:** C
Adrenalin Chloride Solution, Bronkaid Mist, Bronkaid Mistometer ✦, EpiE-Z Pen, EpiE-Z Pen Jr., Epipen, Epipen Jr., Primatene Mist Solution, Sus-Phrine (Both Rx and OTC)

# Epinephrine bitartrate
(ep-ih-**NEF**-rin)
**Pregnancy Category:** C
Asthmahaler Mist, Bronitin Mist, Bronkaid Mist Suspension, Epitrate, Primatene Mist Suspension **(OTC)**

# Epinephrine borate
(ep-ih-**NEF**-rin)
**Pregnancy Category:** C
Epinal Ophthalmic Solution **(Rx)**

# Epinephrine hydrochloride
(ep-ih-**NEF**-rin)
**Pregnancy Category:** C
Adrenalin Chloride, AsthmaNefrin, Epifrin, Glaucon, microNefrin, Nephron, S-2 Inhalant, Vaponefrin (Both Rx and OTC)
**Classification:** Adrenergic agent, direct-acting

See also *Sympathomimetic Drugs* and *Nasal Decongestants.*
**Action/Kinetics:** Causes marked stimulation of alpha, beta-1, and beta-2 receptors, causing sympathomimetic stimulation, pressor effects, cardiac stimulation, bronchodilation, and decongestion. It crosses the placenta but not the blood-brain barrier. **Extreme caution must be taken never to inject 1:100 solution intended for inhalation—injection of this concentration has caused death. SC: Onset,** 6–15 min; **duration:** <1–4 hr. **Inhalation: Onset,** 1–5 min; **duration:** 1–3 hr. **IM, Onset:** variable; duration: <1–4 hr. Ineffective when given PO.
**Uses:** Cardiac arrest, Stokes-Adams syndrome, low CO following ECB. To prolong the action of local anesthetics. As a hemostatic during ocular surgery; treatment of conjunctival congestion during surgery; to induce mydriasis during surgery; treat ocular hypertension during surgery. Topically to control bleeding. Acute bronchial asthma, bronchospasms due to emphysema, chronic bronchitis, or other pulmonary diseases. Treatment of anaphylaxis, angioedema, anaphylactic shock, drug-induced allergic reactions, transfusion reactions, insect bites or stings. As an adjunct in the treatment of open-angle glaucoma (may be used with miotics, beta blockers, hyperosmotic agents, or carbonic anhydrase inhibitors). To produce mydriasis; to treat conjunctivitis. *NOTE:* Autoinjectors are available for emergency self-administration of first aid for anaphylactic reactions due to insect stings or bites, foods, drugs, and other allergens

as well as idiopathic or exercise-induced anaphylaxis.

**Additional Contraindications:** Narrow-angle glaucoma. Use when wearing soft contact lenses (may discolor lenses). Aphakia. Lactation.

**Special Concerns:** May cause anoxia in the fetus. Safety and efficacy of ophthalmic products have not been determined in children; administer parenteral epinephrine to children with caution. Syncope may occur if epinephrine is given to asthmatic children. Administration of the SC injection by the IV route may cause severe or fatal hypertension or cerebrovascular hemorrhage. Epinephrine may temporarily increase the rigidity and tremor of parkinsonism. Use with caution and in small quantities in the toes, fingers, nose, ears, and genitals or in the presence of peripheral vascular disease as vasoconstriction-induced tissue sloughing may occur.

**Additional Side Effects:** *CV:* **Fatal ventricular fibrillation, cerebral or subarachnoid hemorrhage,** obstruction of central retinal artery. *A rapid and large increase in BP may cause aortic rupture, cerebral hemorrhage, or angina pectoris.* *GU:* Decreased urine formation, urinary retention, painful urination. *CNS:* Anxiety, fear, pallor. Parenteral use may cause or aggravate disorientation, memory impairment, psychomotor agitation, panic, hallucinations, **suicidal or homicidal tendencies,** schizophrenic-type behavior. *Miscellaneous:* Prolonged use or overdose may cause elevated serum lactic acid with severe metabolic acidosis. *At injection site:* Bleeding, urticaria, wheal formation, pain. Repeated injections at the same site may cause necrosis from vascular constriction. *Ophthalmic:* Transient stinging or burning when administered, conjunctival hyperemia, brow ache, headache, blurred vision, photophobia, allergic lid reaction, ocular hypersensitivity, poor night vision, eye ache, eye pain. Prolonged ophthalmic use may cause deposits of pigment in the cornea, lids, or conjunctiva. When used for glaucoma in aphakic clients, reversible cystoid macular edema.

**Additional Drug Interactions**
*Beta-adrenergic blocking agents* / Initial effectiveness in treating glaucoma of this combination may ↓ over time
*Chymotrypsin* / Epinephrine, 1:100, will inactivate chymotrypsin in 60 min

**How Supplied:** Epinephrine: *Metered dose inhaler:* 0.25 mg/inh, 0.22 mg/inh; *Injection:* 1 mg/mL, 5 mg/mL; *Kit:* 0.5 mg/mL, 1 mg/mL. Epinephrine bitartrate: *Metered dose inhaler:* 0.3 mg/inh. Epinephrine borate: *Opthalmic solution:* 0.5%, 1%. Epinephrine hydrochloride: *Injection:* 0.1 mg/mL, 1 mg/mL; *Solution:* 1:100, 1:1000; *Ophthalmic solution:* 0.5%, 1%, 2%

**Dosage** ────────────
- **Metered Dose Inhaler**
  *Bronchodilation.*

**Adults and children over 4 years of age:** 0.2–0.275 mg (1 inhalation) of the Aerosol or 0.16 mg (1 inhalation) of the Bitartrate Aerosol; may be repeated after 1–2 min if needed. At least 3 hr should elapse before subsequent doses. Dosage not established in children less than 4 years of age.

- **Inhalation Solution**
  *Bronchodilation.*

**Adults and children over 6 years of age:** 1 inhalation of the 1% solution (of the base); may be repeated after 1–2 min.

- **IM, IV, SC**
  *Bronchodilation using the solution (1:1,000).*

**Adults:** 0.3–0.5 mg SC or IM repeated q 20 min–4 hr as needed; dose may be increased to 1 mg/dose. **Infants and children (except premature infants and full-term newborns):** 0.01 mg/kg (0.3 mg/m$^2$) SC up to a maximum of 0.5 mg/dose; may be repeated q 15 min for two doses and then q 4 hr as needed.

*Bronchodilation using the sterile suspension (1:200).*

**Adults:** 0.5–1.5 mg SC. **Infants and children, 1 month–12 years:** 0.025 mg/kg SC; **children less than 30 kg:** 0.75 mg as a single dose.

*Anaphylaxis.*

**Adults:** 0.2–0.5 mg SC q 10–15 min as needed, up to a maximum of 1 mg/dose if needed. **Pediatric:** 0.01 mg/kg (0.3 mg/m$^2$) up to a maximum of 0.5 mg/dose; may be repeated q 15 min for two doses and then q 4 hr as needed.

- **Autoinjector, IM**

*First aid for anaphylaxis.*

The autoinjectors deliver a single dose of either 0.3 mg or 0.15 mg (for children) of epinephrine. In cases of a severe reaction, repeat injections may be necessary.

*Vasopressor.*

**Adults, IM or SC, initial:** 0.5 mg repeated q 5 min if needed; **then,** give 0.025–0.050 mg IV q 5–15 min as needed. **Adults, IV, initial:** 0.1–0.25 mg given slowly. May be repeated q 5–15 min as needed. Or, use IV infusion beginning with 0.001 mg/min and increasing the dose to 0.004 mg/min if needed. **Pediatric, IM, SC:** 0.01 mg/kg, up to a maximum of 0.3 mg repeated q 5 min if needed. **Pediatric, IV:** 0.01 mg/kg/5–15 min if an inadequate response to IM or SC administration is observed.

*Cardiac stimulant.*

**Adults, intracardiac or IV:** 0.1–1 mg repeated q 5 min if needed. **Pediatric, intracardiac or IV:** 0.005–0.01 mg/kg (0.15–0.3 mg/m$^2$) repeated q 5 min if needed; this may be followed by IV infusion beginning at 0.0001 mg/kg/min and increased in increments of 0.0001 mg/kg/min up to a maximum of 0.0015 mg/kg/min.

*Adjunct to local anesthesia.*

**Adults and children:** 0.1–0.2 mg in a 1:200,000–1:20,000 solution.

*Adjunct with intraspinal anesthetics.*

**Adults:** 0.2–0.4 mg added to the anesthetic spinal fluid.

- **Solution**

*Antihemorrhagic, mydriatic.*

**Adults and children, intracameral or subconjunctival:** 0.01%–0.1% solution.

*Topical antihemorrhagic.*

**Adults and children:** 0.002%–0.1% solution.

*Nasal decongestant.*

**Adults and children over 6 years of age:** Apply 0.1% solution as drops or spray or with a sterile swab as needed.

- **Borate Ophthalmic Solution, Hydrochloride Ophthalmic Solution**

*Glaucoma.*

**Adults:** 1–2 gtt into affected eye(s) 1–2 times/day. Determine frequency of use by tonometry. Dosage has not been established in children.

## DENTAL CONCERNS

See also *Dental Concerns* for *Sympathomimetic Drugs* and *Nasal Decongestants.*

# Erythromycin base

(eh-**rih**-throw-**MY**-sin)

**Pregnancy Category:** B (A/T/S, Erymax, Staticin, and T-Stat are C)

**Capsules/Tablets:** Alti-Erythromycin ✳, Apo-Erythro Base ✳, Apo-Erythro-EC ✳, Diomycin ✳, E-Base Caplets, E-Base Tablets, E-Mycin, Erybid ✳, Eryc, Ery-Tab, Erythro-Base ✳, Erythromid ✳, Erythromycin Base Film-Tabs, Novo–Rythro EnCap ✳, PCE Dispertab, PMS-Erythromycin ✳, Robimycin Robitabs. **Gel, topical:** A/T/S, Erygel. **Ointment, topical:** Akne-mycin. **Ointment, ophthalmic:** Ilotycine Ophthalmic, **Pledgets:** Erycette, T-Stat. **Solution:**, Del-Mycin, Eryderm 2%, Erymax, Erythra-Derm, Staticin, Theramycin Z, T-Stat **(Rx)**

**Classification:** Antibiotic, erythromycin

See also *Erythromycins* and *Anti-Infective Agents.*

**Uses:** See *Erythromycins.* **Ophthalmic solution:** Treatment of ocular infections (along with PO therapy) due to *Streptococcus pneumoniae, Staphylococcus aureus, S. pyogenes, Corynebacterium* species, *Hae-*

*mophilus influenzae,* and *Bacteroides* infections. Also prophylaxis of ocular infections due to *Neisseria gonorrhoeae* and *Chlamydia trachomatis.* **Topical solution:** Acne vulgaris. **Topical ointment:** Prophylaxis of infection in minor skin abrasions; treatment of superficial infections of the skin. Acne vulgaris. **Contraindications:** Use of topical preparations in the eye or near the nose, mouth, or any mucous membrane. Ophthalmic use in dendritic keratitis, vaccinia, varicella, myobacterial infections of the eye, fungal diseases of the eye. Use with steroid combinations following uncomplicated removal of a corneal foreign body.

**Special Concerns:** Use of other drugs for acne may result in a cumulative irritant effect.

**Additional Side Effects:** *When used topically:* Erythema, desquamation, burning sensation, eye irritation, tenderness, dryness, pruritus, oily skin, generalized urticaria.

**Drug Interactions:** Antagonism has been observed when topical erythromycin is used with clindamycin.

**How Supplied:** *Enteric coated capsule:* 250 mg; *Enteric coated tablet:* 250 mg, 333 mg, 500 mg; *Gel/Jelly:* 2%; *Ointment:* 2%; *Ophthalmic ointment:* 5 mg/g; *Pad:* 2%; *Solution:* 1.5%, 2%; *Swab:* 2%; *Tablet:* 250 mg, 500 mg; *Tablet, Coated particles:* 333 mg, 500 mg

## Dosage
• **Delayed-Release Capsules, Enteric-Coated Tablets, Delayed-Release Tablets, Film-Coated Tablets, Suspension**
*Respiratory tract infections due to* Mycoplasma pneumoniae.
500 mg q 6 hr for 5–10 days (up to 3 weeks for severe infections).
*URTIs (mild to moderate) due to* S. pyogenes and S. pneumoniae.
250–500 mg q.i.d. (or 20–50 mg/kg/day in divided doses) for 10 days.
*URTIs due to* H. influenzae.

Erythromycin ethylsuccinate, 50 mg/kg/day, plus sulfisoxazole, 150 mg/kg/day, given together for 10 days.
*Lower respiratory tract infections (mild to moderate) due to* S. pyogenes *and* S. pneumoniae.
250–500 mg q.i.d. (or 20–50 mg/kg/day in divided doses) for 10 days.
*Intestinal amebiasis due to* Entamoeba histolytica.
**Adults:** 250 mg q.i.d. for 10–14 days; **pediatric:** 30–50 mg/kg/day in divided doses for 10–14 days.
*Legionnaire's disease.*
500–1,000 mg q.i.d. for 3 weeks (or 1–4 g/day in divided doses).
Bordetella pertussis.
500 mg q.i.d. for 10 days (or 40–50 mg/kg/day in divided doses for 5–14 days).
*Infections due to* Corynebacterium diphtheriae.
500 mg q.i.d. for 10 days.
*Erythrasma.*
250 mg t.i.d. for 3 weeks.
*Primary syphilis.*
20 g in divided doses over 10 days.
*Chlamydial infections.*
**Infants:** 50 mg/kg/day in four divided doses for 14 (conjunctivitis) to 21 (pneumonia) days; **adults:** 500 mg q.i.d. for 7 days or 250 mg q.i.d. for 14 days for urogenital infections.
*Mild to moderate skin and skin structure infections due to* S. pyogenes *and* S. aureus.
250–500 mg q 6 hr (or 50 mg/kg/day in divided doses—to a maximum of 4 g/day) for 10 days.
Listeria monocytogenes *infections.*
500 mg q 12 hr (or 250 mg q 6 hr), up to maximum of 4 g/day.
*Pelvic inflammatory disease, acute* N. gonorrhoeae.
Erythromycin lactobionate, 500 mg IV q 6 hr for 3 days; **then,** 250 mg erythromycin base q 6 hr for 7 days. Alternatively for pelvic inflammatory disease, 500 mg PO q.i.d. for 10–14 days.

**E**

*Prophylaxis of initial or recurrent rheumatic fever.*
250 mg b.i.d.

*Bacterial endocarditis due to alpha-hemolytic streptococcus.*
**Adults:** 1 g 2 hr prior to the procedure; **then,** 500 mg 6 hr after the initial dose. **Pediatric,** 20 mg/kg 2 hr prior to the procedure; **then,** 10 mg/kg 6 hr after the initial dose.

*Pneumonia of infancy, conjunctivitis of the newborn, and urogenital infections during pregnancy due to* C. trachomatis.
500 mg q.i.d. for 7 days (or 250 mg q.i.d. for 14 days).

*Nongonococcal urethritis due to* Ureaplasma urealyticum.
500 mg q.i.d. for at least 7 days.

*Erythrasma due to* Corynebacterium minutissimum.
250 mg t.i.d. for 21 days.

• **Ophthalmic Ointment**
*Mild to moderate infections.*
0.5-in. ribbon b.i.d.–t.i.d.

*Acute infections.*
0.5 in. q 3–4 hr until improvement is noted.

*Prophylaxis of neonatal gonococcal or chlamydial conjunctivitis.*
0.2–0.4 in. into each conjunctival sac.

• **Topical Gel (2%), Ointment (2%), Solution (2%)**
Clean the affected area and apply, using fingertips or applicator, morning and evening, to affected areas. If no improvement is seen after 6 to 8 weeks, discontinue therapy.

## DENTAL CONCERNS

See also *Dental Concerns* for *Anti-Infectives* and *Erythromycins*.
**Client/Family Teaching**
1. Continue entire prescription; do not stop if symptoms subside. Return for follow-up once completed.
2. Report any unusual or intolerable side effects or lack of response.
3. Take on an empty stomach; the delayed-release forms of the base can be taken without regard for meals.
4. Report if no symptom improvement after 48–72 hr.
5. Use an additional nonhormonal form of birth control if taking oral contraceptives because their effectiveness may be diminished.

# Erythromycin estolate
(eh-**rih**-throw-**MY**-sin)
**Pregnancy Category:** B
Ilosone, Novo-Rythro Estolate ✱ **(Rx)**
**Classification:** Antibiotic, erythromycin

See also *Erythromycins*.
**Action/Kinetics:** Most active form of erythromycin, with relatively long-lasting activity.
**Uses:** See *Erythromycins*.
**Additional Contraindications:** Cholestatic jaundice or preexisting liver dysfunction. Treatment of chronic disorders such as acne, furunculosis, or prophylaxis of rheumatic fever.
**Additional Side Effects:** Hepatotoxicity.
**How Supplied:** *Capsule:* 250 mg; *Suspension:* 125 mg/5 mL, 250 mg/5 mL; *Tablet:* 500 mg

## Dosage

• **Capsules, Suspension, Tablets**
See *Erythromycin base.* Similar blood levels are achieved using erythromycin base, estolate, or stearate.

## DENTAL CONCERNS

See also *Dental Concerns* for *Erythromycins*.
**Client/Family Teaching**
1. Shake suspension well before using; do not store for more than 2 weeks at room temperature.
2. Chew or crush chewable tablets.
3. May take without regard to meals.
4. Report if no symptom improvement after 48–72 hr.
5. Use an additional nonhormonal form of birth control if taking oral contraceptives because their effectiveness may be diminished.

# Erythromycin ethylsuccinate
(eh-**rih**-throw-**MY**-sin)

**Pregnancy Category:** B
Apo-Erythro-ES, E.E.S. 200 and 400,
E.E.S. Granules, EryPed, EryPed 200,
EryPed 400, EryPed Drops, Erythro-ES
✹, Novo-Rythro Ethylsuccinate ✹ **(Rx)**
**Classification:** Antibiotic, erythromycin

See also *Erythromycins.*
**Uses:** See *Erythromycins.*
**Additional    Contraindications:**
Preexisting liver disease.
**How Supplied:** *Chew Tablet:* 200
mg; *Granule for reconstitution:* 100
mg/2.5 mL, 200 mg/5 mL, 400 mg/5
mL; *Suspension:* 200 mg/5 mL, 400
mg/5 mL; *Tablet:* 400 mg

**Dosage** ———————————
• **Oral    Suspension,    Tablets,
Chewable Tablets**
See *Erythromycin base. NOTE:* 400
mg of erythromycin ethylsuccinate
will achieve the same blood levels
of erythromycin as 250 mg of the
base, estolate, or stearate forms.
    Hemophilus    influenzae    *infec-
tions.*
Erythromycin    ethylsuccinate,    50
mg/kg/day with sulfisoxazole, 150
mg/kg/day, both for a total of 10
days.

**DENTAL CONCERNS**

See also *Dental Concerns* for *Erythromycins.*
**Client/Family Teaching**
1. Take without regard to meals.
2. Chew or crush chewable tablets.
3. Refrigerate oral suspension; store
for 1 week maximum.
4. Report if no symptom improvement after 48–72 hr.
5. Use an additional nonhormonal
form of birth control if taking oral
contraceptives because their effectiveness may be diminished.

# Erythromycin
# lactobionate
(eh-**rih**-throw-**MY**-sin)
**Pregnancy Category:** B
Erythrocin I.V. ✹, Erythrocin Lactobionate IV **(Rx)**

**Classification:** Antibiotic, erythromycin

See also *Erythromycins.*
**Uses:** For seriously ill or vomiting
clients with infections caused by
susceptible organisms; acute pelvic
inflammatory disease due to gonorrhea. Legionnaire's disease.
**Additional Side Effects:** Transient
deafness.
**Additional Drug Interactions:** Do
not add drugs to IV solutions of
erythromycin lactobionate.
**How Supplied:** *Powder for injection:* 500 mg, 1 g

**Dosage** ———————————
• **IV**
**Adults   and   children:**    15–20
mg/kg/day up to 4 g/day in severe infections.
    *Acute pelvic inflammatory disease
caused by gonorrhea.*
500 mg q 6 hr for 3 days followed by
250 mg erythromycin stearate, **PO,** q
6 hr for 7 days.
    *Legionnaire's disease.*
1–4 g/day in divided doses. Change to
PO therapy as soon as possible.

**DENTAL CONCERNS**

See also *Dental Concerns* for *Erythromycins.*

# Erythromycin stearate
(eh-**rih**-throw-**MY**-sin)
**Pregnancy Category:** B
Apo-Erythro-S ✹, Eramycin, Novo-
Rythro Stearate ✹, Nu-Erythromycin-S
✹ **(Rx)**
**Classification:** Antibiotic, erythromycin

See also *Erythromycins.*
**Uses:** See *Erythromycins.*
**Additional Side Effects:** Causes
more allergic reactions (e.g., skin
rash and urticaria) than other erythromycins. Hepatotoxicity.
**How Supplied:** *Tablet:* 250 mg, 500
mg

**Dosage** ———————————
• **Tablets, Film Coated**

See *Erythromycin base.* Similar blood levels are achieved using erythromycin base, estolate, or stearate forms.

## DENTAL CONCERNS

See also *Dental Concerns* for *Erythromycins.*

**Client/Family Teaching**
1. Take on an empty stomach; food decreases absorption.
2. Report lack of effect or evidence of allergic reaction, i.e., rash or itching.
3. Report if no symptom improvement after 48–72 hr.
4. Use an additional nonhormonal form of birth control if taking oral contraceptives because their effectiveness may be diminished.

# Etanercept
(eh-**TAN**-er-sept)
**Pregnancy Category:** B
Enbrel
**Classification:** Antirheumatic, disease modifying

**Action/Kinetics:** Binds tumor necrosis factor (TNF) and blocks its interaction with cell surface receptors. TNF has a major role in the inflammatory process of rheumatiod arthritis and resulting joint pathology. **Serum half-life:** 115 hours. **Time to peak:** 72 hours.
**Uses:** Patients with moderately to severely active rheumatoid arthritis who have had an inadequate response to one or more disease modifying antirheumatic drugs. *Non-FDA Approved Uses:* Treatment of patients with organ transplants, reduce toxicity associated with aldesleukin, treatment of congestive heart failure.
**Contraindications:** Sepsis, live vaccines, serious infection.
**Special Concerns:** Children under the age of 4, varicella virus
**Side Effects:** *GI:* Abdominal pain, dyspepsia. *CNS:* Headache, dizziness. *Pulmonary:* Respiratory tract infection, upper respiratory tract infection, pharyngitis, respiratory disorder, sinusitis, rhinitis. *Local:* injection site reaction. *Dermatologic:* Rash.

*Neuromuscular:* Weakness. *Miscellaneous:* Infection, positive ANA, positive anti-double stranded DNA antibodies.
**Drug Interactions:** None reported at this time.
**How Supplied:** *Powder for injection:* 25 mg

**Dosage** ─────────────
• **Subcutaneous injection**
  *Moderately to severely active rheumatoid arthritis*
Adults: 25 mg twice weekly. Children: 0.4 mg/kg (not to exceed 25 mg)

## DENTAL CONCERNS
**General**
1. A semisupine position for the dental chair may be necessary to help minimize or avoid GI adverse effects or for patients with rheumatoid arthritis.
**Consultation with Primary Care Provider**
1. Consultation may be required in order to assess extent of disease control.

# Ethosuximide
(eth-oh-**SUCKS**-ih-myd)
Zarontin **(Rx)**
**Classification:** Anticonvulsant, succinimide type

See also *Anticonvulsants.*
**Action/Kinetics: Peak serum levels:** 3–7 hr. **t½, adults:** 40–60 hr; **t½, children:** 30 hr. Steady serum levels reached in 7–10 days. **Therapeutic serum levels:** 40–100 mcg/mL. Not bound to plasma protein. Metabolized in the liver. Both inactive metabolites and unchanged drug are excreted in the urine.
**Uses:** Absence (petit mal) seizures.
**Additional Drug Interactions:** Both isoniazid and valproic acid may ↑ the effects of ethosuximide.
**How Supplied:** *Capsule:* 250 mg; *Syrup:* 250 mg/5 mL

**Dosage** ─────────────
• **Capsules, Syrup**
  *Absence seizures.*

**Adults and children over 6 years, initial:** 250 mg b.i.d.; the dose may be increased by 250 mg/day at 4–7-day intervals until seizures are controlled or until total daily dose reaches 1.5 g.
**Children under 6 years, initial:** 250 mg/day; dosage may be increased by 250 mg/day every 4–7 days until control is established or total daily dose reaches 1 g.

## DENTAL CONCERNS

See also *Dental Concerns* for *Anticonvulsants* .

# Etidocaine hydrochloride
(et-**TEE**-doh-kayn)
**Pregnancy Category:** B
Duranest, Duranest MPF, Duranest with Epinephrine, Durnaest MPF with Epinephrine
**Classification:** Amide local anesthetic

See also *Amide Local Anesthetics*.
**Action/Kinetics:** Blocks nerve action potential by inhibiting ion fluxes across the cell membrane. **Onset:** 2-8 min, **Duration:** 1.5-9 hr. Renally excreted and metabolized by the liver.
**Uses:** Local dental anesthesia, peripheral nerve block, caudal anesthesia, central neural block, vaginal block.
**Contraindications:** Hypersensitivity, children < 12 years of age.
**Special Concerns:** See also *Amide Local Anesthetics*.
**Side Effects:** See also *Amide Local Anesthetics*.
**Drug Interactions:** See also *Amide Local Anesthetics*.
**How Supplied:** *Injection without vasoconstrictor:* 1%, 1.5%. *Injection with vasoconstrictor:* 1%, 1.5% with epinephrine concentration of 1:200,000

## Dosage

• **1.5% injection with 1:200,000 epinephrine**
*Infiltration or conduction block.*

150–300 mg, not to exceed 400 mg. Dose should be adjusted down for medically compromised, debilitated, or elderly patients. (See also *Appendix 9*.)

## DENTAL CONCERNS

See also *Dental Concerns* for *Amide Local Anesthetic Agents*.

# Etoposide (VP-16–213)
(eh-**TOH**-poh-syd)
**Pregnancy Category:** D
Etopophos, VePesid **(Rx)**, Etoposide Phosphate
**Classification:** Antineoplastic, miscellaneous

See also *Antineoplastic Agents*.
**Action/Kinetics:** Acts as a mitotic inhibitor at the $G_2$ portion of the cell cycle to inhibit DNA synthesis. At high doses, cells entering mitosis are lysed, whereas at low doses, cells will not enter prophase. **t½:** biphasic, initial, 1.5 hr; final, 4–11 hr. **Effective plasma levels:** 0.3–10 mcg/mL. Poor CNS penetration. Eliminated through both the urine and bile unchanged and as liver metabolites. Is water soluble.
**Uses:** With combination therapy to treat refractory testicular tumors and small cell lung cancer. *Non-FDA Approved Uses:* Alone or in combination to treat acute monocytic leukemia, non-Hodgkin's lymphoma, Hodgkin's disease, AIDS-associated Kaposi's sarcoma, Ewing's sarcoma. Also, choriocarcinoma; hepatocellular carcinoma; nonsmall cell lung, breast, endometrial, and gastric cancers; acute lymphocytic leukemia; soft tissue carcinoma; rhabdomyosarcoma.
**Contraindications:** Lactation.
**Special Concerns:** Safety and efficacy in children have not been established. Severe myelosuppression may occur.
**Additional Side Effects:** *Anaphylactic-type reactions,* hypotension, peripheral neuropathy, somnolence.

---

**How Supplied:** *Capsule:* 50 mg; *Injection:* 20 mg/mL; *Powder for injection:* 100 mg

## Dosage

- **IV**

*Testicular carcinoma.*
50–100 mg/m²/day on days 1–5 or 100 mg/m²/day on days 1, 3, and 5 q 3–4 weeks (i.e., after recovery from toxic effects). Used in combination with other agents.

*Small cell lung carcinoma.*
35 mg/m²/day for 4 days to 50 mg/m²/day for 5 days, repeated q 3–4 weeks.

- **Capsules**

*Small cell lung carcinoma.*
70 mg/m² (rounded to the nearest 50 mg) daily for 4 days to 100 mg/m² (rounded to the nearest 50 mg) daily for 5 days; repeat q 3–4 weeks.
*NOTE:* Etopophos is given in higher concentrations than VePesid. Doses above are for VePesid.

## DENTAL CONCERNS

See also *Dental Concerns* for *Antineoplastic Agents.*

---

# F

---

# Famciclovir
(fam-**SY**-kloh-veer)
**Pregnancy Category:** B
Famvir **(Rx)**
**Classification:** Antiviral agent

See also *Antiviral Agents.*

**Action/Kinetics:** Undergoes rapid biotransformation to the active compound penciclovir. Inhibits viral DNA synthesis and therefore replication in HSV types 1 (HSV-1) and 2 (HSV-2) and varicella-zoster virus. Penciclovir is further metabolized to inactive compounds that are excreted through the urine. $t\frac{1}{2}$: 2 hr following IV administration and 2.3 hr following PO use. Half-life increased in renal insufficiency.

**Uses:** Management of acute herpes zoster (shingles). Treatment of recurrent herpes simplex (genital herpes) and to prevent outbreaks of recurrent genital herpes.

**Contraindications:** Use during lactation.

**Special Concerns:** The dose should be adjusted in clients with $C_{CR}$ less than 60 mL/min. Safety and efficacy have not been determined in children less than 18 years of age.

**Side Effects:** *GI:* N&V, diarrhea, constipation, anorexia, abdominal pain, dyspepsia, flatulence. *CNS:* Headache, dizziness, paresthesia, somnolence, insomnia. *Body as a whole:* Fatigue, fever, pain, rigors. *Musculoskeletal:* Back pain, arthralgia. *Respiratory:* Pharyngitis, sinusitis, upper respiratory infection. *Dermatologic:* Pruritus; signs, symptoms, and complications of zoster and genital herpes.

**Drug Interactions:** None reported in patients who are healthy and not immunocompromised.

**How Supplied:** *Tablet:* 125 mg, 250 mg, 500 mg

## Dosage

- **Tablets**

*Herpes zoster infections.*
500 mg q 8 hr for 7 days. Dosage reduction is recommended in clients with impaired renal function: for $C_{CR}$ of 40–59 mL/min, the dose should be 500 mg q 12 hr; for $C_{CR}$ of 20–39 mL/min, the dose should be 500 mg q 24 hr; for $C_{CR}$ less than 20 mL/min, the dose should be 250 mg q 48 hr. For hemodialysis clients, the recommended dose is 250 mg given after each dialysis treatment.

*Recurrent genital herpes.*
125 mg b.i.d. for 5 days. Should be taken within 6 hr of symptoms or le-

sion onset. Dosage reduction is as follows for those with impaired renal function: for $C_{CR}$ of 40 mL/min or greater, use the recommended dose of 125 mg b.i.d.; for $C_{CR}$ of 20–39 mL/min, the dose should be 125 mg q 24 hr; for $C_{CR}$ less than 20 mL/min, the dose should be 125 mg q 48 hr. For hemodialysis clients, the recommended dose is 125 mg given after each dialysis treatment.

*Prevent outbreaks of genital herpes.*
250 mg b.i.d.

## DENTAL CONCERNS

See also *Dental Concerns* for *Antiviral Agents.*
**General**
1. Use a semisupine position for dental chair in order to help alleviate or minimize GI discomfort from the drug.
2. Be aware of the general discomfort associated with shingles. Acute symptoms may make it necessary to shorten or postpone the appointment.
**Consultation with Primary Care Provider**
1. Medical consultation may be necessary in order to assess patient's ability to tolerate stress.
2. Medical consultation may be necessary in order to assess patient's disease control.

# Famotidine
(fah-**MOH**-tih-deen)
**Pregnancy Category:** B
Apo-Famotidine ✚, Gen-Famotidine ✚, Novo-Famotidine ✚, Nu-Famotidine ✚, Pepcid, Pepcid AC Acid Controller, Pepcid IV **(Rx)** (Pepcid AC is OTC)
**Classification:** Histamine $H_2$ receptor antagonist

See also *Histamine $H_2$ Antagonists.*
**Action/Kinetics:** Competitive inhibitor of histamine $H_2$ receptors leading to inhibition of gastric acid secretion. **Peak plasma levels:** 1–3 hr. **t½:** 2.5–3.5 hr. **Onset:** 1 hr. **Duration:**

10–12 hr. Does not inhibit the cytochrome P-450 system in the liver; thus, drug interactions due to inhibition of liver metabolism are not expected to occur. From 25% to 30% of a PO dose is eliminated through the kidney unchanged; from 65% to 70% of an IV dose is excreted through the kidney unchanged.
**Uses: Rx:** Treatment of active duodenal ulcers. Maintenance therapy for duodenal ulcer, at reduced dosage, after active ulcer has healed. Pathologic hypersecretory conditions such as Zollinger-Ellison syndrome or multiple endocrine adenomas. GERD, including erosive esophagitis. Treatment of benign gastric ulcer. *Non-FDA Approved Uses:* Prevent aspiration pneumonitis, for prophylaxis of stress ulcers, prevent acute upper GI bleeding, as part of multidrug therapy to eradicate *Helicobacter pylori.*
    **OTC:** Relief of and prevention of the symptoms of heartburn, acid indigestion, and sour stomach.
**Contraindications:** Cirrhosis of the liver, impaired renal or hepatic function, lactation.
**Special Concerns:** Safety and efficacy in children have not been established.
**Side Effects:** *Oral:* Dry mouth. *GI:* Constipation, diarrhea, N&V, anorexia, abdominal discomfort. *CNS:* Dizziness, headache, paresthesias, depression, anxiety, confusion, hallucinations, insomnia, fatigue, sleepiness, agitation, ***grand mal seizure,*** psychic disturbances. *Skin:* Rash, acne, pruritus, alopecia, urticaria, dry skin, flushing. *CV:* Palpitations. *Musculoskeletal:* Arthralgia, asthenia, musculoskeletal pain. *Hematologic:* Thrombocytopenia. *Other:* Fever, orbital edema, conjunctival injection, bronchospasm, tinnitus, taste disorders, decreased libido, impotence, pain at injection site (transient).
**Drug Interactions**
*Antacids* / ↓ Absorption of famotidine from the GI tract

*Diazepam* / ↓ Absorption of diazepam from the GI tract

**How Supplied:** *Injection:* 10 mg/mL; *Powder for reconstitution:* 40 mg/5 mL; *Tablet:* 10 mg, 20 mg, 40 mg

## Dosage

• **Oral Suspension, Tablets**

*Duodenal ulcer, acute therapy.*

**Adults:** 40 mg once daily at bedtime or 20 mg b.i.d. Most ulcers heal within 4 weeks and it is rarely necessary to use the full dosage for 6–8 weeks.

*Duodenal ulcer, maintenance therapy.*

**Adults:** 20 mg once daily at bedtime.

*Benign gastric ulcers, acute therapy.*

**Adults:** 40 mg at bedtime.

*Hypersecretory conditions.*

**Adults, individualized, initial:** 20 mg q 6 hr; **then,** adjust dose to response, although doses of up to 160 mg q 6 hr may be required for severe cases.

*Gastroesophageal reflux disease.*

**Adults:** 20 mg b.i.d. for 6 weeks. For esophagitis with erosions and ulcerations, give 20 or 40 mg b.i.d. for up to 12 weeks.

*Prophylaxis of upper GI bleeding.*

**Adults:** 20 mg b.i.d.

*Prophylaxis of stress ulcers.*

**Adults:** 40 mg/day.

*Relief of and prevention of heartburn, acid indigestion, and sour stomach (OTC).*

**Adults and children over 12 years of age, for relief:** 10 mg (1 tablet) with water. **For prevention:** 10 mg 1 hr before eating a meal that may cause symptoms. **Maximum dose:** 20 mg/24 hr. Not to be used continuously for more than 2 weeks unless medically prescribed.

• **IM, IV, IV Infusion**

*Hospitalized clients with hypersecretory conditions, duodenal ulcers, gastric ulcers; clients unable to take PO medication.*

**Adults:** 20 mg IV q 12 hr.

*Before anesthesia to prevent aspiration of gastric acid.*

**Adults:** 40 mg IM or PO.

## DENTAL CONCERNS

See also *Dental Concerns* for *Histamine $H_2$ Antagonists.*

**Client/Family Teaching**

1. Daily home fluoride treatments for persistent dry mouth.

2. Avoid alcohol-containing mouth rinses and beverages.

3. Avoid caffeine-containing beverages.

4. Dry mouth can be treated with tart, sugarless gum or candy, water, sugar-free beverages, or with saliva substitutes if dry mouth persists.

5. Stress the importance of good oral hygiene in order to prevent gingival inflammation.

# Felbamate

(**FELL**-bah-mayt)

**Pregnancy Category:** C

Felbatol **(Rx)**

**Classification:** Anticonvulsant, miscellaneous (second-line therapy)

See also *Anticonvulsants.*

*NOTE:* In August 1994 it was recommended that felbamate treatment be discontinued for epilepsy clients due to several cases of aplastic anemia. Revised labeling states, "...Felbatol should only be used in patients whose epilepsy is so severe that the risk of aplastic anemia is deemed acceptable in light of the benefits conferred by its use..."

**Action/Kinetics:** Mechanism not known. Felbamate may reduce seizure spread and increase seizure threshold. Has weak inhibitory effects on both GABA and benzodiazepine receptor binding. Well absorbed after PO use. **Terminal t½:** 20–23 hr. Trough blood levels are dose dependent. From 40% to 50% excreted unchanged in the urine.

**Uses:** Alone or as part of adjunctive therapy for the treatment of partial seizures with and without generalization in adults with epilepsy. As an adjunct in the treatment of partial and generalized seizures associated with Lennox-Gastaut syndrome in children. The drug should be used only as second-line therapy.

**Contraindications:** Preexisting liver pathology.

**Special Concerns:** Use with caution in clients who are hypersensitive to carbamates. Aplastic anemia and acute liver failure have been observed in a few clients. Use with caution during lactation. Safety and efficacy have not been established in children other than those with Lennox-Gastaut syndrome.

**Side Effects:** May differ depending on whether the drug is used as monotherapy or adjunctive therapy in adults or for Lennox-Gastaut syndrome in children. *CNS:* Insomnia, headache, anxiety, somnolence, dizziness, nervousness, tremor, abnormal gait, depression, paresthesia, ataxia, stupor, abnormal thinking, emotional lability, agitation, psychologic disturbance, aggressive reaction, hallucinations, euphoria, *suicide attempt,* migraine. *Oral:* Dry mouth, facial edema, buccal mucous membrane swelling (rare), taste perversion. *GI:* Dyspepsia, vomiting, constipation, diarrhea, nausea, anorexia, abdominal pain, hiccoughs, esophagitis, increased appetite. *Respiratory:* Upper respiratory tract infection, rhinitis, sinusitis, pharyngitis, coughing. *CV:* Palpitation, tachycardia, SVT. *Body as a whole:* Fatigue, weight decrease or increase, facial edema, fever, chest pain, pain, asthenia, malaise, flu-like symptoms, *anaphylaxis.* *Ophthalmologic:* Miosis, diplopia, abnormal vision. *GU:* Urinary incontinence, intramenstrual bleeding, UTI. *Hematologic: Aplastic anemia,* purpura, leukopenia, lymphadenopathy, leukopenia, leukocytosis, thrombocytopenia, granulocytopenia, positive antinuclear factor test, *agranulocytosis,* qualitative platelet disorder. *Dermatologic:* Pruritus, urticaria, bullous eruption, *Stevens-Johnson syndrome.* *Miscellaneous:* Otitis media, *acute liver failure,* hypophosphatemia, myalgia, photosensitivity, substernal chest pain, dystonia, allergic reaction.

**Drug Interactions**
*Carbamazepine* / Felbamate ↓ steady-state carbamazepine levels and ↑ steady-state carbamazepine epoxide (metabolite) levels. Also, carbamazepine → 50% ↑ in felbamate clearance
*Phenytoin* / Felbamate ↑ steady-state phenytoin levels necessitating a 40% decrease in phenytoin dose. Also, phenytoin ↑ felbamate clearance
*Valproic acid* / Felbamate ↑ steady-state valproic acid levels

**How Supplied:** *Suspension:* 600 mg/5 mL; *Tablet:* 400 mg, 600 mg

**Dosage** ────────────
• **Suspenion, Tablets**
*Monotherapy, initial therapy.*
**Adults over 14 years of age, initial:** 1,200 mg/day in divided doses t.i.d.–q.i.d. The dose may be increased in 600-mg increments q 2 weeks to 2,400 mg/day based on clinical response and thereafter to 3,600 mg/day, if needed.
*Conversion to monotherapy.*
**Adults:** Initiate at 1,200 mg/day in divided doses t.i.d.–q.i.d. Reduce the dose of concomitant antiepileptic drugs by ⅓ at initiation of felbamate therapy. At week 2, the felbamate dose should be increased to 2,400 mg/day while reducing the dose of other antiepileptic drugs up to another ⅓ of the original dose. At week 3, increase the felbamate dose to 3,600 mg/day and continue to decrease the dose of other antiepileptic drugs as indicated by response.
*Adjunctive therapy.*
**Adults:** Add felbamate at a dose of 1,200 mg/day in divided doses t.i.d.–q.i.d. while reducing current antiepileptic drugs by 20%. Further decreases of concomitant antiepileptic drugs may be needed to minimize side effects due to drug interactions. The dose of felbamate can be increased by 1,200-mg/day incre-

ments at weekly intervals to 3,600 mg/day.

*Lennox-Gastaut syndrome in children, aged 2–14 years.*

As an adjunct, add felbamate at a dose of 15 mg/kg/day in divided doses t.i.d.–q.i.d. while decreasing present antiepileptic drugs by 20%. Further decreases in antiepileptic drug dosage may be needed to minimize side effects due to drug interactions. The dose of felbamate may be increased by 15-mg/kg/day increments at weekly intervals to 45 mg/kg/day.

## DENTAL CONCERNS

See also *Dental Concerns* for *Anticonvulants.*

# Felodipine

(feh-**LOHD**-ih-peen)
**Pregnancy Category:** C
Plendil, Renedil ✳ **(Rx)**
**Classification:** Calcium channel blocking agent

See also *Calcium Channel Blocking Agents.*

**Action/Kinetics: Onset after PO:** 120–300 min. **Peak plasma levels:** 2.5–5 hr. Over 99% bound to plasma protein. **t½, elimination:** 11–16 hr. Metabolized in the liver.

**Uses:** Treatment of mild to moderate hypertension, alone or with other antihypertensives.

**Contraindications:** Hypersensitivity, 2nd or 3rd degree heart block, sick sinus syndrome. Use during lactation.

**Special Concerns:** Use with caution in clients with CHF or compromised ventricular function, especially in combination with a beta-adrenergic blocking agent. Use with caution in impaired hepatic function or reduced hepatic blood flow. Felodipine may cause a greater hypotensive effect in geriatric clients. Safety and effectiveness have not been determined in children.

**Side Effects:** *CV:* Significant hypotension, syncope, angina pectoris, peripheral edema, palpitations, AV block, **MI, arrhythmias,** tachycardia. *CNS:* Dizziness, lightheadedness, headache, nervousness, sleepiness, irritability, anxiety, insomnia, paresthesia, depression, amnesia, paranoia, psychosis, hallucinations. *Body as a whole:* Asthenia, flushing, muscle cramps, pain, inflammation, warm feeling, influenza. *Oral:* Dry mouth, gingival hyperplasia. *GI:* Nausea, abdominal discomfort, cramps, dyspepsia, diarrhea, constipation, vomiting, flatulence. *Dermatologic:* Rash, dermatitis, urticaria, pruritus. *Respiratory:* Rhinitis, rhinorrhea, pharyngitis, sinusitis, nasal and chest congestion, SOB, wheezing, dyspnea, cough, bronchitis, sneezing, respiratory infection. *Miscellaneous:* Anemia, sexual difficulties, epistaxis, back pain, facial edema, erythema, urinary frequency or urgency, dysuria.

**Drug Interactions**
*Anesthetics* / ↑ Effect of felodipine
*Barbiturates* / ↓ Effect of felodipine
*Carbamazepine* / ↑ Effect of felodipine due to ↓ breakdown by liver
*Fentanyl* / Possible severe hypotension or ↑ fluid volume
*Indomethacin* / ↓ Effect of felodipine
*NSAIDs* / ↓ Possible effect of felodipine
*Phenobarbital* / ↓ Effect of felodipine
*Other drugs with hypotensive effects* / ↑ Effect of felodipine

**How Supplied:** *Tablet, extended release:* 2.5 mg, 5 mg, 10 mg

**Dosage**
• **Tablets, Extended Release**
*Hypertension.*
**Initial:** 5 mg once daily (2.5 mg in clients over 65 years of age and in those with impaired liver function); **then:** adjust dose according to response, usually at 2-week intervals with the usual dosage range being 2.5–10 mg once daily. Doses greater than 10 mg increase the rate of peripheral edema and other vasodilatory side effects.

## DENTAL CONCERNS

See also *Dental Concerns* for *Calcium Channel Blocking Agents*.
**General**
1. Frequent visits to assess for gingival hyperplasia.
2. Vasoconstrictors should be used with caution, in low doses, and with careful aspiration. Epinephrine-impregnated gingival retraction cords should be avoided.
**Client/Family Teaching**
1. Practice frequent careful oral hygiene to minimize the incidence and severity of drug-induced gingival hyperplasia.
2. Need for frequent visits with a dental health professional if hyperplasia occurs.

## Fenoprofen calcium

(fen-oh-**PROH**-fen)
**Pregnancy Category:** B
Fenopron, Nalfon **(Rx)**
**Classification:** Nonsteroidal anti-inflammatory analgesic

See also *Nonsteroidal Anti-Inflammatory Drugs*.
**Action/Kinetics: Peak serum levels:** 1–2 hr. **Peak effect:** 2–3 hr. **Duration:** 4–6 hr. **t½:** 2–3 hr. **Onset, as antiarthritic:** Within 2 days; **maximum effect:** 2–3 weeks. Ninety-nine percent protein bound. Food (but not antacids) delays absorption and decreases the total amount absorbed.
**Uses:** Rheumatoid arthritis, osteoarthritis, mild to moderate pain. *Non-FDA Approved Uses:* Juvenile rheumatoid arthritis, prophylaxis of migraine, migraine due to menses, sunburn.
**Contraindications:** Use in pregnancy and children less than 12 years of age.
**Additional Contraindications:** Renal dysfunction.
**Special Concerns:** Safety and efficacy in children have not been established.
**Additional Side Effects:** *GU:* Dysuria, hematuria, cystitis, interstitial nephritis, nephrotic syndrome. Overdosage has caused tachycardia and hypotension.
**How Supplied:** *Capsule:* 200 mg, 300 mg; *Tablet:* 600 mg

**Dosage**
• **Capsules, Tablets**
*Rheumatoid and osteoarthritis.*
**Adults:** 300–600 mg t.i.d.–q.i.d. Adjust dose according to response of client.
*Mild to moderate pain.*
**Adults:** 200 mg q 4–6 hr. Maximum daily dose for all uses: 3,200 mg.

## DENTAL CONCERNS

See also *Dental Concerns* for *Nonsteroidal Anti-Inflammatory Drugs*.

## Fentanyl citrate

(**FEN**-tah-nil)
**Pregnancy Category:** C
Actiq, Fentanyl Oralet, Sublimaze **(C-II) (Rx)**
**Classification:** Opioid analgesic, morphine type

See also *Opioid Analgesics*.
**Action/Kinetics:** Similar to those of morphine and meperidine. **IV. Onset:** 7–8 min. **Peak effect:** Approximately 30 min. **Duration:** 1–2 hr. **t½:** 1.5–6 hr. When the oral lozenge (transmucosal administration) is sucked, fentanyl citrate is absorbed through the mucosal tissues of the mouth and GI tract. **Peak effect, transmucosal:** 20–30 min. Actiq resembles a lollipop; sucking provides a rapid onset of action. Faster-acting and shorter duration than morphine or meperidine.
**Uses: Parenteral:** Preanesthetic medication, induction, and maintenance of anesthesia of short duration and immediate postoperative period. Supplement in general or regional anesthesia. Combined with droperidol for preanesthetic medication, induction of anesthesia, or as adjunct in maintenance of general or regional anesthesia. Combined with oxygen for anesthesia in high-risk clients undergoing open heart sur-

gery, orthopedic procedures, or complicated neurologic procedures.

**Oral (transmucosal):** Anesthetic premedication in children and adults in an operating room setting. To induce conscious sedation before diagnostic or medical procedures (use only in closely monitored situations due to the risk of hypoventilation). Actiq is used for severe pain associated with cancer treatment in those already using an opiate but experience breakthrough pain.

**Contraindications:** The transmucosal form is contraindicated in children who weigh less than 15 kg, for the treatment of acute or chronic pain (safety for this use not established), and for doses in excess of 15 mcg/kg in children and in excess of 5 mcg/kg (maximum of 400 mcg) in adults. Use outside the hospital setting is contraindicated. Myasthenia gravis and other conditions in which muscle relaxants should not be used. Clients particularly sensitive to respiratory depression. Use during labor.

**Special Concerns:** Safety and effectiveness have not been determined in children less than 2 years of age. Use with caution and at reduced dosage in poor-risk clients, children, the elderly, and when other CNS depressants are used. Use of the transmucosal form carries a risk of hypoventilation that may result in death.

**Additional Side Effects:** Skeletal and thoracic muscle rigidity, especially after rapid IV administration. Bradycardia, *seizures,* diaphoresis.

**Additional Drug Interactions:** ↑ Risk of CV depression when high doses of fentanyl are combined with nitrous oxide or diazepam.

**How Supplied:** *Injection:* 0.05 mg/mL; *Lozenge:* 100 mcg, 200 mcg

**Dosage**
- **IM, IV**
  *Preoperatively.*
  **Adults:** 0.05–0.1 mg IM 30–60 min before surgery.
  *Adjunct to anesthesia, induction.*
  **Adults:** 0.002–0.05 mg/kg IV, depending on length and depth of an-

esthesia desired; **maintenance:** 0.025–0.1 mg/kg when indicated.
  *Adjunct to regional anesthesia.*
  **Adults:** 0.05–0.1 mg IM or IV over 1–2 min when indicated.
  *Postoperatively.*
  **Adults:** 0.05–0.1 mg IM q 1–2 hr for control of pain.
  *As general anesthetic with oxygen and a muscle relaxant.*
  0.05–0.1 mg/kg (up to 0.15 mg/kg may be required).
  *Children, induction and maintenance of anesthesia.*
  **Pediatric, 2–12 years:** 2–3 mcg/kg.
  *Children, general anesthetic.*
  0.05–0.1 mg/kg with oxygen and a muscle relaxant when attenuation of the responses to surgical stress is important (e.g., open heart surgery).
- **Transmucosal (Oral Lozenge)**
  Individualize according to weight, age, physical status, general condition and medical status, underlying pathology, use of other drugs, type of anesthetic to be used, and the type and length of the surgical procedure. Doses of 5 mcg/kg are equivalent to IM fentanyl, 0.75–1.25 mcg/kg. Clients receiving more than 5 mcg/kg should be under the direct observation of medical personnel. Children may require up to 15 mcg/kg, provided their body weight is not less than 10 kg. Clients over 65 years of age should receive a dose from 2.5 to 5 mcg/kg. The maximum dose for adults and children, regardless of weight, is 400 mcg.

---

### DENTAL CONCERNS

See also *Dental Concerns* for *Opioid Analgesics.*

---

# Fentanyl Transdermal System
(**FEN**-tah-nil)
**Pregnancy Category:** C
Duragesic-25, -50, -75, and -100 **(C-II) (Rx)**
**Classification:** Opioid analgesic, morphine type

---

See also *Opioid Analgesics* and *Fentanyl citrate*.

**Action/Kinetics:** The system provides continuous delivery of fentanyl for up to 72 hr. The amount of fentanyl released from each system each hour depends on the surface area (25 mcg/hr is released from each 10 cm$^2$). Each system also contains 0.1 mL of alcohol/10 cm$^2$; the alcohol enhances the rate of drug flux through the copolymer membrane and also increases the permeability of the skin to fentanyl. Following application of the system, the skin under the system absorbs fentanyl, resulting in a depot of the drug in the upper skin layers, which is then available to the general circulation. After the system is removed, the residual drug in the skin continues to be absorbed so that serum levels fall 50% in about 17 hr. Metabolized in the liver and excreted mainly in the urine.

**Uses:** Restrict use for the management of severe chronic pain that cannot be managed with less powerful drugs. Only use on clients already on and tolerant to narcotic analgesics and who require continuous narcotic administration.

**Contraindications:** Use for acute or postoperative pain (including out-patient surgeries). To manage mild or intermittent pain that can be managed by acetaminophen-opioid combinations, NSAIDs, or short-acting opioids. Hypersensitivity to fentanyl or adhesives. ICP, impaired consciousness, coma, medical conditions causing hypoventilation. Use during labor and delivery. Use of initial doses exceeding 25 mcg/hr, use in children less than 12 years of age and clients under 18 years of age who weigh less than 50 kg. Lactation.

**Special Concerns:** Use with caution in clients with brain tumors and bradyarrhythmias, as well as in elderly, cachectic, or debilitated individuals. Safety and efficacy have not been determined in children.

**Additional Side Effects:** Sustained hypoventilation.

**How Supplied:** *Film, extended release:* 25 mcg/hr, 50 mcg/hr, 75 mcg/hr, 100 mcg/hr

**Dosage** ────────────────
• **Transdermal System**
  *Analgesia.*
**Adults, usual initial:** 25 mcg/hr unless the client is tolerant to opioids (Duragesic-50, -75, and -100 are intended for use only in clients tolerant to opioids). Initial dose should be based on (1) the daily dose, potency, and characteristics (i.e., pure agonist, mixed agonist/antagonist) of the drug the client has been taking; (2) the reliability of the relative potency estimates used to calculate the dose as estimates vary depending on the route of administration; (3) the degree, if any, of tolerance to narcotics; and (4) the general condition and status of the client.

To convert clients from PO or parenteral opioids to the transdermal system, the following method should be used: (1) the previous 24-hr analgesic requirement should be calculated; (2) convert this amount to the equianalgesic PO morphine dose; (3) find the calculated 24-hr morphine dose and the corresponding transdermal fentanyl dose using the table provided with the product; and (4) initiate treatment using the recommended fentanyl dose. The dose may be increased no more frequently than 3 days after the initial dose or q 6 days thereafter. The ratio of 90 mg/24 hr of PO morphine to 25 mcg/hr increase in transdermal fentanyl dose should be used to base appropriate dosage increments on the daily dose of supplementary opioids.

If the dose of the fentanyl transdermal system exceeds 300 mcg/hr, it may be necessary to change clients to another narcotic analgesic. In such cases, the transdermal system should be removed and treatment initiated with one-half the equianalgesic dose of the new opioid 12–18 hr later. The dose of the new analgesic should be titrated based on the level of pain reported by the client.

## DENTAL CONCERNS

See also *Dental Concerns* for *Opioid Analgesics*.

## Fexofenadine hydrochloride
(fex-oh-**FEN**-ah-deen)
**Pregnancy Category:** C
Allegra **(Rx)**
**Classification:** Antihistamine

See also *Antihistamines*.
**Action/Kinetics:** Fexofenadine, a metabolite of terfenadine, is an $H_1$-histamine receptor blocker. Low to no sedative or anticholinergic effects. **Onset:** Rapid. **Peak plasma levels:** 2.6 hr. **t½, terminal:** 14.4 hr. Approximately 90% of the drug is excreted through the feces (80%) and urine (10%) unchanged.
**Uses:** Seasonal allergic rhinitis in adults and children 12 years of age and older.
**Contraindications:** Hypersensitivity; troglitazone.
**Special Concerns:** Use with care during lactation. Safety and efficacy have not been determined in children less than 12 years of age.
**Side Effects:** *CNS:* Drowsiness, fatigue. *GI:* Nausea, dyspepsia. *Miscellaneous:* Viral infection (flu, colds), dysmenorrhea, sinusitis, throat irritation.
**Drug Interactions:** No differences in side effects or the QTc interval were observed when fexofenadine was given with either erythromycin or ketoconazole.
**How Supplied:** *Capsule:* 60 mg

**Dosage**
• **Capsules**
  *Seasonal allergic rhinitis.*
**Adults and children over 12 years of age:** 60 mg b.i.d. In clients with decreased renal function, the initial dose should be 60 mg once daily.

## DENTAL CONCERNS
**General**
1. Patients taking this drug may require a semisupine position of the dental chair in order to avoid or minimize GI adverse effects.

## Flecainide acetate
(fleh-**KAY**-nyd)
**Pregnancy Category:** C
Tambocor **(Rx)**
**Classification:** Antiarrhythmic, class IC

See also *Antiarrhythmic Agents*.
**Action/Kinetics:** The antiarrhythmic effect is due to a local anesthetic action, especially on the His-Purkinje system in the ventricle. Drug decreases single and multiple PVCs and reduces the incidence of ventricular tachycardia. **Peak plasma levels:** 3 hr.; **steady state levels:** 3–5 days. **Effective plasma levels:** 0.2–1 mcg/mL (trough levels). **t½:** 20 hr (12–27 hr). Forty percent is bound to plasma protein. Approximately 30% is excreted in urine unchanged. Impaired renal function decreases rate of elimination of unchanged drug. Food or antacids do not affect absorption.
**Uses:** Life-threatening arrhythmias manifested as sustained ventricular tachycardia. Prevention of paroxysmal supraventricular tachycardias (PSVT) and paroxysmal atrial fibrillation or flutter (PAF) associated with disabling symptoms but not structural heart disease. Antiarrhythmic drugs have not been shown to improve survival in clients with ventricular arrhythmias.
**Contraindications:** Cardiogenic shock, preexisting second- or third-degree AV block, right bundle branch block when associated with bifascicular block (unless pacemaker is present to maintain cardiac rhythm). Recent MI. Cardiogenic shock. Chronic atrial fibrillation. Frequent premature ventricular complexes and symptomatic nonsustained ventricular arrhythmias. Lactation.

**Special Concerns:** Use with caution in sick sinus syndrome, in clients with a history of CHF or MI, in disturbances of potassium levels, in clients with permanent pacemakers or temporary pacing electrodes, renal and liver impairment. Safety and efficacy in children less than 18 years of age are not established. The incidence of proarrhythmic effects may be increased in geriatric clients.

**Side Effects:** *CV: New or worsened ventricular arrhythmias, increased risk of death in clients with non-life-threatening cardiac arrhythmias,* new or worsened CHF, palpitations, chest pain, sinus bradycardia, sinus pause, sinus arrest, *ventricular fibrillation, ventricular tachycardia that cannot be resuscitated,* second- or third-degree AV block, tachycardia, hypertension, hypotension, bradycardia, angina pectoris. *CNS:* Dizziness, faintness, syncope, lightheadedness, neuropathy, unsteadiness, headache, fatigue, paresthesia, paresis, hypoesthesia, insomnia, anxiety, malaise, vertigo, depression, *seizures,* euphoria, confusion, depersonalization, apathy, morbid dreams, speech disorders, stupor, amnesia, weakness, somnolence. *Oral:* Dry mouth, change in taste. *GI:* Nausea, constipation, abdominal pain, vomiting, anorexia, dyspepsia, diarrhea, flatulence. *Ophthalmic:* Blurred vision, difficulty in focusing, spots before eyes, diplopia, photophobia, eye pain, nystagmus, eye irritation, photophobia. *Hematologic:* Leukopenia, thrombocytopenia. *GU:* Decreased libido, impotence, urinary retention, polyuria. *Musculoskeletal:* Asthenia, tremor, ataxia, arthralgia, myalgia. *Dermatologic:* Skin rashes, urticaria, exfoliative dermatitis, pruritus, alopecia. *Other:* Edema, dyspnea, fever, *bronchospasm,* flushing, sweating, tinnitus, swollen mouth, lips, and tongue.

**Drug Interactions**

No specific interactions have been reported with drugs that are used in dentistry. However, lowest effective dose should be used, such as a local anesthetic, vasoconstrictor, or anticholinergic, if required.

**How Supplied:** *Tablet:* 50 mg, 100 mg, 150 mg

**Dosage** ⎯⎯⎯⎯⎯⎯⎯⎯⎯⎯
• **Tablets**

*Sustained ventricular tachycardia.*

**Initial:** 100 mg q 12 hr; **then,** increase by 50 mg b.i.d. q 4 days until effective dose reached. **Usual effective dose:** 150 mg q 12 hr; dose should not exceed 400 mg/day.

*PSVT, PAF.*

**Initial:** 50 mg q 12 hr; **then,** dose may be increased in increments of 50 mg b.i.d. q 4 days until effective dose reached. Maximum recommended dose: 300 mg/day. *NOTE:* For PAF clients, increasing the dose from 50 to 100 mg b.i.d. may increase efficacy without a significant increase in side effects.

*NOTE:* For clients with a $C_{CR}$ less than 35 mL/min/1.73 m$^2$, the starting dose is 100 mg once daily (or 50 mg b.i.d.). For less severe renal disease, the initial dose may be 100 mg q 12 hr.

## DENTAL CONCERNS

See also *Dental Concerns* for *Antiarrhythmic Agents.*

# Fluconazole

(flew-**KON**-ah-zohl)
**Pregnancy Category:** C
Diflucan, Difulcan-150 ✿ **(Rx)**
**Classification:** Antifungal agent

**Action/Kinetics:** Inhibits the enzyme cytochrome P-450 in the organism, which results in a decrease in cell wall integrity and extrusion of intracellular material, leading to death. Apparently does not affect the cytochrome P-450 enzyme in animals or humans. **Peak plasma levels:** 1–2 hr. **t½:** 30 hr, which allows for once daily dosing. Penetrates all body fluids at steady state. Bioavailability is not affected by agents that increase gastric pH. Eighty percent of the drug is excreted unchanged by the kidneys.

**Uses:** Oropharyngeal and esophageal candidiasis. Serious systemic candidal infection (including UTIs, peritonitis, and pneumonia). Cryptococcal meningitis. Maintenance therapy to prevent cryptococcal meningitis in AIDS clients. Vaginal candidiasis. To decrease the incidence of candidiasis in clients undergoing a bone marrow transplant who receive cytotoxic chemotherapy or radiation therapy. Treatment of cryptococcal meningitis and candidal infections in children.

**Contraindications:** Hypersensitivity to fluconazole.

**Special Concerns:** Use with caution if client shows hypersensitivity to other azoles. Care should be used when fluconazole is prescribed during lactation. The effectiveness of the drug has not been adequately assessed in children. Use with caution in clients taking either astemizole or terfenadine. The risk for dysrhythmias is unknown.

**Side Effects: Following single doses.** *GI:* Nausea, abdominal pain, diarrhea, dyspepsia, taste perversion. *CNS:* Headache, dizziness. *Other:* Angioedema, **anaphylaxis (rare).**

**Following multiple doses.** Side effects are more frequently reported in HIV-infected clients than in non-HIV-infected clients. *GI:* N&V, abdominal pain, diarrhea, **serious hepatic reactions.** *CNS:* Headache, **seizures.** *Dermatologic:* Skin rash, exfoliative skin disorders (including **Stevens-Johnson syndrome,** and toxic epidermal necrolysis), alopecia. *Hematologic:* Leukopenia, thrombocytopenia. *Other:* Hypercholesterolemia, hypertriglyceridemia, hypokalemia.

**Drug Interactions**
*Benzodiazepines* / ↓ Metabolism of benzodiazepines
*Cimetidine* / ↓ Plasma levels of fluconazole
*Cyclosporine* / Fluconazole may ↑ cyclosporine levels in renal transplant clients with or without impaired renal function

*Hydrochlorothiazide* / ↑ Plasma levels of fluconazole due to ↓ renal clearance
*Glipizide* / ↑ Plasma levels of glipizide due to ↓ breakdown by the liver
*Glyburide* / ↑ Plasma levels of glyburide due to ↓ breakdown by the liver
*Phenytoin* / Fluconazole ↑ plasma levels of phenytoin
*Rifampin* / ↓ Plasma levels of fluconazole due to ↑ breakdown by the liver
*Theophylline* / ↑ Plasma levels of theophylline
*Tolbutamide* / ↑ Plasma levels of tolbutamide due to ↓ breakdown by the liver
*Warfarin* / ↑ PT
*Zidovudine* / ↑ Plasma levels of AZT

**How Supplied:** *Injection:* 2 mg/mL, 200 mg/100 mL, 400 mg/200 mL; *Powder for reconstitution:* 50 mg/5 mL, 200 mg/5 mL; *Tablet:* 50 mg, 100 mg, 150 mg, 200 mg

**Dosage** ─────────────
• **Tablets, Oral Suspension, IV**
*Vaginal candidiasis.*
150 mg as a single oral dose.

*Oropharyngeal or esophageal candidiasis.*
**Adults, first day:** 200 mg; **then,** 100 mg/day for a minimum of 14 days (for oropharyngeal candidiasis) or 21 days (for esophageal candidiasis). Up to 400 mg/day may be required for esophageal candidiasis. **Children, first day:** 6 mg/kg; **then,** 3 mg/kg once daily for a minimum of 14 days (for oropharyngeal candidiasis) or 21 days (for esophageal candidiasis).

*Candidal UTI and peritonitis.*
50–200 mg/day.

*Systemic candidiasis (e.g., candidemia, disseminated candidiasis, and pneumonia).*
Optimal dosage and duration in adults have not been determined although doses up to 400 mg/day have been used. **Children:** 6–12 mg/kg/day.

*Acute cryptococcal meningitis.*

**Adults, first day:** 400 mg; **then,** 200 mg/day (up to 400 mg may be required) for 10 to 12 weeks after CSF culture is negative. **Children, first day:** 12 mg/kg; **then,** 6 mg/kg once daily for 10 to 12 weeks after CSF culture is negative.

*Maintenance to prevent relapse of cryptococcal meningitis in AIDS clients.*
**Adults:** 200 mg once daily. **Pediatric:** 6 mg/kg once daily.

*Prevention of candidiasis in bone marrow transplant.*
400 mg once daily. In clients expected to have severe granulocytopenia (less than 500 neutrophils/mm³), fluconazole should be started several days before the anticipated onset of neutropenia and continued for 7 days after the neutrophil count rises about 1,000 cells/mm³. In clients with renal impairment, an initial loading dose of 50–400 mg can be given; daily dose is based then on $C_{CR}$.

## DENTAL CONCERNS

See also *General Dental Concerns for All Anti-Infectives.*
**Client/Family Teaching**
1. Replace toothbrush or other oral hygiene devices used during treatment of oral infection in order to prevent reinfection.
2. Long-term therapy may be necessary. Complete the full course of antifungal therapy.

# Fluorouracil
# (5-Fluorouracil, 5-FU)
(flew-roh-**YOUR**-ah-sill)
**Pregnancy Category:** X
Adrucil, Efudex, Fluoroplex (Abbreviation: 5-FU) **(Rx)**
**Classification:** Antineoplastic, antimetabolite

**Action/Kinetics:** Pyrimidine antagonist that inhibits the methylation reaction of deoxyuridylic acid to thymidylic acid. Thus, synthesis of DNA and, to a lesser extent, RNA is inhibited.

**t½, initial:** 5–20 min; **final:** 20 hr. From 60% to 80% eliminated as respiratory $CO_2$ (8–12 hr); small amount (15%) excreted unchanged in urine (1–6 hr). Highly toxic; initiate use in hospital. When used topically, the following response occurs:
• Early inflammation: erythema for several days (minimal reaction)
• Severe inflammation: burning, stinging, vesiculation
• Disintegration: erosion, ulceration, necrosis, pain, crusting, reepithelialization
• Healing: within 1–2 weeks with some residual erythema and temporary hyperpigmentation

**Uses: Systemic:** Palliative management of certain cancers of the rectum, stomach, colon, pancreas, and breast. In combination with levamisole for Dukes' stage C colon cancer after surgical resection. In combination with leucovorin for metastatic colorectal cancer. *Non-FDA Approved Uses:* Cancer of the bladder, ovaries, prostate, cervix, endometrium, lung, liver, head, and neck. Also, malignant pleural, peritoneal, and pericardial effusions. **Topical (as solution or cream):** Multiple actinic or solar keratoses. Superficial basal cell carcinoma. *Non-FDA Approved Uses:* Condylomata acuminata (1% solution in 70% ethanol or the 5% cream).

**Contraindications:** Hypersensitivity. Pregnancy.

**Special Concerns:** Safety and efficacy of topical products have not been established in children. Occlusive dressings may result in increased inflammation in adjacent normal skin when topical products are used.

**Side Effects: Topical:** *Dermatologic:* Pain, pruritus, hyperpigmentation, irritation, inflammation, burning at site of application, scarring, soreness, allergic contact dermatitis, tenderness, scaling, swelling, suppuration, alopecia, photosensitivity, urticaria. *CNS:* Insomnia, irritability. *Oral:* Stomatitis, medicinal taste. *Miscellane-*

*ous:* Lacrimation, telangiectasia, toxic granulation.

**Drug Interactions:** None reported for topical dose form. Use caution with drugs that may cause photosensitivity.

**How Supplied:** *Cream:* 1%, 5%; *Solution:* 1%, 2%, 5%

**Dosage** ⎯⎯⎯⎯⎯⎯⎯⎯⎯⎯⎯

• **Cream, Topical Solution**
*Actinic or solar keratoses.*
Apply 1%–5% cream or solution to cover lesion 1–2 times/day for 2–6 weeks.
*Superficial basal cell carcinoma.*
Apply 5% cream or solution to cover lesion b.i.d. for 3–6 weeks (up to 10–12 weeks may be required).

## DENTAL CONCERNS

1. Topical dose form: Be aware of the patient's disease and avoid the affected area in order to prevent further irritation.

**Client/Family Teaching**

1. Review and demonstrate appropriate method for topical administration.

2. Affected area may appear much worse before healing takes place in 1–2 months.

3. Avoid exposure to sunlight. If exposed, wear protective clothing, sunglasses, and sunscreen.

# Fluoxetine hydrochloride

(flew-**OX**-eh-teen)
**Pregnancy Category:** B
Apo-Fluoxetine ✶, Dom-Fluoxetine ✶, Novo-Fluoxetine ✶, Nu-Fluoxetine ✶, PMS-Fluoxetine ✶, Prozac, STCC-Fluoxetine ✶ **(Rx)**
**Classification:** Antidepressant, selective serotonin reuptake inhibitor

See also *Selective Serotonin Reuptake Inhibitors.*

**Action/Kinetics:** Effect thought to be due to inhibition of uptake of serotonin into CNS neurons. Slight to no anticholinergic, sedative, or orthostatic hypotensive effects. Also binds to muscarinic, histaminergic, and alpha-1-adrenergic receptors, accounting for many of the side effects. Metabolized in the liver to norfluoxetine, a metabolite with equal potency to fluoxetine. Norfluoxetine is further metabolized by the liver to inactive metabolites that are excreted by the kidneys. **Time to peak plasma levels:** 6–8 hr. **Peak plasma concentrations:** 15–55 ng/mL. **t½, fluoxetine:** 2–7 days; **t½, norfluoxetine:** 7–9 days. **Time to steady state:** 2–4 weeks. Active drug maintained in the body for weeks after withdrawal.

**Uses:** Depression, obsessive-compulsive disorders (as defined in the current edition of DSM), bulimia nervosa. *Non-FDA Approved Uses:* Many (see *Dosage*).

**Contraindications:** Use with or within 14 days of discontinuing an MAO inhibitor.

**Special Concerns:** Use with caution during lactation and in clients with impaired liver or kidney function. Safety and efficacy have not been determined in children. A lower initial dose may be necessary in geriatric clients. Use in hospitalized clients, use for longer than 5–6 weeks for depression, or use for more than 13 weeks for obsessive-compulsive disorder has not been studied adequately.

**Side Effects:** A large number of side effects have been reported for this drug. Listed are those with a reported frequency of greater than 1%. *CNS:* Headache (most common), activation of mania or hypomania, insomnia, anxiety, nervousness, dizziness, fatigue, sedation, decreased libido, drowsiness, lightheadedness, decreased ability to concentrate, tremor, disturbances in sensation, agitation, abnormal dreams. Although less frequent than 1%, *some clients may experience seizures or attempt suicide.* Oral: Dry mouth, alteration in taste. *GI:* Nausea (most common), diarrhea, vomiting, constipation, dyspepsia, anorexia, abdominal pain, flatulence, gastroenteritis, increased appetite. *CV:* Hot flashes, palpitations. *GU:* Sexual dysfunction, impotence, anorgasmia, frequent urination, infection of the urinary tract, dysmenorrhea. *Respiratory:*

Upper respiratory tract infections, pharyngitis, cough, dyspnea, rhinitis, bronchitis, nasal congestion, sinusitis, sinus headache, yawn. *Skin:* Rash, pruritus, excessive sweating. *Musculoskeletal:* Muscle, joint, or back pain. *Miscellaneous:* Flu-like symptoms, asthenia, fever, chest pain, allergy, visual disturbances, blurred vision, weight loss, bacterial or viral infection, limb pain, chills.

**Drug Interactions**
*Alprazolam* / ↑ Alprazolam levels and ↓ psychomotor performance
*Carbamazepine* / ↑ Serum levels of carbamazepine → toxicity
*Diazepam* / Fluoxetine ↑ half-life of diazepam → excessive sedation or impaired psychomotor skills
*MAO inhibitors* / MAO inhibitors should be discontinued 14 days before initiation of fluoxetine therapy due to the possibility of symptoms resembling a neuroleptic malignant syndrome or fatal reactions
*Phenytoin* / Fluoxetine may ↑ phenytoin levels
*Tricyclic antidepressants* / ↑ Pharmacologic and toxicologic effects of tricyclics due to ↓ breakdown by liver

**How Supplied:** *Capsule:* 10 mg, 20 mg; *Solution:* 20 mg/5 mL

**Dosage**
• **Capsules, Liquid**
*Antidepressant.*
**Adults, initial:** 20 mg/day in the morning. If clinical improvement is not observed after several weeks, the dose may be increased to a maximum of 80 mg/day in two equally divided doses.
*Obsessive-compulsive disorder.*
**Initial:** 20 mg/day in the morning. If improvement is not significant after several weeks, the dose may be increased. **Usual dosage range:** 20–60 mg/day; the total daily dosage should not exceed 80 mg.
*Treatment of bulimia nervosa.*
60 mg/day given in the morning. May be necessary to titrate up to this dose over several days.

*Alcoholism.*
40–80 mg/day.
*Anorexia nervosa, bipolar II affective disorder, trichotillomania.*
20–80 mg/day.
*Attention deficit hyperactivity disorder, obesity, schizophrenia.*
20–60 mg/day.
*Borderline personality disorder.*
5–80 mg/day.
*Cataplexy and narcolepsy, Tourette's syndrome.*
20–40 mg/day.
*Kleptomania.*
60–80 mg/day.
*Migraine, chronic daily headaches, tension headaches.*
20 mg every other day to 40 mg/day.
*Posttraumatic stress disorder.*
10–80 mg/day.
*Premenstrual syndrome, recurrent syncope.*
20 mg/day.
*Levodopa-induced dyskinesia.*
40 mg/day.
*Social phobia.*
10–60 mg/day.

## DENTAL CONCERNS

See also *Dental Concerns* for *Antidepressants, Tricyclic* and *Selective Serotonin Reuptake Inhibitors.*

# Fluphenazine decanoate
(flew-**FEN**-ah-zeen)
Modecate Decanoate ✤, PMS-Fluphenazine ✤, Prolixin Decanoate, Rho-Fluphenazine Decanoate ✤ **(Rx)**

# Fluphenazine enanthate
(flew-**FEN**-ah-zeen)
Moditen Enanthate ✤, Prolixin Enanthate **(Rx)**

# Fluphenazine hydrochloride
(flew-**FEN**-ah-zeen)
Apo-Fluphenazine ✤, Permitil, Prolixin, Moditen HCl ✤, PMS-Fluphenazine ✤ **(Rx)**
**Classification:** Antipsychotic, piperazine-type phenothiazine

See also *Antipsychotic Agents, Phenothiazines.*

**Action/Kinetics:** High incidence of extrapyramidal symptoms and a low incidence of sedation, anticholinergic effects, antiemetic effects, and orthostatic hypotension. The enanthate and decanoate esters dramatically increase the duration of action. *Decanoate:* **Onset,** 24–72 hr; **peak plasma levels,** 24–48 hr; **t½** (approximate), 14 days; **duration,** up to 4 weeks. *Enanthate:* **Onset,** 24–72 hr; **peak plasma levels,** 48–72 hr; **t½** (approximate), 3.6 days; **duration,** 1–3 weeks.

Fluphenazine hydrochloride can be cautiously administered to clients with known hypersensitivity to other phenothiazines.

Fluphenazine enanthate may replace fluphenazine hydrochloride if desired response occurs with hypersensitivity reaction to fluphenazine.

**Uses:** Psychotic disorders. Adjunct to tricyclic antidepressants for chronic pain states (e.g., diabetic neuropathy, and clients trying to withdraw from narcotics).

**How Supplied:** Fluphenazine decanoate: *Injection:* 25 mg/mL Fluphenazine enanthate: *Injection:* 25 mg/mL. Fluphenazine hydrochloride: *Concentrate:* 5 mg/mL; *Elixir:* 2.5 mg/5 mL; *Injection:* 2.5 mg/mL; *Tablet:* 1 mg, 2.5 mg, 5 mg

**Dosage** ————————————
Fluphenazine hydrochloride is administered **PO and IM.** Fluphenazine enanthate or decanoate is administered **SC and IM.**

*Hydrochloride.*
• **Elixir, Oral Solution, Tablets**
*Psychotic disorders.*

**Adults and adolescents, initial:** 2.5–10 mg/day in divided doses q 6–8 hr; **then,** reduce gradually to maintenance dose of 1–5 mg/day (usually given as a single dose, not to exceed 20 mg/day). **Geriatric, emaciated, debilitated clients, initial:** 1–2.5 mg/day; **then,** dosage determined by response. **Pediatric:** 0.25–0.75 mg 1–4 times/day.

*Hydrochloride.*

• **IM**
*Psychotic disorders.*

**Adults and adolescents:** 1.25–2.5 mg q 6–8 hr as needed. Maximum daily dose: 10 mg. Elderly, debilitated, or emaciated clients should start with 1–2.5 mg/day.

*Decanoate.*
• **IM, SC**
*Psychotic disorders.*

**Adults, initial:** 12.5–25 mg; **then,** the dose may be repeated or increased q 1–3 weeks. The usual maintenance dose is 50 mg/1–4 weeks. Maximum adult dose: 100 mg/dose. **Pediatric, 12 years and older:** 6.25–18.75 mg/week; the dose can be increased to 12.5–25 mg given q 1–3 weeks. **Pediatric, 5–12 years:** 3.125–12.5 mg with this dose being repeated q 1–3 weeks.

*Enanthate.*
• **IM, SC**
*Psychotic disorders.*

**Adults and adolescents:** 25 mg; dose can be repeated or increased q 1–3 weeks. For doses greater than 50 mg, increases should be made in increments of 12.5 mg. Maximum adult dose: 100 mg.

## DENTAL CONCERNS

See also *Dental Concerns* for *Antipsychotic Agents, Phenothiazines.*

# Flurazepam hydrochloride
(flur-**AYZ**-eh-pam)
Apo-Flurazepam ✤, Dalmane, Durapam, Novo-Flupam ✤, PMS-Flurazepam ✤, Somnol ✤, Som Pam ✤
**(C-IV) (Rx)**
**Classification:** Benzodiazepine sedative-hypnotic

See also *Sedative-Hypnotics* (Antianxiety)/*Antimanic Drugs.*

**Action/Kinetics:** Combines with benzodiazepine receptors, which are part of the benzodiazepine-GABA receptor-chloride ionophore complex. Results in enhanced inhibitory action of GABA leading to interference of transmission of nerve impulses in the reticular activating system. **Onset:** 17 min. The major active metabolite, *N*-desalkyl-flu-razepam, is active and has a **t½** of 47–100 hr. **Time to peak plasma levels, flurazepam:** 0.5–1 hr; **active metabolite:** 1–3 hr. **Duration:** 7–8 hr. **Maximum effectiveness:** 2–3 days (due to slow accumulation of active metabolite). Significantly bound to plasma protein. Elimination is slow because metabolites remain in the blood for several days. Exceeding the recommended dose may result in development of tolerance and dependence.

**Uses:** Insomnia (all types). Flurazepam is increasingly effective on the second or third night of consecutive use and for one or two nights after the drug is discontinued.

**Contraindications:** Hypersensitivity. Pregnancy or in women wishing to become pregnant. Depression, renal or hepatic disease, chronic pulmonary insufficiency, children under 15 years.

**Special Concerns:** Use during the last few weeks of pregnancy may result in CNS depression of the neonate. Use during lactation may cause sedation and feeding problems in the infant. Geriatric clients may be more sensitive to the effects of flurazepam.

**Side Effects:** *CNS:* Ataxia, dizziness, drowsiness/sedation, headache, disorientation. Symptoms of stimulation including nervousness, apprehension, irritability, and talkativeness. *Oral:* Dry mouth. *GI:* N&V, diarrhea, gastric upset or pain, heartburn, constipation. *Miscellaneous:* Arthralgia, chest pains, or palpitations. Rarely, symptoms of allergy, SOB, jaundice, anorexia, blurred vision.

**Drug Interactions**
*Cimetidine* / ↑ Effect of flurazepam due to ↓ breakdown by liver
*CNS depressants* / Addition or potentiation of CNS depressant effects—drowsiness, lethargy, stupor, respiratory depression or collapse, coma, and possible death

*Ethanol* / Additive depressant effects up to the day following flurazepam administration

**How Supplied:** *Capsule:* 15 mg, 30 mg

**Dosage** ────────────
• **Capsules**
**Adults:** 15–30 mg at bedtime; 15 mg for geriatric and/or debilitated clients.

## DENTAL CONCERNS

See also *Dental Concerns* for *Sedative-Hypnotics* (Anti-anxiety)/*Antimanic Drugs*.
1. Elderly clients may experience adverse reactions more quickly than younger clients; use a lower dose in this group.

# Flutamide
(**FLOO**-tah-myd)
**Pregnancy Category:** D
Euflex ✿, Eulexin **(Rx)**
**Classification:** Antineoplastic, hormonal agent

See also *Antineoplastic Agents*.
**Action/Kinetics:** Acts either to inhibit uptake of androgen or to inhibit nuclear binding of androgen in target tissues. Thus, the effect of androgen is decreased in androgen-sensitive tissues. Rapidly metabolized to active (alpha-hydroxylated derivative) and inactive metabolites in the liver and mainly excreted in the urine. **t½ of active metabolite:** 6 hr (8 hr in geriatric clients). Ninety-four percent to 96% is bound to plasma proteins.

**Uses:** In combination with leuprolide acetate (i.e., a LHRH agonist) to treat stage $D_2$ metastatic prostatic carcinoma as well as locally confined stage $B_2$-C prostate cancer.

**Contraindications:** Use during pregnancy.

**Side Effects:** Side effects are listed for treatment of flutamide with LHRH agonist. *GU:* Loss of libido, impotence. *CV:* Hot flashes, hypertension. *Oral:* Dry mouth, stomatitis. *GI:* N&V, diarrhea, GI disturbances, anorexia. *CNS:* Confusion, depression, drowsiness, anxiety, nervousness. *Hematologic:* Anemia, leukopenia, thrombocytopenia, **hemolytic anemia,** macrocytic anemia, methemoglobinemia. *Hepatic:* Hepatitis, cholestatic jaundice, hepatic encephalopathy, **hepatic necrosis.** *Dermatologic:* Rash, injection site irritation, erythema, ulceration, bullous eruptions, *epidermal necrolysis. Miscellaneous:* Gynecomastia, edema, neuromuscular symptoms, pulmonary symptoms, GU symptoms, malignant breast tumors.

**How Supplied:** *Capsule:* 125 mg

## Dosage

* **Capsules**
    *Locally confined stage B₂-C and stage D₂ metastatic cancer of the prostate.*
    250 mg (2 capsules) t.i.d. q 8 hr for a total daily dose of 750 mg.

## DENTAL CONCERNS

See also *Dental Concerns* for *Antineoplastic Agents.*

---

# Fluticasone propionate
(flu-**TIH**-kah-sohn)
**Pregnancy Category:** C
Flonase, Flovent **(Rx)**
**Classification:** Corticosteroid

See also *Corticosteroids.*
**Action/Kinetics:** Following intranasal use, a small amount is absorbed into the general circulation. **Onset:** Approximately 12 hr. **Maximum effect:** May take several days. Absorbed drug is metabolized in the liver and excreted in the urine.
**Uses:** Maintenance treatment of asthma in adults and children over four years of age. To manage seasonal and perennial allergic rhinitis in adults and children over four years of age.
**Contraindications:** Use for nonallergic rhinitis. Use following nasal septal ulcers, nasal surgery, or nasal trauma until healing has occurred.
**Special Concerns:** Safety and efficacy in children less than 12 years of age

have not been determined. Clients on immunosuppressant drugs, such as corticosteroids, are more susceptible to infections. Use with caution, if at all, in active or quiescent tuberculosis infections; untreated fungal, bacterial, or systemic viral infections; or ocular herpes simplex. Use with caution during lactation.
**Side Effects:** *Allergic:* Rarely, immediate hypersensitivity reactions or contact dermatitis. *Respiratory:* Epistaxis, nasal burning, blood in nasal mucus, pharyngitis, irritation of nasal mucous membranes, sneezing, runny nose, nasal dryness, sinusitis, nasal congestion, bronchitis, nasal ulcer, nasal septum excoriation. *CNS:* Headache, dizziness. *Ophthalmologic:* Eye disorder, cataracts, glaucoma, increased intraocular pressure. *Oral:* Dry mouth, candidiasis. *GI:* N&V, xerostomia. *Miscellaneous:* Unpleasant taste, urticaria. High doses have resulted in hypercorticism and adrenal suppression.
**How Supplied:** *Metered dose inhaler:* 0.11 mg/inh, 0.22 mg/inh, 0.44 mg/inh; *Nasal spray:* 0.05 mg/inh; *Ointment:* 0.005%; *Cream:* 0.05%

## Dosage

* **Metered Dose Inhaler**
    *Treatment of asthma.*
**Adults and children over 4 years of age, initial:** 100 mcg b.i.d. For oral steroid sparing, the recommended dose is 1,000 mcg b.i.d.
* **Nasal Spray**
    *Allergic rhinitis.*
**Adults and children over 4 years of age, initial:** One 50-mcg spray in each nostril once a day, for a total daily dose of 100 mcg/day. Maximum dose is two sprays (200 mcg) in each nostril once a day.
* **Ointment, Cream**
Apply sparingly to affected area 2–4 times daily.

## DENTAL CONCERNS
**General**
1. Examine the patient for the presence of oral candidiasis, especially in patients using the oral spray.
2. Allergic rhinitis may cause dry

mouth because the patient mouth breathes in an attempt to compensate for nasal congestion.

**Client/Family Teaching**

1. Daily home fluoride treatments for persistent dry mouth.
2. Avoid alcohol-containing mouth rinses and beverages.
3. Avoid caffeine-containing beverages.
4. Dry mouth can be treated with tart, sugarless gum or candy, water, sugar-free beverages, or with saliva substitutes if dry mouth persists.
5. Review use, care, and storage of inhaler. Rinse out mouth and wash the mouth piece, spacer, sprayer and dry after each use.
6. Review technique for use and care of prescribed inhalers and respiratory equipment. Rinsing of equipment and of mouth after use is imperative in preventing oral fungal infections.

## Fluvastatin sodium

(flu-vah-**STAH**-tin)
**Pregnancy Category:** X
Lescol **(Rx)**
**Classification:** Antihyperlipidemic agent

See also *Antihyperlipidemic Agents—HMG-CoA Reductase Inhibitors.*

**Action/Kinetics:** t½: 1.2 hr. Undergoes extensive first-pass metabolism. Significantly bound (greater than 98%) to plasma protein. Metabolized in the liver with 90% excreted through the feces and 5% through the urine.

**Uses:** Adjunct to diet for the reduction of elevated total and LDL cholesterol levels in clients with primary hypercholesterolemia. The lipid-lowering effects of fluvastatin are enhanced when it is combined with a bile-acid binding resin or with niacin. To slow the progression of coronary atherosclerosis in coronary heart disease.

**Contraindications:** Hypersensitivity, active liver disease, pregnancy, lactation, children under the age of 18.

**Special Concerns:** Use with caution in clients with severe renal impairment.

**Side Effects:** Side effects listed are those most common with fluvastatin. A complete list of possible side effects is provided under *Antihyperlipidemic Agents—HMG-CoA Reductase Inhibitors. GI:* N&V, diarrhea, abdominal pain or cramps, constipation, flatulence, dyspepsia, tooth disorder. *Musculoskeletal:* Muscle cramps or pain, back pain, arthropathy. *CNS:* Headache, dizziness, insomnia. *Respiratory:* Upper respiratory infection, rhinitis, cough, pharyngitis, sinusitis, bronchitis. *Miscellaneous:* Rash, pruritus, fatigue, influenza, allergy, accidental trauma.

**Drug Interactions**
No specific interactions have been reported with drugs that are used in dentistry. However, this drug should not be used with erythromycin or cyclosporine.

**How Supplied:** *Capsule:* 20 mg, 40 mg

**Dosage** —————————

• **Capsules**

*Antihyperlipidemic to slow progression of coronary atherosclerosis.*
**Adults:** 20 mg once daily at bedtime. **Dose range:** 20–40 mg/day as a single dose in the evening. Splitting the 40-mg dose into a twice-daily regimen results in a modest improvement in LDL cholesterol.

## DENTAL CONCERNS

See also *Dental Concerns* for *Antihyperlipidemic Agents—HMG-CoA Reductase Inhibitors.*

## Fluvoxamine maleate

(flu-**VOX**-ah-meen)
**Pregnancy Category:** C
Luvox **(Rx)**
**Classification:** Antidepressant, selective serotonin uptake inhibitor

See also *Antidepressants, Tricyclic* and *Selective Serotonin Reuptake Inhibitors.*

**F**

---

**Action/Kinetics:** Mechanism in obsessive-compulsive disorders is likely due to inhibition of serotonin reuptake in the CNS. Produces few if any anticholinergic, sedative, or orthostatic hypotensive effects. **Maximum plasma levels:** 3–8 hr. About 80% if bound to plasma proteins. **t½:** 13.6–15.6 hr. **Peak plasma concentration:** 88–546 ng/mL. **Time to reach steady state:** 3–8 hr. Elderly clients manifest higher mean plasma levels and a decreased clearance. Metabolized in the liver and excreted through the urine.

**Uses:** Obsessive-compulsive disorder (as defined in DSM-III-R) for adults, adolescents, and children. *Non-FDA Approved Uses:* Treatment of depression.

**Contraindications:** Concomitant use with astemizole or terfenadine. Alcohol ingestion. Use with MAO inhibitors or within 14 days of discontinuing treatment with an MAO inhibitor. Lactation.

**Special Concerns:** Use with caution in clients with a history of mania, seizure disorders, and liver dysfunction and in those with diseases that could affect hemodynamic responses or metabolism. Safety and efficacy have not been determined in children less than 18 years of age.

**Side Effects:** Side effects listed occur at an incidence of 0.1% or greater. *CNS:* Somnolence, insomnia, nervousness, dizziness, tremor, anxiety, hypertonia, agitation, decreased libido, depression, CNS stimulation, amnesia, apathy, hyperkinesia, hypokinesia, manic reaction, myoclonus, psychoses, fatigue, malaise, agoraphobia, akathisia, ataxia, *convulsion,* delirium, delusion, depersonalization, drug dependence, dyskinesia, dystonia, emotional lability, euphoria, extrapyramidal syndrome, unsteady gait, hallucinations, hemiplegia, hostility, hypersomnia, hypochondriasis, hypotonia, hysteria, incoordination, increased libido, neuralgia, paralysis, paranoia, phobia, sleep disorders, stupor, twitching, vertigo. *Oral:* Dry mouth, dysphagia, toothache, tooth caries, gingivitis, glossitis, stomatitis. *GI:* Nausea, diarrhea, constipation, dyspepsia, anorexia, vomiting, flatulence, dysphagia, colitis, eructation, esophagitis, gastritis, gastroenteritis, *GI hemorrhage,* GI ulcer, hemorrhoids, melena, rectal hemorrhage. *CV:* Palpitations, hypertension, postural hypotension, vasodilation, syncope, tachycardia, angina pectoris, bradycardia, *cardiomyopathy,* CV disease, cold extremities, conduction delay, *heart failure, MI,* pallor, irregular pulse, ST segment changes. *Respiratory:* Upper respiratory infection, dyspnea, yawn, increased cough, sinusitis, asthma, bronchitis, epistaxis, hoarseness, hyperventilation. *Body as a whole:* Headache, asthenia, flu syndrome, chills, malaise, edema, weight gain or loss, dehydration, hypercholesterolemia, allergic reaction, neck pain, neck rigidity, photosensitivity, *suicide attempt. Dermatologic:* Excessive sweating, acne, alopecia, dry skin, eczema, exfoliative dermatitis, furunculosis, seborrhea, skin discoloration, urticaria. *Musculoskeletal:* Arthralgia, arthritis, bursitis, generalized muscle spasm, myasthenia, tendinous contracture, tenosynovitis. *GU:* Delayed ejaculation, urinary frequency, impotence, anorgasmia, urinary retention, anuria, breast pain, cystitis, delayed menstruation, dysuria, female lactation, hematuria, menopause, menorrhagia, metrorrhagia, nocturia, polyuria, PMS, urinary incontinence, UTI, urinary urgency, impaired urination, *vaginal hemorrhage,* vaginitis. *Hematologic:* Anemia, ecchymosis, leukocytosis, lymphadenopathy, thrombocytopenia. *Ophthalmic:* Amblyopia, abnormal accommodation, conjunctivitis, diplopia, dry eyes, eye pain, mydriasis, photophobia, visual field defect. *Otic:* Deafness, ear pain, otitis media. *Miscellaneous:* Taste perversion or loss, parosmia, hypothyroidism, hypercholesterolemia, dehydration.

**Drug Interactions**
*Astemisole* / ↑ Risk of severe cardiovascular effects, including QT prolongation, ventricular tachycardia,

and torsades de pointes (may be fatal)

*Carbamazepine* / ↑ Risk of carbamazepine toxicity

*Diazepam* / ↑ Effect of diazepam due to ↓ clearance

*MAO inhibitors* / Serious and possibly fatal reactions, including hyperthermia, rigidity, myoclonus, rapid fluctuations of VS, changes in mental status (agitation, delirium, coma)

*Methadone* / ↑ Risk of methadone toxicity

*Midazolam* / ↑ Effect of midazolam due to ↓ clearance

*Terfenadine* / ↑ Risk of severe cardiovascular effects, including QT prolongation, ventricular tachycardia, and torsades de pointes (may be fatal)

*Triazolam* / ↑ Effect of triazolam due to ↓ clearance

*Tricyclic antidepressants* / Significant ↑ in plasma levels of tricyclic antidepressants

**How Supplied:** *Tablet:* 50 mg, 100 mg

**Dosage** ———————
- **Tablets**

  *Obsessive-compulsive disorder.*

**Adults, initial:** 50 mg at bedtime; **then,** increase the dose in 50-mg increments q 4–7 days, as tolerated, until a maximum benefit is reached, not to exceed 300 mg/day. **Children and adolescents:** 25 mg at bedtime; **then,** increase the dose in 25-mg increments q 4–7 days until a maximum benefit is reached, not to exceed 200 mg/day.

**DENTAL CONCERNS**

See also *Dental Concerns* for *Antidepressants, Tricyclic* and *Selective Serotonin Reuptake Inhibitors.*

## Fosfomycin tromethamine
(fos-foh-**MY**-sin)
**Pregnancy Category:** B
Monurol **(Rx)**

**Classification:** Anti-infective, antibiotic

See also *Anti-Infective Agents.*

**Action/Kinetics:** Bactericidal drug that inactivates enzyme enolpyruvyl transferase, irreversibly blocking condensation of uridine diphosphate-N-acetylglucosamine with p-enolpyruvate. This is one of first steps in bacterial wall synthesis. Also reduces adherence of bacteria to uroepithelial cells. Rapidly absorbed from GI tract and converted to fosfomycin. **Maximum serum levels:** 2 hr. **t½, elimination:** 5.7 hr. Excreted unchanged in both urine and feces.

**Uses:** Treatment of uncomplicated urinary tract infections (acute cystitis) in women due to *Escherichia coli* and *Enterococcus faecalis.*

**Contraindications:** Lactation.

**Special Concerns:** Safety and efficacy have not been determined in children 12 years and younger.

**Side Effects:** *Oral:* Dry mouth. *GI:* Diarrhea, nausea, dyspepsia, abdominal pain, abnormal stools, anorexia, constipation, flatulence, vomiting. *CNS:* Headache, dizziness, insomnia, migraine, nervousness, paresthesia, somnolence. *GU:* Vaginitis, dysmenorrhea, dysuria, hematuria, menstrual disorder. *Respiratory:* Rhinitis, pharyngitis. *Miscellaneous:* Asthenia, back pain, pain, rash, ear disorder, fever, flu syndrome, infection, lymphadenopathy, myalgia, pruritus, skin disorder.

**Drug Interactions**

*Metoclopramide* / ↓ Serum levels and urinary excretion of fosfomycin

**Dosage** ———————
- **Sachet**

  *Acute cystitis.*

**Women, 18 years and older:** One sachet of fosfomycin mixed with water before ingesting.

**DENTAL CONCERNS**

See also *Dental Concerns* for *Anti-Infective Agents.*

# Fosinopril sodium
(foh-**SIN**-oh-prill)
**Pregnancy Category:** D
Monopril **(Rx)**
**Classification:** Angiotensin-converting enzyme inhibitor

See also *Angiotensin-Converting Enzyme Inhibitors.*

**Action/Kinetics:** **Onset:** 1 hr. **Time to peak serum levels:** About 3 hr. Metabolized in the liver to the active fosinoprilat. Significantly bound to plasma proteins. **t½:** 12 hr for fosinoprilat (prolonged in impaired renal function) following IV administration. **Duration:** 24 hr. Approximately 50% excreted through the urine and 50% in the feces. Food decreases the rate, but not the extent, of absorption of fosinopril.

**Uses:** Alone or in combination with other antihypertensive agents (especially thiazide diuretics) for the treatment of hypertension. Adjunct in treating CHF in clients not responding adequately to diuretics and digitalis.

**Contraindications:** Hypersensitivity to ACE inhibitors. Use during lactation and in children.

**Side Effects:** *CV:* Orthostatic hypotension, chest pain, hypotension, palpitations, angina pectoris, **CVA, MI,** rhythm disturbances, hypertensive crisis, claudication. *CNS:* Headache, dizziness, fatigue, confusion, memory disturbance, tremors, drowsiness, mood change, insomnia, vertigo, sleep disturbances. *Oral:* Dry mouth, taste disturbances. *GI:* N&V, diarrhea, abdominal pain, constipation, dysphagia, abdominal distention, flatulence, heartburn, appetite changes, weight changes. *Respiratory:* Cough, sinusitis, **bronchospasm,** asthma, pharyngitis, laryngitis. *Hematologic:* Leukopenia, eosinophilia, decreases in hemoglobin (mean of 0.1 g/dL) or hematocrit, neutropenia. *Dermatologic:* Diaphoresis, photosensitivity, flushing, pruritus, rash, urticaria. *Body as a whole:* Angioedema, muscle cramps, syncope, myalgia, arthralgia, edema, weakness, musculoskeletal pain. *GU:* Decreased libido, sexual dysfunction, renal insufficiency, urinary frequency. *Miscellaneous:* Paresthesias, hepatitis, pancreatitis, syncope, tinnitus, gout, lymphadenopathy, rhinitis, epistaxis, vision disturbances, eye irritation, laryngitis.

**Drug Interactions:** See also *Angiotensin-Converting Enzyme Inhibitors.*

**How Supplied:** *Tablet:* 10 mg, 20 mg, 40 mg

**Dosage**
• **Tablets**
*Hypertension.*
**Initial:** 10 mg once daily; **then,** adjust dose depending on BP response at peak (2–6 hr after dosing) and trough (24 hr after dosing) blood levels. **Maintenance:** Usually 20–40 mg/day, although some clients manifest beneficial effects at doses up to 80 mg.
*In clients taking diuretics.*
Discontinue diuretic 2–3 days before starting fosinopril. If diuretic cannot be discontinued, use an initial dose of 10 mg fosinopril.
*Congestive heart failure.*
**Initial:** 10 mg once daily; **then,** following initial dose, observe the client for at least 2 hr for the presence of hypotension or orthostasis (if either is present, monitor until BP stabilizes). An initial dose of 5 mg is recommended in heart failure with moderate to severe renal failure or in those who have had significant diuresis. The dose is increased over several weeks, not to exceed a maximum of 40 mg daily (usual effective range is 20–40 mg once daily).

## DENTAL CONCERNS

See also *Dental Concerns* for *Angiotensin-Converting Enzyme Inhibitors* and *Antihypertensive Agents.*

# Fosphenytoin sodium
(**FOS**-fen-ih-toyn)
**Pregnancy Category:** D
Cerebyx **(Rx)**
**Classification:** Anticonvulsant

See also *Anticonvulsants* and *Phenytoin.*

**Action/Kinetics:** Fosphenytoin is a prodrug of phenytoin; thus, its anticonvulsant effects are due to phenytoin. For every millimole of fosphenytoin administered, 1 mmol of phenytoin is produced. **t½, fosphenytoin:** 15 min after IV infusion. **Peak plasma levels, after IM:** 30 min. Significantly bound (95% to 99%) to plasma protein. Fosphenytoin displaces phenytoin from plasma protein binding sites. Fosphenytoin is better tolerated at the infusion site than is phenytoin (i.e., pain and burning associated with IV phenytoin is decreased). The IV infusion rate for fosphenytoin is three times faster than for IV phenytoin. IM use results in systemic phenytoin concentrations that are similar to PO phenytoin, thus allowing interchangeable use. Phenytoin derived from fosphenytoin is extensively metabolized in the liver and excreted in the urine.

**Uses:** Short-term parenteral use for the control of generalized convulsive status epilepticus and prophylaxis and treatment of seizures occurring during neurosurgery. It can be substituted, short term, for PO phenytoin when PO administration is not possible.

**Contraindications:** Hypersensitivity to fosphenytoin, phenytoin, or other hydantoins. Use in clients with sinus bradycardia, SA block, second- and third-degree AV block, and Adams-Stokes syndrome. Use to treat absence seizures. Use during lactation.

**Special Concerns:** The safety and efficacy of fosphenytoin have not been determined for longer than 5 days. The safety has not been determined in pediatric clients. After administration of fosphenytoin to those with renal and/or hepatic dysfunction or in those with hypoalbuminemia, fosphenytoin clearance to phenytoin may be increased without a similar increase in phenytoin clearance, thus increasing the potential for serious side effects.

**Side Effects:** See *Phenytoin.* The most common side effects include ataxia, dizziness, headache, nystagmus, paresthesia, pruritus, and somnolence.

**Drug Interactions:** See *Phenytoin.*

**How Supplied:** *Injection:* 75 mg/mL

**Dosage** ─────────

*NOTE:* Doses of fosphenytoin are expressed as phenytoin sodium equivalents (PE = phenytoin sodium equivalent). Thus, adjustments in the recommended doses should not be made when substituting fosphenytoin for phenytoin sodium or vice versa.

- **IV**
  *Status epilepticus.*
**Loading dose:** 15–20 mg PE/kg given at a rate of 100–150 mg PE/min. The loading dose is followed by maintenance doses of either fosphenytoin or phenytoin, either PO or parenterally.
- **IM, IV**
  *Nonemergency loading and maintenance dosing.*
**Loading dose:** 15–20 mg PE/kg given at a rate of 100–150 mg PE/min.
**Maintenance:** 4–6 mg PE/kg/day.
  *Temporary substitution for PO phenytoin.*
Use the same daily PO dose of phenytoin in milligrams given at a rate not to exceed 150 mg PE/min.

─────────

## DENTAL CONCERNS
**General**
1. This drug is for hospital or emergency room use. Patients will convert to oral phenytoin upon discharge from the hospital or emergency room.
2. Precaution is necessary if a general anesthetic or sedation is required. There is an increased risk of hypotension.

**Consultation with Primary Care Provider**
1. Consultation may be required in or-

der to assess the extent of disease control and the patient's ability to tolerate stress.

# Furosemide

(fur-**OH**-seh-myd)
**Pregnancy Category:** C
Apo-Furosemide ✺, Furoside ✺, Lasix, Myrosemide, Novo-Semide ✺, Uritol ✺ **(Rx)**
**Classification:** Loop diuretic

See also *Diuretics, Loop.*

**Action/Kinetics:** Inhibits the reabsorption of sodium and chloride in the ascending loop of Henle; this results in the excretion of sodium, chloride, and, to a lesser degree, potassium and bicarbonate ions. The resulting urine is more acid. Diuretic action is independent of changes in clients' acid-base balance. Has a slight antihypertensive effect. **Onset: PO, IM:** 30–60 min; **IV:** 5 min. **Peak: PO, IM:** 1–2 hr; **IV:** 20–60 min. **t½:** About 2 hr after PO use. **Duration: PO, IM:** 6–8 hr; **IV:** 2 hr. Metabolized in the liver and excreted through the urine. May be effective for clients resistant to thiazides and for those with reduced GFRs.

**Uses:** Edema associated with CHF, nephrotic syndrome, hepatic cirrhosis, and ascites. IV for acute pulmonary edema. Furosemide can be used orally to treat hypertension in conjunction with spironolactone, triamterene, and other diuretics *except* ethacrynic acid. *Non-FDA Approved Uses:* Hypercalcemia.

**Contraindications: Never use with ethacrynic acid.** Anuria, hypersensitivity to drug, severe renal disease associated with azotemia and oliguria, hepatic coma associated with electrolyte depletion. Lactation.

**Special Concerns:** Use with caution in premature infants and neonates due to prolonged half-life in these clients (dosing interval must be extended). Geriatric clients may be more sensitive to the usual adult dose. Allergic reactions may be seen in clients who show hypersensitivity to sulfonamides.

**Side Effects:** *Electrolyte and fluid effects:* Fluid and electrolyte depletion leading to dehydration, hypovolemia, thromboembolism. Hypokalemia and hypochloremia may cause metabolic alkalosis. Hyperuricemia, azotemia, hyponatremia. *Oral:* Dry mouth, increased thirst, lichenoid drug reaction. *GI:* Nausea, oral and gastric irritation, vomiting, anorexia, diarrhea (especially in children) or constipation, cramps, pancreatitis, jaundice, ischemic hepatitis. *Otic:* Tinnitus, hearing impairment (may be reversible or permanent), reversible deafness. Usually following rapid IV or IM administration of high doses. *CNS:* Vertigo, headache, dizziness, blurred vision, restlessness, paresthesias, xanthopsia. *CV:* Orthostatic hypotension, thrombophlebitis, chronic aortitis. *Hematologic:* Anemia, thrombocytopenia, neutropenia, leukopenia, *agranulocytosis,* purpura. *Rarely, aplastic anemia. Allergic:* Rashes, pruritus, urticaria, photosensitivity, exfoliative dermatitis, vasculitis, erythema multiforme. *Miscellaneous:* Interstitial nephritis, fever, weakness, hyperglycemia, glycosuria, exacerbation of, aggravation of, or worsening of SLE, increased perspiration, muscle spasms, urinary bladder spasm, urinary frequency.

*Following IV use:* Thrombophlebitis, *cardiac arrest. Following IM use:* Pain and irritation at injection site, *cardiac arrest.*

Because this drug is resistant to the effects of pressor amines and potentiates the effects of muscle relaxants, it is recommended that the PO drug be discontinued 1 week before surgery and the IV drug 2 days before surgery.

**Drug Interactions:** See also *Diuretics, Loop.*

**How Supplied:** *Injection:* 10 mg/mL; *Solution:* 10 mg/ mL, 40 mg/5 mL; *Tablet:* 20 mg, 40 mg, 80 mg

**Dosage** ————————————
• **Oral Solution, Tablets**
  *Edema.*

**Adults, initial:** 20–80 mg/day as a single dose. For resistant cases, dosage can be increased by 20–40 mg q 6–8 hr until desired diuretic response is attained. Maximum daily dose should not exceed 600 mg. **Pediatric, initial:** 2 mg/kg as a single dose; **then,** dose can be increased by 1–2 mg/kg q 6–8 hr until desired response is attained (up to 5 mg/kg may be required in children with nephrotic syndrome; maximum dose should not exceed 6 mg/kg). A dose range of 0.5–2 mg/kg b.i.d. has also been recommended.

*Hypertension.*
**Adults, initial:** 40 mg b.i.d. Adjust dosage depending on response.
*CHF and chronic renal failure.*
**Adults:** 2–2.5 g/day.
*Antihypercalcemic.*
**Adults:** 120 mg/day in one to three doses.

• **IV, IM**
*Edema.*
**Adults, initial:** 20–40 mg; if response inadequate after 2 hr, increase dose in 20-mg increments.
**Pediatric, initial:** 1 mg/kg given slowly; if response inadequate after 2 hr, increase dose by 1 mg/kg. Doses greater than 6 mg/kg should not be given.
*Antihypercalcemic.*
**Adults:** 80–100 mg for severe cases; dose may be repeated q 1–2 hr if needed.

• **IV**
*Acute pulmonary edema.*
**Adults:** 40 mg slowly over 1–2 min; if response inadequate after 1 hr, give 80 mg slowly over 1–2 min. Concomitant oxygen and digitalis may be used.
*CHF, chronic renal failure.*
**Adults:** 2–2.5 g/day. For IV bolus injections, the maximum should not exceed 1 g/day given over 30 min.
*Hypertensive crisis, normal renal function.*
**Adults:** 40–80 mg.
*Hypertensive crisis with pulmonary edema or acute renal failure.*
**Adults:** 100–200 mg.

**DENTAL CONCERNS**

See also *Dental Concerns* for *Diuretics, Loop.*

# G

## Gabapentin
(gab-ah-**PEN**-tin)
**Pregnancy Category:** C
Neurontin **(Rx)**
**Classification:** Anticonvulsant

See also *Anticonvulsants.*
**Action/Kinetics:** Anticonvulsant mechanism is not known. Food has no effect on the rate and extent of absorption; however, as the dose increases, the bioavailability decreases. **t½:** 5–7 hr. Excreted unchanged through the urine.
**Uses:** In adults as an adjunct in the treatment of partial seizures with and without secondary generalization.

**Contraindications:** Hypersensitivity
**Special Concerns:** Use during lactation only if benefits outweigh risks. Plasma clearance is reduced in geriatric clients and in those with impaired renal function. Safety and efficacy have not been determined in children less than 12 years of age.
**Side Effects:** Side effects listed are those with an incidence of 0.1% or greater.
*CNS:* Most commonly: somnolence, ataxia, dizziness, and fatigue. Also, nystagmus, tremor, nervousness, dysarthria, amnesia, depression, abnormal thinking, twitching, abnormal coordination, headache, *convulsions (including the possibility*

*of precipitation of status epilepticus),* confusion, insomnia, emotional lability, vertigo, hyperkinesia, paresthesia, decreased/increased/absent reflexes, anxiety, hostility, CNS tumors, syncope, abnormal dreaming, aphasia, hypesthesia, *intracranial hemorrhage,* hypotonia, dysesthesia, paresis, dystonia, hemiplegia, facial paralysis, stupor, cerebellar dysfunction, positive Babinski sign, decreased position sense, subdural hematoma, apathy, hallucinations, decreased or loss of libido, agitation depersonalization, euphoria, "doped-up" sensation, *suicidal tendencies,* psychoses. *Oral:* Dry mouth and throat, dental abnormalities, gingivitis, glossitis, gum hemorrhage, stomatitis, taste loss, unusual taste, increased salivation. *GI:* Most commonly: N&V. Also, dyspepsia, constipation, increased appetite, abdominal pain, diarrhea, anorexia, flatulence, thirst, gastroenteritis, hemorrhoids, bloody stools, fecal incontinence, hepatomegaly. *CV:* Hypertension, vasodilation, hypotension, angina pectoris, peripheral vascular disorder, palpitation, tachycardia, migraine, murmur. *Musculoskeletal:* Myalgia, fracture, tendinitis, arthritis, joint stiffness or swelling, positive Romberg test. *Respiratory:* Rhinitis, pharyngitis, coughing, pneumonia, epistaxis, dyspnea, apnea. *Dermatologic:* Pruritus, abrasion, rash, acne, alopecia, eczema, dry skin, increased sweating, urticaria, hirsutism, seborrhea, cyst, herpes simplex. *Body as a whole:* Weight increase, back pain, peripheral edema, asthenia, facial edema, allergy, weight decrease, chills. *GU:* Hematuria, dysuria, frequent urination, cystitis, urinary retention, urinary incontinence, vaginal hemorrhage, amenorrhea, dysmenorrhea, menorrhagia, breast cancer, inability to climax, abnormal ejaculation, impotence. *Hematologic:* Leukopenia, decreased WBCs, purpura, anemia, thrombocytopenia, lymphadenopathy. *Ophthalmologic:* Diplopia, amblyopia, abnormal vision, cataract, conjunctivitis, dry eyes, eye pain, visual field defect, photophobia, bilateral or unilateral ptosis, eye hemorrhage, hordeolum, eye twitching. *Otic:* Hearing loss, earache, tinnitus, inner ear infection, otitis, ear fullness.

**Drug Interactions**
*Antacids* / Antacids ↓ bioavailability of gabapentin
*Cimetidine* / Cimetidine ↓ renal excretion of gabapentin
**How Supplied:** *Capsule:* 100 mg, 300 mg, 400 mg

## Dosage
- **Capsules**
  *Anticonvulsant.*
**Adults:** Dose range of 900–1,800 mg/day in three divided doses. Titration to an effective dose can begin on day 1 with 300 mg followed by 300 mg b.i.d. on day 2 and 300 mg t.i.d. on day 3. If necessary, the dose may be increased to 300–400 mg t.i.d., up to 1,800 mg/day. In clients with a creatinine clearance of 30–60 mL/min, the dose is 300 mg b.i.d.; if the creatinine clearance is 15–30 mL/min, the dose is 300 mg/day; if the creatinine clearance is less than 15 mL/min, the dose is 300 mg every other day.

## DENTAL CONCERNS

See also *Dental Concerns* for *Anticonvulsants.*

# Gemfibrozil
(jem-**FIH**-broh-zill)
**Pregnancy Category:** B
Apo-Gemfibrozil ✶, Gemcor, Lopid, Novo-Gemfibrozil ✶, Nu-Gemfibrozil ✶ **(Rx)**
**Classification:** Antihyperlipidemic

**Action/Kinetics:** Gemfibrozil, which resembles clofibrate, decreases triglycerides, cholesterol, and VLDL and increases HDL; LDL levels either decrease or do not change. Also, decreases hepatic triglyceride production by inhibiting peripheral lipolysis and decreasing extraction of free fatty acids by the liver. Also, gemfibrozil decreases VLDL synthesis by inhibiting synthesis of VLDL carrier apolipoprotein B as well as inhibits peripheral lipolysis and decreases hepatic extraction of free fatty acids (thus decreasing hepatic triglyceride production). May be beneficial in inhibiting development of atherosclerosis. **Onset:** 2–5 days. **Peak plasma levels:** 1–2 hr; **t½:** 1.5 hr. Nearly 70% is excreted unchanged.

**Uses:** Hypertriglyceridemia (type IV and type V hyperlipidemia) unresponsive to dietary control or in clients who are at risk of pancreatitis and abdominal pain. Reduce risk of coronary heart disease in clients with type IIb hyperlipidemia who have not responded to diet, weight loss, exercise, and other drug therapy.

**Contraindications:** Gallbladder disease, primary biliary cirrhosis, hepatic or renal dysfunction.

**Special Concerns:** Use with caution during lactation. Safety and efficacy have not been established in children. The dose may have to be reduced in geriatric clients due to age-related decreases in renal function.

**Side Effects:** *GI:* Cholelithiasis, abdominal or epigastric pain, N&V, diarrhea, dyspepsia, constipation, acute appendicitis, colitis, pancreatitis, cholestatic jaundice, hepatoma. *CNS:* Dizziness, headache, fatigue, vertigo, somnolence, paresthesia, hypesthesia, depression, confusion, syncope, *seizures.* *CV:* Atrial fibrillation, extrasystole, peripheral vascular disease, *intracerebral hemorrhage.* *Hematopoietic:* Anemia, leukopenia, eosinophilia, thrombocytopenia, bone marrow hypoplasia. *Musculoskeletal:* Painful extremities, arthralgia, myalgia, myopathy, myasthenia, rhabdomyolysis, synovitis. *Allergic:* Urticaria, lupus-like syndrome, angioedema, *laryngeal edema,* vasculitis, *anaphylaxis.* *Dermatologic:* Eczema, dermatitis, pruritus, skin rashes, exfoliative dermatitis, alopecia. *Ophthalmic:* Blurred vision, retinal edema, cataracts. *Miscellaneous:* Increased chance of viral and bacterial infections, taste perversion, impotence, decreased male fertility, weight loss.

**Drug Interactions:** No drug interactions reported of concern to dentistry.

**How Supplied:** *Tablet:* 600 mg

## Dosage
- **Tablets**

**Adults:** 600 mg 30 min before the morning and evening meal (range: 900–1,500 mg/day). Dosage has not been established in children. Discontinue if significant improvement not observed within 3 months.

### DENTAL CONCERNS
**General**
1. Patients on chronic drug therapy may develop blood dyscrasias. Symptoms include fever, sore throat, bleeding, and poor wound healing.

**Consultation with Primary Care Provider**
1. Patients with symptoms of blood dyscrasias should be referred to their primary care provider for complete blood counts. Treatment should be postponed until the results are known.

# Gentamicin sulfate
(jen-tah-**MY**-sin)
**Pregnancy Category:** C
Alcomicin ✹, Cidomycin ✹, Diogent ✹, Garamycin, Garamycin Cream or Ointment, Garamycin Intrathecal, Garamycin IV Piggyback, Garamycin Ophthalmic Ointment, Garamycin Ophthalmic Solution, Garamycin Pediatric, Garatec ✹, Genoptic Ophthalmic Liquifilm, Genoptic S.O.P. Ophthalmic, Gentacidin Ophthalmic, Gentafair, Gentak Ophthalmic, Gentamicin, Gentamicin Ophthalmic, Gentamicin Sulfate IV Piggyback, Gentrasul Ophthalmic, G-myticin Cream or Ointment, Jenamicin, Minims Gentamicin ✹, Ocugram ✹, Pediatric Gentamicin Sulfate, PMS-Gentamicin Sulfate ✹, Schwinpharm Gentamicin ✹ **(Rx)**
**Classification:** Antibiotic, aminoglycoside

---

See also *Aminoglycosides.*
**Action/Kinetics:     Therapeutic serum levels: IM,** 4–8 mcg/mL. **Toxic serum levels:** >12 mcg/mL (peak) and >2 mcg/mL (trough). Prolonged serum levels above 12 mcg/mL should be avoided. **t½:** 2 hr. Can be used with carbenicillin to treat serious *Pseudomonas* infections; do not mix these drugs in the same flask as carbenicillin will inactivate gentamicin.

**Uses: Systemic:** Prevention of bacterial endocarditis in high-risk patients. Serious infections caused by *Pseudomonas aeruginosa, Proteus, Klebsiella, Enterobacter, Serratia, Citrobacter,* and *Staphylococcus.* Infections include bacterial neonatal sepsis, bacterial septicemia, and serious infections of the skin, bone, soft tissue (including burns), urinary tract, GI tract (including peritonitis), and CNS (including meningitis). Should be considered as initial therapy in suspected or confirmed gramnegative infections. In combination with carbenicillin for treating life-threatening infections due to *P. aeruginosa.* In combination with penicillin for treating endocarditis caused by group D streptococci. In combination with penicillin for treating suspected bacterial sepsis or staphylococcal pneumonia in the neonate. Intrathecal administration is used in combination with systemic gentamicin for treating meningitis, ventriculitis, or other serious CNS infections due to *Pseudomonas. Investigational:* Pelvic inflammatory disease.

**Ophthalmic:** Ophthalmic infections due to *Staphylococcus, S. aureus, Streptococcus pneumoniae,* beta-hemolytic streptococci, *Corynebacterium* species, *Streptococcus pyogenes, Escherichia coli, Haemophilus influenzae, H. aegyptius, H. ducreyi, Klebsiella pneumoniae, Neisseria gonorrhoeae, Proteus* species, *Acinetobacter calcoaceticus, Enterobacter aerogenes, P. aeruginosa, Serratia marcescens, Moraxella lacunata.*

**Topical:** Prevention of infections following minor cuts, wounds, burns, and skin abrasions. Treatment of primary or secondary skin infections. Treatment of infected skin cysts and other skin abscesses when preceded by incision and drainage to permit adequate contact between the drug and the infecting bacteria, infected stasis and other skin ulcers, infected superficial burns, paronychia, infected insect bites and stings, infected lacerations and abrasions and wounds from minor surgery.

**Contraindications:**    Ophthalmic use to treat dendritic keratitis, vaccinia, varicella, mycobacterial infections of the eye, fungal diseases of the eye, use with steroids after uncomplicated removal of a corneal foreign body.

**Special Concerns:** Use with caution in premature infants and neonates. Ophthalmic ointments may retard corneal epithelial healing.

**Side Effects:** See also *Aminoglycosides.*

**Additional Side Effects:** Muscle twitching, numbness, *seizures,* increased BP, alopecia, purpura, pseudotumor cerebri. Photosensitivity when used topically. *After ophthalmic use:* Transient irritation, burning, stinging, itching, inflammation, angioneurotic edema, urticaria, vesicular and maculopapular dermatitis, mydriasis, conjunctival paresthesia, conjunctival hyperemia, nonspecific conjunctivitis, conjunctival epithelial defects, lid itching and swelling, bacterial/fungal corneal ulcers.

**Drug   Interactions:**    See   also *Aminoglycosides.*

**Additional   Drug   Interactions:** With carbenicillin or ticarcillin, gentamicin may result in increased effect when used for *Pseudomonas* infections.

**How Supplied:** *Cream:* 0.1%; *Injection:* 10 mg/mL, 40 mg/mL; *Ointment:* 1%; *Ophthalmic ointment:* 3

mg/g;  *Ophthalmic solution:*  3 mg/mL

**Dosage** ───────────────
• **IM (usual), IV**
**Adults with normal renal function.**
*Infections.*
1 mg/kg q 8 hr, up to 5 mg/kg/day in life-threatening infections; **children:** 2–2.5 mg/kg q 8 hr; **infants and neonates:** 2.5 mg/kg q 8 hr; **premature infants or neonates less than 1 week of age:** 2.5 mg/kg q 12 hr. Therapy may be required for 7–10 days.

*Prevention of bacterial endocarditis, dental or respiratory tract procedures.*
**Adults:** 1.5 mg/kg gentamicin (not to exceed 80 mg) plus 1 g ampicillin, each IM or IV, 30–60 min before the procedure; one additional dose of each can be given 8 hr later (alternative: penicillin V, 1 g PO, 6 hr after initial dose).

*Prophylaxis of bacterial endocarditis in GI or GU tract procedures or surgery.*
**Adults:** 1.5 mg/kg gentamicin (not to exceed 80 mg) plus 2 g ampicillin, each IM or IV, 30–60 min before procedure; dose should be repeated 8 hr later. **Children:** 2 mg/kg gentamicin plus penicillin G, 30,000 units/kg, or ampicillin, 50 mg/kg in same dosage interval as for adults. Pediatric dosage should not exceed single or 24-hr adult doses.

*NOTE:* In clients allergic to penicillin, vancomycin, 1 g IV given slowly over 1 hr, may be substituted; the dose of vancomycin should be repeated 8–12 hr later. **Adults with impaired renal function:** To calculate interval (hr) between doses, multiply serum creatinine level (mg/100 mL) by 8.
• **IV**
*Septicemia.*
**Initially:** 1–2 mg/kg infused over 30–60 min; **then,** maintenance doses may be administered.
• **Intrathecal**

*Meningitis.*
**Use only the intrathecal preparation. Adults, usual:** 4–8 mg/day; **children and infants 3 months and older:** 1–2 mg/day
*Pelvic inflammatory disease.*
**Initial:** 2 mg/kg IV; **then,** 1.5 mg/kg t.i.d. plus clindamycin, 500 mg IV q.i.d. Continue for at least 4 days and at least 48 hr after client improves. Continue clindamycin, 450 mg PO q.i.d. for 10–14 days.
• **Ophthalmic Solution (0.3%)**
*Acute infections.*
**Initially:** 1–2 gtt in conjunctival sac q 15–30 min; **then,** as infection improves, reduce frequency.
*Moderate infections.*
1–2 gtt in conjunctival sac 4–6 times/day.
*Trachoma.*
2 gtt in each eye b.i.d.–q.i.d.; treatment should be continued for up to 1–2 months.
• **Ophthalmic Ointment (0.3%)**
Depending on the severity of infection, ½-in. ribbon from q 3–4 hr to 2–3 times/day.
• **Topical      Cream/Ointment (0.1%)**
Apply 3–4 times/day to affected area. The area may be covered with a sterile bandage.

─────────────────────────
**DENTAL CONCERNS**

See also *Dental Concerns* for *Aminoglycosides.*

# Glimepiride
(**GLYE**-meh-pye-ride)
**Pregnancy Category:** C
Amaryl **(Rx)**
**Classification:** Antidiabetic agent, sulfonylurea
─────────────────────────

See also *Hypoglycemic Agents.*
**Action/Kinetics:** Lowers blood glucose by stimulating the release of insulin from functioning pancreatic beta cells and by increasing the sensitivity of peripheral tissues to insulin. Completely absorbed from the GI tract within 1 hr. **Time to maxi-**

**mum effect:** 2–3 hr. Completely metabolized in the liver and metabolites are excreted through both the urine and feces.

**Uses:** As an adjunct to diet and exercise to lower blood glucose in non-insulin-dependent diabetes mellitus (Type II diabetes mellitus). In combination with insulin to decrease blood glucose in those whose hyperglycemia cannot be controlled by diet and exercise in combination with an oral hypoglycemic drug.

**Contraindications:** Diabetic ketoacidosis with or without coma. Use during lactation.

**Special Concerns:** The use of oral hypoglycemic drugs has been associated with increased CV mortality compared with treatment with diet alone or diet plus insulin. Safety and efficacy have not been determined in children.

**Side Effects:** The most common side effect is hypoglycemia. *GI:* N&V, GI pain, diarrhea, cholestatic jaundice (rare). *CNS:* Dizziness, headache. *Dermatologic:* Pruritus, erythema, urticaria, morbilliform or maculopapular eruptions. *Hematologic:* Leukopenia, agranulocytosis, thrombocytopenia, hemolytic anemia, aplastic anemia, pancytopenia. *Miscellaneous:* Hyponatremia, increased release of ADH, changes in accommodation and/or blurred vision.

**Drug Interactions:** See *Hypoglycemic Agents.*

**How Supplied:** *Tablet:* 1 mg, 2 mg, 4 mg

**Dosage** ——————————

• **Tablets**

*Non-insulin-dependent diabetes mellitus (Type II diabetes).*

**Adults, initial:** 1–2 mg once daily, given with breakfast or the first main meal. The initial dose should be 1 mg in those sensitive to hypoglycemic drugs, in those with impaired renal or hepatic function, and in elderly, debilitated, or malnourished clients. The maximum initial dose is 2 mg or less daily. **Maintenance:** 1–4 mg once daily up to a maximum of 8 mg once daily. After a dose of 2 mg is reached, the dose should be increased in increments of 2 mg or less at 1- to 2-week intervals (determined by the blood glucose response). **When combined with insulin therapy:** 8 mg once daily with the first main meal with low-dose insulin. The fasting glucose level for beginning combination therapy is greater than 150 mg/dL glucose in the plasma or serum.

*Type II diabetes—transfer from other hypoglycemic agents.*

When transferring clients to glimipiride, no transition period is required. However, clients should be observed closely for 1 to 2 weeks for hypoglycemia when being transferred from longer half-life sulfonylureas (e.g., chlorpropamide) to glimepiride.

## DENTAL CONCERNS

See also *Dental Concerns* for *Antidiabetic Agents: Hypoglycemic Agents.*

# Glipizide

(**GLIP**-ih-zyd)
**Pregnancy Category:** C
Glucotrol, Glucotrol XL **(Rx)**
**Classification:** Sulfonylurea (anti-diabetic), second-generation

See also *Antidiabetic Agents: Hypoglycemic Agents.*

**Action/Kinetics:** Also has mild diuretic effects. **Onset:** 1–1.5 hr. **t½:** 2–4 hr. **Time to peak levels:** 1–3 hr. **Duration:** 10–16 hr. Metabolized in liver to inactive metabolites, which are excreted through the kidneys.

**Uses:** Adjunct to diet for control of hyperglycemia in clients with non-insulin-dependent diabetes.

**Additional Drug Interactions:** Cimetidine may ↑ effect of glipizide due to ↓ breakdown by liver.

**How Supplied:** *Tablet:* 5 mg, 10 mg; *Tablet, extended release:* 5 mg, 10 mg

**Dosage** ——————————

• **Tablets, Extended Release Tablets**

*Diabetes.*

**Adults, initial:** 5 mg 30 min before breakfast; **then,** adjust dosage by 2.5–5 mg every few days, depending on the blood glucose response, until adequate control is achieved. **Maintenance:** 15–40 mg/day. Older clients should begin with 2.5 mg. The extended release tablets are taken once daily (usually at breakfast) in doses of either 5 or 10 mg.

**DENTAL CONCERNS**

See also *Dental Concerns* for *Antidiabetic Agents: Hypoglycemic Agents.*
**Client/Family Teaching**
1. Skin reactions may occur and should be reported. Avoid sun exposure; when in the sun, use sunscreen and wear sunglasses and protective clothing.

# Glyburide

(**GLYE**-byou-ryd)
**Pregnancy Category:** B
Albert Glyburide ✹, Apo-Glyburide ✹, Diabeta, Euglucon ✹, Gen-Glybe ✹, Glynase PresTab, Med-Glybe ✹, Micronase, Novo-Glyburide ✹, Nu-Glyburide ✹ **(Rx)**
**Classification:** Sulfonylurea (anti-diabetic), second-generation

See also *Antidiabetic Agents.*
**Action/Kinetics:** Has a mild diuretic effect. **Onset, nonmicronized:** 2–4 hr; **micronized:** 1 hr. **t½, nonmicronized:** 10 hr; **micronized:** Approximately 4 hr. **Time to peak levels:** 4 hr. **Duration, both forms:** 24 hr. Metabolized in liver to weakly active metabolites. Excreted in bile (50%) and through the kidneys (50%).
**How Supplied:** *Tablet:* 1.25 mg, 1.5 mg, 2.5 mg, 3 mg, 5 mg, 6 mg

**Dosage**
• **Tablets, Nonmicronized (DiaBeta/Micronase)**
*Diabetes.*
**Adults, initial:** 2.5–5 mg/day given with breakfast (or the first main meal); **then,** increase by 2.5 mg at weekly intervals to achieve the desired response. **Maintenance:** 1.25–20 mg/day. Clients sensitive to sulfonylureas should start with 1.25 mg/day.
• **Tablets, Micronized (Glynase)**
*Diabetes.*
**Adults, initial:** 1.5–3 mg/day given with breakfast (or the first main meal); **then,** increase by no more than 1.5 mg at weekly intervals to achieve the desired response. **Maintenance:** 0.75–12 mg/day.

**DENTAL CONCERNS**

See also *Dental Concerns* for *Antidiabetic Agents* and *Glipizide.*

# Guaifenesin (Glyceryl guaiacolate)

(gwye-**FEN**-eh-sin)
**Pregnancy Category:** C
Anti-Tuss, Balminil Expectorant ✹, Benylin-E ✹, Breonesin, Fenesin, Gee-Gee, Genatuss, GG-Cen, Glyate, Glycotuss, Glytuss, Guiatuss, Halotussin, Humibid L.A., Humibid Sprinkle, Hytuss, Hytuss-2X, Mytussin, Naldecon Senior EX, Robitussin, Scot-tussin, Sinumist-SR Capsulets, Uni-tussin **(OTC)**
**Classification:** Expectorant

**Action/Kinetics:** May increase the output of fluid of the respiratory tract by reducing the viscosity and surface tension of respiratory secretions, thereby facilitating their expectoration. Data on efficacy are lacking.
**Uses:** Dry, nonproductive cough due to colds and minor upper respiratory tract infections when there is mucus in the respiratory tract.
**Contraindications:** Chronic cough (e.g., due to smoking, asthma, or emphysema), cough accompanied by excess secretions. Use in children under age 12 for persistent or chronic cough due to asthma or cough accompanied by excessive mucus (unless prescribed by a provider).
**Special Concerns:** Persistent cough may indicate a serious infection; thus, the provider should be con-

sulted if cough lasts for more than 1 week, is recurring, or is accompanied by high fever, rash, or persistent headache.

**Side Effects:** *GI:* N&V, GI upset. *CNS:* Dizziness, headache. *Dermatologic:* Rash, urticaria.

**Drug Interactions:** Inhibition of platelet adhesiveness by guaifenesin may result in bleeding tendencies.

**How Supplied:** *Capsule:* 200 mg; *Capsule, extended release:* 300 mg; *Liquid:* 100 mg/5 mL, 200 mg/5 mL; *Syrup:* 50 mg/5 mL, 100 mg/5 mL; *Tablet:* 100 mg, 200 mg; *Tablet, extended release:* 600 mg, 800 mg, 1,200 mg

**Dosage**
• **Capsules, Tablets, Oral Liquid, Syrup**
*Expectorant.*
**Adults and children over 12 years:** 100–400 mg q 4 hr, not to exceed 2.4 g/day; **pediatric, 6–12 years:** 100–200 mg q 4 hr, not to exceed 1.2 g/day; **pediatric, 2–6 years:** 50–100 mg q 4 hr, not to exceed 600 mg/day. If less than 2 years of age, the dosage must be individualized by the provider.

• **Sustained-Release Capsules, Sustained-Release Tablets**
*Expectorant.*
**Adults and children over 12 years:** 600–1,200 mg q 12 hr, not to exceed 2.4 g/day; **pediatric, 6–12 years:** 600 mg q 12 hr, not to exceed 1.2 g/day; **pediatric, 2–6 years:** 300 mg q 12 hr, not to exceed 600 mg/day. *NOTE:* The liquid dosage forms may be more suitable for children less than 6 years of age.

### DENTAL CONCERNS
**General**
1. Local hemostatic measures may be necessary to prevent excessive bleeding.
**Client/Family Teaching**
1. Use caution when using oral hygiene aids.
2. Brush teeth with a soft-bristle toothbrush.
3. Avoid OTC agents especially aspirin and NSAIDs.
4. Report any unusual bruising or bleeding; advise others esp. dentist of prescribed therapy, before surgery or new meds added.

# Haloperidol
(hah-low-**PAIR**-ih-dohl)
**Pregnancy Category:** C
Apo-Haloperidol ✿, Haldol, Novo–Peridol ✿, Peridol ✿, PMS Haloperidol ✿ **(Rx)**

# Haloperidol decanoate
(hah-low-**PAIR**-ih-dohl)
**Pregnancy Category:** C (decanoate form)
Haldol Decanoate 50 and 100, Haldol LA ✿ **(Rx)**

# Haloperidol lactate
(hah-low-**PAIR**-ih-dohl)
**Pregnancy Category:** C

Haldol Lactate **(Rx)**
**Classification:** Antipsychotic, butyrophenone

**Action/Kinetics:** Precise mechanism not known. Haloperidol competitively blocks dopamine receptors to cause sedation. Also causes alpha-adrenergic blockade, decreases release of growth hormone, and increases prolactin release by the pituitary. Causes significant extrapyramidal effects, as well as a low incidence of sedation, anticholinergic effects, and orthostatic hypotension. Narrow margin between the therapeutically effective dose and that causing extrapyramidal symptoms.

Also has antiemetic effects. **Peak plasma levels: PO,** 3–5 hr; **IM,** 20 min; **IM, decanoate:** approximately 6 days. **Therapeutic serum levels:** 3–10 ng/mL. **t½, PO:** 12–38 hr; **IM:** 13–36 hr; **IM, decanoate:** 3 weeks; **IV:** approximately 14 hr. **Plasma protein binding:** 90%. Metabolized in liver, slowly excreted in urine and bile.

**Uses:** Psychotic disorders including manic states, drug-induced psychoses, and schizophrenia. Aggressive and agitated clients, including chronic brain syndrome or mental retardation. Severe behavior problems in children (those with combative, explosive hyperexcitability not accounted for by immediate provocation). Short-term treatment of hyperactive children. Control of tics and vocal utterances associated with Gilles de la Tourette's syndrome in adults and children. The decanoate is used for prolonged therapy in chronic schizophrenia.

*Non-FDA Approved Uses:* Antiemetic for cancer chemotherapy, phencyclidine (PCP) psychosis, infantile autism. IV for acute psychiatric conditions.

**Contraindications:** Use with extreme caution, or not at all, in clients with parkinsonism. Lactation.

**Special Concerns:** PO dosage has not been determined in children less than 3 years of age; IM dosage is not recommended in children. Geriatric clients are more likely to exhibit orthostatic hypotension, anticholinergic effects, sedation, and extrapyramidal side effects (such as parkinsonism and tardive dyskinesia).

**Side Effects:** Extrapyramidal symptoms, especially akathisia and dystonias, occur more frequently than with the phenothiazines. Overdosage is characterized by severe extrapyramidal reactions, hypotension, or sedation. The drug does not elicit photosensitivity reactions like those of the phenothiazines.

**Drug Interactions**

*Amphetamine* / ↓ Effect of amphetamine by ↓ uptake of drug at its site of action

*Anticholinergics* / ↓ Effect of haloperidol

*Antidepressants, tricyclic* / ↑ Effect of antidepressants due to ↓ breakdown by liver

*Barbiturates* / ↓ Effect of haloperidol due to ↑ breakdown by liver

*Phenytoin* / ↓ Effect of haloperidol due to ↑ breakdown by liver

**How Supplied:** Haloperidol: *Tablet:* 0.5 mg, 1 mg, 2 mg, 5 mg, 10 mg, 20 mg. Haloperidol decanoate: *Injection:* 50 mg/mL, 100 mg/mL. Haloperidol lactate: *Concentrate:* 2 mg/mL; *Injection:* 5 mg/mL; *Solution:* 1 mg/mL

**Dosage** ———————————
- **Oral Solution, Tablets**
  *Psychoses.*

**Adults:** 0.5–2 mg b.i.d.–t.i.d. up to 3–5 mg b.i.d.–t.i.d. for *severe* symptoms; **maintenance:** reduce dosage to lowest effective level. Up to 100 mg/day may be required in some. **Geriatric or debilitated clients:** 0.5–2 mg b.i.d.–t.i.d. **Pediatric, 3–12 years or 15–40 kg:** 0.5 mg/day in two to three divided doses; if necessary the daily dose may be increased by 0.5-mg increments q 5–7 days for a total of 0.15 mg/kg/day for psychotic disorders and 0.075 mg/kg for nonpsychotic behavior disorders and Tourette's syndrome. Doses for children 3–6 years of age are 0.01–0.03 mg/kg/day PO for agitation and hyperkinesia and 0.5–4 mg/day for infantile autism.

- **IM, Lactate**
  *Acute psychoses.*

**Adults and adolescents, initial:** 2–5 mg; may be repeated if necessary q 4–8 hr to a total of 100 mg/day. Switch to **PO** therapy as soon as possible.

- **IM, Decanoate**
  *Chronic therapy.*

**Adults, initial dose:** 10–15 times the daily PO dose, not to exceed 100 mg initially, regardless of the previous oral antipsychotic dose; **then,** repeat q 4 weeks (decanoate is not to be given IV).

## DENTAL CONCERNS

See also *Dental Concerns* for *Antipsychotic Agents, Phenothiazines.*

---

# Hydralazine hydrochloride
(hy-**DRAL**-ah-zeen)
**Pregnancy Category:** C
Apo-Hydralazine ✿, Apresoline, Novo-Hylazin ✿, Nu-Hydral ✿ **(Rx)**
**Classification:** Antihypertensive, direct action on vascular smooth muscle

---

See also *Antihypertensive Agents.*
**Action/Kinetics:** Exerts a direct vasodilating effect on vascular smooth muscle. Because there is a reflex increase in cardiac function, hydralazine is commonly used with drugs that inhibit sympathetic activity (e.g., beta blockers, clonidine, methyldopa). Rapidly absorbed after PO use. Food increases bioavailability of the drug. **PO: Onset:** 45 min; **peak plasma level:** 1–2 hr; **duration:** 3–8 hr. **t½:** 3–7 hr. **IM: Onset:** 10–30 min; **peak plasma level:** 1 hr; **duration:** 2–4 hr. **IV: Onset:** 10–20 min; **maximum effect:** 10–80 min; **duration:** 2–4 hr. Metabolized in the liver and excreted through the kidney (2%–5% unchanged after PO use and 11%–14% unchanged after IV administration).
**Uses: PO:** In combination with other drugs for essential hypertension. **Parenteral:** Severe essential hypertension when PO use is not possible or when there is an urgent need to lower BP. Hydralazine is the drug of choice for eclampsia. *Non-FDA Approved Uses:* To reduce afterload in CHF, severe aortic insufficiency, and after valve replacement.
**Contraindications:** Coronary artery disease, angina pectoris, advanced renal disease (as in chronic renal hypertension), rheumatic heart disease (e.g., mitral valvular) and chronic glomerulonephritis.

**Special Concerns:** Use with caution in stroke clients and in those with pulmonary hypertension. Use with caution during lactation, in clients with advanced renal disease, and in clients with tartrazine sensitivity. Safety and efficacy have not been established in children. Geriatric clients may be more sensitive to the hypotensive and hypothermic effects of hydralazine; also, a decrease in dose may be necessary in these clients due to age-related decreases in renal function.
**Side Effects:** *CV:* Orthostatic hypotension, hypotension, *MI,* angina pectoris, palpitations, paradoxical pressor reaction, tachycardia. *CNS:* Headache, dizziness, psychoses, tremors, depression, anxiety, disorientation. *GI:* N&V, diarrhea, anorexia, constipation, paralytic ileus. *Allergic:* Rash, urticaria, fever, chills, arthralgia, pruritus, eosinophilia. Rarely, hepatitis, obstructive jaundice. *Hematologic:* Decrease in hemoglobin and RBCs, purpura, agranulocytosis, leukopenia. *Other:* Peripheral neuritis (paresthesias, numbness, tingling), dyspnea, impotence, nasal congestion, edema, muscle cramps, lacrimation, flushing, conjunctivitis, difficulty in urination, lupus-like syndrome, lymphadenopathy, splenomegaly. Side effects are less severe when dosage is increased slowly. *NOTE:* Hydralazine may cause symptoms resembling system lupus erythematosus (e.g., arthralgia, dermatoses, fever, splenomegaly, glomerulonephritis). Residual effects may persist for several years and long-term treatment with steroids may be necessary.
**Drug Interactions**
Benzodiazepines / ↑ CNS effects
*Indomethacin* / ↓ Effect of hydralazine
*NSAIDs* / ↓ Effect of hydralazine.
Also, potential for increased GI adverse effects.
*Opioid analgesics* / ↑ CNS effects
*Sympathomimetics* / ↑ Risk of tachycardia and angina
**How Supplied:** *Injection:* 20 mg/mL; *Tablet:* 10 mg, 25 mg, 50 mg, 100 mg

**Dosage**
- **Tablets**
  *Hypertension.*
**Adult, initial:** 10 mg q.i.d for 2–4 days; **then,** increase to 25 mg q.i.d. for rest of first week. For second and following weeks, increase to 50 mg q.i.d. **Maintenance:** individualized to lowest effective dose; maximum daily dose should not exceed 300 mg. **Pediatric, initial:** 0.75 mg/kg/day (25 mg/m²/day) in two to four divided doses; dosage may be increased gradually up to 7.5 mg/kg/day (or 300 mg/day). Food increases the bioavailability of the drug.
- **IV, IM**
  *Hypertensive crisis.*
**Adults, usual:** 20–40 mg, repeated as necessary. BP may fall within 5–10 min, with maximum response in 10–80 min. Usually switch to PO medication in 1–2 days. Dosage should be decreased in clients with renal damage. **Pediatric:** 0.1–0.2 mg/kg q 4–6 hr as needed.
  *Eclampsia.*
5–10 mg q 20 min as an IV bolus. If no effect after 20 mg, another drug should be tried.

## DENTAL CONCERNS

See also *Dental Concerns* for *Antihypertensive Agents.*
1. Patients on chronic drug therapy may develop blood dyscrasias. Symptoms include fever, sore throat, bleeding, and poor wound healing.
2. Patients on sodium restricted diets should receive sodium-containing fluids (i.e., saline solution) with caution.

# Hydrochlorothiazide
(**hy**-droh-klor-oh-**THIGH**-ah-zyd)
**Pregnancy Category:** B
Apo-Hydro ✸, Diuchlor H ✸, Esidrex, Ezide, Hydro-DIURIL, Hydro-Par, Microzide, Neo-Codema ✸, Novo-Hydrazide ✸, Oretic, Urozide ✸ **(Rx)**
**Classification:** Diuretic, thiazide type

See also *Diuretics, Thiazide.*
**Action/Kinetics: Onset:** 2 hr. **Peak effect:** 4–6 hr. **Duration:** 6–12 hr. **t½:** 5.6–14.8 hr.
**Uses:** Diuresis, edema, hypertension, treatment of CHF.
**Additional Uses:** Microzide is available for once-daily, low-dose treatment for hypertension.
**Contraindications:** Hypersensitivity to thiazides or sulfonamides, anuria, renal decomposition, hypomagnesemia.
**Special Concerns:** Geriatric clients may be more sensitive to the usual adult dose.
**Side Effects:** See also *Diuretics, Thiazide.*
**Additional Side Effects:** *CV:* Allergic myocarditis, hypotension. *Dermatologic:* Alopecia, exfoliative dermatitis, **toxic epidermal necrolysis,** erythema multiforme, **Stevens-Johnson syndrome.** *Miscellaneous:* **Anaphylactic reactions, respiratory distress including pneumonitis and pulmonary edema.**
**Drug Interactions:** See also *Diuretics, Thiazide.*
**How Supplied:** *Capsule:* 12.5 mg; *Solution:* 50 mg/5 mL; *Tablet:* 25 mg, 50 mg, 100 mg

**Dosage**
- **Oral Solution, Tablets**
  *Diuretic.*
**Adults, initial:** 25–200 mg/day for several days until dry weight is reached; **then,** 25–100 mg/day or intermittently. Some clients may require up to 200 mg/day.
  *Antihypertensive.*
**Adults, initial:** 25 mg/day as a single dose. The dose may be increased to 50 mg/day in one to two doses. Doses greater than 50 mg may cause significant reductions in serum potassium. **Pediatric, under 6 months:** 3.3 mg/kg/day in two doses; **up to 2 years of age:** 12.5–37.5 mg/day in two doses; **2–12 years of age:** 37.5–100 mg/day in two doses.

**H**

---

**DENTAL CONCERNS**

See also *Dental Concerns* for *Diuretics, Thiazide.*

————COMBINATION DRUG————

# Hydrocodone bitartrate and Acetaminophen

(**high**-droh-**KOH**-dohn, ah-**seat**-ah-**MIN**-oh-fen)
**Pregnancy Category:** C
Anexia 5/500, Anexia 7.5/650, Anexsia 10 mg Hydrocodone bitartrate, Anexsia 660 mg Acetaminophen, Lorcet 10/650, Lorcet Plus, Lortab 10/500 10 mg Hydrocodone bitartrate, Lortab 500 mg Acetaminophen, Vicodin, Vicoprofen **(Rx) (C-III)**
**Classification:** Analgesic

See also *Opioid Analgesics* and *Acetaminophen.*

**Content:** Anexia 5/500: *Opioid analgesic:* Hydrocodone bitartrate, 5 mg, and *Nonopioid analgesic:* Acetaminophen, 500 mg.

Anexia 10/650 and Lorcet 10/650: *Opioid analgesic:* Hydrocodone bitartrate, 10 mg, and *Nonopioid analgesic:* Acetaminophen, 650 mg. Anexia 7.5/650 and Lorcet Plus: *Opioid analgesic:* Hydrocodone bitartrate, 7.5 mg, and *Nonopioid analgesic:* Acetaminophen, 650 mg. Lortab 10/500: *Opioid analgesic:* Hydrocodone bitartrate, 10 mg, and *Nonopioid analgesic:* Acetaminophen, 500 mg.

**Action/Kinetics:** Hydrocodone produces its analgesic activity by an action on the CNS via opiate receptors. The analgesic action of acetaminophen is produced by both peripheral and central mechanisms.
**Uses:** Relief of moderate to moderately severe pain.
**Contraindications:** Hypersensitivity to acetaminophen or hydrocodone. Lactation.
**Special Concerns:** Use with caution, if at all, in clients with head injuries as the CSF pressure may be increased further. Use with caution in geriatric or debilitated clients; in those with impaired hepatic or renal function; in hypothyroidism, Addison's disease, prostatic hypertrophy, or urethral stricture; and in clients with pulmonary disease. Use shortly before delivery may cause respiratory depression in the newborn. Safety and efficacy have not been determined in children.
**Side Effects:** *CNS:* Lightheadedness, dizziness, sedation, drowsiness, mental clouding, lethargy, impaired mental and physical performance, anxiety, fear, dysphoria, psychologic dependence, mood changes. *Oral:* Dry mouth. *GI:* N&V. *Respiratory:* Respiratory depression (dose-related), irregular and periodic breathing. *GU:* Ureteral spasm, spasm of vesical sphincters, urinary retention.
**Drug Interactions**
*Anticholinergics* / ↑ Risk of paralytic ileus
*CNS depressants, including other opioid analgesics, antianxiety agents, antipsychotics, alcohol* / Additive CNS depression
*MAO inhibitors* / ↑ Effect of either the narcotic or the antidepressant
*Tricyclic antidepressants* / ↑ Effect of either the narcotic or the antidepressant
**How Supplied:** See Content

**Dosage** ————
• **Tablets**
  *Analgesia.*
1 tablet of Anexsia 7.5/650, Lorcet 10/650, or Lorcet Plus q 4–6 hr as needed for pain. The total 24-hr dose should not exceed 6 tablets. 1–2 tablets of Anexia 5/500 q 4–6 hr as needed for pain. The total 24-hr dose should not exceed 8 tablets.

**DENTAL CONCERNS**

See also *Dental Concerns* for *Opioid Analgesics* and *Acetaminophen.*

# Hydrocortisone (Cortisol)

(hy-droh-**KOR**-tih-zohn)
**Pregnancy Category:** C (topical and dental products)
**Parenteral:** Sterile Hydrocortisone Suspension. **Rectal:** Dermolate Anal-Itch, Cortenema ✿, Proctocort, ProctoCream.HC 2.5%, Rectocort ✿. **Retention Enema:** Cortenema, Hycort

✹, Rectocort ✹. **Roll-on Applicator:** Cortaid FastStick, Maximum Strength Cortaid Faststick, **Tablets:** Cortef, Hydrocortone. **Topical Cream:** Ala-Cort, Allercort, Alphaderm, Bactine, Cortate ✹, Cort-Dome, Cortifair, Dermacort, DermiCort, Dermolate Anti-Itch, Dermtex HC, Emo-Cort ✹, H₂Cort, Hi-Cor 1.0 and 2.5, Hydro-Tex, Hytone, Nutracort, Penecort, Prevex HC ✹, Synacort. **Topical Gel:** Extra Strength CortaGel, **Topical Liquid:** Scalpicin, T/Scalp, **Topical Lotion:** Acticort 100, Ala-Cort, Ala-Scalp, Allercort, Aquacort ✹, Cetacort, Cortate ✹, Cort-Dome, Delacort, Dermacort, Dermolate Scalp-Itch, Emo-Cort ✹, Gly-Cort, Hytone, LactiCare-HC, Lemoderm, Lexocort Forte, My Cort, Nutracort, Pentacort, Rederm, Sarna HC ✹, S-T Cort. **Topical Ointment:** Allercort, Cortoderm ✹, Cortril, Hytone, Lemoderm, Penecort. **Topical Solution:** Penecort, Emo-Cort Scalp Solution, Texacort Scalp Solution. **Topical Spray:** Cortaid, Dermolate Anti-Itch, Maximum Strength Coraid, Procort **(OTC) (Rx)**

## Hydrocortisone acetate
(hy-droh-**KOR**-tih-zohn)
**Pregnancy Category:** C (topical and dental products)
**Dental Paste:** Orabase-HCA. **Intrarectal Foam:** Cortifoam. **Ophthalmic/Otic:** Cortamed ✹. **Parenteral:** Hydrocortone Acetate. **Rectal:** Cort-Dome High Potency, Cortenema, Corticaine, Cortifoam. **Suppository:** Cortiment ✹, Rectocort ✹, **Topical Cream:** CaldeCORT Light, Carmol-HC, Cortaid, Cortef Feminine Itch, Corticaine, Corticreme ✹, FoilleCort, Gynecort, Gynecort Female Cream, Hyderm ✹, Lanacort, Lanacort 10, Lanacort 5, Maximum Strength Cortaid, Pharma-Cort, Rhulicort. **Topical Lotion:** Cortaid, Rhulicort. **Topical Ointment:** Anusol HC-1, Cortef Acetate, Dermaflex HC 1% ✹, Lanacort, Lanacort 5, Nov–Hydrocort, Maximum Strength Cortaid **(OTC) (Rx)**

## Hydrocortisone buteprate
(hy-droh-**KOR**-tih-zohn)
**Pregnancy Category:** C

**Topical Cream:** Pandel **(Rx)**

## Hydrocortisone butyrate
(hy-droh-**KOR**-tih-zohn)
**Pregnancy Category:** C (topical products)
**Topical Cream, Ointment, Solution:** Locoid **(Rx)**

## Hydrocortisone cypionate
(hy-droh-**KOR**-tih-zohn)
**Pregnancy Category:** C
**Oral Suspension:** Cortef **(Rx)**

## Hydrocortisone sodium phosphate
(hy-droh-**KOR**-tih-zohn)
**Pregnancy Category:** C
**Parenteral:** Hydrocortone Phosphate **(Rx)**

## Hydrocortisone sodium succinate
(hy-droh-**KOR**-tih-zohn)
**Pregnancy Category:** C
**Parenteral:** A-hydroCort, Solu-Cortef **(Rx)**

## Hydrocortisone valerate
(hy-droh-**KOR**-tih-zohn)
**Pregnancy Category:** C (topical products)
**Topical Cream/Ointment:** Westcort **(Rx)**
**Classification:** Corticosteroid, naturally occurring; glucocorticoid-type

See also *Corticosteroids.*
**Action/Kinetics:** Short-acting. **t½:** 80–118 min. Topical products are available without a prescription in strengths of 0.5% and 1%.
**How Supplied:** Hydrocortisone Cortisol: *Balm:* 1%; *Cream:* 0.25%, 0.5%, 1%, 2.5%; *Enema:* 100 mg/60 mL; *Gel/jelly:* 1%; *Liquid:* 1%; *Lotion:* 0.25%, 0.5%, 1%, 2%, 2.5%; *Ointment:* 0.5%, 1%, 2.5%; *Pad:* 0.5%, 1%; *Solution:* 1%, 2.5%; *Spray:* 0.5%, 1%; *Tablet:* 5 mg, 10 mg, 20 mg. Hydrocortisone acetate: *Cream:* 0.5%, 1%; *Foam:* 10%; *Injection:* 25 mg/mL, 50 mg/mL; *Lotion:* 1%; *Oint-*

*ment:* 0.5%, 1%; *Paste:* 0.5%; *Spray:* 0.5%; *Suppository:* 25 mg. Hydrocortisone butyrate: *Cream:* 0.1%; *Ointment:* 0.1%; *Solution:* 0.1%. Hydrocortisone cypionate: *Suspension:* 10 mg/5 mL. Hydrocortisone sodium phosphate: *Injection:* 50 mg/mL. Hydrocortisone sodium succinate: *Powder for injection:* 100 mg, 250 mg, 500 mg, 1 g. Hydrocortisone valerate: *Cream:* 0.2%; *Ointment:* 0.2%.

## Dosage

HYDROCORTISONE
- **Tablets**
20–240 mg/day, depending on disease.
- **IM Only**
One-third to one-half the PO dose q 12 hr.
- **Rectal**
100 mg in retention enema nightly for 21 days (up to 2 months of therapy may be needed; discontinue gradually if therapy exceeds 3 weeks).
- **Topical Ointment, Cream, Gel, Lotion, Solution, Spray**
Apply sparingly to affected area and rub in lightly t.i.d.–q.i.d.
HYDROCORTISONE ACETATE
- **Intralesional, Intra-articular, Soft Tissue**
5–50 mg, depending on condition.
- **Intrarectal Foam**
1 applicatorful (90 mg) 1–2 times/day for 2–3 weeks; **then** every second day.
- **Topical**
See *Hydrocortisone.*
HYDROCORTISONE BUTEPRATE
- **Topical Cream**
Apply a thin film to the affected area 1–2 times/day.
HYDROCORTISONE BUTYRATE
- **Topical Cream, Ointment, Solution**
Apply a thin film to the affected area b.i.d.–t.i.d.
HYDROCORTISONE CYPIONATE
- **Suspension**
20–240 mg/day, depending on the severity of the disease.
HYDROCORTISONE SODIUM PHOSPHATE
- **IV, IM, SC**

*General uses.*
**Initial:** 15–240 mg/day depending on use and on severity of the disease. Usually, one-half to one-third of the PO dose is given q 12 hr.
*Adrenal insufficiency, acute.*
**Adults, initial:** 100 mg IV; **then,** 100 mg q 8 hr in an IV fluid; **older children, initial:** 1–2 mg/kg by IV bolus; **then,** 150–250 mg/kg/day **IV** in divided doses; **infants, initial:** 1–2 mg/kg by IV bolus; **then,** 25–150 mg/kg/day in divided doses.
HYDROCORTISONE SODIUM SUCCINATE
- **IM, IV**
**Initial:** 100–500 mg; **then,** may be repeated at 2-, 4-, and 6-hr intervals depending on response and severity of condition.
HYDROCORTISONE VALERATE
- **Topical Cream**
See *Hydrocortisone.*

## DENTAL CONCERNS

See also *Dental Concerns* for *Corticosteroids.*

# Hydroxyurea
(hy-**DROX**-ee-you-**ree**-ah)
**Pregnancy Category:** D
Hydrea (Abbreviation: HYD)
**Classification:** Antineoplastic, antimetabolite

See also *Antineoplastic Agents.*
**Action/Kinetics:** Inhibits DNA synthesis but not synthesis of RNA or protein. As an antimetabolite, it interferes with the conversion of ribonucleotides to deoxyribonucleotides due to blockade of the ribonucleotide reductase system. May also inhibit incorporation of thymidine into DNA. Rapidly absorbed from GI tract. **Peak serum concentration:** 1–2 hr. t½: 3–4 hr. Crosses the blood-brain barrier. Degraded in liver; 80% excreted through the urine with 50% unchanged; also excreted as respiratory $CO_2$.
**Uses:** Chronic, resistant, myelocytic leukemia. Carcinoma of the ovary (recurrent, inoperable, or metastatic). Melanoma. With irradiation to treat primary squamous cell carcino-

ma of the head and neck (but not the lip). *Non-FDA Approved Uses:* Sickle cell anemia, thrombocytopenia, HIV, psoriasis.

**Contraindications:** Leukocyte count less than 2,500/mm³ or thrombocyte count less than 100,000/mm³. Severe anemia.

**Special Concerns:** Use during pregnancy only if benefits clearly outweigh risks. Give with caution to clients with marked renal dysfunction. Geriatric clients may be more sensitive to the effects of hydroxyurea necessitating a lower dose. Dosage has not been established in children.

**Additional Side Effects:** Erythrocyte abnormalities including megaloblastic erythropoiesis. Constipation, redness of the face, maculopapular rash.

**How Supplied:** *Capsule:* 500 mg

**Dosage**—————————
• **Capsules**

*Solid tumors, intermittent therapy or when used together with irradiation.*
**Dose individualized. Usual:** 80 mg/kg as a single dose every third day. Intermittent dosage offers advantage of reduced toxicity. If effective, maintain client on drug indefinitely unless toxic effects preclude such a regimen.
*Solid tumors, continuous therapy.*
20–30 mg/kg/day as a single dose.
*Resistant chronic myelocytic leukemia.*
20–30 mg/kg/day in a single dose or two divided daily doses.
*Concomitant therapy with irradiation for carinoma of the head and neck.*
80 mg/kg as a single dose every third day.

## DENTAL CONCERNS

See also *Dental Concerns* for *Antineoplastic Agents.*

---

# Ibuprofen
(eye-byou-**PROH**-fen)
**Pregnancy Category:** not established
**Rx:** Actiprofen ✦, Alti-Ibuprofen ✦, Apo-Ibuprofen ✦, Children's Advil, Children's Motrin, IBU, Ibuprohm, Motrin, Novo-Profen ✦, Nu-Ibuprofen ✦, Saleto-400, -600, and -800.
**OTC:** Advil Caplets and Tablets, Bayer Select Pain Relief Formula Caplets, Children's Advil Suspension, Children's Motrin Liquid Suspension, Children's Motrin Drops, Genpril Caplets and Tablets, Haltran, Ibuprin, Ibuprohm Caplets and Tablets, Junior Strength Motrin Caplets, Menadol, Midol IB, Motrin-IB Caplets and Tablets, Nuprin Caplets and Tablets, PediaCare Fever Drops, Saleto-200
**Classification:** Nonsteroidal anti-inflammatory drug (NSAID)

See also *Nonsteroidal Anti-Inflammatory Drugs.*
**Action/Kinetics: Time to peak levels:** 1–2 hr. **Onset:** 30 min for analgesia and approximately 1 week for anti-inflammatory effect. **Peak serum levels:** 1–2 hr. **t½:** 2 hr. **Duration:** 4–6 hr for analgesia and 1–2 weeks for anti-inflammatory effect. Food delays absorption rate but not total amount of drug absorbed.
**Uses:** Analgesic for mild to moderate pain. Primary dysmenorrhea, rheumatoid arthritis, osteoarthritis, antipyretic. *Non-FDA Approved Uses:* Resistant acne vulgaris (with tetracyclines); inflammation due to ultraviolet-B exposure (sunburn), juvenile rheumatoid arthritis. High doses to

---

✦ = Available in Canada                    ***bold italic*** = life-threatening side effect

treat progressive lung deterioration in cystic fibrosis. OTC products are used for the relief of fever and minor aches and pains due to colds, flu, sore throats, headaches, and toothaches.

**Contraindications:** Use of ibuprofen is not recommended during pregnancy, especially during the last trimester.

**Special Concerns:** The dosage must be individually determined for children less than 12 years of age as safety and effectiveness have not been established.

**Additional Side Effects:** Dermatitis (maculopapular type), rash. Hypersensitivity reaction consisting of abdominal pain, fever, headache, *meningitis,* N&V, signs of liver damage; especially seen in clients with SLE.

**Additional Drug Interactions**
*Furosemide* / Ibuprofen ↓ diuretic effect of furosemide due to ↓ renal prostaglandin synthesis
*Lithium* / Ibuprofen ↑ plasma levels of lithium
*Thiazide diuretics* / Ibuprofen ↓ diuretic effect of furosemide due to ↓ renal prostaglandin synthesis

**How Supplied:** *Chew Tablet:* 50 mg, 100 mg; *Suspension:* 50 mg/1.25 mL, 100 mg/5 mL; *Tablet:* 50 mg, 100 mg, 200 mg, 300 mg, 400 mg, 600 mg, 800 mg

**Dosage** ———————
• **Suspension, Chewable Tablets, Tablets**
*Rheumatoid arthritis, osteoarthritis.*
Either 300 mg q.i.d. or 400, 600, or 800 mg t.i.d.–q.i.d.; adjust dosage according to client response. Full therapeutic response may not be noted for 2 or more weeks.
*Juvenile arthritis.*
30–70 mg/kg/day in three to four divided doses (20 mg/kg/day may be adequate for mild cases).
*Mild to moderate pain.*
**Adults:** 400 mg q 4–6 hr, as needed.
*Antipyretic.*
**Pediatric, 2–12 years of age:** 5 mg/kg if baseline temperature is 102.5°F (39.1°C) or below or 10 mg/kg if baseline temperature is

greater than 102.5°F (39.1°C). Maximum daily dose: 40 mg/kg.
*Primary dysmenorrhea.*
**Adults:** 400 mg q 4 hr, as needed.
• **Tablets for OTC Use**
*Mild to moderate pain, antipyretic, dysmenorrhea.*
200 mg q 4–6 hr; dose may be increased to 400 mg if pain or fever persist. Dose should not exceed 1,200 mg/day.
• **Suspension for OTC Use**
*Pain, fever.*
**Children, 2–11 years:** 7.5 mg/kg, up to q.i.d., to a maximum of 30 mg/kg/day.

## DENTAL CONCERNS

See also *Dental Concerns* for *Nonsteroidal Anti-Inflammatory Drugs.*

# Indapamide
(in-**DAP**-ah-myd)
**Pregnancy Category:** B
Lozol **(Rx)**

# Indapamide hemihydrate
(in-**DAP**-ah-myd)
**Pregnancy Category:** B
Gen-Indapamide ✤, Lozide ✤ **(Rx)**
**Classification:** Diuretic, thiazide type

See also *Diuretics, Thiazide.*
**Action/Kinetics: Onset:** 1–2 weeks after multiple doses. **Peak levels:** 2 hr. **Duration:** Up to 8 weeks with multiple doses. **t½:** 14 hr. Nearly 100% is absorbed from the GI tract. Excreted through the kidneys (70% with 7% unchanged) and the GI tract (23%).
**Uses:** Alone or in combination with other drugs for treatment of hypertension. Edema in CHF.
**Contraindications:** Hypersensitivity, asthma, severe hepatic disease, severe renal disease.
**Special Concerns:** Dosage has not been established in children. Geriatric clients may be more sensitive to the hypotensive and electrolyte effects.
**Side Effects:** See also *Diuretics, Thiazide.*
**Drug Interactions:** See also *Diuretics, Thiazide.*

**How Supplied:** *Tablet:* 1.25 mg, 2.5 mg

Dosage ─────────────────
• **Tablets**
*Edema of CHF.*
**Adults:** 2.5 mg as a single dose in the morning. If necessary, may be increased to 5 mg/day after 1 week.
*Hypertension.*
**Adults:** 1.25 mg as a single dose in the morning. If the response is not satisfactory after 4 weeks, the dose may be increased to 2.5 mg taken once daily. If the response to 2.5 mg is not satisfactory after 4 weeks, the dose may be increased to 5 mg taken once daily (however, consideration should be given to adding another antihypertensive).

## DENTAL CONCERNS

See also *Dental Concerns* for *Diuretics, Thiazide* and *Antihypertensive Agents.*

# Indinavir sulfate

(in-**DIN**-ah-veer)
**Pregnancy Category:** C
Crixivan **(Rx)**
**Classification:** Antiviral drug, protease inhibitor

See also *Antiviral Drugs.*
**Action/Kinetics:** Binds to active sites on the HIV protease enzyme resulting in inhibition of enzyme activity. Inhibition prevents cleavage of the viral polyproteins resulting in the formation of immature noninfectious viral particles. Varying degrees of cross resistance have been noted between indinavir and other HIV-protease inhibitors. Rapidly absorbed in fasting clients; **time to peak plasma levels:** Approximately 0.8 hr. Administration with a meal high in calories, fat, and protein results in a significant decrease in the amount absorbed and in the peak plasma concentration. Approximately 60% bound to plasma proteins. **t½:** 1.8 hr. Metabolized in the liver with both parent drug and metab-olites excreted through the feces (over 80%) and the urine.
**Uses:** Treatment of HIV infection in adults when antiretroviral therapy is indicated. May be used with other anti-HIV drugs.
**Contraindications:** Lactation. Do not take with astemizole, cisapride, midazolam, rifampin, terfenadine, and triazolam. Mild to moderate liver or kidney disease.
**Special Concerns:** Not a cure for HIV infections; clients may continue to develop opportunistic infections and other complications of HIV disease. Not been shown to reduce the risk of transmission of HIV through sexual contact or blood contamination. No data on the effect of indinavir therapy on clinical progression of HIV infection, including survival or the incidence of opportunistic infections. Hemophiliacs treated for HIV infections with protease inhibitors may manifest spontaneous bleeding episodes. Safety and efficacy have not been determined in children.
**Side Effects:** *Oral:* Dry mouth, aphthous stomatitis, cheilitis, gingivitis, gingival hemorrhage, glossodynia. *GI:* N&V, diarrhea, abdominal pain, abdominal distention, acid regurgitation, anorexia, cholecystitis, cholestasis, constipation, dyspepsia, eructation, flatulence, gastritis, increased appetite, infectious gastroenteritis, jaundice, liver cirrhosis. *CNS:* Headache, insomnia, dizziness, somnolence, agitation, anxiety, bruxism, decreased mental acuity, depression, dream abnormality, dysesthesia, excitement, fasciculation, hypesthesia, nervousness, neuralgia, neurotic disorder, paresthesia, peripheral neuropathy, sleep disorder, tremor, vertigo. *CV:* CV disorder, palpitation. *Musculoskeletal:* Back pain, arthralgia, leg pain, myalgia, muscle cramps, muscle weakness, musculoskeletal pain, shoulder pain, stiffness. *Body as a whole:* Asthenia, fatigue, flank pain, malaise, chest pain, chills, fever, flu-like illness, fungal infection, malaise, pain, syn-

cope. *Hematologic:* Anemia, lymphadenopathy, spleen disorder. *Respiratory:* Cough, dyspnea, halitosis, pharyngeal hyperemia, pharyngitis, pneumonia, rales, rhonchi, **respiratory failure,** sinus disorder, sinusitis, URI. *Dermatologic:* Body odor, contact dermatitis, dermatitis, dry skin, flushing, folliculitis, herpes simplex, herpes zoster, night sweats, pruritus, seborrhea, skin disorder, skin infection, sweating, urticaria. *GU:* Nephrolithiasis, dysuria, hematuria, hydronephrosis, nocturia, PMS, proteinuria, renal colic, urinary frequency, UTI, uterine abnormality, urine sediment abnormality, urolithiasis. *Ophthalmic:* Accommodation disorder, blurred vision, eye pain, eye swelling, orbital edema. *Miscellaneous:* Asymptomatic hyperbilirubinemia, food allergy, taste disorder.

**Drug Interactions**
*Astemizole* / ↓ Metabolism of astemizole → possibility of cardiac arrhythmias and prolonged sedation
*Clarithromycin* / ↑ Plasma levels of both indinavir and clarithromycin
*Fluconazole* / ↓ Plasma levels of indinavir
*Ketoconazole* / ↑ Plasma levels of indinavir
*Midazolam* / ↓ Metabolism of midazolam → possibility of cardiac arrhythmias and prolonged sedation
*Terfenadine* / ↓ Metabolism of terfenadine → possibility of cardiac arrhythmias and prolonged sedation
*Triazolam* / ↓ Metabolism of triazolam → possibility of cardiac arrhythmias and prolonged sedation
*Trimethoprim/Sulfamethoxazole* / ↑ Plasma levels of trimethoprim (no change in levels of sulfamethoxazole

**How Supplied:** *Capsules:* 200 mg, 400 mg

**Dosage** ⎯⎯⎯⎯⎯⎯⎯⎯⎯⎯
• **Capsules**
  *HIV infections.*
**Adults:** 800 mg (two 400-mg capsules) q 8 hr ATC. The dosage is the same whether the drug is used alone or in combination with other retroviral agents. Reduce the dose to 600 mg

q 8 hr with mild to moderate hepatic insufficiency due to cirrhosis.

---

## DENTAL CONCERNS

See also *Dental Concerns* for *Antiviral Drugs.*
**General**
1. Semisupine position for dental chair in order to help alleviate or minimize GI discomfort from the drug.
2. Monitor vital signs at every appointment because of cardiovascular side effects.
3. Decreased saliva flow can put the patient at risk for dental caries, periodontal disease, and candidiasis.
4. Examine patient for oral signs and symptoms of opportunistic infection.
5. Burning mouth, secondary candidiasis, and tooth erosion may be symptoms of gastroesophageal disease which can occur simultaneously.

**Consultation with Primary Care Provider**
1. Medical consultation may be necessary in order to assess patient's disease control.

**Client/Family Teaching**
1. Review the importance of good oral hygiene in order to prevent soft tissue inflammation.
2. Review the proper use of oral hygiene aids in order to prevent injury.
3. Daily home fluoride treatments for persistent dry mouth.
4. Avoid alcohol-containing mouth rinses and beverages.
5. Avoid caffeine-containing beverages.
6. Dry mouth can be treated with tart, sugarless gum or candy, water, sugar-free beverages, or with saliva substitutes if dry mouth persists.
7. Report oral sores, lesions, or bleeding to the dentist.
8. Update patient's dental record (medication/health history) as needed.

---

# Indomethacin
(in-doh-**METH**-ah-sin)

Apo-Indomethacin ✿, Indochron E-R, Indocid ✿, Indocid Ophthalmic Suspension ✿, Indocid SR ✿, Indocin, Indocin SR, Indocollyre ✿, Indotec ✿, Novo–Methacin ✿, Nu-Indo ✿, Pro-Indo ✿, Rhodacine ✿ **(Rx)**

# Indomethacin sodium trihydrate

(in-doh-**METH**-ah-sin)

Indocin I.V. **(Rx)**

**Classification:** Nonsteroidal anti-inflammatory drug, analgesic, antipyretic

See also *Nonsteroidal Anti-Inflammatory Drugs.*

**Action/Kinetics: PO. Onset:** 30 min for analgesia and up to 1 week for anti-inflammatory effect. **Peak plasma levels:** 1–2 hr (2–4 hr for sustained-release). **Peak action for gout:** 24–36 hr; swelling gradually disappears in 3–5 days. **Peak activity for antirheumatic effect:** About 4 weeks. **Duration:** 4–6 hr for analgesia and 1–2 weeks for anti-inflammatory effect. **Therapeutic plasma levels:** 10–18 mcg/mL. **t½:** Approximately 5 hr (up to 6 hr for sustained-release). **Plasma t½ following IV in infants:** 12–20 hr, depending on age and dose. Approximately 90% plasma protein bound. Metabolized in the liver and excreted in both the urine and feces.

**Uses:** Not a simple analgesic; use only for the conditions listed. Moderate to severe rheumatoid arthritis, osteoarthritis, and ankylosing spondylitis (drug of choice). Acute gouty arthritis and acute painful shoulder (tendinitis, bursitis). *IV:* Pharmacologic closure of persistent patent ductus arteriosus in premature infants. *Non-FDA Approved Uses:* Topically to treat cystoid macular edema (0.5% and 1% drops), sunburn, primary dysmenorrhea, prophylaxis of migraine, cluster headache, polyhydramnios.

**Additional Contraindications:** Pregnancy and lactation. PO indomethacin in children under 14 years of age. GI lesions or history of recurrent GI lesions. *IV use:* GI or intracranial bleeding, thrombocytopenia, renal disease, defects of coagulation, necrotizing enterocolitis. *Suppositories:* Recent rectal bleeding, history of proctitis.

**Special Concerns:** Use in children should be restricted to those unresponsive to or intolerant of other anti-inflammatory agents; efficacy has not been determined in children less than 14 years of age. Geriatric clients are at greater risk of developing CNS side effects, especially confusion. To be used with caution in clients with history of epilepsy, psychiatric illness, or parkinsonism and in the elderly. Indomethacin should be used with extreme caution in the presence of existing, controlled infections.

**Additional Side Effects:** Reactivation of latent infections may mask signs of infection. More marked CNS manifestations than for other drugs of this group. Aggravation of depression or other psychiatric problems, epilepsy, and parkinsonism.

**Additional Drug Interactions**

*Captopril* / Indomethacin ↓ effect of captopril, probably due to inhibition of prostaglandin synthesis

*Diflunisal* / ↑ Plasma levels of indomethacin; also, possible fatal GI hemorrhage

*Diuretics (loop, potassium-sparing, thiazide)* / Indomethacin may reduce the antihypertensive and natriuretic action of diuretics

*Lisinopril* / Possible ↓ effect of lisinopril

*Prazosin* / Indomethacin ↓ antihypertensive effects of prazosin

**How Supplied:** Indomethacin: *Capsule:* 25 mg, 50 mg; *Capsule, extended release:* 75 mg; *Suppository:* 50 mg; *Suspension:* 25 mg/5 mL Indomethacin sodium trihydrate: *Powder for injection:* 1 mg

## Dosage

• **Capsules, Oral Suspension**

---

*Moderate to severe arthritis, osteo-arthritis, ankylosing spondylitis.*

**Adults, initial:** 25 mg b.i.d.–t.i.d.; may be increased by 25–50 mg at weekly intervals, according to condition and, if tolerated, until satisfactory response is obtained. With persistent night pain or morning stiffness, a maximum of 100 mg of the total daily dose can be given at bedtime. **Maximum daily dosage:** 150–200 mg. In acute flares of chronic rheumatoid arthritis, the dose may need to be increased by 25–50 mg/day until the acute phase is under control.

*Acute gouty arthritis.*

**Adults, initial:** 50 mg t.i.d. until pain is tolerable; **then,** reduce dosage rapidly until drug is withdrawn. Pain relief usually occurs within 2–4 hr, tenderness and heat subside in 24–36 hr, and swelling disappears in 3–4 days.

*Acute painful shoulder (bursitis/tendinitis).*

75–150 mg/day in three to four divided doses for 1–2 weeks.

- **Sustained-Release Capsules**
  *Antirheumatic, anti-inflammatory.*

**Adults:** 75 mg, of which 25 mg is released immediately, 1–2 times/day.

- **Suppositories**
  *Anti-inflammatory, antirheumatic, antigout.*

**Adults:** 50 mg up to q.i.d. **Pediatric:** 1.5–2.5 mg/kg/day in three to four divided doses (up to a maximum of 4 mg/kg or 250–300 mg/day, whichever is less).

- **IV Only**
  *Patent ductus arteriosus.*

3 IV doses, depending on age of the infant, are given at 12–24-hr intervals. **Infants less than 2 days:** first dose, 0.2 mg/kg, followed by two doses of 0.1 mg/kg each; **infants 2–7 days:** three doses of 0.2 mg/kg each; **infants more than 7 days:** first dose, 0.2 mg/kg, followed by two doses of 0.25 mg/kg each. If patent ductus arteriosus reopens, a second course of one to three doses may be given. Surgery may be required if there is no response after two courses of therapy.

## DENTAL CONCERNS

See also *Dental Concerns* for *Nonsteroidal Anti-Inflammatory Drugs.*

# Insulin injection (crystalline zinc insulin, unmodified insulin, regular insulin)

(IN-sue-lin)

**Pork:** Iletin II ✿, Insulin-Toronto ✿, Regular Iletin II, Regular Purified Pork Insulin. **Beef/Pork:** Iletin ✿, Regular Iletin I. **Human:** Humulin-R ✿, Novolin R, Novolin R PenFill, Novolin R Prefilled, Velosulin Human BR **(OTC)**

**Classification:** Rapid-acting insulin

See also *Antidiabetic Agents: Insulins.*

**Action/Kinetics:** Rarely administered as the sole agent due to its short duration of action. Injections of 100 units/mL are clear; cloudy, colored solutions should not be used. Regular insulin is the only preparation suitable for IV administration. Available only as 100 units/mL. **Onset, SC:** 30–60 min; **IV:** 10–30 min. **Peak, SC:** 2–4 hr; **IV:** 15–30 min. **Duration, SC:** 6–8 hr; **IV:** 30–60 min.

**Uses:** Suitable for treatment of diabetic coma, diabetic acidosis, or other emergency situations. Especially suitable for the client suffering from labile diabetes. During acute phase of diabetic acidosis or for the client in diabetic crisis, client is monitored by serum glucose and serum ketone levels.

**How Supplied:** Insulin injection: *Injection:* 100 U/mL.

## Dosage

- **SC**
  *Diabetes.*

**Adults, individualized, usual, initial:** 5–10 units; **pediatric:** 2–4 units. Injection is given 15–30 min before meals and at bedtime.

*Diabetic ketoacidosis.*

**Adults:** 0.1 unit/kg/hr given by continuous IV infusion.

## DENTAL CONCERNS

See also *Dental Concerns* for *Antidiabetic Agents: Insulins.*

# Insulin injection, concentrated

(**IN**-sue-lin)
**Pregnancy Category:** C
Regular (Concentrated) Iletin II U-500 **(Rx)**
**Classification:** Insulin, concentrated

See also *Antidiabetic Agents: Insulins.*

**Action/Kinetics:** Concentrated insulin injection (500 U/mL). Depending on response, may be given SC or IM as a single or as two or three divided doses. Not suitable for IV administration because of possible allergic or anaphylactoid reactions.

**Uses:** Insulin resistance requiring more than 200 units insulin/day.

**Contraindications:** Allergy to pork or mixed pork/beef insulin (unless client has been desensitized).

**Special Concerns:** Use with caution during lactation.

**Additional Side Effects:** Deep secondary hypoglycemia 18 24 hr after administration.

**Drug Interactions:** Do not use together with PO hypoglycemic agents.

**How Supplied:** *Injection:* 500 U/mL

**Dosage** —————
• **SC, IM**

   ***Individualized,*** depending on severity of condition. Clients must be kept under close observation until dosage is established.

## DENTAL CONCERNS

See also *Dental Concerns* for *Antidiabetic Agents: Insulins.*

# Insulin lispro injection (rDNA origin)

(**IN**-sue-lin **LYE**-sproh)
**Pregnancy Category:** B

Humalog **(Rx)**
**Classification:** Insulin, rDNA origin

See also *Antidiabetic Agents: Insulins.*

**Action/Kinetics:** Absorbed faster than regular human insulin. Compared with regular insulin, has a more rapid onset of glucose-lowering activity, an earlier peak for glucose lowering, and a shorter duration of glucose-lowering activity. However, is equipotent to human regular insulin (i.e., one unit of insulin lispro has the same glucose-lowering capacity as one unit of regular insulin). May lower the risk of nocturnal hypoglycemia in clients with type I diabetes. **Onset:** 15 min. **Peak effect:** 30–90 min. **t½:** 1 hr. **Duration:** 5 hr or less.

**Uses:** Diabetes mellitus.

**Contraindications:** Use during episodes of hypoglycemia. Hypersensitivity to insulin lispro.

**Special Concerns:** Since insulin lispro has a more rapid onset and shorter duration of action than regular insulin, clients with type I diabetes also require a longer acting insulin to maintain glucose control. Requirements may be decreased in impaired renal or hepatic function. Use with caution during lactation. Safety and efficacy have not been determined in children less than 12 years of age.

**Side Effects:** See *Antidiabetic Agents: Insulins.*

**Drug Interactions:** See *Antidiabetic Agents: Insulins.*

**How Supplied:** *Injection:* 100 U/mL

**Dosage** —————
• **SC**
   *Diabetes.*
Individualized, depending on severity of the condition.

## DENTAL CONCERNS

See also *Dental Concerns* for *Antidiabetic Agents: Insulins.*

---

# Insulin zinc suspension (Lente)

(**IN**-sue-lin)
**Pork:** Iletin II ✤, Lente Iletin II, Lente L.
**Beef/Pork:** Iletin ✤, Lentin Iletin I. **Human:** Humulin L, Novolin ge Lente ✤, Novolin L **(OTC)**
**Classification:** Intermediate-acting insulin

See also *Antidiabetic Agents: Insulins.*
**Action/Kinetics:** Contains 70% crystalline and 30% amorphous insulin suspension. Considered intermediate-acting. Principal advantage is the absence of a sensitizing agent such as protamine. **Onset:** 1–2.5 hr. **Peak:** 7–15 hr. **Duration:** About 22 hr.
**Uses:** Allergy to other types of insulin and in clients disposed to thrombotic phenomena in which protamine may be a factor. Zinc insulin is not a replacement for regular insulin and is not suitable for emergency use.
**How Supplied:** *Injection:* 100 U/mL

**Dosage** ————————
• **SC**
*Diabetes.*
**Adults, initial:** 7–26 units 30–60 min before breakfast. Dosage is then increased by daily or weekly increments of 2–10 units until satisfactory readjustment is established. A second smaller dose may be given prior to the evening meal or at bedtime. Clients on NPH can be transferred to insulin zinc suspension on a unit-for-unit basis. Clients being transferred from regular insulin should begin zinc insulin at two-thirds to three-fourths the regular insulin dosage. If the client is being transferred from protamine zinc insulin, the dose of zinc insulin should be about 50% of that required for protamine zinc insulin.

## DENTAL CONCERNS

See *Dental Concerns* for *Antidiabetic Agents: Insulins.*

# Insulin zinc suspension, extended (Ultralente)

(**IN**-sue-lin)
**Human:** Humulin-U ✤, Humulin U Ultralente, Novolin ge Ultralente ✤ **(OTC)**
**Classification:** Long-acting insulin

See also *Antidiabetic Agents: Insulins.*
**Action/Kinetics:** Large crystals of insulin and a high content of zinc are responsible for the slow-acting properties of this preparation. Products containing both 40 units/mL and 100 units/mL are available. **Onset:** 4–8 hr. **Peak:** 10–30 hr. **Duration:** 36 hr or longer.
**Uses:** Mild to moderate hyperglycemia in stabilized diabetics. Not suitable for the treatment of diabetic coma or emergency situations.
**How Supplied:** *Injection:* 100 U/mL

**Dosage** ————————
• **SC**
*Individualized.*
**Usual, initial:** 7–26 units as a single dose 30–60 min before breakfast.
**Do not administer IV.**

## DENTAL CONCERNS

See *Dental Concerns* for *Antidiabetic Agents: Insulins.*

# Ipratropium bromide

(eye-prah-**TROH**-pee-um)
**Pregnancy Category:** B
Alti-Ipratropium Bromide ✤, Apo-Ipravent ✤, Atrovent, Novo-Ipramide ✤ **(Rx)**
**Classification:** Anticholinergic, quaternary ammonium compound

See also *Cholinergic Blocking Agents.*
**Action/Kinetics:** Chemically related to atropine. Antagonizes the action of acetylcholine in bronchial smooth muscle; this leads to bronchodilation which is primarily a local, site-specific effect. Not easily absorbed into the systemic circulation; excreted through the feces. **t½, elimination:** 2 hr after inhalation.

**Uses: Aerosol or solution:** Bronchodilation in COPD, including chronic bronchitis and emphysema. **Nasal spray:** Symptomatic relief (using 0.06%) of rhinorrhea associated with allergic and nonallergic perennial ·rhinitis in clients over 12 years of age. Symptomatic relief (using 0.06%) of rhinorrhea associated with the common cold in those over 12 years of age. *NOTE:* The use of ipratropium with sympathomimetic bronchodilators, methylxanthines, steroids, or cromolyn sodium (all of which are used in treating COPD) are without side effects.

**Contraindications:** Hypersensitivity to atropine, ipratropium, or derivatives. Hypersensitivity to soya lecithin or related food products, including soy bean or peanut (inhalation aerosol).

**Special Concerns:** Use with caution in clients with narrow-angle glaucoma, prostatic hypertrophy, or bladder neck obstruction and during lactation. Safety and efficacy have not been determined in children. Use of ipratropium as a single agent for the relief of bronchospasm in acute COPD has not been studied adequately.

**Side Effects:** *Inhalation aerosol. CNS:* Cough, nervousness, dizziness, headache, fatigue, insomnia, drowsiness, difficulty in coordination, tremor. *Oral:* Dry mouth, dryness of oropharynx. *GI:* GI distress, nausea, constipation. *CV:* Palpitations, tachycardia, flushing. *Dermatologic:* Itching, hives, alopecia. *Miscellaneous:* Irritation from aerosol, worsening of symptoms, rash, hoarseness, blurred vision, difficulty in accommodation, drying of secretions, urinary difficulty, paresthesias, mucosal ulcers.

*Inhalation solution. CNS:* Dizziness, insomnia, nervousness, tremor, headache. *Oral:* Dry mouth, stomatitis, metallic taste. *GI:* Nausea, constipation. *CV:* Hypertension, aggravation of hypertension, tachycardia, palpitations. *Respiratory:* Worsening of COPD symptoms, coughing, dyspnea, bronchitis, bronchospasm, increased sputum, URI, pharyngitis, rhinitis, sinusitis. *Miscellaneous:* Urinary retention, UTIs, urticaria, pain, flu-like symptoms, back or chest pain, arthritis.

*Nasal spray. CNS:* Headache, dizziness. *Oral:* Dry mouth, taste perversion. *GI:* Nausea. *CV:* Palpitation, tachycardia. *Respiratory:* URI, epistaxis, pharyngitis, nasal dryness, miscellaneous nasal symptoms, nasal irritation, blood-tinged mucus, dry throat, cough, nasal congestion, nasal burning, coughing. *Ophthalmic:* Ocular irritation, blurred vision, conjunctivitis. *Miscellaneous:* Hoarseness, thirst, tinnitis, urinary retention.

*All products. Allergic:* Skin rash; angioedema of the tongue, throat, lips, and face; urticaria, laryngospasm, **anaphylaxis.** *Anticholinergic reactions:* Precipitation or worsening of narrow angle glaucoma, prostatic disorders, tachycardia, urinary retention, constipation, and bowel obstruction.

**How Supplied:** *Aerosol:* 0.018 mg/inh; *Nasal spray:* 0.03%; *Solution for inhalation:* 0.02%

## Dosage

• **Respiratory Aerosol**
*Treat bronchospasms.*
**Adults:** 2 inhalations (36 mcg) q.i.d. Additional inhalations may be required but should not exceed 12 inhalations/day.

• **Solution for Inhalation**
*Treat bronchospasms.*
**Adults:** 500 mcg (1-unit-dose vial) administered t.i.d.–q.i.d. by oral nebulization with doses 6–8 hr apart.

• **Nasal Spray, 0.03%**
*Perennial rhinitis.*
2 sprays (42 mcg) per nostril b.i.d.–t.i.d. for a total daily dose of 168–252 mcg/day.

• **Nasal Spray, 0.06%**
*Rhinitis due to the common cold.*
2 sprays (84 mcg) per nostril t.i.d.–q.i.d. for a total daily dose of 504–672 mcg/day. The safety and ef-

ficacy for use for the common cold for more than 4 days have not been determined.

## DENTAL CONCERNS

See also *Dental Concerns* for *Cholinergic Blocking Agents*.
1. Dental visits may precipitate acute asthma attacks. Have the patient keep his short-acting sympathomimetic inhaler available or make sure that the inhaler in the emergency kit is available.

**Client/Family Teaching**
1. May experience a bitter taste and dry mouth; use frequent mouth rinses with water after each use and suck on hard, sugarless candy to relieve bitter taste and dry mouth.

---

# Irbesartan

(ihr-beh-**SAR**-tan)
**Pregnancy Category:** C (first trimester), D (second and third trimesters)
Avapro **(Rx)**
**Classification:** Antihypertensive, angiotensin II receptor antagonist

See also *Antihypertensive Drugs*.
**Action/Kinetics:** By binding to $AT_1$ angiotensin II receptor, blocks vasoconstrictor and aldosterone-secreting effects of angiotensin II. Rapid absorption after PO use. **Peak plasma levels:** 1.5–2 hr. Food does not affect bioavailability. **$t\frac{1}{2}$, terminal elimination:** 11–15 hr. Over 90% bound to plasma proteins. Metabolized in liver and both unchanged drug and metabolites excreted through urine and feces.
**Uses:** Treat hypertension alone or in combination with other antihypertensives.
**Contraindications:** Hypersensitivity to the drug or any of its components.
**Special Concerns:** Safety and efficacy have not been determined in children. Should not be used during the second and third trimesters of pregnancy.
**Side Effects:** *Oral:* Oral lesion. *GI:* Diarrhea, dyspepsia, heartburn, abdominal pain, N&V, constipation,

gastroenteritis, flatulence, abdominal distention. *CV:* Tachycardia, syncope, orthostatic hypotension, hypotension (especially in volume- or salt-depletion), flushing, hypertension, cardiac murmur, *MI, cardio-respiratory arrest, heart failure, hypertensive crisis, CVA,* angina pectoris, arrhythmias, conduction disorder, transient ischemic attack. *CNS:* Sleep disturbance, anxiety, nervousness, dizziness, numbness, somnolence, emotional disturbance, depression, paresthesia, tremor. *Musculoskeletal:* Extremity swelling, muscle cramp, arthritis, muscle ache, musculoskeletal pain, musculoskeletal chest pain, joint stiffness, bursitis, muscle weakness. *Respiratory:* Epistaxis, tracheobronchitis, congestion, pulmonary congestion, dyspnea, wheezing, upper respiratory infection, rhinitis, pharyngitis, sinus abnormality. *GU:* Abnormal urination, prostate disorder, urinary tract infection, sexual dysfunction, libido change. *Dermatologic:* Pruritus, dermatitis, ecchymosis, facial erythema, urticaria. *Ophthalmic:* Vision disturbance, conjunctivitis, eyelid abnormality. *Otic:* Hearing abnormality, ear infection, ear pain, ear abnormality. *Miscellaneous:* Gout, fever, fatigue, chills, facial edema, upper extremity edema, headache, influenza, rash, chest pain.
**Drug Interactions:** No specific interactions have been reported with drugs that are used in dentistry. However, lowest effective dose should be used, such as a local anesthetic, vasoconstrictor, or anticholinergic, if required.
**How Supplied:** Tablets: 75 mg, 150 mg, 300 mg

## Dosage
• **Tablets**
  *Hypertension.*
150 mg once daily, up to 300 mg once daily. Lower initial dose of 75 mg is recommended for clients with depleted intravascular volume or salt. If BP is not controlled by irbesartan alone, hydrochlorothiazide may have an additive effect. Clients not ad-

equately treated by 300 mg irbesartan are unlikely to get benefit from higher dose or b.i.d. dosing.

## DENTAL CONCERNS

See also *Dental Concerns* for *Antihypertensive Drugs.*

# Isosorbide dinitrate chewable tablets
(eye-so-**SOR**-byd)
**Pregnancy Category:** C
Sorbitrate **(Rx)**

# Isosorbide dinitrate extended-release capsules
(eye-so-**SOR**-byd)
**Pregnancy Category:** C
Dilatrate-SR, Isordil Tembids **(Rx)**

# Isosorbide dinitrate extended-release tablets
(eye-so-**SOR**-byd)
**Pregnancy Category:** C
Cedocard-SR ✸, Coradur ✸, Isordil Tembids **(Rx)**

# Isosorbide dinitrate sublingual tablets
(eye-so-**SOR**-byd)
**Pregnancy Category:** C
Apo-ISDN ✸, Isordil, Sorbitrate **(Rx)**

# Isosorbide dinitrate tablets
(eye-so-**SOR**-byd)
**Pregnancy Category:** C
Apo-ISDN ✸, Isordil Titradose, Sorbitrate **(Rx)**
**Classification:** Coronary vasodilator, antianginal drug

See also *Antianginal Drugs—Nitrates/Nitrites.*
**Action/Kinetics:**    **Sublingual, chewable. Onset:** 2–5 min; **duration:** 1–3 hr. **Oral Capsules/Tablets. Onset:** 20–40 min; **duration:** 4–6 hr. **Extended-release. Onset:** up to 4 hr; **duration:** 6–8 hr.

**Additional Uses:** Diffuse esophageal spasm. Oral tablets are only for prophylaxis while sublingual and chewable forms may be used to terminate acute attacks of angina.
**Special Concerns:** Use with caution during lactation. Safety and efficacy have not been established in children.
**Additional Side Effects:** Vascular headaches occur especially frequently.
**Additional Drug Interactions**
*Acetylcholine* / Isosorbide antagonizes the effect of acetylcholine
*Norepinephrine* / Isosorbide antagonizes the effect of norepinephrine
**How Supplied:** *Chew tablet:* 5 mg, 10 mg; *Capsule, extended release:* 40 mg; *Tablet, extended release:* 40 mg; *Sublingual tablet:* 2.5 mg, 5 mg, 10 mg; *Tablet:* 2.5 mg, 5 mg, 10 mg, 20 mg, 30 mg, 40 mg

**Dosage** ────────────
• **Tablets**
  *Antianginal.*
**Initial:** 5–20 mg q 6 hr; **maintenance:** 10–40 mg q 6 hr (usual: 20–40 mg q.i.d.
• **Chewable Tablets**
  *Antianginal, acute attack.*
**Initial:** 5 mg q 2–3 hr. The dose can be titrated upward until angina is relieved or side effects occur.
  *Prophylaxis.*
5–10 mg q 2–3 hr.
• **Extended-Release Capsules**
  *Antianginal.*
**Initial:** 40 mg; **maintenance:** 40–80 mg q 8–12 hr.
• **Extended-Release Tablets**
  *Antianginal.*
**Initial:** 40 mg; **maintenance:** 40–80 mg q 8–12 hr.
• **Sublingual**
  *Acute attack.*
2.5–5 mg q 2–3 hr as required. The dose can be titrated upward until angina is relieved or side effects occur.
  *Prophylaxis.*
5–10 mg q 2–3 hr.

────────────────────────────

## DENTAL CONCERNS

See also *Dental Concerns* for *Antianginal Drugs—Nitrates/Nitrites.*

---

# Isosorbide mononitrate, oral

(eye-so-**SOR**-byd)
**Pregnancy Category:** C
Imdur, ISMO, Monoket **(Rx)**
**Classification:** Coronary vasodilator, antianginal drug

---

See also *Antianginal Drugs—Nitrates/Nitrites* and *Isosorbide dinitrate.*

**Action/Kinetics:** Isosorbide mononitrate is the major metabolite of isosorbide dinitrate. The mononitrate is not subject to first-pass metabolism. Bioavailability is nearly 100%. **Onset:** 30–60 min. **t½:** About 5 hr.

**Uses:** Prophylaxis of angina pectoris.

**Contraindications:** To abort acute anginal attacks. Use in acute MI or CHF.

**Special Concerns:** Use with caution in clients who may be volume depleted or who are already hypotensive. Use with caution during lactation. Safety and effectiveness have not been determined in children. The benefits have not been established in acute MI or CHF.

**Side Effects:** *CV:* Hypotension (may be accompanied by paradoxical bradycardia and increased angina pectoris). *CNS:* Headache, lightheadedness, dizziness. *GI:* N&V. *Miscellaneous:* Possibility of methemoglobinemia.

**Drug Interactions**
*Ethanol* / Additive vasodilation
*Sildenafil citrate* / ↑ Risk for adverse cardiovascular events

**How Supplied:** *Tablet:* 10 mg, 20 mg; *Tablet, extended release:* 30 mg, 60 mg, 120 mg

## Dosage

IMDUR TABLETS
*Prophylaxis of angina.*
**Initial:** 30 mg (given as one-half of the 60-mg tablet) or 60 mg once daily; **then,** dosage may be increased to 120 mg given as 2–60-mg tablets once daily. Rarely, 240 mg daily may be needed.

ISMO, MONOKET TABLETS
*Prevention and treatment of angina.*
**Adults:** 20 mg b.i.d. with the doses 7 hr apart (it is preferable that first dose be given on awakening). An initial dose of 5 mg may be best for clients of small stature; the dose should then be increased to at least 10 mg by the second or third day of therapy.

## DENTAL CONCERNS

See also *Dental Concerns* for *Antianginal Drugs—Nitrates/Nitrites* and *Isosorbide dinitrate.*

---

# Isradipine

(iss-**RAD**-ih-peen)
**Pregnancy Category:** C
DynaCirc, DynaCirc CR **(Rx)**
**Classification:** Calcium channel blocking agent

---

See also *Calcium Channel Blocking Agents.*

**Action/Kinetics:** Binds to calcium channels resulting in the inhibition of calcium influx into cardiac and smooth muscle and subsequent arteriolar vasodilation. Reduced systemic resistance leads to a decrease in BP with a small increase in resting HR. In clients with normal ventricular function, the drug reduces afterload leading to some increase in CO. Well absorbed from the GI tract, although it undergoes significant first-pass metabolism. **Peak plasma levels:** 1 ng/mL after 1.5 hr. **Onset:** 2–3 hr. Food increases the time to peak effect by about 1 hr, although the total bioavailability does not change. **t½, initial:** 1.5–2 hr; **terminal,** 8 hr. Completely metabolized in the liver with 60%–65% excreted through the kidneys and 25%–30% through the feces. Maximum effect may not be observed for 2–4 wks.

**Uses:** Alone or with thiazide diuretics in the management of essential hypertension. *Non-FDA Approved Uses:* Chronic stable angina.

**Contraindications:** Hypersensitivity, hypotension < 90 mm Hg, 2nd or 3rd degree heart block, sick sinus syndrome. Lactation.

**Special Concerns:** Safety and effectiveness have not been determined in children. Use with caution in clients with CHF, especially those taking a beta-adrenergic blocking agent. Bioavailability increases in those over 65 years of age, in impaired hepatic function, and in mild renal impairment.

**Side Effects:** *CV:* Palpitations, edema, flushing, tachycardia, SOB, hypotension, transient ischemic attack, *stroke,* atrial fibrillation, *ventricular fibrillation, MI,* CHF, angina. *CNS:* Headache, dizziness, fatigue, drowsiness, insomnia, lethargy, nervousness, depression, syncope, amnesia, psychosis, hallucinations, weakness, jitteriness, paresthesia. *Oral:* Dry mouth, gingival hyperplasia. *GI:* Nausea, abdominal discomfort, diarrhea, constipation, dry mouth. *Respiratory:* Dyspnea, cough. *Dermatologic:* Pruritus, urticaria. *Miscellaneous:* Chest pain, rash, pollakiuria, cramps of the legs and feet, nocturia, polyuria, hyperhidrosis, visual disturbances, numbness, throat discomfort, leukopenia, sexual difficulties.

**Drug Interactions**
*Anesthetics* / ↑ Effect of isradipine
*Barbiturates* / ↓ Effect of isradipine
*Carbamazepine* / ↑ Effect of isradipine due to ↓ breakdown by liver
*Fentanyl* / Possible severe hypotension or ↑ fluid volume
*Indomethacin* / ↓ Effect of isradipine
*NSAIDs* / ↓ Possible effect of isradipine
*Phenobarbital* / ↓ Effect of isradipine
*Other drugs with hypotensive effects* / ↑ Effect of isradipine
**How Supplied:** *Capsule:* 2.5 mg, 5 mg; *Tablet, extended release:* 5 mg, 10 mg

**Dosage** ───────────
• **Capsules**
*Hypertension.*
**Adults, initial:** 2.5 mg b.i.d. alone or in combination with a thiazide diuretic. If BP is not decreased satisfactorily after 2–4 weeks, the dose may be increased in increments of 5 mg/day at 2– to 4-week intervals up to a maximum of 20 mg/day. Adverse effects increase, however, at doses above 10 mg/day.
• **Tablets, Controlled-Release**
*Hypertension.*
**Adults:** 5–10 mg once daily.

## DENTAL CONCERNS

See also *Dental Concerns* for *Calcium Channel Blocking Agents.*
**General**
1. Frequent visits to assess for gingival hyperplasia.
2. Vasoconstrictors should be used with caution, in low doses, and with careful aspiration. Epinephrine-impregnated gingival retraction cords should be avoided.
3. Patients on chronic drug therapy may develop blood dyscrasias. Symptoms include fever, sore throat, and bleeding, and poor wound healing.
**Consultation with Primary Care Provider**
1. Patients with symptoms of blood dyscrasias should be referred to their primary care provider for complete blood counts. Treatment should be postponed until the results are known.
**Client/Family Teaching**
1. Practice frequent careful oral hygiene to minimize the incidence and severity of drug-induced gingival hyperplasia.
2. Need for frequent visits with a dental health professional if hyperplasia occurs.

# Itraconazole
(ih-trah-**KON**-ah-zohl)
**Pregnancy Category:** C

## Sporanox (Rx)
**Classification:** Antifungal

**Action/Kinetics:** Believed to inhibit cytochrome P-450-dependent synthesis of ergosterol, a necessary component of fungal cell membranes. Absorption appears to increase when taken with a cola beverage. Concentrates in fatty tissues, omentum, liver, kidney, and skin. **t½, at steady-state:** 64 hr. Extensively metabolized by the liver; the major metabolite is hydroxyitraconazole, which also has antifungal activity. The drug and major metabolite are extensively bound (over 99%) to plasma proteins. Metabolites are excreted in both the urine and feces.

**Uses:** Treatment of blastomycosis (pulmonary and extrapulmonary) and histoplasmosis (including chronic cavitary pulmonary disease and disseminated, nonmeningeal histoplasmosis) in both immunocompromised and nonimmunocompromised clients. To treat aspergillus infections (pulmonary and extrapulmonary) in clients intolerant or refractory to amphotericin B. Onychomycosis due to tinea unguium of the toenail with or without fingernail involvement. The drug is effective against *Blastomyces dermatitidis, Histoplasma capsulatum* and *H. duboisii, Aspergillus flavus* and *A. fumigatis,* and *Cryptococcus neoformans.* Oropharyngeal and esophageal candidiasis. In vitro activity has also been found for a number of other organisms, including *Sporothirx scheneckii, Trochophyton* species, *Candida albicans,* and *Candida* species. *Investigational:* (1) Superficial mycoses including dermatophytoses (tinea capitis, tinea corporis, tinea cruris, tinea pedis, and tinea manum), pityriasis versicolor, candidiasis (vaginal, oral, chronic mucocutaneous), and sebopsoriasis. (2) Systemic mycoses including dimorphic infections (paracoccidioidomycosis, coccidioidomycosis), cryptococcal infections (meningitis, disseminated), and candidiasis. (3) Miscellaneous mycoses including fungal keratitis, alternariosis, leishmaniasis (cutaneous), subcutaneous mycoses (chromomycosis, sporotrichosis), and zygomycosis.

**Contraindications:** Concomitant use of astemizole, cisapride, triazolam, oral midazolam, or terfenadine. Hypersensitivity to the drug or its excipients. Lactation. Use for the treatment of onychomycosis in pregnant women or in women wishing to become pregnant.

**Special Concerns:** Safety and efficacy have not been determined in children although pediatric clients have been treated for systemic fungal infections.

**Side Effects:** *GI:* N&V, diarrhea, abdominal pain, anorexia, general GI disorders, flatulence, constipation, gastritis. *CNS:* Headache, dizziness, vertigo, insomnia, decreased libido, somnolence, depression. *CV:* Hypertension, orthostatic hypotension, vasculitis. *Dermatologic:* Rash (occurs more frequently in immunocompromised clients also taking immunosuppressant drugs), pruritus. *Allergic:* Rash, pruritus, urticaria, angioedema, and rarely, **anaphylaxis and Stevens-Johnson syndrome.** *Miscellaneous:* Edema, fatigue, fever, malaise, abnormal hepatic function, hypokalemia, albuminuria, tinnitus, impotence, adrenal insufficiency, gynecomastia, breast pain in males, menstrual disorder, hepatitis (rare), neuropathy (rare).

**Drug Interactions**
*Astemizole* / ↑ Astemizole levels → serious CV toxicity including ventricular tachycardia, torsades de pointes, and death
*Calcium blockers (especially amlodipine and nifedipine)* / Development of edema
*Cisapride* / Cisapride levels serious CV toxicity including ventricular tachycardia, torsades de pointes, and death.
*Cyclosporine and HMG-CoA reductase inhibitors* / Possible development of rhabdomyolysis. ↑ Cyclosporine levels (dose of cyclosporine should be ↓ by 50% if itraconazole

doses are much greater than 100 mg/day)

*Digoxin* / ↑ Digoxin levels

*H₂ Antagonists* / ↓ Plasma levels of itraconazole

*Midazolam, oral* / ↑ Levels of oral midazolam → potentiation of sedative and hypnotic effects

*Isoniazid* / ↓ Plasma levels of itraconazole

*Phenytoin* / ↓ Plasma levels of itraconazole; also, metabolism of phenytoin may be altered

*Rifampin* / ↓ Plasma levels of itraconazole

*Quinidine* / Tinnitus and decreased hearing

*Sulfonylureas* / ↑ Risk of hypoglycemia

*Tacrolimus* / ↑ Levels of tacrolimus

*Terfenadine* / ↑ Terfenadine levels → serious CV toxicity including **ventricular tachycardia, torsades de pointes, and death**

*Triazolam* / Levels of triazolam potentiation of sedative and hypnotic effects

*Warfarin* / ↑ Anticoagulant effect of warfarin

**How Supplied:** *Capsule:* 100 mg

**Dosage**

• **Capsules**

*Blastomycosis or histoplasmosis.*

**Adults:** 200 mg once daily. If there is no improvement or the disease is progressive, the dose may be increased in 100-mg increments to a maximum of 400 mg/day. **Children, 3–16 years of age:** 100 mg/day (for systemic fungal infections).

*Aspergilliosis.*

200–400 mg daily.

*Life-threatening infections.*

**Adults:** A loading dose of 200 mg t.i.d. for the first 3 days should be given.

*Onychomycosis.*

200 mg once a day for 12 consecutive weeks. Alternatively, for fingernail fungus, 200 mg b.i.d. for 1 week, followed by a 3-week rest and then a second 1-week pulse of 200 mg b.i.d.

*Unlabeled uses.*

**Adults:** 50–400 mg/day for 1 day to more than 6 months, depending on the condition and the response.

• **Oral Solution**

*Oropharyngeal candidiasis.*

200 mg/day for 1–2 weeks.

*Esophageal candidiasis.*

100 mg/day for a minimum of 3 weeks.

## DENTAL CONCERNS

**General**

1. Semisupine position for dental chair in order to help alleviate or minimize GI discomfort from the drug.

2. Monitor vital signs at every appointment because of cardiovascular side effects.

3. Determine why the patient is taking this drug.

**Consultation with Primary Care Provider**

1. Medical consultation may be necessary in order to assess patient's ability to tolerate stress.

# Ketoconazole

(kee-toe-**KON**-ah-zohl)

**Pregnancy Category:** C

Nizoral **(Rx)**, Nizoral AD **(OTC)**

**Classification:** Broad-spectrum antifungal

See also *Anti-Infectives.*

**Action/Kinetics:** Inhibits synthesis of sterols (e.g., ergosterol), damaging the cell membrane and resulting in loss of essential intracellular material. Also inhibits biosynthesis of triglycerides and phospholipids and inhibits oxidative and peroxidative enzyme activity. When used to treat *Candida albicans,* it inhibits transformation of blastospores into the invasive mycelial form. Use in Cushing's syndrome is due to its ability to inhibit adrenal steroidogenesis. **Peak plasma levels:** 3.5 mcg/mL after 1–2 hr after a 200-mg dose. t½ [biphasic]: first, 2 hr; second, 8 hr. Requires acidity for dissolution. Metabolized in liver to inactive metabolites and most excreted through feces.

**Uses: PO:** Candidiasis, chronic mucocutaneous candidiasis, candiduria, histoplasmosis, chromomycosis, oral thrush, blastomycosis, coccidioidomycosis, paracoccidioidomycosis. Recalcitrant cutaneous dermatophyte infections not responding to other therapy. **Cream:** Tinea pedis. Tinea corporis and tinea cruris due to *Trichophyton rubrum, T. mentagrophytes,* and *Epidermophyton floccosum.* Tinea versicolor caused by *Microsporum furfur;* cutaneous candidiasis caused by *Candida* species; seborrheic dermatitis. **Shampoo:** To reduce scaling due to dandruff and tinea versicolor. *Non-FDA Approved Uses:* Onychomycosis due to *Candida* and *Trichophyton.* High doses to treat CNS fungal infections. Advanced prostate cancer, Cushing's syndrome.

**Contraindications:** Hypersensitivity, fungal meningitis. Topical product not for ophthalmic use. Use during lactation.

**Special Concerns:** Use tablets with caution in children less than 2 years of age. The safety and effectiveness of the shampoo and cream have not been determined in children. Use with caution during lactation.

**Side Effects:** *GI:* N&V, abdominal pain, diarrhea. *CNS:* Headache, dizziness, somnolence, fever, chills. *Hematologic:* Thrombocytopenia, leukopenia, *hemolytic anemia. Miscellaneous:* Hepatotoxicity, photophobia, pruritus, gynecomastia, impotence, bulging fontanelles, urticaria, decreased serum testosterone levels, anaphylaxis (rare). *Topical cream:* Stinging, irritation, pruritus. *Shampoo:* Increased hair loss, irritation, abnormal hair texture, itching, oiliness or dryness of the scalp and hair, scalp pustules.

**Drug Interactions**

*Antacids* / ↓ Absorption of ketoconazole due to ↑ pH induced by these drugs

*Anticoagulants* / ↓ Effect of anticoagulants

*Anticholinergics* / ↓ Absorption of ketoconazole due to ↑ pH induced by these drugs

*Astemizole* / ↑ Plasma levels of astemizole → serious CV effects

*Corticosteroids* / ↑ Risk of corticosteroid toxicity due to ↑ bioavailability

*Cyclosporine* / ↑ Levels of cyclosporine (may be used therapeutically to decrease the dose of cyclosporine)

*Histamine H₂ antagonists* / ↓ Absorption of ketoconazole due to ↑ pH induced by these drugs

*Isoniazid* / ↓ Bioavailability of ketoconazole

*Rifampin* / ↓ Serum levels of both drugs

*Terfenadine* / ↑ Plasma levels of terfenadine → serious CV effects

*Theophyllines* / ↓ Serum levels of theophylline

**How Supplied:** *Cream:* 2%; *Shampoo:* 2%; *Tablet:* 200 mg

**Dosage** ————————
• **Tablets**
  *Fungal infections.*
**Adults:** 200–400 mg once daily. **Pediatric, over 2 years:** 3.3–6.6 mg/kg once daily.
  *CNS fungal infections.*
**Adults:** 800–1,200 mg/day.
  *Advanced prostate cancer.*
400 mg q 8 hr.
  *Cushing's syndrome.*
800–1,200 mg/day.
• **Topical Cream (2%)**

*Tinea corporis, tinea cruris, tinea versicolor, tinea pedis, cutaneous candidiasis.*
Cover the affected and immediate surrounding areas once daily (twice daily for more resistant cases). Duration of treatment is usually 2 weeks.
*Seborrheic dermatitis.*
Apply to affected area b.i.d. for 4 weeks or until symptoms clear.

• **Shampoo (1%, 2%)**
Use twice a week for 4 weeks with at least 3 days between each shampooing. **Then,** use as required to maintain control.

## DENTAL CONCERNS

See also *General Dental Concerns for All Anti-Infectives.*
1. Decreased saliva flow can put the patient at risk for dental caries, periodontal disease, and candidiasis.
2. Replace toothbrush or other oral hygiene devices used during treatment of oral infection in order to prevent reinfection.
3. Frequent recall may be necessary in order to evaluate the healing process.
4. Determine if the medication is effective in controlling the disease.
**Client/Family Teaching**
1. Take tablets with food to decrease GI upset. Take 2 hr before drugs that alter gastric pH.
2. Report persistent fever, pain, or diarrhea.
3. With lack of stomach acid, dissolve each tablet in 4 mL aqueous solution of 0.2 N HCl; use a straw to avoid contact with teeth. This is followed by drinking a glass of tap water.
4. Use caution when driving or when performing hazardous tasks; may cause headaches, dizziness, and drowsiness.
5. Avoid alcohol or alcohol-containing products.
6. Wear sunglasses, sunscreen, and protective clothing, avoid sun exposure to prevent photosensitivity reactions.

# Ketoprofen
(kee-toe-**PROH**-fen)
**Pregnancy Category:** B
**Rx:** Apo-Keto ✦, Apo-Keto-E ✦, Apo-Keto-SR ✦, Novo-Keto ✦, Novo-Keto-EC ✦, Nu-Ketoprofen ✦, Nu-Ketoprofen-E ✦, Orafen ✦, Orudis, Orudis-E ✦, Orudis-SR ✦, Oruvail, PMS-Ketoprofen ✦, PMS-Ketoprofen-E ✦, Rhodis ✦, Rhodis-EC ✦, Rhodis SR ✦, Rhovail ✦, **OTC:** Actron, Orudis KT.
**Classification:** Nonsteroidal anti-inflammatory drug

See also *Nonsteroidal Anti-Inflammatory Drugs.*
**Action/Kinetics:** Possesses anti-inflammatory, antipyretic, and analgesic properties. Known to inhibit both prostaglandin and leukotriene synthesis, to have antibradykinin activity, and to stabilize lysosomal membranes. **Onset:** 15–30 min. **Peak plasma levels:** 0.5–2 hr. **Duration:** 4–6 hr. t½: 2–4 hr. t½, **geriatrics:** Approximately 5 hr. Is 99% bound to plasma proteins. Food does not alter the bioavailability; however, the rate of absorption is reduced.

**Uses: Rx:** Acute or chronic rheumatoid arthritis and osteoarthritis (both capsules and sustained-release capsules). Primary dysmenorrhea. Analgesic for mild to moderate pain.
**OTC:** Temporary relief of aches and pains associated with the common cold, toothache, headache, muscle aches, backache, menstrual cramps, reduction of fever, and minor pain of arthritis.
*Non-FDA Approved Uses:* Juvenile rheumatoid arthritis, sunburn, prophylaxis of migraine, migraine due to menses.
**Contraindications:** Should not be used during late pregnancy. Use should be avoided during lactation and in children. Use of the extended-release product for acute pain.
**Special Concerns:** Safety and effectiveness have not been established in children. Geriatric clients may manifest increased and prolonged serum levels due to decreased protein

K

---

binding and clearance. Use with caution in clients with a history of GI tract disorders, in fluid retention, hypertension, and heart failure.

**Additional Side Effects:** *GI:* Peptic ulcer, *GI bleeding,* dyspepsia, nausea, diarrhea, constipation, abdominal pain, flatulence, anorexia, vomiting, stomatitis. *CNS:* Headache. *CV:* Peripheral edema, fluid retention.

**Additional Drug Interactions**
*Acetylsalicylic acid* / ↑ Plasma ketoprofen levels due to ↓ plasma protein binding
*Hydrochlorothiazide* / ↓ Chloride and potassium excretion
*Methotrexate* / Concomitant use → toxic plasma levels of methotrexate
*Probenecid* / ↓ Plasma clearance of ketoprofen and ↓ plasma protein binding
*Warfarin* / Additive effect to cause bleeding

**How Supplied:** *Capsule:* 25 mg, 50 mg, 75 mg; *Capsule, extended release:* 100 mg, 150 mg, 200 mg; *Tablet:* 12.5 mg

**Dosage** ———————————

• **Rx: Extended Release Capsules, Capsules**
*Rheumatoid arthritis, osteoarthritis.*
**Adults, initial:** 75 mg t.i.d. or 50 mg q.i.d.; **maintenance:** 150–300 mg in three to four divided doses daily. Doses above 300 mg/day are not recommended. Alternatively, 200 mg once daily using the sustained-release formulation (Oruvail). Dosage should be decreased by one-half to one-third in clients with impaired renal function or in geriatric clients.
*Mild to moderate pain, dysmenorrhea.*
**Adults:** 25–50 mg q 6–8 hr as required, not to exceed 300 mg/day. Dosage should be reduced in smaller or geriatric clients and in those with liver or renal dysfunction. Doses greater than 75 mg do not provide any added therapeutic effect.

• **OTC: Tablets**
**Adults, over 16 years of age:** 12.5 mg with a full glass of liquid every 4 to 6 hr. If pain or fever persists after 1 hr follow with an additional 12.5

mg. Experience may determine that an initial dose of 25 mg gives a better effect. Dosage should not exceed 25 mg in a 4- to 6-hr period or 75 mg in a 24-hr period.

---

## DENTAL CONCERNS

See also *Dental Concerns* for *Nonsteroidal Anti-Inflammatory Drugs.*

---

# Ketorolac tromethamine
(kee-toh-**ROH**-lack)
**Pregnancy Category:** C
Acular, Acular PF, Toradol, Toradol IM **(Rx)**
**Classification:** Nonsteroidal anti-inflammatory drug

---

See also *Nonsteroidal Anti-Inflammatory Drugs.*

**Action/Kinetics:** Possesses anti-inflammatory, analgesic, and antipyretic effects. Completely absorbed following IM use. **Onset:** Within 30 min. **Maximum effect:** 1–2 hr after IV or IM dosing. **Duration:** 4–6 hr. **Peak plasma levels:** 2.2–3.0 mcg/mL 50 min after a dose of 30 mg. **t½, terminal:** 3.8–6.3 hr in young adults and 4.7–8.6 hr in geriatric clients. Over 99% is bound to plasma proteins. Metabolized in the liver with over 90% excreted in the urine and the remainder excreted in the feces.

**Uses: PO:** Short-term (up to 5 days) management of severe, acute pain that requires analgesia at the opiate level. Always initiate therapy with IV or IM followed by PO only as continuation treatment, if necessary. **IM/IV:** Ketorolac has been used with morphine and meperidine and shows an opioid-sharing effect. The combination can be used for breakthrough pain. **Ophthalmic:** Relieve itching caused by seasonal allergic conjunctivitis. Reduce ocular pain and photo phobia following incisional refractive surgery.

**Contraindications:** Hypersensitivity to the drug, incomplete or partial syndrome of nasal polyps, angioedema, and bronchospasm due to aspirin or other NSAIDs. Use in clients with advanced renal impairment or in those at risk for renal failure due to volume depletion. Use in suspected or confirmed cardiovascular bleeding, hemorrhagic diathesis, or incomplete hemostasis and in those with a high risk of bleeding. Use as an obstetric preoperative medication or for obstetric analgesia. Routine use with other NSAIDs. Intrathecal or epidural administration. Use in labor and delivery. The ophthalmic solution should not be used in clients wearing soft contact lenses.

**Special Concerns:** Use with caution in impaired hepatic or renal function, during lactation, in geriatric clients, and in clients on high-dose salicylate regimens. The age, dosage, and duration of therapy should receive special consideration when using this drug. Safety and effectiveness have not been determined in children.

**Additional Side Effects:** *CV:* Vasodilation, pallor. *Oral:* Dry mouth, stomatitis. *GI:* GI pain, peptic ulcers, nausea, dyspepsia, flatulence, GI fullness, excessive thirst, GI bleeding (higher risk in geriatric clients), *perforation. CNS:* Headache, nervousness, abnormal thinking, depression, euphoria. *Hypersensitivity:* **Bronchospasm, anaphylaxis.** *Miscellaneous:* Purpura, asthma, abnormal vision, abnormal liver function.

*Use of the ophthalmic solution:* Transient stinging and burning following instillation, ocular irritation, allergic reactions, superficial ocular infections, superficial keratitis.

**Drug Interactions:** Ketorolac may ↑ plasma levels of salicylates due to ↓ plasma protein binding.

**How Supplied:** *Injection:* 15 mg/mL, 30 mg/mL; *Ophthalmic solution:* 0.5%; *Tablet:* 10 mg

**Dosage** ————————————
• **IM**
*Analgesic, single dose.*
**Adults: less than 65 years of age:** One 60-mg dose. **Adults, over 65 years of age, in renal impair-**

**ment, or weight less than 50 kg:** One 30-mg dose.
*Analgesic, multiple dose.*
**Adults, less than 65 years of age:** 30 mg q 6 hr, not to exceed 120 mg daily. **Adults, over 65 years of age, in renal impairment, or weight less than 50 kg:** 15 mg q 6 hr, not to exceed 60 mg daily.
• **IV**
*Analgesic, single dose.*
**Adults, less than 65 years of age:** One 30-mg dose. **Adults, over 65 years of age, in renal impairment, or weight less than 50 kg:** One 15-mg dose.
• **Tablets**
*Transition from IV/IM to PO.*
**Adults less than 65 years of age:** 20 mg as a first PO dose for clients who received 60 mg IM single dose, 30 mg IV single dose, or 30 mg multiple dose IV/IM; **then,** 10 mg q 4–6 hr, not to exceed 40 mg in a 24-hr period. **Adults, over 65 years of age, in renal impairment, or weight less than 50 kg:** 10 mg as a first PO dose for those who received a 30-mg IM single dose, a 15-mg IV single dose, or a 15-mg multiple dose IV/IM; **then,** 10 mg q 4–6 hr, not to exceed 40 mg in a 24-hr period.
• **Ophthalmic Solution**
*Seasonal allergic conjunctivitis.*
1 gtt (0.25 mg) q.i.d. Efficacy has not been determined beyond 1 week of use.
*Following cataract extraction.*
1 gtt to the affected eye(s) q.i.d. beginning 24 hr after surgery and continuing for 2 weeks postoperatively.

## DENTAL CONCERNS
### General
1. Decreased saliva flow can put the patient at risk for dental caries, periodontal disease, and candidiasis.
2. Avoid dental use during pregnancy.
3. The patient should not take prescription and over-the-counter aspirin-containing drug products.
4. Avoid long-term use. Combined

use of IM/IV and oral dose forms should not exceed 5 days.

**Consultation with Primary Care Provider**

1. Consultation with appropriate health care provider may be necessary in order to assess level of disease control.

**Client/Family Teaching**

1. Take NSAIDs with a full glass of water or milk, with meals, or with a prescribed antacid and remain upright 30 min following administration to reduce gastric irritation or ulcer formation.

2. Use caution in operating machinery or in driving a car; may cause dizziness or drowsiness.

3. Avoid alcohol, aspirin, acetaminophen, and any other OTC preparations without approval because of increased risk for GI bleeding.

# L

# Labetalol hydrochloride
(lah-**BET**-ah-lohl)
**Pregnancy Category:** C
Normodyne, Trandate **(Rx)**
**Classification:** Alpha- and beta-adrenergic blocking agent

See also *Beta-Adrenergic Blocking Agents* and *Antihypertensive Agents*.

**Action/Kinetics:** Decreases BP by blocking both alpha- and beta-adrenergic receptors. Standing BP is lowered more than supine. Significant reflex tachycardia and bradycardia do not occur although AV conduction may be prolonged. **Onset: PO,** 2–4 hr; **IV,** 5 min. **Peak plasma levels, PO:** 1–2 hr. **Peak effects, PO:** 2–4 hr. **Duration: PO,** 8–12 hr. **t½: PO,** 6–8 hr; **IV,** 5.5 hr. Significant first-pass effect; metabolized in liver. Food increases bioavailability of the drug.

**Uses: PO:** Alone or in combination with other drugs for hypertension. **IV:** Hypertensive emergencies. *Non-FDA Approved Uses:* Pheochromocytoma, clonidine withdrawal hypertension.

**Contraindications:** Cardiogenic shock, cardiac failure, bronchial asthma, bradycardia, greater than first-degree heart block.

**Special Concerns:** Use with caution during lactation, in impaired renal and hepatic function, in chronic bronchitis and emphysema, and in diabetes (may prevent premonitory signs of acute hypoglycemia). Safety and efficacy in children have not been established.

**Side Effects:** See also *Beta-Adrenergic Blocking Agents*. **After PO Use.** *GI:* Diarrhea, cholestasis with or without jaundice. *CNS:* Fatigue, drowsiness, paresthesias, headache, syncope (rare). *GU:* Impotence, priapism, ejaculation failure, difficulty in micturition, Peyronie's disease, acute urinary bladder retention. *Respiratory:* Dyspnea, bronchospasm. *Musculoskeletal:* Muscle cramps, asthenia, toxic myopathy. *Dermatologic:* Generalized maculopapular, lichenoid, or urticarial rashes; bullous lichen planus, psoriasis, facial erythema, reversible alopecia. *Ophthalmic:* Abnormal vision, dry eyes. *Miscellaneous:* SLE, positive antinuclear factor, antimitochondrial antibodies, fever, edema, nasal stuffiness.

**After parenteral use.** *CV:* Ventricular arrhythmias. *CNS:* Numbness, somnolence, yawning. *Miscellaneous:* Pruritus, flushing, wheezing.

**After PO or parenteral use.** *GI:* N&V, dyspepsia, taste distortion. *CNS:* Dizziness, tingling of skin or scalp, vertigo. *Miscellaneous:* Postural hypotension, increased sweating.

**Drug Interactions**

*Epinephrine* / ↑ Chance for hypertension, bradycardia

*Halothane* / ↑ Risk of severe myo-cardial depression → hypotension
*Indomethacin* / ↓ Hypotensive effects of labetolol
*Lidocaine* / ↓ Metabolism of labetol
*NSAIDs* / ↓ Hypotensive effects of labetolol
*Sympathomimetics* / ↓ Effects of labetolol, ↑ chance of hypertension, bradycardia
**How Supplied:** *Injection:* 5 mg/mL; *Tablet:* 100 mg, 200 mg, 300 mg

**Dosage** ————————————
• **Tablets**
*Hypertension.*
**Individualize. Initial:** 100 mg b.i.d. alone or with a diuretic; **maintenance:** 200–400 mg b.i.d. up to 1,200–2,400 mg/day for severe cases.
• **IV**
*Hypertension.*
**Individualize. Initial:** 20 mg slowly over 2 min; **then,** 40–80 mg q 10 min until desired effect occurs or a total of 300 mg has been given.
• **IV Infusion**
*Hypertension.*
**Initial:** 2 mg/min; **then,** adjust rate according to response. **Usual dose range:** 50–300 mg.
*Transfer from IV to PO therapy.*
**Initial:** 200 mg; **then,** 200–400 mg 6–12 hr later, depending on response. Thereafter, dosage based on response.

**DENTAL CONCERNS**

See also *Dental Concerns* for *Beta-Adrenergic Blocking Agents, Alpha-1 Adrenergic Blocking Agents,* and *Antihypertensive Agents.*

## Lamivudine (3TC)

(lah-**MIH**-vyou-deen)
**Pregnancy Category:** C
3TC ✶, Epivir **(Rx)**
**Classification:** Antiviral drug

See also *Antiviral Drugs.*
**Action/Kinetics:** Synthetic nucleoside analog effective against HIV. Converted to active 5'-triphosphate (L-TP) metabolite which inhibits HIV

reverse transcription via viral DNA chain termination. L-TP also inhibits the RNA- and DNA-dependent DNA polymerase activities of reverse transcriptase. Rapidly absorbed after PO administration. Most eliminated unchanged through the urine.
**Uses:** In combination with AZT for the treatment of HIV infection, based on clinical or immunologic evidence of progression of the disease. There are no data on the effect of lamivudine and AZT on clinical progression of HIV infection, such as the incidence of opportunistic infections or survival.
**Contraindications:** Lactation.
**Special Concerns:** Clients taking lamivudine and AZT may continue to develop opportunistic infections and other complications of HIV infection. Use with caution and at a reduced dose in those with impaired renal function. Data on the use of lamivudine and AZT in pediatric clients are lacking; however, use the combination with extreme caution in children with pancreatitis.
**Side Effects:** Side effects are for the combination of lamivudine plus AZT. *GI:* N&V, diarrhea, anorexia, or decreased appetite, abdominal pain, abdominal cramps, dyspepsia. *CNS:* Neuropathy, insomnia or other sleep disorders, dizziness, depressive disorders, paresthesias, peripheral neuropathies. *Respiratory:* Nasal signs and symptoms, cough. *Musculoskeletal:* Musculoskeletal pain, myalgia, arthralgia. *Body as a whole:* Headache, malaise, fatigue, fever or chills, skin rashes. *NOTE:* Pediatric clients have an increased risk to develop *pancreatitis.*
**Drug Interactions:** Use of lamivudine with trimethoprim-sulfamethoxazole resulted in a significant increase in lamivudine levels.
**How Supplied:** *Tablet:* 150 mg; *Solution:* 10 mg/mL

**Dosage** ————————————
• **Oral Solution, Tablets**
*HIV infection.*

**Adults and adolescents, aged 12–16 years:** 150 mg b.i.d. in combination with AZT. For adults with low body weight (less than 50 kg), the recommended dose is 2 mg/kg b.i.d. in combination with AZT. **Children, 3 months to 12 years of age:** 4 mg/kg b.i.d. (up to a maximum of 150 mg b.i.d.) in combination with AZT. In clients over 16 years of age, the dose should be adjusted, as follows, in impaired renal function. Creatinine clearance ($C_{CR}$) less than 50 mL/min: 150 mg b.i.d., $C_{CR}$ 30–49 mL/min: 150 mg once daily. $C_{CR}$ 15–29 mL/min: 150 mg for the first dose followed by 100 mg once daily. $C_{CR}$ 5–14 mL/min: 150 mg for the first dose followed by 50 mg once daily. $C_{CR}$ less than 5 mL/min: 50 mg for the first dose followed by 25 mg once daily.

## DENTAL CONCERNS

See also *Dental Concerns* for *Antiviral Drugs.*
**General**
1. Patients on chronic drug therapy may develop blood dyscrasias. Symptoms include fever, sore throat, bleeding, and poor wound healing.
2. Examine patient for oral signs and symptoms of opportunistic infection.
**Consultation with Primary Care Provider**
1. Patients with symptoms of blood dyscrasias should be referred to their primary care provider for complete blood counts. Treatment should be postponed until the results are known.
2. Medical consultation may be necessary in order to assess patient's ability to tolerate stress and level of disease control.
**Client/Family Teaching**
1. Review the importance of good oral hygiene in order to prevent soft tissue inflammation.
2. Review the proper use of oral hygiene aids in order to prevent injury.
3. Secondary oral infection may occur. Seek dental treatment immediately if this happens.

# Lamivudine/Zidovudine
((lah-**MIH**-vyou-deen, zye-**DOH**-vyou-deen))
**Pregnancy Category:** C
Combivir **(Rx)**
**Classification:** Antiviral drug combination

See also *Lamivudine, Zidovudine,* and *Antiviral Drugs.*
**Content:** Each Combivir tablet contains: *Antiviral:* Lamivudine, 150 mg and *Antiviral:* Zidovudine, 300 mg.
**Action/Kinetics:** Both drugs are reverse transcriptase inhibitors with activity against HIV. Combination results in synergistic antiretroviral effect. Each drug is rapidly absorbed.
**Uses:** Treatment of HIV infection.
**Contraindications:** Use in clients requiring dosage reduction, children less than 12 years of age, $C_{CR}$ less than 50 mL/min, body weight less than 50 kg, and in those experiencing dose-limiting side effects.
**Side Effects:** See individual drugs.
**Drug Interactions:** See individual drugs.

**Dosage**
• **Tablets**
  *HIV infection.*
**Adults and children over 12 years of age:** One combination tablet—150 mg lamivudine/300 mg zidovudine—b.i.d.

## DENTAL CONCERNS

See also *Dental Concerns* for *Lamivudine, Zidovudine,* and *Antiviral Drugs.*
**Client/Family Teaching:** See individual drugs.

# Lamotrigine
(lah-**MAH**-trih-jeen)
**Pregnancy Category:** C
Lamictal **(Rx)**
**Classification:** Anticonvulsant

See also *Anticonvulsants.*
**Action/Kinetics:** Mechanism of anticonvulsant action not known. May act to inhibit voltage-sensitive sodium channels. This effect stabiliz-

es neuronal membranes and modulates presynaptic transmitter release of excitatory amino acids such as glutamate and aspartate. Rapidly and completely absorbed after PO use. **Peak plasma levels:** 1.4–4.8 hr. **t½, after repeated doses: About 33 hr.** Metabolized by the liver with metabolites and unchanged drug excreted mainly through the urine (94%). Lamotrigine induces its own metabolism. Eliminated more rapidly in clients who have been taking antiepileptic drugs that induce liver enzymes. However, valproic acid decreases the clearance of lamotrigine.

**Uses:** Adjunct in the treatment of partial seizures in adults with epilepsy. *Non-FDA Approved Uses:* Adults with generalized clonic-tonic, absence, atypical absence, and myoclonic seizures. Infants and children with Lennox-Gastaut syndrome.

**Contraindications:** Use during lactation and in children less than 16 years of age.

**Special Concerns:** Use with caution in clients with diseases or conditions that could affect metabolism or elimination of the drug, such as in impaired renal, hepatic, or cardiac function.

**Side Effects:** Side effects listed are those with an incidence of 0.1% or greater. *CNS:* Dizziness, ataxia, somnolence, headache, incoordination, insomnia, tremor, depression, anxiety, irritability, decreased memory, speech disorder, confusion, disturbed concentration, sleep disorder, emotional lability, vertigo, mind racing, amnesia, nervousness, abnormal thinking, abnormal dreams, agitation, akathisia, aphasia, CNS depression, depersonalization, dyskinesia, dysphoria, euphoria, faintness, hallucinations, hostility, hyperkinesia, hypesthesia, myoclonus, panic attack, paranoid reaction, personality disorder, psychosis, stupor. *Oral:* Dry mouth, tooth disorder, gingivitis, gum hyperplasia, increased salivation, mouth ulceration,

stomatitis. *GI:* N&V, diarrhea, dyspepsia, constipation, anorexia, abdominal pain, dysphagia, flatulence, increased appetite, abnormal liver function tests, thirst. *CV:* Hot flashes, palpitations, flushing, migraine, syncope, tachycardia, vasodilation. *Musculoskeletal:* Arthralgia, joint disorder, myasthenia, dysarthria, muscle spasm, twitching. *Hematologic:* Anemia, ecchymosis, leukocytosis, leukopenia, lymphadenopathy, petechiae. *Respiratory:* Rhinitis, pharyngitis, increased cough, dyspnea, epistaxis, hyperventilation. *Dermatologic:* **Stevens-Johnson syndrome, toxic epidermal necrolysis,** pruritus, alopecia, acne, dry skin, eczema, erythema, hirsutism, maculopapular rash, sweating, urticaria. *Ophthalmologic:* Diplopia, blurred vision, nystagmus, abnormal vision, abnormal accommodation, conjunctivitis, oscillopsia, photophobia. *GU:* Dysmenorrhea, vaginitis, amenorrhea, female lactation, hematuria, polyuria, urinary frequency or incontinence, UTI, vaginal moniliasis. *Body as a whole:* **Possibility of sudden unexplained death in epilepsy,** flu syndrome, fever, infection, neck pain, malaise, **seizure exacerbation,** chills, halitosis, facial edema, weight gain or loss, peripheral edema, hyperglycemia. *Miscellaneous:* Ear pain, tinnitus, taste perversion.

**Drug Interactions**
*Acetaminophen /* ↓ Serum lamotrigine levels
*Carbamazepine /* Lamotrigine concentration is ↓ by about 40%
*Phenobarbital /* Lamotrigine concentration is ↓ by about 40%

**How Supplied:** *Tablet:* 25 mg, 100 mg, 150 mg, 200 mg

**Dosage** ─────────────
• **Tablets**
*Treatment of partial seizures.*
**Adults and children over 16 years of age who are taking enzyme-inducing antiepileptic drugs, but not valproate:** 50 mg once a day for weeks 1 and 2, followed by 100

mg/day in two divided doses for weeks 3 and 4. **Maintenance dose:** 300–500 mg/day given in two divided doses. The dose should be increased by 100 mg/day every week until maintenance levels are reached. **Adults and children over 16 years of age who are taking enzyme-inducing antiepileptic drugs plus valproic acid:** 25 mg every other day for weeks 1 and 2, followed by 25 mg once daily for weeks 3 and 4. **Maintenance dose:** 100–150 mg/day in two divided doses. The dose should be increased by 25–50 mg/day every 1–2 weeks.

## DENTAL CONCERNS

See also *Dental Concerns* for *Anticonvulsants*.

# Lansoprazole

(lan-**SAHP**-rah-zohl)
**Pregnancy Category:** B
Prevacid **(Rx)**
**Classification:** GI drug, proton pump inhibitor

**Action/Kinetics:** Suppresses gastric acid secretion by inhibition of the $(H^+, K^+)$-ATPase system located at the secretory surface of the parietal cells in the stomach. Drug is a gastric acid (proton) pump inhibitor in that it blocks the final step of acid production. Both basal and stimulated gastric acid secretion are inhibited, regardless of the stimulus. May have antimicrobial activity against *Helicobacter pylori*. Absorption begins only after lansoprazole granules leave the stomach, but absorption is rapid. **Peak plasma levels:** 1.7 hr. **Mean plasma $t\frac{1}{2}$:** 1.5 hr. Over 97% bound to plasma proteins. Food does not appear to affect the rate of absorption, if given before meals. Metabolized in the liver with metabolites excreted through both the urine (33%) and feces (66%).

**Uses:** Short-term treatment (up to 4 weeks) for healing and symptomatic relief of active duodenal ulcer. With clarithromycin and amoxicillin as triple therapy to eradicate *H. pylori* in-

fection in active or recurrent duodenal ulcers. Short-term treatment (up to 8 weeks) for healing and symptomatic relief of all grades of erosive esophagitis. Maintenance treatment of healed erosive esophagitis. Long-term treatment of pathologic hypersecretory conditions, including Zollinger-Ellison syndrome.

**Contraindications:** Lactation.

**Special Concerns:** Reduce dosage in impaired hepatic function. Symptomatic relief does not preclude the presence of gastric malignancy. Safety and efficacy have not been determined in children less than 18 years of age.

**Side Effects:** *Oral:* Dry mouth, increased salivation, stomatitis. *GI:* Diarrhea, abdominal pain, nausea, melena, anorexia, bezoar, cardiospasm, cholelithiasis, constipation, thirst, dyspepsia, dysphagia, eructation, esophageal stenosis, esophageal ulcer, esophagitis, fecal discoloration, flatulence, gastric nodules, fundic gland polyps, gastroenteritis, **GI hemorrhage, rectal hemorrhage,** hematemesis, increased appetite, tenesmus, vomiting, ulcerative colitis. *CV:* Angina, hypertension or hypotension, **CVA, MI, shock,** palpitations, vasodilation. *CNS:* Headache, agitation, amnesia, anxiety, apathy, confusion, depression, syncope, dizziness, hallucinations, hemiplegia, aggravated hostility, decreased libido, nervousness, paresthesia, abnormal thinking. *GU:* Abnormal menses, breast enlargement, gynecomastia, breast tenderness, hematuria, albuminuria, glycosuria, impotence, kidney calculus. *Respiratory:* Asthma, bronchitis, increased cough, dyspnea, epistaxis, hemoptysis, hiccoughs, pneumonia, upper respiratory inflammation or infection. *Endocrine:* Diabetes mellitus, goiter, hypoglycemia or hyperglycemia. *Hematologic:* Anemia, eosinophilia, hemolysis. *Musculoskeletal:* Arthritis, arthralgia, musculoskeletal pain, myalgia. *Dermatologic:* Acne, alopecia, pruritus, rash, urticaria. *Ophthalmologic:* Amblyopia, eye pain, visual field defect. *Otic:* Deafness, otitis media, tinnitus. *Miscellaneous:* Gout, weight loss or gain, taste perversion, asthenia, candidiasis, chest pain, edema, fever, flu syndrome, halitosis, infection, malaise.

**Drug Interactions**
*Ampicillin /* ↓ Effect of ampicillin due to ↓ absorption
*Ketoconazole /* ↓ Effect of ketoconazole due to ↓ absorption
*Sucralfate /* Delayed absorption of lansoprazole

**How Supplied:** *Enteric-coated capsule:* 15 mg, 30 mg

**Dosage** ⸻

• **Capsules, Delayed Release**
*Duodenal ulcer.*
**Adults:** 15 mg daily before breakfast for 4 weeks.
*Maintenance of healed duodenal ulcer.*
**Adults:** 15 mg once daily.
*Duodenal ulcers associated with H. pylori.*
**Triple therapy:** Lansoprazole, 30 mg, plus clarithromycin, 500 mg, and amoxicilin, 1 g, b.i.d. for 14 days. **Double therapy:** Lansoprazole, 30 mg, plus amoxicillin, 1 g, t.i.d. for 14 days in those intolerant or resistant to clarithromycin.
*Erosive esophagitis.*
30 mg before eating for up to 8 weeks. If the client does not heal in 8 weeks, an additional 8 weeks of therapy may be given. If there is a recurrence, an additional 8-week course may be considered.
*Maintenance of healed erosive esophagitis.*
15 mg once daily for up to 12 months.
*Pathologic hypersecretory conditions.*
**Initial:** 60 mg once daily. Adjust the dose to client need. Dosage may be continued as long as necessary. Doses up to 90 or 120 mg (in divided doses) daily have been given.

**DENTAL CONCERNS**
**General**
1. A semisupine position for the dental chair may be necessary to help minimize or avoid GI effects of the disease.
2. Determine the patient's ability to tolerate aspirin or NSAID-related products.
3. Decreased saliva flow can put the patient at risk for dental caries, periodontal disease, and candidiasis.

**Client/Family Teaching**
1. Review the importance of good oral hygiene in order to prevent soft tissue inflammation.
2. Review the proper use of oral hygiene aids in order to prevent injury.
3. Daily home fluoride treatments for persistent dry mouth.
4. Avoid alcohol-containing mouth rinses and beverages.
5. Avoid caffeine-containing beverages.
6. Dry mouth can be treated with tart, sugarless gum or candy, water, sugar-free beverages, or with saliva substitutes if dry mouth persists.

# Leflunomide
(leh-**FLOON**-oh-myd)
**Pregnancy Category:** X
Avara
**Classification:** Antimetabolite

**Action/Kinetics:** Inhibits pyrimidine synthesis which results in antiproliferative and anti-inflammatory effects. **Serum half-life:** 14-15 days. **Time to peak:** 6-12 hours.

**Uses:** Reduce the signs and symptoms of active rheumatoid arthritis and to retard structural damage as demonstrated by x-ray erosions and joint space narrowing.

**Contraindications:** Pregnancy or women who may become pregnant.

**Special Concerns:** Significant hepatic impairment, positive hepatitis B or C virus serologies.

**Side Effects:** *Oral:* Stomatitis, gingivitis, candidiasis, enlarged salivary gland, tooth disorder, dry mouth, taste disturbances. *GI:* Diarrhea, nausea, abdominal pain, dyspepsia, weight loss, anorexia, gastroenteritis, vomiting, cholelithiasis, colitis, constipation, esophagitis, flatulence, gastritis, melena. *GU:* Urinary tract infection, albuminuria, cystitis, dysuria, hematuria, vaginal candidiasis, prostate disorder, urinary frequency. *CNS:* Headache, dizziness, pain, fever, malaise, migraine, anxiety, depression, insomnia, sleep disorders. *CV:* Hypertension, chest pain, palpitations, tachycardia, vasculitis, vasodilation, varicose veins, edema. *Dermatologic:* Alopecia, rash, pruritis, dry skin, eczema, acne, dermatitis, hair discoloration, hematoma, herpes infection, nail disorder, subcutaneous nodule, skin disorder/discoloration, skin ulcer, bruising. *Endocrine and metabolic:* Hypokalemia, diabetes mellitus, hyperglycemia, hyperlipidemia, hyperthyroidism, menstrual disorders. *Hematologic:* Anemia. *Hepatic:* Abnormal liver function tests. *Neuromuscular and skeletal:* Back pain, joint disorder, weakness, tenosynovitis, synovitis, arthralgias, paresthesia, muscle cramps, neck pain, pelvic pain, increased CPK, arthrosis, bursitis, myalgia, bone necrosis, bone pain, tendon rupture, neuralgia, neuritis. *Ocular:* Blurred vision, cataracts, conjunctivitis, eye disorders. *Pulmonary:* Bronchitis, cough, pharyngitis, pneumonia, rhinitis, sinusitis, asthma, dyspnea, epistaxis, lung disorder. *Miscellaneous:* Infection, accidental injury, allergic reactions, diaphoresis.

**Drug Interactions:** None have been reported at this time with dental significance.

**How Supplied:** *Tablets:* 10 mg, 20 mg, 100 mg

## Dosage
- **Tablets**

   *Active rheumatiod arthritis.*

**Adults:** Loading dose of 100 mg/day for 3 days, followed by 20 mg QD. This can be lowered to 10 mg/day.

## DENTAL CONCERNS
### General
1. A semisupine position for the dental chair may be necessary to help minimize or avoid GI adverse effects or for patients with rheumatoid arthritis.

### Consultation with Primary Care Provider
1. Consultation may be required in order to assess extent of disease control.

### Client/Family Teaching
1. Take with a full glass of water or milk, with meals, or with a prescribed antacid and remain upright 30 min following administration to reduce gastric irritation or ulcer formation.
2. Review the importance of good oral hygiene in order to prevent soft tissue inflammation.
3. Review the proper use of oral hygiene aids in order to prevent injury.
4. Daily home fluoride treatments for persistent dry mouth.
5. Avoid alcohol-containing mouth rinses or beverages.
6. Avoid caffeine-containing beverages.
7. Dry mouth can be treated with tart, sugarless gum or candy, water, sugarless beverages, or with saliva substitutes if dry mouth persists.

# Levodopa
(lee-voh-**DOH**-pah)
Dopar, Larodopa, L-Dopa **(Rx)**
**Pregnancy Category:** C
**Classification:** Antiparkinson agent

**Action/Kinetics:** Levodopa, a dopamine precursor, is able to cross the blood-brain barrier to enter the CNS. It is decarboxylated (broken down) to dopamine in the basal ganglia, thus replenishing depleted dopamine stores. **Peak plasma levels:** 0.5–2 hr (may be delayed if ingested with food). **t½, plasma:** 1–3 hr. Onset occurs in 2–3 weeks although some clients may require up to 6 months. Extensively metabolized both in the GI tract and the liver; metabolites are excreted in the urine.

**Uses:** Idiopathic, arteriosclerotic, or postencephalitic parkinsonism. Parkinsonism due to carbon monoxide or manganese intoxication. Levodopa only provides symptomatic relief and does not alter the course of the disease. When effective, it relieves rigidity, bradykinesia, tremors, dysphagia, seborrhea, sialorrhea, and postural instability. Used in combination with carbidopa. *Non-FDA Approved Uses:* Pain from herpes zoster; restless legs syndrome.

**Contraindications:** Concomitant use with MAO inhibitors. History of melanoma or in clients with undiagnosed skin lesions. Lactation. Hypersensitivity to drug, narrow-angle glaucoma, blood dyscrasias, hypertension, coronary sclerosis.

**Special Concerns:** Use with extreme caution in clients with history of MIs, convulsions, arrhythmias, bronchial asthma, emphysema, active peptic ulcer, psychosis or neurosis, wide-angle glaucoma, and renal, hepatic, or endocrine diseases. Use during pregnancy only if benefits clearly outweigh risks. Safety has not been established in children less than 12 years of age. Geriatric clients may require a lower dose as they have a reduced tolerance for the drug and its side effects (including cardiac effects). Clients may experience an "on-off" phenomenon in which they experience an improved clinical status followed by loss of therapeutic effect.

**Side Effects:** The side effects of levodopa are numerous and usually dose related. Some may abate with usage. *CNS:* Choreiform and/or dystonic movements, paranoid ideation, psychotic episodes, ***depression (with possibility of suicidal tendencies),*** dementia, ***seizures (rare),*** dizziness, headache, faintness, confusion, insomnia, nightmares, hallucinations, delusions, agitation, anxiety, malaise, fatigue, euphoria. *Oral:* Dry mouth, sialorrhea, dysgeusia, burning sensation of tongue, bitter taste. *GI:* N&V, anorexia, abdominal pain, dysphagia, hiccups, diarrhea, constipation, flatulence, weight gain or loss, GI bleeding (rare), duodenal ulcer (rare). *CV:* Cardiac irregularities, palpitations, orthostatic hypotension, hypertension, phlebitis, hot flashes. *Ophthalmologic:* Diplopia, dilated pupils, blurred vision, development of Horner's syndrome, oculogyric crisis. *Hematologic:* ***Hemolytic anemia, agranulocytosis,*** leukopenia. *Musculoskeletal:* Muscle twitching (early sign of overdose), tonic contraction of the muscles of mastication, increased hand tremor, ataxia. *Miscellaneous:* Blepharospasm (early sign of overdose), urinary retention, urinary incontinence, increased sweating, unusual breathing patterns, weakness, numbness, bruxism, alopecia, priapism, hoarseness, edema, dark sweat and/or urine, flushing, skin rash, sense of stimulation. Levodopa interacts with many other drugs (see what follows) and must be administered cautiously.

**Drug Interactions**

*Antacids* / ↑ Effect of levodopa due to ↑ absorption from GI tract

*Anticholinergic drugs* / Possible ↓ effect of levodopa due to ↑ breakdown of levodopa in stomach (due to delayed gastric emptying time)

*Antidepressants, tricyclic* / ↓ Effect of levodopa due to ↓ absorption from GI tract; also, ↑ risk of hypertension

*Benzodiazepines* / ↓ Effect of levodopa

*Ephedrine* / Levodopa potentiates the effect of indirectly acting sympathomimetics

*MAO inhibitors* / Concomitant administration may result in hypertension, lightheadedness, and flushing due to ↓ breakdown of dopamine and norepinephrine formed from levodopa

*Phenothiazines* / ↓ Effect of levodopa due to ↓ uptake of dopamine into neurons

*Phenytoin* / Antagonizes the effect of levodopa

*Pyridoxine* / Reverses levodopa-induced improvement in Parkinson's disease

*Thioxanthines* / ↓ Effect of levodopa in Parkinson clients

*Tricyclic antidepressants* / ↓ Absorption of levodopa → ↓ effect

**How Supplied:** *Capsule:* 100 mg, 250 mg, 500 mg; *Tablet:* 100 mg, 250 mg, 500 mg

## Dosage

• **Capsules, Tablets**
*Parkinsonism.*

**Adults, initial:** 250 mg b.i.d.–q.i.d. taken with food; **then,** increase total daily dose by 100–750 mg/3–7 days until optimum dosage reached (should not exceed 8 g/day). Up to 6 months may be required to achieve a significant therapeutic effect.

## DENTAL CONCERNS

### General

1. Have the patient sit up slowly and remain seated for at least two minutes after being supine in order to minimize the risk of orthostatic hypotension.
2. Decreased saliva flow can put the patient at risk for dental caries, periodontal disease, and candidiasis.
3. Patients on chronic drug therapy may develop blood dyscrasias. Symptoms include fever, sore throat, bleeding, and poor wound healing.
4. Dark glasses may be necessary because the dental light can be irritating.

### Consultation with Primary Care Provider

1. Patients with symptoms of blood dyscrasias should be referred to their primary care provider for complete blood counts. Treatment should be postponed until the results are known.
2. Consultation may be required in order to assess the extent of disease control.
3. Use caution if dental surgery and anesthetics are necessary.

### Client/Family Teaching

1. Daily home fluoride treatments for persistent dry mouth.
2. Avoid alcohol-containing mouth rinses and beverages.
3. Avoid caffeine-containing beverages.
4. Dry mouth can be treated with tart, sugarless gum or candy, water, sugar-free beverages, or with saliva substitutes if dry mouth persists.

# Levothyroxine sodium ($T_4$)

(lee-voh-thigh-**ROX**-een)
**Pregnancy Category: A**
Eltroxin, Levo-T, Levothroid, Levoxyl, Synthroid, L-Thyroxine Sodium **(Rx)**
Classification: Thyroid preparation

See also *Thyroid Drugs.*

**Action/Kinetics:** Levothyroxine is the synthetic sodium salt of the levoisomer of $T_4$ (tetraiodothyronine). Levothyroxine, 0.05–0.6 mg equals approximately 60 mg (1 grain) of thyroid. Absorption from the GI tract is incomplete and variable, especially when taken with food. Has a slower onset but a longer duration than sodium liothyronine. More active on a weight basis than thyroid. Is usually the drug of choice. Effect is predictable as thyroid content is standard. **Time to peak therapeutic effect:** 3–4 weeks. **t½:** 6–7 days in a euthyroid person, 9–10 days in a hypothyroid client, and 3–4 days in a hyperthyroid client. Is 99% protein bound. **Duration:** 1–3 weeks after withdrawal of chronic therapy. *NOTE:* All levothyroxine products are not bioequivalent; thus, changing brands is not recommended.

**Drug Interactions:** Concurrent use of aluminum hydroxide and levothyroxine may result in adsorption of levothyroxine to the aluminum and increased fecal elimination of levothyroxine.

**How Supplied:** *Powder for injection:* 0.2 mg, 0.5 mg; *Tablet:* 0.025 mg, 0.05 mg, 0.075 mg, 0.088 mg, 0.1 mg, 0.112 mg, 0.125 mg, 0.137 mg, 0.15 mg, 0.175 mg, 0.2 mg, 0.3 mg, 0.5 mg

## Dosage

• **Tablets**
*Mild hypothyroidism.*

**Adults, initial:** 50 mcg once daily; **then,** increase by 25–50 mcg q 2–3 weeks until desired clinical response is attained; **maintenance, usual:** 75–125 mcg/day (although doses up to 200 mcg/day may be required in some clients).

*Severe hypothyroidism.*
**Adults, initial:** 12.5–25 mcg once daily; **then,** increase dose, as necessary, in increments of 25 mcg at 2- to 3-week intervals.
*Congenital hypothyroidism.*
**Pediatric, 12 years and older:** 2–3 mcg/kg once daily until the adult daily dose (usually 150 mcg) is reached. **6–12 years of age:** 4–5 mcg/kg/day or 100–150 mcg once daily. **1–5 years of age:** 5–6 mcg/kg/day or 75–100 mcg once daily. **6–12 months of age:** 6–8 mcg/kg/day or 50–75 mcg once daily. **Less than 6 months of age:** 8–10 mcg/kg/day or 25–50 mcg once daily.
• **IM, IV**
*Myxedematous coma.*
**Adults, initial:** 400 mcg by rapid IV injection, even in geriatric clients; **then,** 100–200 mcg/day, IV. **Maintenance:** 100–200 mcg/day, IV. Smaller daily doses should be given until client can tolerate PO medication.
*Hypothyroidism.*
**Adults:** 50–100 mcg once daily; **pediatric, IV, IM:** A dose of 75% of the usual PO pediatric dose should be given.

## DENTAL CONCERNS

See also *Dental Concerns* for *Thyroid Drugs.*

# Lidocaine hydrochloride
(**LYE**-doh-kayn)
**Pregnancy Category:** B
Dalcaine, Dilocaine, Duo-Trach Kit, L-Caine, Lidoject, Nervocaine, Octocaine, Ultracaine, Xylocaine, Xylocaine-MPF, Octocaine with Epinephrine, Xylocaine with Epinephrine
**Classification:** Amide local anesthetics

See also *Amide Local Anesthetic Agents.*
**Action/Kinetics:** Blocks nerve action potential by inhibiting ion fluxes across the cell membrane. **Onset:** 2-10 min; **Duration:** 20 min-4 hours. Renally excreted and metabolized by the liver. Metabolites may contribute to toxicity in a single dose.
**Uses:** Local dental anesthesia, peripheral nerve block, caudal anesthesia, epidural anesthesia, spinal anesthesia, surgical anesthesia.
**Contraindications:** See also *Amide Local Anesthetic Agents.*
**Special Concerns:** Elderly, large doses of lidocaine in patients with myasthenia gravis.
**Side Effects:** See also *Amide Local Anesthetic Agents.*
**Drug Interactions:** See also *Amide Local Anesthetic Agents.*
**How Supplied:** *Injection without epinephrine:* 0.5%, 1%, 1.5%, 2%, 4%, 5% *Injection with epinephrine:* 0.5%, 1%, 1.5%, 2% with epinephrine concentrations of 1:50,000, 1:100,000, 1:200,000. Usual dental use is 2% lidocaine with 1:100,000 epinephrine

## Dosage
• **2% Lidocaine Injection Without Vasconstrictor**
*Dental anesthesia.*
20–300 mg per dental appointment. Dose should be adjusted down for medically compromised, debilitated, or elderly patients. (See also *Appendix 9.*)
• **2% Lidocaine Injection with 1:50,000 Epinephrine**
*Dental anesthesia.*
20–100 mg not to exceed 500 mg per dental appointment. Dose should be adjusted down for medically compromised, debilitated, or elderly patients. (See also *Appendix 9.*)
• **2% Lidocaine Injection with 1:100,000 Epinephrine**
*Dental anesthesia.*
20–100 mg not to exceed 500 mg per dental appointment. Dose should be adjusted down for medically compromised, debilitated, or elderly patients. (See also *Appendix 9.*)
• **2% Lidocaine Injection with 1:200,000 Epinephrine**
*Dental anesthesia.*
20–100 mg not to exceed 500 mg per dental appointment. Dose

**L**

should be adjusted down for medically compromised, debilitated, or elderly patients. (See also *Appendix 9*.)

## DENTAL CONCERNS

See also *Dental Concerns* for *Amide Local Anesthetic Agents*.

# Lidocaine hydrochloride (topical)
(**LYE**-doh-kayn)
**Pregnancy Category:** B
Xylocaine Viscous
**Classification:** Topical, amide local anesthetic

**Action/Kinetics:** Promotes anesthesia by inhibiting sensory nerve impulses.
**Uses:** Topical anesthesia for inflamed or ulcerated mucosa, to reduce the gag reflex in patients undergoing dental radiologic examinations or dental impressions.
**Contraindications:** Hypersensitivity, application over a large area.
**Special Concerns:** Sepsis, denuded skin.
**Side Effects:** *Skin:* Rash, irritation, sensitization
**Drug Interactions:** None reported.
**How Supplied:** *Topical solution:* 2% in 100- and 450- mL bottles

## Dosage
• **Topical Solution**
*Irritated or inflamed mucosa.*
**Adults:** Rinse with 5–15 mL prior to meals or as needed to reduce pain of aphthous ulcers. Expectorate after rinsing.

## DENTAL CONCERNS
**General**
1. Do not apply to infected areas.
2. Do not overuse.
**Client/Family Teaching**
1. Use just before eating to reduce pain.
2. Do not overuse.
3. Report any rash, redness, or swelling to the dentist.

# Lidocaine hydrochloride
(**LYE**-doh-kayn)

**Pregnancy Category:** B
**IM:** LidoPen Auto-Injector **(Rx)**. **Direct IV or IV Admixtures:** Lidocaine HCl for Cardiac Arrhythmias, Xylocaine HCl IV for Cardiac Arrhythmias, Xylocard ✿ **(Rx)**. **IV Infusion:** Lidocaine HCl in 5% Dextrose **(Rx)**
**Classification:** Antiarrhythmic, class IB

See also *Antiarrhythmic Agents*.
**Action/Kinetics:** Shortens the refractory period and suppresses the automaticity of ectopic foci without affecting conduction of impulses through cardiac tissue. Increases the electrical stimulation threshold of the ventricle during diastole. It does not affect BP, CO, or myocardial contractility. **IV: Onset**, 45–90 sec; **duration:** 10–20 min. **IM, Onset**, 5–15 min; **duration,** 60–90 min. **t½:** 1–2 hr. **Therapeutic serum levels:** 1.5–6 mcg/mL. **Time to steady-state plasma levels:** 3–4 hr (8–10 hr in clients with AMI). **Protein-binding:** 40%–80%. Ninety percent is rapidly metabolized in the liver to active metabolites. Since lidocaine has little effect on conduction at normal antiarrhythmic doses, use in acute situations (instead of procainamide) in instances in which heart block might occur.
**Uses: IV:** Treatment of acute ventricular arrhythmias such as those following MIs or occurring during surgery. The drug is ineffective against atrial arrhythmias. **IM:** Certain emergency situations (e.g., ECG equipment not available; mobile coronary care unit, under advice of a physician).
*Non-FDA Approved Uses:* IV in children who develop ventricular couplets or frequent premature ventricular beats.
**Contraindications:** Hypersensitivity to amide-type local anesthetics, Stokes-Adams syndrome, Wolff-Parkinson-White syndrome, severe SA, AV, or intraventricular block (when no pacemaker is present).
**Special Concerns:** Use with caution during labor and delivery, during lactation, and in the presence of liver or severe kidney disease, CHF, marked hypoxia, digitalis toxicity

with AV block, severe respiratory depression, or shock. In geriatric clients, the rate and dose for IV infusion should be decreased by one-half and slowly adjusted. Safety and efficacy have not been determined in children; the IM autoinjector product should not be used for children.

**Side Effects:** *Body as a whole:* Malignant hyperthermia characterized by tachycardia, tachypnea, labile BP, metabolic acidosis, temperature elevation. *CV: Precipitation or aggravation of arrhythmias (following IV use),* hypotension, *bradycardia (with possible cardiac arrest), CV collapse. CNS:* Dizziness, apprehension, euphoria, lightheadedness, nervousness, drowsiness, confusion, changes in mood, hallucinations, twitching, "doom anxiety," *convulsions,* unconsciousness. *Respiratory:* Difficulties in breathing or swallowing, *respiratory depression or arrest. Allergic:* Rash, cutaneous lesions, urticaria, edema, *anaphylaxis. Other:* Tinnitus, blurred or double vision, vomiting, numbness, sensation of heat or cold, twitching, tremors, soreness at IM injection site, fever, *venous thrombosis or phlebitis (extending from site of injection),* extravasation. During anesthesia, CV depression may be the first sign of lidocaine toxicity. During other usage, convulsions are the first sign of lidocaine toxicity.

**Drug Interactions**
*Aminoglycosides* / ↑ Neuromuscular blockade
*Beta-adrenergic blockers* / ↑ Lidocaine levels with possible toxicity
*Cimetidine* / ↓ Clearance of lidocaine → possible toxicity
*Phenytoin* / IV phenytoin → excessive cardiac depression
*Procainamide* / Additive cardiodepressant effects
*Succinylcholine* / ↑ Action of succinylcholine by ↓ plasma protein binding
*Tocainide* / ↑ Risk of side effects
*Tubocurarine* / ↑ Neuromuscular blockade

**How Supplied:** *Dextrose/lidocaine hydrochloride—injection:* 5%-0.2%, 5%-0.4%, 5%-0.8%, 7.5%-5%; *Lidocaine hydrochloride—injection:* 0.5%, 1%, 1.5%, 2%, 4%, 10%, 20%

**Dosage** ————————
• **IV Bolus**
    *Antiarrhythmic.*
**Adults:** 50–100 mg at rate of 25–50 mg/min. Bolus is used to establish rapid therapeutic plasma levels. Repeat if necessary after 5-min interval. Onset of action is 10 sec. **Maximum dose/hr:** 200–300 mg.
• **Infusion**
    *Antiarrhythmic.*
20–50 mcg/kg at a rate of 1–4 mg/min. No more than 200–300 mg/hr should be given. **Pediatric, loading dose:** 1 mg/kg IV or intratracheally q 5–10 min until desired effect reached (maximum total dose: 5 mg/kg).
• **IV Continuous Infusion**
    *Maintain therapeutic plasma levels following loading doses.*
**Adults:** Give at a rate of 1–4 mg/min (20–50 mcg/kg/min). Dose should be reduced in clients with heart failure, with liver disease, or who are taking drugs that interact with lidocaine. **Pediatric:** 20–50 mcg/kg/min (usual is 30 mcg/kg/min).
• **IM**
    *Antiarrhythmic.*
**Adults:** 4.5 mg/kg (approximately 300 mg for a 70-kg adult). Switch to IV lidocaine or oral antiarrhythmics as soon as possible although an additional IM dose may be given after 60–90 min.

————————

## DENTAL CONCERNS

See also *Dental Concerns* for *Antiarrhythmic Agents.*

# Lidocaine transoral delivery system
(**LYE**-doh-kayn)
**Pregnancy Category:** B
DentiPatch

L

---

*bold italic* = life-threatening side effect

**Classification:** Amide local anesthetic

**Action/Kinetics:** Promotes anesthesia by inhibiting sensory nerve impulses.

**Uses:** Apply to mucous membranes of the mouth prior to superficial dental therapy.

**Contraindications:** Hypersensitivity.

**Special Concerns:** Contains phenylalanine (caution phenylketonurics), local anesthetic toxicity, children < 12 years of age, elderly, liver dysfunction, onset longer for maxilla, lactation.

**Side Effects:** *Oral:* Erythema, mucous irritation, stomatitis, taste alteration. *GI:* Nausea. *CNS:* Excitatory or depressive effects, headache, dizziness, nervousness, confusion, tinnitus, twitching, tremors. *CV:* Bradycardia, hypotension, *cardiovascular collapse.* *Miscellaneous:* Allergic reaction.

**Drug Interactions:** None reported with dental drugs.

**How Supplied:** *Patch:* 2 cm$^2$ (46.1 mg)

**Dosage**
- **Patch**
  *Dental procedure.*
Apply patch to area of application after drying it with gauze. Leave in place for no more than 15 mins.

## DENTAL CONCERNS
**Client/Family Teaching**
1. Have the patient report any oral lesions that fail to heal.
2. Advise the patient to refrain from eating or chewing gum following application of this drug.

# Lisinopril
(lie-**SIN**-oh-prill)
**Pregnancy Category:** C
Prinivil, Zestril **(Rx)**
**Classification:** Antihypertensive, ACE inhibitor

See also *Angiotensin-Converting Enzyme Inhibitors.*

**Action/Kinetics:** Both supine and standing BPs are reduced, although the drug is less effective in blacks than in Caucasians. Although food does not alter the bioavailability of lisinopril, only 25% of a PO dose is absorbed. **Onset:** 1 hr. **Peak serum levels:** 7 hr. **Duration:** 24 hr. **t½:** 12 hr. 100% of the drug is excreted unchanged in the urine.

**Uses:** Alone or in combination with a diuretic (usually a thiazide) to treat hypertension (step I therapy). In combination with digitalis and a diuretic for treating CHF not responding to other therapy. Use within 24 hr of acute MI to improve survival in hemodynamically stable clients (clients should receive the standard treatment, including thrombolytics, aspirin, and beta blockers).

**Contraindications:** See also *Angiotensin-Converting Enzyme Inhibitors.*

**Special Concerns:** Use with caution during lactation. Safety and efficacy have not been established in children. Geriatric clients may manifest higher blood levels. Dosage should be reduced in clients with impaired renal function.

**Side Effects:** *CNS:* Dizziness, headache, fatigue, vertigo, insomnia, depression, sleepiness, paresthesias, malaise, nervousness, confusion. *Oral:* Dysgeusia, dry mouth. *GI:* Diarrhea, N&V, dyspepsia, anorexia, constipation, abdominal pain, flatulence. *Respiratory:* Cough, dyspnea, bronchitis, upper respiratory symptoms, nasal congestion, sinusitis, pharyngeal pain, *bronchospasm, asthma.* *CV:* Hypotension, orthostatic hypotension, angina, tachycardia, palpitations, rhythm disturbances, *stroke,* chest pain, orthostatic effects, peripheral edema, *MI, CVA. Musculoskeletal:* Asthenia, muscle cramps, joint pain, shoulder and back pain, myalgia, arthralgia, arthritis. *Hepatic:* Hepatitis, cholestatic jaundice, pancreatitis. *Dermatologic:* Rash, pruritus, flushing, increased sweating, urticaria. *GU:* Impotence, oliguria, progressive azotemia, acute renal failure, UTI. *Miscellaneous:* **Angioedema (may be fatal if laryngeal edema oc-**

*curs),* hyperkalemia, neutropenia, anemia, **bone marrow depression,** decreased libido, chest pain, fever, blurred vision, syncope, vasculitis of the legs, gout.

**Drug Interactions:** See also *Angiotensin-Converting Enzyme Inhibitors.*

**How Supplied:** *Tablet:* 2.5 mg, 5 mg, 10 mg, 20 mg, 40 mg

**Dosage** ─────────────

• **Tablets**

*Essential hypertension, used alone.*

10 mg once daily. Adjust dosage depending on response (range: 20–40 mg/day given as a single dose). Doses greater than 80 mg/day do not give a greater effect.

*Essential hypertension in combination with a diuretic.*

**Initial:** 5 mg. The BP-lowering effects of the combination are additive. Dosage should be reduced in clients with renal impairment.

*CHF.*

**Initial:** 5 mg once daily (2.5 mg/day in clients with hyponatremia) in combination with diuretics and digitalis. **Dosage range:** 5–20 mg/day as a single dose.

*Acute MI.*

**First dose:** 5 mg; **then,** 5 mg after 24 hr, 10 mg after 48 hr, and then 10 mg daily. Continue dosing for 6 weeks. In clients with a systolic pressure less than 120 mm Hg when treatment is started or within 3 days after the infarct should be given 2.5 mg. If hypotension occurs (systolic BP less than 100 mm Hg), the dose may be temporarily reduced to 2.5 mg. If prolonged hypotension occurs, the drug should be withdrawn.

─────────────

**DENTAL CONCERNS**

See also *Dental Concerns* for *Angiotensin-Converting Enzyme Inhibitors* and *Antihypertensive Agents.*

─────────────

# Lithium carbonate
(**LITH**-ee-um)

**Pregnancy Category:** D
Carbolith ✹, Duralith ✹, Eskalith, Eskalith CR, Lithane, Lithizine ✹, Lithobid, Lithonate, Lithotabs **(Rx)**

# Lithium citrate
(**LITH**-ee-um)
**Pregnancy Category:** D
PMS-Lithium ✹
**Classification:** Antipsychotic agent, miscellaneous

**Action/Kinetics:** Mechanism for the antimanic effect of lithium is unknown. May alter sodium, potassium, and potassium ion transportation across cell membranes in nerve and muscle cells; may affect norepinephrine and serotonin in the CNS.

Affects the distribution of calcium, magnesium, and sodium ions and affects glucose metabolism. **Peak serum levels** (regular release): 1–4 hr; (slow-release): 4–6 hr. **Onset:** 5–14 days. **Therapeutic serum levels:** 0.4–1.0 mEq/L (must be carefully monitored because toxic effects may occur at these levels and significant toxic reactions occur at serum lithium levels of 2 mEq/L). **t½ (plasma):** 24 hr (longer in presence of renal impairment and in the elderly). Lithium and sodium are excreted by the same mechanism in the proximal tubule. Thus, to reduce the danger of lithium intoxication, sodium intake must remain at normal levels.

**Uses:** Control of manic and hypomanic episodes in manic-depressive clients. Prophylaxis of bipolar depression. *Non-FDA Approved Uses:* To reverse neutropenia induced by cancer chemotherapy and in children with chronic neutropenia. Prophylaxis of cluster headaches and cyclic migraine headaches. Treatment of certain types of mental depression (e.g., schizoaffective disorder, augment the antidepressant effect of tricyclic or MAO drugs in treating unipolar depression). Also for premenstrual tension, alcoholism accompanied by depression, tardive dyskinesia, bulimia, hyperthyroidism, excess ADH secretion. Lithium

L

─────────────

succinate, in a topical form, has been used for the treatment of genital herpes and seborrheic dermatitis. **Contraindications:** Cardiovascular or renal disease. Brain damage. Dehydration, sodium depletion, clients receiving diuretics. Lactation.

**Special Concerns:** Safety and efficacy have not been established for children less than 12 years of age. Use with caution in geriatric clients because lithium is more toxic to the CNS in these clients; also, geriatric clients are more likely to develop lithium-induced goiter and clinical hypothyroidism and are more likely to manifest excessive thirst and larger volumes of urine.

**Side Effects:** These are related to the blood lithium level. *CNS:* Fainting, drowsiness, slurred speech, confusion, dizziness, tiredness, lethargy, ataxia, dysarthria, aphasia, vertigo, stupor, restlessness, **coma, seizures.** Pseudotumor cerebri leading to papilledema and increased ICP. *Oral:* Dry mouth, increased thirst. *GI:* Anorexia, N&V, diarrhea, bloated stomach. *Muscular:* Tremors (especially of hand), muscle weakness, fasciculations and/or twitching, clonic movements of limbs, increased deep tendon reflexes, choreoathetoid movements, cogwheel rigidity. *Renal:* Nephrogenic diabetes insipidus (polyuria, polydipsia), oliguria, albuminuria. *Endocrine:* Hypothyroidism, goiter, hyperparathyroidism. *CV:* Changes in ECG, edema, hypotension, *CV collapse,* irregular pulse, tachycardia. *Ophthalmologic:* Blurred vision, downbeat nystagmus. *Dermatologic:* Acneform eruptions, pruritic-maculopapular rashes, drying and thinning of hair, alopecia, paresthesia, cutaneous ulcers, lupus-like symptoms. *Miscellaneous:* Hoarseness; swelling of feet, lower legs, or neck; cold sensitivity; leukemia; leukocytosis; dyspnea on exertion.

**Drug Interactions**

*Carbamazepine* / ↑ Risk of lithium toxicity
*Diazepam* / ↑ Risk of hypothermia
*Haloperidol* / ↑ Risk of neurologic toxicity
*Ibuprofen* / ↑ Chance of lithium toxicity due to ↓ renal clearance
*Indomethacin* / ↑ Chance of lithium toxicity due to ↓ renal clearance
*Naproxen* / ↑ Chance of lithium toxicity due to ↑ serum levels
*Neuromuscular blocking agents* / Lithium ↑ effect of these agents → respiratory depression and apnea
*Phenothiazines* / ↓ Levels of phenothiazines and ↑ neurotoxicity
*Phenylbutazone* / ↑ Chance of lithium toxicity due to ↓ renal clearance
*Piroxicam* / ↑ Chance of lithium toxicity due to ↓ renal clearance
*Probenecid* / ↑ Chance of lithium toxicity due to ↑ serum levels
*Sodium bicarbonate* / ↓ Lithium effect by ↑ renal excretion
*Sodium chloride* / Excretion of lithium is proportional to amount of sodium chloride ingested; if client is on salt-free diet, may develop lithium toxicity since less lithium excreted
*Succinylcholine* / ↑ Muscle relaxation
*Sympathomimetics* / ↓ Pressor effect of sympathomimetics
*Tetracyclines* / ↑ Chance of lithium toxicity due to ↑ serum levels
*Tricyclic antidepressants* / ↑ Effect of tricyclic antidepressants

**How Supplied:** Lithium carbonate: *Capsule:* 150 mg, 300 mg, 600 mg; *Tablet:* 300 mg; *Tablet, extended release:* 300 mg, 450 mg; Lithium citrate: *Syrup:* 300 mg/5 mL

## Dosage

• **Capsules, Tablets, Extended-Release Tablets, Syrup**
    *Acute mania.*
**Adults:** Individualized and according to lithium serum level (not to exceed 1.4 mEq/L) and clinical response. **Usual initial:** 300–600 mg t.i.d. or 600–900 mg b.i.d. of slow-release form; **elderly and debilitated clients:** 0.6–1.2 g/day in three doses. **Maintenance:** 300 mg t.i.d.–q.i.d.

Administration of drug is discontinued when lithium serum level exceeds 1.2 mEq/L and resumed 24 hr after it has fallen below that level.
    *To reverse neutropenia.*

300–1,000 mg/day (to achieve serum levels of 0.5–1.0 mEq/L) for 7–10 days.

*Prophylaxis of cluster headaches.* 600–900 mg/day.

## DENTAL CONCERNS

See also *Dental Concerns* for *Sedative Hypnotics (Anti-anxiety)/Antimanic Drugs.*

**Client/Family Teaching**
1. Avoid any caffeinated beverages/foods because these may aggravate mania.
2. Report any episodes of persistent diarrhea; may indicate need for supplemental fluids or salt.
3. Maintain a constant level of salt intake to avoid fluctuations in lithium activity. Weight gain and edema may be related to sodium retention; report if excessive.
4. Drink 10–12 glasses of water each day; avoid dehydration (e.g., vigorous exercise, sunbathing, sauna) to prevent increased concentrations of lithium in urine.
5. Carry name and telephone number of persons to contact if needed or if family members note behavioral changes or physical changes contrary to expectations. Carry ID, noting diagnosis and prescribed meds.

# Lomefloxacin hydrochloride
(**loh**-meh-**FLOX**-ah-sin)
**Pregnancy Category:** C
Maxaquin **(Rx)**
**Classification:** Antibacterial, fluoroquinolone derivative

See also *Fluoroquinolones.*

**Action/Kinetics: Mean peak plasma levels:** 4.2 mcg/mL after a 400-mg dose. The rate and extent of absorption are decreased if taken with food. **t½:** 8 hr. Metabolized in the liver with 65% excreted unchanged through the urine and 10% excreted unchanged in the feces.

**Uses:** Acute bacterial exacerbation of chronic bronchitis caused by *Hae-*

*mophilus influenzae* or *Moraxella catarrhalis.* Uncomplicated UTIs due to *Escherichia coli, Klebsiella pneumoniae, Proteus mirabilis,* or *Staphylococcus saprophyticus.* Complicated UTIs due to *E. coli, K. pneumoniae, P. mirabilis, Pseudomonas aeruginosa, Citrobacter diversus,* or *Enterobacter cloacae.* Preoperatively to decrease the incidence of UTIs 3–5 days after surgery in clients undergoing transurethral procedures. Uncomplicated gonococcal infections. Prevent infection in preoperative transrectal prostate biopsy.

**Contraindications:** Use in minor urologic procedures for which prophylaxis is not indicated (e.g., simple cystoscopy, retrograde pyelography). Use for the empiric treatment of acute bacterial exacerbation of chronic bronchitis due to *Streptococcus pneumoniae.* Lactation.

**Special Concerns:** Plasma clearance is reduced in the elderly. Safety and efficacy have not been determined in children less than 18 years of age. Serious hypersensitivity reactions that are occasionally fatal have occurred, even with the first dose. No dosage adjustment is needed for elderly clients with normal renal function. Not efficiently removed from the body by hemodialysis or peritoneal dialysis.

**Additional Side Effects:** *CNS:* Confusion, tremor, vertigo, nervousness, anxiety, hyperkinesia, anorexia, agitation, increased appetite, depersonalization, paranoia, ***coma.*** *Oral:* Tongue discoloration, bad taste in mouth, dry mouth, candidiasis, stomatitis, glossitis. *GI:* GI inflammation or bleeding, dysphagia. *GU:* Dysuria, hematuria, micturition disorder, anuria, strangury, leukorrhea, intermenstrual bleeding perineal pain, vaginal moniliasis, orchitis, epididymitis, proteinuria, albuminuria. *Hypersensitivity Reactions:* Urticaria, itching, pharyngeal or facial edema, ***CV collapse,*** tingling, loss of consciousness, dyspnea. *CV:* Hypotension, tachycardia, bradycardia, extrasystoles, cyanosis, *arrhythmia, cardiac failure,* angina pectoris, *MI, pulmonary embolism, cardiomyopathy,* phlebitis, cerebrovascular disorder. *Respiratory:* Dyspnea, respiratory infection, epistaxis, *bronchospasm,* cough, increased sputum, respiratory disorder, stridor. *Hematologic:* Eosinophilia, leukopenia, increase or decrease in platelets, increase in ESR, lymphocytopenia, decreased hemoglobin, anemia, bleeding, increased PT, increase in monocytes. *Dermatologic:* Urticaria, eczema, skin exfoliation, skin disorder. *Ophthalmologic:* Conjunctivitis, eye pain. *Otic:* Earache, tinnitus. *Musculoskeletal:* Back or chest pain, asthenia, leg cramps, arthralgia, myalgia. *Miscellaneous:* Increase or decrease in blood glucose, flushing, increased sweating, facial edema, influenza-like symptoms, decreased heat tolerance, purpura, lymphadenopathy, increased fibrinolysis, thirst, gout, hypoglycemia, phototoxicity.

**Drug Interactions**
*Antacids* / ↓ Effects of lomefloxacin
*Caffeine* / ↑ Levels of caffeine
*Cyclosporine* / ↑ Levels of cyclosporine

**How Supplied:** *Tablet:* 400 mg

**Dosage** —————————
• **Tablets**
  *Acute bacterial exacerbation of chronic bronchitis. Cystitis.*
**Adults:** 400 mg once daily for 10 days.
  *Complicated UTIs.*
**Adults:** 400 mg once daily for 14 days.
  *Uncomplicated UTIs.*
400 mg once daily for 3 days.
  *Prophylaxis of infection before surgery for transurethral procedures.*
Single 400-mg dose 2–6 hr before surgery.
  *Uncomplicated gonococcal infections.*
400 mg as a single dose (as an alternative to ciprofloxacin or ofloxacin).

—————————

**DENTAL CONCERNS**

See also *General Dental Concerns*

*for All Anti-Infectives* and *Fluoroquinolones.*
**General**
1. Ingestible sodium bicarbonate products (i.e., air polishing systems) can only be used 2 hours after taking lomefloxin.
2. Use caution when prescribing caffeine-containing prescription and nonprescription drugs.
3. Determine why the patient is taking the medication.
**Consultation with Primary Care Provider**
1. Consult with the patient's health care provider if an acute dental infection occurs and the patient requires another anti-infective.
**Client/Family Teaching**
1. Review the importance of good oral hygiene in order to prevent soft tissue inflammation.
2. Daily home fluoride treatments for persistent dry mouth.
3. Avoid alcohol-containing mouth rinses and beverages.
4. This medication can cause photosensitivity. Use a sunscreen/sunblock and limit sun exposure.
5. You may want to wear dark glasses in order to avoid photophobia, which can occur with the dental light.
6. Discontinue treatment and inform dentist immediately if the patient experiences pain or inflammation in his or her tendons. Rest and avoid exercise.

—————————

# Loperamide hydrochloride
(loh-**PER**-ah-myd)
**Pregnancy Category:** B
Alti-Loperamide ✽, Apo-Loperamide ✽, Imodium, Imodium A-D Caplets, Kaopectate II Caplets, Maalox Anti-Diarrheal Caplets, Novo-Loperamide ✽, Pepto Diarrhea Control, PMS-Loperamide Hydrochloride ✽ (Imodium is Rx, all others are OTC)
**Classification:** Antidiarrheal agent, systemic

—————————

**Action/Kinetics:** Slows intestinal motility by acting on opiate receptors on nerve endings and/or intramural ganglia embedded in the intestinal wall. **Time to peak effect, capsules:** 5 hr; **PO solution:** 2.5 hr. **t½:** 9.1–14.4 hr. Twenty-five percent excreted unchanged in the feces.

**Uses: Rx:** Symptomatic relief of acute nonspecific diarrhea and of chronic diarrhea associated with inflammatory bowel disease. Decrease the volume of discharge from ileostomies.

**OTC:** Control symptoms of diarrhea, including traveler's diarrhea. *Non-FDA Approved Uses:* With trimethoprim-sulfamethoxazole to treat traveler's diarrhea.

**Contraindications:** Discontinue drug promptly if abdominal distention develops in clients with acute ulcerative colitis. In clients in whom constipation should be avoided. OTC if body temperature is over 101°F (38°C) and in presence of bloody diarrhea. Use in acute diarrhea associated with organisms that penetrate the intestinal mucosa, such as *E. coli, Salmonella,* and *Shigella.*

**Special Concerns:** Safe use in children under 2 years of age and during lactation has not been established. Fluid and electrolyte depletion may occur in clients with diarrhea. Children less than 3 years of age are more sensitive to the narcotic effects of loperamide.

**Side Effects:** *Oral:* Dry mouth. *GI:* Abdominal pain, distention, or discomfort. Constipation, N&V, epigastric distress. Toxic megacolon in clients with acute colitis. *CNS:* Drowsiness, dizziness, fatigue. *Other:* Allergic skin rashes.

**Drug Interactions**
*Opioid analgesics* / ↑ Actions of opioid analgesics

**How Supplied:** *Capsule:* 2 mg; *Liquid:* 1 mg/5 mL; *Tablet:* 2 mg

**Dosage** ——————
• **Rx Capsules, Liquid**
*Acute diarrhea.*
**Adults, initial:** 4 mg, followed by 2 mg after each unformed stool, up to maximum of 16 mg/day. **Pediatric:**

D*ay 1 doses:* **8–12 years:** 2 mg t.i.d.; **6–8 years:** 2 mg b.i.d.; **2–5 years:** 1 mg t.i.d. using only the liquid. *After day 1:* 1 mg/10 kg after a loose stool (total daily dosage should not exceed day 1 recommended doses).
*Chronic diarrhea.*
**Adults:** 4–8 mg/day as a single or divided dose. Dosage not established for chronic diarrhea in children.
• **OTC Oral Solution, Tablets**
*Acute diarrhea.*
**Adults:** 4 mg after the first loose bowel movement followed by 2 mg after each subsequent bowel movement to a maximum of 8 mg/day for no more than 2 days. **Pediatric, 9–11 years:** 2 mg after the first loose bowel movement followed by 1 mg after each subsequent loose bowel movement, not to exceed 6 mg/day for no more than 2 days. **Pediatric, 6–8 years:** 1 mg after the first bowel movement followed by 1 mg after each subsequent loose bowel movement, not to exceed 4 mg/day for no more than 2 days.

## DENTAL CONCERNS
**General**
1. Decreased saliva flow can put the patient at risk for dental caries, periodontal disease, and candidiasis.
2. A semisupine position for the dental chair may be necessary to help minimize or avoid GI adverse effects.
3. This drug is usually used on a short-term basis. Some patients may require it for longer periods of time.
**Client/Family Teaching**
1. Daily home fluoride treatments for persistent dry mouth.
2. Avoid alcohol-containing mouth rinses and beverages.
3. Avoid caffeine-containing beverages.
4. Dry mouth can be treated with tart, sugarless gum or candy, water, sugar-free beverages, or with saliva substitutes if dry mouth persists.

# Loracarbef
(**lor**-ah-**KAR**-bef)
Pregnancy Category: B
Lorabid **(Rx)**
Classification: Beta-lactam antibiotic

See also *Anti-Infectives.*

**Action/Kinetics:** Related chemically to cephalosporins. Acts by inhibiting cell wall synthesis. Stable in the presence of certain bacterial beta-lactamases. **Average peak plasma levels:** 8 mcg/mL following a single 200-mg dose in a fasting subject after 90 min and 14 mcg/mL following a single 400-mg dose in a fasting subject after 90 min. Following doses of 7.5 mg/kg and 15 mg/kg of the oral suspension to children, average peak plasma levels were 13 and 19 mcg/mL, respectively, within 40–60 min. **Elimination t½:** 1 hr (increased to 5.6 hr in clients with a $C_{CR}$ from 10 to 50 mL/min/1.73 m² and to 32 hr in clients with a $C_{CR}$ of less than 10 mL/min/1.73 m²). Not metabolized in humans.

**Uses:** Secondary bacterial infections of acute bronchitis caused by *Streptococcus pneumoniae, Haemophilus influenzae,* or *Moraxella catarrhalis* (including beta-lactamase-producing strains of both organisms). Acute bacterial exacerbations of chronic bronchitis caused by *S. pneumoniae, H. influenzae,* or *M. catarrhalis* (including beta-lactamase-producing strains of both organisms). Pneumonia caused by *S. pneumoniae* or *H. influenzae* (only non-beta-lactamase-producing strains). Otitis media caused by *S. pneumoniae, Streptococcus pyogenes, H. influenzae,* or *M. catarrhalis* (including beta-lactamase-producing strains of both organisms). Acute maxillary sinusitis caused by *S. pneumoniae, H. influenzae* (only non-beta-lactamase-producing strains), or *M. catarrhalis* (including beta-lactamase-producing strains). Pharyngitis and tonsillitis caused by *S. pyogenes.* Uncomplicated skin and skin structure infections caused by *Staphylococcus aureus* (including penicillinase-producing strains) or *S. pyogenes.* Uncomplicated UTIs caused by *Escherichia coli* or *Staphylococcus saprophyticus.* Uncomplicated pyelonephritis caused by *E. coli.*

**Contraindications:** Hypersensitivity to loracarbef or cephalosporin-class antibiotics.

**Special Concerns:** Use during labor and delivery only if clearly needed. Pseudomembranous colitis is possible with most antibacterial agents. Use with caution and at reduced dosage in clients with impaired renal function, in those with a history of colitis, in clients receiving concurrent treatment with potent diuretics, during lactation, and in clients with known penicillin allergies. Safety and efficacy in children less than 6 months of age have not been determined.

**Side Effects:** The incidence of certain side effects is different in the pediatric population compared with the adult population. *Oral:* Candidiasis, glossitits. *GI:* Diarrhea, N&V, abdominal pain, anorexia, pseudomembranous colitis. *Hypersensitivity:* Skin rashes, urticaria, pruritus, erythema multiforme. *CNS:* Headache, somnolence, nervousness, insomnia, dizziness. *Hematologic:* Transient thrombocytopenia, leukopenia, eosinophilia. *Miscellaneous:* Vasodilation, vaginitis, vaginal moniliasis, rhinitis.

**Drug Interactions**
*Erythromycin* / ↓ Effects of erythromycin
*Lincomyicn* / ↓ Effects of lincomycin
*Oral contraceptives* / ↓ Effects of OCs
*Tetracyclines* / ↓ Effects of tetracyclines

**How Supplied:** *Capsule:* 200 mg, 400 mg; *Powder for reconstitution:* 100 mg/5 mL, 200 mg/5 mL

**Dosage** ————————
• **Capsules, Oral Suspension**
  *Secondary bacterial infection of acute bronchitis.*
**Adults 13 years of age and older:** 200–400 mg q 12 hr for 7 days.

*Acute bacterial exacerbation of chronic bronchitis.*
**Adults 13 years of age and older:** 400 mg q 12 hr for 7 days.
*Pneumonia.*
**Adults 13 years of age and older:** 400 q 12 hr for 14 days.
*Pharyngitis, tonsillitis.*
**Adults 13 years of age and older:** 200 mg q 12 hr for 10 days. **Infants and children, 6 months–12 years:** 15 mg/kg/day in divided doses q 12 hr for 10 days.
*Sinusitis.*
**Adults 13 years of age and older:** 400 mg q 12 hr for 10 days.
*Acute otitis media.*
**Infants and children, 6 months–12 years:** 30 mg/kg/day in divided doses q 12 hr for 10 days. Use the suspension as it is more rapidly absorbed than the capsules, resulting in higher peak plasma levels when given at the same dose.
*Skin and skin structure infections (impetigo).*
**Infants and children, 6 months–12 years:** 15 mg/kg/day in divided doses q 12 hr for 7 days.

### DENTAL CONCERNS

See also *Dental Concerns for All Anti-Infectives.*
**Client/Family Teaching**
1. Take at least 1 hr before or at least 2 hr after meals. Complete entire prescription.
2. Report persistent diarrhea, which may be secondary to pseudomembranous colitis and requires medical intervention.

# Loratidine

(loh-**RAH**-tih-deen)
**Pregnancy Category:** B
Claritin, Claritin Reditabs **(Rx)**
**Classification:** Antihistamine

See also *Antihistamines.*
**Action/Kinetics:** Metabolized in the liver to active metabolite descarboethoxyloratidine. Has low to no sedative and anticholinergic effects.

Does not alter cardiac repolarization and has not been linked to development of torsades de pointes as seen with astemizole and terfenadine. **Onset:** 1–3 hr. **Maximum effect:** 8–12 hr. Food delays absorption. **t½, loratidine:** 8.4 hr; **t½, descarboethoxyloratidine:** 28 hr. **Duration:** 24 hr. Excreted through both the urine and feces.
**Uses:** Relief of nasal and nonnasal symptoms of seasonal allergic rhinitis, including runny nose, itchy and watery eyes, itchy palate, and sneezing. Treatment of chronic idiopathic urticaria.
**Special Concerns:** Use with caution, if at all, during lactation. Give a lower initial dose in liver impairment. Safety and efficacy have not been determined in children less than 2 years of age.
**Side Effects:** Most commonly, headache, somnolence, fatigue, and dry mouth. *GI:* Altered salivation, gastritis, dyspepsia, stomatitis, tooth ache, thirst, altered taste, flatulence. *CNS:* Hypoesthesia, hyperkinesia, migraine, anxiety, depression, agitation, paroniria, amnesia, impaired concentration. *Ophthalmologic:* Altered lacrimation, conjunctivitis, blurred vision, eye pain, blepharospasm. *Respiratory:* Upper respiratory infection, epistaxis, pharyngitis, dyspnea, coughing, rhinitis, sinusitis, sneezing, bronchitis, ***bronchospasm,*** hemoptysis, laryngitis. *Body as a whole:* Asthenia, increased sweating, flushing, malaise, rigors, fever, dry skin, aggravated allergy, pruritus, purpura. *Musculoskeletal:* Back/chest pain, leg cramps, arthralgia, myalgia. *GU:* Breast pain, menorrhagia, dysmenorrhea, vaginitis. *Miscellaneous:* Earache, dysphonia, dry hair, urinary discoloration.
**How Supplied:** *Syrup:* 5 mg/5 mL; *Tablet:* 10 mg

**Dosage**
• **Syrup, Tablets**
  *Allergic rhinitis, chronic idiopathic urticaria.*

**Adults and children 6 years and older:** 10 mg once daily on an empty stomach. *In clients with impaired liver function (GFR less than 30 mL/min):* 10 mg every other day.

## DENTAL CONCERNS

See also *Dental Concerns* for *Antihistamines.*
1. May have increased sedation with drugs used for conscious sedation.

---

## Lorazepam
(lor-**AYZ**-eh-pam)
**Pregnancy Category:** D
Apo-Lorazepam ✿, Ativan, Lorazepam Intensol, Novo-Lorazem ✿, Nu-Loraz ✿, PMS-Lorazepam ✿, Pro-Lorazepam ✿ **(C-IV) (Rx)**
**Classification:** Antianxiety agent, benzodiazepine

---

See also *Sedative-Hypnotics (Anti-anxiety)/Antimanic Drugs.*
**Action/Kinetics:** Absorbed and eliminated faster than other benzodiazepines. **Peak plasma levels: PO,** 1–6 hr; **IM,** 1–1.5 hr. **t½:** 10–20 hr. Metabolized to inactive compounds, which are excreted through the kidneys.
**Uses: PO:** Anxiety, tension, anxiety with depression, insomnia, acute alcohol withdrawal symptoms. **Parenteral:** Amnesic agent, anticonvulsant, antitremor drug, adjunct to skeletal muscle relaxants, preanesthetic medication, adjunct prior to endoscopic procedures, treatment of status epilepticus, relief of acute alcohol withdrawal symptoms. *Non-FDA Approved Uses:* Antiemetic in cancer chemotherapy.
**Additional Contraindications:** Narrow-angle glaucoma. Use cautiously in presence of renal and hepatic disease. Parenterally in children less than 18 years.
**Special Concerns:** PO dosage has not been established in children less than 12 years of age and IV dosage has not been established in children less than 18 years of age.
**Additional Drug Interactions:** With parenteral lorazepam, scopola-

mine → sedation, hallucinations, and behavioral abnormalities.
**How Supplied:** *Concentrate:* 2 mg/mL; *Injection:* 2 mg/mL, 4 mg/mL; *Tablet:* 0.5 mg, 1 mg, 2 mg

### Dosage
• **Tablets, Concentrate**
*Anxiety.*
**Adults:** 1–3 mg b.i.d.–t.i.d.
*Hypnotic.*
**Adults:** 2–4 mg at bedtime. **Geriatric/debilitated clients, initial:** 0.5–2 mg/day in divided doses. Dose can be adjusted as required.
• **IM**
*Preoperatively.*
**Adults:** 0.05 mg/kg up to maximum of 4 mg 2 hr before surgery for maximum amnesic effect.
• **IV**
*Preoperatively.*
**Adults, initial:** 0.044 mg/kg or a total dose of 2 mg, whichever is less.
*Amnesic effect.*
**Adults:** 0.05 mg/kg up to a maximum of 4 mg administered 15–20 min prior to surgery.
*Antiemetic in cancer chemotherapy.*
**Initial:** 2 mg 30 min before beginning chemotherapy; **then,** 2 mg q 4 hr as needed.

## DENTAL CONCERNS

See also *Dental Concerns* for *Sedative-Hypnotics (Anti-anxiety)/Antimanic Drugs.*
1. Review anxiety level and identify any contributing factors.
2. Elderly clients may experience adverse reactions more quickly than younger clients; use a lower dose in this group.
3. Have someone drive the patient to and from the dental appointment if this drug is used for conscious sedation.
4. Assist the patient to and from the dental chair because of the possibility of dizziness.

---

## Losartan potassium
(loh-**SAR**-tan)
**Pregnancy Category:** C (first trimes-

ter), D (second and third trimesters)
Cozaar **(Rx)**
**Classification:** Antihypertensive,
angiotensin II receptor antagonist

See also *Antihypertensive Agents.*

**Action/Kinetics:** Angiotensin II, a potent vasoconstrictor, is the primary vasoactive hormone of the renin-angiotensin system; it is involved in the pathophysiology of hypertension. Angiotensin II increases systemic vascular resistance, causes sodium and water retention, and leads to increased heart rate and vasoconstriction. Losartan competitively blocks the angiotensin $AT_1$ receptor located in vascular smooth muscle and the adrenal glands, which is involved in mediating the effects of angiotensin II. Thus, BP is reduced. No significant effects on heart rate, has minimal orthostatic effects, and does not affect potassium levels significantly. Also, losartan does act on the $AT_2$ receptor. Undergoes significant first-pass metabolism in the liver, where it is converted to an active carboxylic acid metabolite that is responsible for most of the angiotensin receptor blockade. Rapidly absorbed after PO administration, although food slows absorption. **Peak plasma levels of losartan and metabolite:** 1 hr and 3–4 hr, respectively. **t½, losartan:** 2 hr; **t½, metabolite:** 6–9 hr. The drug and metabolite are highly bound to plasma proteins. Maximum effects are usually seen within 1 week, although from 3 to 6 weeks may be required in some clients. Drug and metabolites are excreted through both the urine (35%) and feces (60%).

**Uses:** Treatment of hypertension, alone or in combination with other antihypertensive agents.

**Contraindications:** Lactation. Use after pregnancy is discouraged.

**Special Concerns:** When used alone, the effect to decease BP in blacks was less than in non-blacks. Dosage adjustments are not required in clients with renal impairment, un-

less they are volume depleted. In clients with severe CHF, there is a risk of oliguria and/or progressive azotemia with acute renal failure and/or death (which are rare). In those with unilateral or bilateral renal artery stenosis, there is a risk of increased serum creatinine or BUN. Lower doses are recommended in those with hepatic insufficiency. Safety and efficacy have not been determined in children less than 18 years of age.

**Side Effects:** *Oral:* Dental pain, dry mouth. *GI:* Diarrhea, dyspepsia, anorexia, constipation, flatulence, gastritis, vomiting, taste perversion. *CV:* Angina pectoris, second-degree AV block, **CVA, MI, ventricular tachycardia, ventricular fibrillation,** hypotension, palpitation, sinus bradycardia, tachycardia, orthostatic effects. *CNS:* Dizziness, insomnia, anxiety, anxiety disorder, ataxia, confusion, depression, abnormal dreams, hypesthesia, decreased libido, impaired memory, migraine, nervousness, paresthesia, peripheral neuropathy, panic disorder, sleep disorder, somnolence, tremor, vertigo. *Respiratory:* Upper respiratory infection, cough, nasal congestion, sinus infection, sinusitis, dyspnea, bronchitis, pharyngeal discomfort, epistaxis, rhinitis, respiratory congestion. *Musculoskeletal:* Muscle cramps, myalgia, joint swelling, musculoskeletal pain, stiffness, arthralgia, arthritis, fibromyalgia, muscle weakness; pain in the back, legs, arms, hips, knees, shoulders. *Dermatologic:* Alopecia, dermatitis, dry skin, ecchymosis, erythema, flushing, photosensitivity, pruritus, rash, sweating, urticaria. *GU:* Impotence, nocturia, urinary frequency, UTI. *Ophthalmologic:* Blurred vision, burning/stinging in the eye, conjunctivitis, decrease in visual acuity. *Miscellaneous:* Gout, anemia, tinnitus, facial edema, fever, syncope.

**Drug Interactions:** No specific interactions have been reported with drugs that are used in dentistry.

L

---

However, lowest effective dose should be used, such as a local anesthetic, vasoconstrictor, or anticholinergic, if required.

**How Supplied:** *Tablet:* 25 mg, 50 mg

**Dosage** ───────────

• **Tablets**

*Hypertension.*

**Adults:** 50 mg once daily. In those with possible depletion of intravascular volume (e.g., clients treated with a diuretic, use 25 mg once daily. If the antihypertensive effect (measured at trough) is inadequate, a twice-a-day regimen, using the same dose, may be tried; or an increase in dose may give a more satisfactory result. If BP is not controlled by losartan alone, a diuretic (e.g., hydrochlorothiazide) may be added.

## DENTAL CONCERNS

See also *Dental Concerns* for *Antihypertensive Agents.*

# Lovastatin (Mevinolin)
(**LOW**-vah-**STAT**-in, me-**VIN**-oh-lin)
**Pregnancy Category:** X
Mevacor **(Rx)**
**Classification:** Antihyperlipidemic

See also *Antihyperlipidemic Agents—HMG-CoA Reductase Inhibitors.*

**Action/Kinetics:** It specifically inhibits HMG–coenzyme A reductase enzyme, which reduces cholesterol synthesis. Approximately 35% of a dose is absorbed. Extensive first-pass effect—less than 5% reaches the general circulation. Absorption is decreased by about one-third if the drug is given on an empty stomach rather than with food. **Onset:** within 2 weeks using multiple doses. **Time to peak plasma levels:** 2–4 hr. **Time to peak effect:** 4–6 weeks using multiple doses. **Duration:** 4–6 weeks after termination of therapy. Over 95% is bound to plasma proteins. Metabolized in the liver (its main site of action) to active metabolites. Over 80% of a PO dose is excreted in the feces, via the bile, and approximately 10% is excreted through the urine.

**Uses:** As an adjunct to diet in primary hypercholesterolemia (types IIa and IIb) in clients with a significant risk of CAD and who have not responded to diet or other measures. May also be useful in clients with combined hypercholesterolemia and hypertriglyceridemia. To slow the progression of coronary atherosclerosis in clients with CAD in order to lower total and LDL cholesterol levels. *Non-FDA Approved Uses:* Diabetic dyslipidemia, nephrotic hyperlipidemia, familial dysbetalipoproteinemia, and familial combined hyperlipidemia.

**Contraindications:** During pregnancy and lactation, active liver disease, persistent unexplained elevations of serum transaminases. Use in children less than 18 years of age.

**Special Concerns:** Use with caution in clients who have a history of liver disease or who are known heavy consumers of alcohol. Carefully monitor clients with impaired renal function.

**Side Effects:** *GI:* Flatus (most common), abdominal pain, cramps, diarrhea, constipation, dyspepsia, N&V, heartburn, anorexia, stomatitis, acid regurgitation, dry mouth. *CNS:* Headache, dizziness, tremor, vertigo, memory loss, paresthesia, anxiety, depression, insomnia. *Musculoskeletal:* Myalgia, muscle cramps, localized pain, arthralgia, myopathy, rhabdomyolysis with renal dysfunction secondary to myoglobinuria. *Hypersensitivity reaction:* Vasculitis, purpura, polymyalgia rheumatica, angioedema, lupus erythematosus-like syndrome, thrombocytopenia, *hemolytic anemia,* leukopenia, eosinophilia, positive ANA, arthritis, arthralgia, urticaria, asthenia, ESR increase, fever, chills, flushing, photosensitivity, malaise, dyspnea, *toxic epidermal necrolysis, anaphylaxis, erythema multiforme including Stevens-Johnson syndrome. Dermatologic:* Alopecia, pruritus, rash, skin changes, including nodules, discoloration, dryness, changes to hair and nails. *Hepatic:* Hepatitis (including chronic active hepatitis), cholestatic jaundice, fatty change in liver, cirrhosis, **fulminant hepatic necrosis,** hepatoma, pancreatitis. *GU:* Gynecomastia, loss of libido, erectile dysfunction. *Ophthalmic:* Blurred vision, progression of cataracts, lens opacities, ophthalmoplegia. *Hematologic:* Anemia, leukopenia, transient asymptomatic eosinophilia, thrombocytopenia. *Miscellaneous:* Cardiac chest pain, dysgeusia, edema, alteration of taste, impairment of extraocular movement, facial paresis, peripheral neuropathy, peripheral nerve palsy.

**Drug Interactions**
*Cyclosporine /* ↑ Risk of rhabdomyolysis or severe myopathy

*Erythromycin /* ↑ Risk of rhabdomyolysis or severe myopathy

**How Supplied:** *Tablet:* 10 mg, 20 mg, 40 mg

## Dosage
• **Tablets**
**Adults/adolescents, initial:** 20 mg once daily with the evening meal. Dose range: 10–80 mg/day in single or two divided doses with meals. If serum cholesterol levels are greater than 300 mg/dL, initial dose should be 40 mg/day. Adjust dose at intervals of every 4 weeks, if necessary.

## DENTAL CONCERNS

See also *Dental Concerns* for *Antihyperlipidemic Agents—HMG-CoA Reductase Inhibitors.*

# Mepivacaine hydrochloride
(meh-**PIV**-ah-kayn)
**Pregnancy Category:** C
Carbocaine, Carbocaine with Neo-Cobefrin, Isocaine, Polocaine, Polocaine MPF, Polocaine/Levonordefrin, Isocaine/Levonordefrin
**Classification:** Amide local anesthetic

See also *Amide Local Anesthetic Agents.*
**Action/Kinetics:** Blocks nerve action potential by inhibiting ion fluxes across the cell membrane. **Onset:** 2-10 min, **Duration:** 20 min-4 hr, Renally excreted and metabolized by the liver.
**Uses:** Local dental anesthesia, nerve block, caudal anesthesia, epidural, pain relief, paracervical block, transvaginal block or infiltration.
**Contraindications:** See also *Amide Local Anesthetic Agents.*

**Special Concerns:** See also *Amide Local Anesthetic Agents.*
**Side Effects:** See also *Amide Local Anesthetic Agents.*
**Drug Interactions:** See also *Amide Local Anesthetic Agents.*
**How Supplied:** *Injection without vasoconstrictor:* 1%, 1.5%, 2%, 3%; *Injection with vasoconstrictor:* 2% with levonordefrin 1:20,000

## Dosage
• **3% injection without vasoconstrictor**
*Dental anesthesia.*
54-270 mg not to exceed 300 mg per dental appointment. Dose should be adjusted down for medically compromised, debilitated, or elderly patients. (See also *Appendix 9.*)
• **2% injection with 1:20,000 levonordefrin**
*Dental anesthesia.*
36-180 mg not to exceed 400 mg per dental appointment. Dose should be adjusted down for medical-

ly compromised, debilitated, or elderly patients. (See also *Appendix 9*.)

## DENTAL CONCERNS

See also *Dental Concerns* for *Amide Local Anesthetic Agents*.

## Metformin hydrochloride
(met-**FOR**-min)
**Pregnancy Category:** B
Apo-Metformin ✿, Gen-Metformin ✿, Glucophage, Novo-Metformin ✿, Nu-Metformin ✿ **(Rx)**
**Classification:** Oral antidiabetic

**Action/Kinetics:** Decreases hepatic glucose production, decreases intestinal absorption of glucose, and increases peripheral uptake and utilization of glucose. Food decreases and slightly delays the absorption of metformin. Negligibly bound to plasma protein; steady-state plasma levels (less than 1 mcg/mL) are reached within 24–48 hr. Excreted unchanged in the urine; no biliary excretion. $t^{1/2}$, **plasma elimination:** 6.2 hr. The plasma and blood half-lives are prolonged in decreased renal function.

**Uses:** Alone as an adjunct to diet to lower blood glucose in clients having non-insulin-dependent diabetes mellitus whose blood glucose cannot be managed satisfactorily via diet alone. Also, metformin may be used concomitantly with a sulfonylurea when diet and metformin or a sulfonylurea alone do not result in adequate control of blood glucose.

**Contraindications:** Renal disease or dysfunction (serum creatinine levels greater than 1.5 mg/dL in males and greater than 1.4 mg/dL in females) or abnormal $C_{CR}$ due to cardiovascular collapse, acute MI, or septicemia. In clients undergoing radiologic studies using iodinated contrast media, because use of such products may cause alteration of renal function, leading to acute renal failure and lactic acidosis. Acute or chronic metabolic acidosis, including diabetic ketoacidosis, with or without coma. Lactation.

**Special Concerns:** Cardiovascular collapse, acute CHF, acute MI, and other conditions characterized by hypoxia have been associated with lactic acidosis, which may also be caused by metformin. Use of oral hypoglycemic agents may increase the risk of cardiovascular mortality. Although hypoglycemia does not usually occur with metformin, it may result with deficient caloric intake, with strenuous exercise not supplemented by increased intake of calories, or when metformin is taken with sulfonylureas or alcohol. Because of age-related decreases in renal function, use with caution as age increases. Safety and efficacy have not been determined in children.

**Side Effects:** *Metabolic:* Lactic acidosis (fatal in approximately 50% of cases). *Oral:* Unpleasant or metallic taste. *GI:* Diarrhea, N&V, abdominal bloating, flatulence, anorexia. *Hematologic:* Asymptomatic subnormal serum vitamin $B_{12}$ levels.

**Drug Interactions:** None reported that would interact with dental therapy or oral health.

**How Supplied:** *Tablet:* 500 mg, 850 mg

## Dosage
• **Tablets**

*Non-insulin-dependent diabetes mellitus.*

**Adults, using 500-mg tablet:** Starting dose is one 500-mg tablet b.i.d. given with the morning and evening meals. Dosage increases may be made in increments of 500 mg every week, given in divided doses, up to a maximum of 2,500 mg/day. If a 2,500-mg daily dose is required, it may be better tolerated when given in divided doses t.i.d. with meals. **Adults, using 850-mg tablet:** Starting dose is 850 mg once daily given with the morning meal. Dosage increases may be made in increments of 850 mg every other week, given in divided doses, up to a maximum of 2,550 mg/day. **Usual maintenance dose:** 850 mg b.i.d. with the morning and evening meals. However, some clients may require 850 mg t.i.d. with meals.

## DENTAL CONCERNS

See also *Dental Concerns* for *Antidiabetic Agents.*
**General**
1. Place dental chair in semisupine position to help eliminate or minimize GI adverse effects of the drug.
**Consultation with Primary Care Provider**
1. Immediately notify health care provider if symptoms of lactic acidosis are observed; myalgia, respiratory distress, weakness, diarrhea, malaise, muscle cramps, somnolence.
2. Those oral and maxillofacial surgical procedures that require the patient to significantly restrict food intake require medical consultation in order to temporarily hold the metformin.
**Client/Family Teaching**
1. Review the importance of good oral hygiene in order to prevent soft tissue inflammation.
2. Drug may cause a metallic taste; should subside.

# Methotrexate, Methotrexate sodium

(meth-oh-**TREKS**-ayt)
**Pregnancy Category:** D (X for pregnant psoriatic or rheumatoid arthritis clients)
Amethopterin, Folex PFS, Rheumatrex Dose Pack (Abbreviation: MTX) **(Rx)**
**Classification:** Antineoplastic, antimetabolite (folic acid analog)

See also *Antineoplastic Agents.*
**Action/Kinetics:** Cell-cycle specific for the S phase of cell division. Acts by inhibiting dihydrofolate reductase, which prevents reduction of dihydrofolate to tetrahydrofolate; this results in decreased synthesis of purines and consequently DNA. The most sensitive cells are bone marrow, fetal cells, dermal epithelium, urinary bladder, buccal mucosa, intestinal mucosa, and malignant cells.

When used for rheumatoid arthritis it may affect immune function. Variable absorption from GI tract. **Peak serum levels, IM:** 30–60 min; **PO:** 1–2 hr. **t½:** initial, 1 hr; intermediate, 2–3 hr; final, 8–12 hr. May accumulate in the body. Excreted by kidney (55%–92% in 24 hr). Renal function tests are recommended before initiation of therapy; perform daily leukocyte counts during therapy.

**Uses:** Uterine choriocarcinoma (curative), chorioadenoma destruens, hydatidiform mole, acute lymphocytic and lymphoblastic leukemia, lymphosarcoma, and other disseminated neoplasms in children; meningeal leukemia, some beneficial effect in regional chemotherapy of head and neck tumors, breast tumors, and lung cancer. In combination for advanced stage non-Hodgkin's lymphoma. Advanced mycosis fungoides. High doses followed by leucovorin rescue in combination with other drugs for prolonging relapse-free survival in nonmetastatic osteosarcoma in individuals who have had surgical resection or amputation for the primary tumor. Severe, recalcitrant, disabling psoriasis. Rheumatoid arthritis (severe, active, classical, or definite) in clients who have had inadequate response to NSAIDs and at least one or more antirheumatic drugs (disease modifying). *Investigational:* Severe corticosteroid-dependent asthma to reduce corticosteroid dosage; adjunct to treat osteosarcoma. Psoriatic arthritis and Reiter's disease.

**Contraindications:** Psoriasis clients with kidney or liver disease; blood dyscrasias as hypoplasia, thrombocytopenia, anemia, or leukopenia. Alcoholism, alcoholic liver disease, or other chronic liver disease. Immunodeficiency syndromes. Pregnancy and lactation.

**Special Concerns:** Use with caution in impaired renal function and elderly clients. Use with extreme caution in the presence of active infection and in debilitated clients.

M

*bold italic* = life-threatening side effect

Safety and efficacy have not been established for juvenile rheumatoid arthritis.

**Additional Side Effects:** *Severe bone marrow depression.* Hepatotoxicity, fibrosis, cirrhosis. *Hemorrhagic enteritis, intestinal ulceration or perforation,* acne, ecchymosis, hematemesis, melena, increased pigmentation, diabetes, leukoencephalopathy, chronic interstitial obstructive pulmonary disease, acute renal failure. Intrathecal use may result in chemical arachnoiditis, transient paresis, or *seizures.* Concomitant exposure to sunlight may aggravate psoriasis.

**Drug Interactions**

*Alcohol, ethyl* / Additive hepatotoxicity; combination can result in coma

*Aminoglycosides, oral* / ↓ Absorption of PO methotrexate

*Anticoagulants, oral* / Additive hypoprothrombinemia

*Folic acid–containing vitamin preparations* / ↓ Response to methotrexate

*Ibuprofen* / ↑ Effect of methotrexate by ↓ renal secretion

*NSAIDs* / Possible fatal interaction

*PABA* / ↑ Effect of methotrexate by ↓ plasma protein binding

*Phenylbutazone* / ↑ Effect of methotrexate by ↓ renal secretion

*Phenytoin* / ↑ Effect of methotrexate by ↓ plasma protein binding

*Probenecid* / ↑ Effect of methotrexate by ↓ renal clearance

*Procarbazine* / Possible ↑ nephrotoxicity

*Pyrimethamine* / ↑ Methotrexate toxicity

*Salicylates (aspirin)* / ↑ Effect of methotrexate by ↓ plasma protein binding; also, salicylates ↓ renal excretion of methotrexate

*Sulfonamides* / ↑ Effect of methotrexate by ↓ plasma protein binding

*Tetracyclines* / ↑ Effect of methotrexate by ↓ plasma protein binding

**How Supplied:** *Injection:* 25 mg/mL; *Powder for injection:* 20 mg, 1 g; *Tablet:* 2.5 mg

**Dosage** ─────────────────

• **Tablets (Methotrexate). IM, IV,**

**IA, Intrathecal (Methotrexate Sodium)**

*Choriocarcinoma and similar trophoblastic diseases.*

**Dose individualized. PO, IM:** 15–30 mg/day for 5 days. May be repeated 3–5 times with 1-week rest period between courses.

*Acute lymphatic (lymphoblastic) leukemia.*

**Initial:** 3.3 mg/m$^2$ (with 60 mg/m$^2$ prednisone daily); **maintenance: PO, IM,** 30 mg/m$^2$ 2 times/week or **IV,** 2.5 mg/kg q 14 days.

*Meningeal leukemia.*

**Intrathecal:** 12 mg/m$^2$ q 2–5 days until cell count returns to normal.

*Lymphomas.*

**PO:** 10–25 mg/day for 4–8 days for several courses of treatment with 7- to 10-day rest periods between courses.

*Mycosis fungoides.*

**PO:** 2.5–10 mg/day for several weeks or months; **alternatively, IM:** 50 mg once weekly or 25 mg twice weekly.

*Lymphosarcoma.*

0.625–2.5 mg/kg/day in combination with other drugs.

*Osteosarcoma.*

Used in combination with other drugs, including doxorubicin, cisplatin, bleomycin, cyclophosphamide, and dactinomycin. **Usual IV starting dose for methotrexate:** 12 g/m$^2$; dose may be increased to 15 g/m$^2$ to achieve a peak serum level of 10$^{-3}$ mol/L at the end of the methotrexate infusion.

*Psoriasis.*

**Adults, usual: PO, IM, IV,** 10–25 mg/week, continued until beneficial response observed. Weekly dose should not exceed 50 mg. **Alternate regimens: PO,** 2.5 mg q 12 hr for three doses or q 8 hr for four doses each week (not to exceed 30 mg/week); **or PO,** 2.5 mg daily for 5 days followed by 2 days of rest (dose should not exceed 6.25 mg/day). Once beneficial effects are noted, reduce dose to lowest possible level with longest rest periods between doses.

*Rheumatoid arthritis.*

**Initial:** Single PO doses of 7.5 mg/week or divided PO doses of 2.5 mg at 12-hr intervals for three doses given once a week; **then,** adjust dosage to achieve optimum response, not to exceed a total weekly dose of 20 mg. Once response has been reached, the dose should be reduced to the lowest possible effective dose.

## DENTAL CONCERNS

See also *Dental Concerns* for *Antineoplastic Agents.*

# Methyldopa

(meth-ill-**DOH**-pah)
**Pregnancy Category:** B (PO)
Aldomet, Apo-Methyldopa ✤, Dopamet ✤, Medimet ✤, Novo–Medopa ✤, Nu-Medopa ✤ **(Rx)**

# Methyldopate hydrochloride

(meth-ill-**DOH**-payt)
**Pregnancy Category:** B (PO), C (IV)
Aldomet Hydrochloride **(Rx)**
**Classification:** Antihypertensive, centrally acting antiadrenergic

See also *Antihypertensive Agents.*
**Action/Kinetics:** The active metabolite, alpha-methylnorepinephrine, lowers BP by stimulating central inhibitory alpha-adrenergic receptors, false neurotransmission, and/or reduction of plasma renin. Little change in CO. **PO: Onset:** 7–12 hr. **Duration:** 12–24 hr. All effects terminated within 48 hr. Absorption is variable. **IV: Onset:** 4–6 hr. **Duration:** 10–16 hr. Seventy percent of drug excreted in urine. **Full therapeutic effect:** 1–4 days. **t½:** 1.7 hr. Metabolites excreted in the urine.
**Uses:** Moderate to severe hypertension. Particularly useful for clients with impaired renal function, renal hypertension, resistant cases of hypertension complicated by stroke, CAD, or nitrogen retention, and for hypertensive crisis (parenterally).

**Contraindications:** Sensitivity to drug (including sulfites), labile and mild hypertension, pregnancy, active hepatic disease, use with MAO inhibitors, or pheochromocytoma.
**Special Concerns:** Use with caution in clients with a history of liver or kidney disease. A decrease in dose in geriatric clients may prevent syncope.
**Side Effects:** *CNS:* Sedation (transient), weakness, headache, asthenia, dizziness, paresthesias, Parkinson-like symptoms, psychic disturbances, symptoms of CV impairment, choreoathetotic movements, Bell's palsy, decreased mental acuity, verbal memory impairment. *CV:* Bradycardia, orthostatic hypotension, hypersensitivity of carotid sinus, worsening of angina, paradoxical hypertensive response (after IV), myocarditis, CHF, pericarditis, vasculitis. *Oral:* Dry mouth, bleeding, lichenoid drug reaction, sore or "black tongue," sialoadenitis. *GI:* N&V, abdominal distention, diarrhea or constipation, flatus, colitis, pancreatitis. *Hematologic:* **Hemolytic anemia,** leukopenia, granulocytopenia, thrombocytopenia, **bone marrow depression.** *Endocrine:* Gynecomastia, amenorrhea, galactorrhea, lactation, hyperprolactinemia. *GU:* Impotence, failure to ejaculate, decreased libido. *Dermatologic:* Rash, **toxic epidermal necrolysis.** *Hepatic:* Jaundice, hepatitis, liver disorders, abnormal liver function tests. *Miscellaneous:* Edema, fever, lupus-like symptoms, nasal stuffiness, arthralgia, myalgia, **septic shock-like syndrome.**
**Drug Interactions**
*Anesthetics, general* / Additive hypotension
*Antidepressants, tricyclic* / Tricyclic antidepressants may block hypotensive effect of methyldopa
*Haloperidol* / Methyldopa ↑ toxic effects of haloperidol
*NSAIDs, including indomethacin* / ↓ Effects
*Phenothiazines* / ↑ Risk of serious ↑ BP

**M**

*bold italic* = life-threatening side effect

*Sympathomimetics, including epinephrine* / Potentiation of hypertensive effect of sympathomimetics

*Thioxanthenes* / Additive hypotensive effect

*Tricyclic antidepressants* / ↓ Effect of methyldopa

**How Supplied:** Methyldopa: *Suspension:* 250 mg/5 mL; *Tablet:* 125 mg, 250 mg, 500 mg. Methyldopate hydrochloride: *Injection:* 50 mg/mL

**Dosage**

• **Methyldopa. Oral Suspension, Tablets**

*Hypertension.*

**Initial:** 250 mg b.i.d.–t.i.d. for 2 days. Adjust dose q 2 days. If increased, start with evening dose. **Usual maintenance:** 0.5–3.0 g/day in two to four divided doses; **maximum:** 3 g/day. Transfer to and from other antihypertensive agents should occur gradually, with initial dose of methyldopa not exceeding 500 mg. *NOTE:* Do not use combination medication to initiate therapy. **Pediatric, initial:** 10 mg/kg/day in two to four divided doses, adjusting maintenance to a maximum of 65 mg/kg/day (or 3 g/day, whichever is less).

• **Methyldopate HCl. IV Infusion**

*Hypertension.*

**Adults:** 250–500 mg q 6 hr; **maximum:** 1 g q 6 hr for hypertensive crisis.

Switch to PO methyldopa, at same dosage level, when BP is brought under control. **Pediatric:** 20–40 mg/kg/day in divided doses q 6 hr; **maximum:** 65 mg/kg/day (or 3 g/day, whichever is less).

## DENTAL CONCERNS

See also *Dental Concerns* for *Antihypertensive Agents.*

# Metoprolol succinate
(me-toe-**PROH**-lohl)
**Pregnancy Category:** C
Toprol XL **(Rx)**

# Metoprolol tartrate
(me-toe-**PROH**-lohl)

**Pregnancy Category:** B
Apo-Metoprolol ✿, Apo-Metoprolol (Type L) ✿, Betaloc ✿, Betaloc Durules ✿, Gen-Metoprolol ✿, Lopressor, Novo–Metoprol ✿, Nu-Metop ✿, PMS-Metoprolol-B ✿ **(Rx)**
**Classification:** Beta-adrenergic blocking agent

See also *Beta-Adrenergic Blocking Agents.*

**Action/Kinetics:** Exerts mainly beta-1-adrenergic blocking activity although beta-2 receptors are blocked at high doses. Has no membrane stabilizing or intrinsic sympathomimetic effects. Moderate lipid solubility. **Onset:** 15 min. **Peak plasma levels:** 90 min. **t½:** 3–7 hr. Effect of drug is cumulative. Food increases bioavailability. Exhibits significant first-pass effect. Metabolized in liver and excreted in urine.

**Uses: Metoprolol Succinate:** Alone or with other drugs to treat hypertension. Chronic management of angina pectoris.

**Metoprolol Tartrate:** Hypertension (either alone or with other antihypertensive agents, such as thiazide diuretics). Acute MI in hemodynamically stable clients. Angina pectoris. *Non-FDA Approved Uses:* IV to suppress atrial ectopy in COPD, aggressive behavior, prophylaxis of migraine, ventricular arrhythmias, enhancement of cognitive performance in geriatric clients, essential tremors.

**Contraindications:** Hypersensitivity to metoprolol, cardiogenic shock, 2nd or 3rd degree heart block, sinus bradycardia, CHF, bronchial asthma

**Special Concerns:** CAD, COPD, diabetes mellitus, heart failure, major surgery, nonallergic bronchospams, renal disease, thyroid disease. Safety and effectiveness have not been established in children. Use with caution in impaired hepatic function and during lactation.

**Side Effects:** *Oral:* Dry mouth. *CV:* AV block, bradycardia, cardiac arrest, CHF, dysrhythmias, hypotension, palpitations. *CNS:* Anxiety, confusion, depression, dizziness, fatigue, hallucinations, insomnia, mental changes. *GI: **Diarrhea,*** colitis, constipation, cramps, flatulence, ***hiccups,*** nausea, vomiting. *Hematologic: **Agranulocytosis, eosinophilia, thrombocytopenia purpura.*** *Allergic:* fever, Sore throat, respiratory distress, rash, pharyngitis, ***laryngospasm, anaphylaxis.*** *Skin:* Pruritus, rash, increased skin pigmentation, sweating, dry skin, alopecia, skin irritation, psoriasis. *Ophthalmic:* Dry, burning eyes. *GU:* Impotence. *Respiratory: **Bronchospasm,*** dyspnea, wheezing.

**Drug Interactions:** See also *Drug Interactions* for *Beta-Adrenergic Blocking Agents* and *Antihypertensive Agents.*

**How Supplied:** Metoprolol succinate: *Tablet, extended release:* 50 mg, 100 mg, 200 mg. Metoprolol tartrate: *Injection:* 1 mg/mL; *Tablet:* 50 mg, 100 mg

**Dosage**
- **Metoprolol Succinate Tablets**
  *Angina pectoris.*
**Individualized. Initial:** 100 mg/day in a single dose. Dose may be increased slowly, at weekly intervals, until optimum effect is reached or there is a pronounced slowing of HR. Doses above 400 mg/day have not been studied.
  *Hypertension.*
**Initial:** 50–100 mg/day in a single dose with or without a diuretic. Dosage may be increased in weekly intervals until maximum effect is reached. Doses above 400 mg/day have not been studied.
- **Metoprolol Tartrate Tablets**
  *Hypertension.*
**Initial:** 100 mg/day in single or divided doses; **then,** dose may be increased weekly to maintenance level of 100–450 mg/day. A diuretic may also be used.
  *Aggressive behavior.*
200–300 mg/day.
  *Essential tremors.*
50–300 mg/day.
  *Prophylaxis of migraine.*
50–100 mg b.i.d.

*Ventricular arrhythmias.*
200 mg/day.
- **Metoprolol Tartrate Injection (IV) and Tablets**
  *Early treatment of MI.*
3 IV bolus injections of 5 mg each at approximately 2-min intervals. If clients tolerate the full IV dose, give 50 mg q 6 hr PO beginning 15 min after the last IV dose (or as soon as client's condition allows). This dose is continued for 48 hr followed by **late treatment:** 100 mg b.i.d. as soon as feasible; continue for 1–3 months (although data suggest treatment should be continued for 1–3 years). In clients who do not tolerate the full IV dose, begin with 25–50 mg q 6 hr PO beginning 15 min after the last IV dose or as soon as the condition allows.

## DENTAL CONCERNS

See also *Dental Concerns* for *Beta-Adrenergic Blocking Agents* and *Antihypertensive Agents.*

**Client/Family Teaching**
1. Review the importance of good oral hygiene in order to prevent soft tissue inflammation.
2. Review the proper use of oral hygiene aids in order to prevent injury.
3. Daily home, fluoride treatments for persistent dry mouth.
4. Avoid alcohol-containing mouth rinses.
5. Dry mouth can be treated with tart, sugarless gum or candy, water, or with saliva substitutes if dry mouth persists.

# Metronidazole
(meh-troh-**NYE**-dah-zohl)
**Pregnancy Category:** B
Apo-Metronidazole ✿, Femazole, Flagyl, Flagyl ER, Flagyl I.V., Flagyl I.V. RTU, Metric 21, Metro-Cream Topical, MetroGel Topical, MetroGel-Vaginal, Metro I.V., Metryl, Metryl-500, Metryl I.V., NidaGel ✿, Novo–Nidazol ✿, PMS-Metronidazole ✿, Protostat, Satric, Satric 500, Trikacide ✿ **(Rx)**
**Classification:** Systemic trichomonacide, amebicide

See also *Anti-Infectives*.

**Action/Kinetics:** Effective against anaerobic bacteria and protozoa. Specifically inhibits growth of trichomonae and amoebae by binding to DNA, resulting in loss of helical structure, strand breakage, inhibition of nucleic acid synthesis, and cell death. Well absorbed from GI tract and widely distributed in body tissues. **Peak serum concentration: PO,** 6–40 mcg/mL, depending on the dose, after 1–2 hr. **t½: PO,** 6–12 hr average: 8 hr. Eliminated primarily in urine (20% unchanged), which may be red-brown in color following either PO or IV use. The mechanism for its effectiveness in reducing the inflammatory lesions of acne rosacea are not known.

**Uses: Systemic:** Amebiasis. Symptomatic and asymptomatic trichomoniasis; to treat asymptomatic partner. Amebic dysentery and amebic liver abscess. To reduce postoperative anaerobic infection following colorectal surgery, elective hysterectomy, and emergency appendectomy. Anaerobic bacterial infections of the abdomen, female genital system, skin or skin structures, bones and joints, lower respiratory tract, and CNS. Also, septicemia, endocarditis, hepatic encephalopathy. PO for Crohn's disease and pseudomembranous colitis. *Non-FDA Approved Uses:* giardiasis, *Gardnerella vaginalis.*

**Topical:** Inflammatory papules, pustules, and erythema of rosacea. *Investigational:* Infected decubitus ulcers (use 1% solution prepared from oral tablets).

**Vaginal:** Bacterial vaginosis.

**Contraindications:** Blood dyscrasias; active organic disease of the CNS. Not recommended for trichomoniasis during the first trimester of pregnancy. During lactation. For topical use: hypersensitivity to parabens or other ingredients of the formulation. Consumption of alcohol during use.

**Special Concerns:** Safety and efficacy have not been established in children.

**Side Effects: Systemic Use.** *Oral:* Dry mouth, metallic taste, furry tongue, glossitis, stomatitis (due to overgrowth of *Candida*). *GI:* Nausea, vomiting, diarrhea, abdominal discomfort, constipation. *CNS:* Headache, dizziness, vertigo, incoordination, ataxia, confusion, irritability, depression, weakness, insomnia, syncope, seizures, peripheral neuropathy including paresthesias. *Hematologic:* Leukopenia, **bone marrow aplasia.** *GU:* Burning, dysuria, cystitis, polyuria, incontinence, dryness of vagina or vulva, dyspareunia, decreased libido. *Allergic:* Urticaria, pruritus, erythematous rash, flushing, nasal congestion, fever, joint pain. *Miscellaneous:* ECG abnormalities, thrombophlebitis.

**Topical Use:** Watery eyes if gel applied too closely to this area; transient redness; mild burning, dryness, and skin irritation.

**Vaginal Use:** Symptomatic candida vaginitis, N&V.

**Drug Interactions**

*Barbiturates* / Possible therapeutic failure of metronidazole

*Ethanol or ethanol-containing products* / Possible disulfiram-like reaction, including flushing, palpitations, tachycardia, and N&V

**How Supplied:** *Capsule:* 375 mg; *Cream:* 0.75%; *Gel/jelly:* 0.75%; *Injection:* 500 mg/100 mL; *Tablet:* 250 mg, 500 mg

---

**Dosage** ————————————

• **Capsules, Tablets**

*Amebiasis: Acute amebic dysentery or amebic liver abscess.*

**Adult:** 500–750 mg t.i.d. for 5–10 days; **pediatric:** 35–50 mg/kg/day in three divided doses for 10 days.

*Trichomoniasis, female.*

250 mg t.i.d. for 7 days, 2 g given on 1 day in single or divided doses, or 375 mg b.i.d. for 7 days. **Pediatric:** 5 mg/kg t.i.d. for 7 days. An interval of 4–6 weeks should elapse between courses of therapy. *NOTE:* Do not treat pregnant women during the first trimester. *Male:* Individualize dosage; usual, 250 mg t.i.d. for 7 days.

*Giardiasis.*
250 mg t.i.d. for 7 days.
*G. vaginalis.*
500 mg b.i.d. for 7 days.
• **Tablets, Extended-Release**
*Bacterial vaginosis.*
One 750-mg tablet per day for 7 days.
• **IV**
*Anaerobic bacterial infections.*
**Adults, initially:** 15 mg/kg infused over 1 hr; **then,** after 6 hr, 7.5 mg/kg q 6 hr for 7–10 days (daily dose should not exceed 4 g). Treatment may be necessary for 2–3 weeks, although PO therapy should be initiated as soon as possible.
*Prophylaxis of anaerobic infection during surgery.*
**Adults:** 15 mg/kg given over a 30- to 60-min period, with completion 1 hr prior to surgery and 7.5 mg/kg infused over 30–60 min 6 and 12 hr after the initial dose.
• **Topical (0.75%)**
*Rosacea.*
After washing, apply a thin film and rub in well in the morning and evening for 9 weeks.
• **Vaginal (0.75%)**
*Bacterial vaginosis.*
One applicatorful (5 g) in the morning and evening for 5 days. Metro-Gel Vaginal allows for once-daily dosing at bedtime.

## DENTAL CONCERNS

See also *General Dental Concerns* for *All Anti-Infectives.*
**General**
1. Determine why the patient is taking the drug.
2. Decreased saliva flow can put the patient at risk for dental caries, periodontal disease, and candidiasis.
3. Patients on chronic drug therapy may develop blood dyscrasias. Symptoms include fever, sore throat, and bleeding, and poor wound healing.
**Consultation with Primary Care Provider**
1. Patients with symptoms of blood dyscrasias should be referred to

their primary care provider for complete blood counts. Treatment should be postponed until the results are known.
2. Medical consultation may be necessary in order to assess disease control.
**Client/Family Teaching**
1. No alcohol; a disulfiram-like reaction may occur. Symptoms include abdominal cramps, vomiting, flushing, and headache.
2. Taste perversion may occur.
3. Review the importance of good oral hygiene in order to prevent soft tissue inflammation.
4. Review the proper use of oral hygiene aids in order to prevent injury.
5. Daily home fluoride treatments for persistent dry mouth.
6. Avoid alcohol-containing mouth rinses.
7. Dry mouth can be treated with tart, sugarless gum or candy, water, or with saliva substitutes if dry mouth persists.

**M**

# Midazolam hydrochloride
(my-**DAYZ**-oh-lam)
**Pregnancy Category:** D
Versed **(C-IV) (Rx)**
**Classification:** Benzodiazepine sedative; adjunct to general anesthesia

See also *Sedative-Hypnotics (Antianxiety)/Antimanic Drugs.*
**Action/Kinetics:** Short-acting benzodiazepine with sedative–general anesthetic properties. Depresses the response of the respiratory system to carbon dioxide stimulation, which is more pronounced in clients with COPD. Possible mild to moderate decreases in CO, mean arterial BP, SV, and systemic vascular resistance. HR may rise somewhat in those with slow HRs (< 65/min) and decrease in others (especially those with HRs more than 85/min). **Onset, IM:** 15 min; **IV:** 2–2.5 min for induction (if combined with a preanesthetic narcotic, induction is about 1.5 min). If preanesthetic medication (morphine) is given, the **Peak plasma**

**levels, IM:** 45 min. **Maximum effect:** 30–60 min. **Time to recovery:** Usually within 2 hr, although up to 6 hr may be required. About 97% bound to plasma protein. **t½, elimination:** 1.2–12.3 hr. Rapidly metabolized in the liver to inactive compounds; excreted through the urine.

**Uses: IV, IM:** Preoperative sedation, anxiolysis, and amnesia. **IV:** Sedation, anxiolysis, and amnesia prior to or during short diagnostic, therapeutic, or endoscopic procedures (either alone or with other CNS depressants). Induction of general anesthesia before administration of other anesthetics. Supplement to nitrous oxide and oxygen in balanced anesthesia. Sedation of intubated and mechanically ventilated clients as a component of anesthesia or during treatment in a critical care setting. *Non-FDA Approved Uses:* Treat epileptic seizures. Alternative to terminate refractory status epilepticus.

**Contraindications:** Hypersensitivity to benzodiazepines. Acute narrow-angle glaucoma. Use in obstetrics. Use in coma, shock, or acute alcohol intoxication where VS are depressed. IA injection.

**Special Concerns:** Use with caution during lactation. Pediatric clients may require higher doses than adults. Hypotension may be more common in conscious sedated clients who have received a preanesthetic narcotic. Geriatric and debilitated clients require lower doses to induce anesthesia and they are more prone to side effects. Use IV with extreme caution in severe fluid or electrolyte disturbances.

**Side Effects:** Fluctuations in VS, including decreased respiratory rate and tidal volume, apnea, variations in BP and pulse rate are common. The following are general side effects regardless of the route of administration. *CV:* Hypotension, cardiac arrest. *CNS:* Oversedation, headache, drowsiness, grogginess, confusion, retrograde amnesia, euphoria, nervousness, agitation, anxiety, argumentativeness, restlessness, emergence delirium, increased time for emer-

gence, dreaming during emergence, nightmares, insomnia, tonic-clonic movements, ataxia, muscle tremor, involuntary or athetoid movements, dizziness, dysphoria, dysphonia, slurred speech, paresthesia. *GI:* Hiccoughs, N&V, acid taste, retching, excessive salivation. *Ophthalmologic:* Double vision, blurred vision, nystagmus, pinpoint pupils, visual disturbances, cyclic eyelid movements, difficulty in focusing. *Dermatologic:* Hives, swelling or feeling of burning, warmth or cold feeling at injection site, hive-like wheal at injection site, pruritus, rash. *Miscellaneous:* Blocked ears, loss of balance, chills, weakness, faint feeling, lethargy, yawning, toothache, hematoma.

**More common following IM use:** Pain at injection site, headache, induration and redness, muscle stiffness.

**More common following IV use:** *Respiratory:* ***Bronchospasm,*** coughing, dyspnea, laryngospasm, hyperventilation, shallow respirations, tachypnea, airway obstruction, wheezing, respiratory depression and ***respiratory arrest*** when used for conscious sedation. *CV:* PVCs, bigeminy, bradycardia, tachycardia, vasovagal episode, nodal rhythm. *At injection site:* Tenderness, pain, redness, induration, phlebitis.

**Drug Interactions**

*Alcohol* / ↑ Risk of apnea, airway obstruction, desaturation or hypoventilation

*Anesthetics, inhalation* / ↓ Dose if midazolam used as an induction agent

*CNS Depressants* / ↑ Risk of apnea, airway obstruction, desaturation or hypoventilation

*Droperidol* / ↑ Hypnotic effect of midazolam when used as a premedication

*Fentanyl* / ↑ Hypnotic effect of midazolam when used as a premedication

*Indinavir* / Possible prolonged sedation and respiratory depression

*Meperidine* / See *Narcotics;* also, ↑ Risk of hypotension

*Narcotics* / ↑ Hypnotic effect of midazolam when used as premedications

*Propofol* / ↑ Effect of propofol

*Ritonavir* / Possible prolonged sedation and respiratory depression

*Thiopental* / ↓ Dose if midazolam used as an induction agent

**How Supplied:** *Injection:* 1 mg/mL, 5 mg/mL

Dosage
─────────────

• **IM**

*Preoperative sedation, anxiolysis, amnesia.*

**Adults:** 0.07–0.08 mg/kg IM (average: 5 mg) 1 hr before surgery. **Children:** 0.1–0.15 mg/kg (up to 0.5 mg/kg may be needed for more anxious clients).

• **IV**

*Conscious sedation, anxiolysis, amnesia for endoscopic or CV procedures in healthy adults less than 60 years of age.*

Using the 1 mg/mL (can be diluted with 0.9% sodium chloride or D5W) product, titrate slowly to the desired effect (usually slurred speech); initial dose should be no higher than 2.5 mg IV (may be as low as 1 mg IV) within a 2-min period, after which an additional 2 min should be waited to evaluate the sedative effect. If additional sedation is necessary, small increments should be given waiting an additional 2 min or more after each increment to evaluate the effect. Total doses greater than 5 mg are usually not required. **Children:** Dosage must be individualized by the physician.

*Conscious sedation for endoscopic or CV procedures in debilitated or chronically ill clients or clients aged 60 or over.*

Slowly titrate to the desired effect using no more than 1.5 mg initially IV (may be as little as 1 mg IV) given over a 2-min period after which an additional 2 min or more should be waited to evaluate the effect. If additional sedation is needed, no more than 1 mg should be given over 2 min; wait an additional 2 min or more after each increment in dose. Total doses greater than 3.5 mg are usually not needed.

*Induction of general anesthesia, before use of other general anesthetics, in unmedicated clients.*

**Adults, unmedicated clients up to 55 years of age, IV, initial:** 0.3–0.35 mg/kg given over 20–30 sec, waiting 2 min for effects to occur. If needed, increments of about 25% of the initial dose can be used to complete induction; or, induction can be completed using a volatile liquid anesthetic. Up to 0.6 mg/kg may be used but recovery will be prolonged. **Adults, unmedicated clients over 55 years of age who are good risk surgical clients, initial IV:** 0.15–0.3 mg/kg given over 20–30 sec. **Adults, unmedicated clients over 55 years of age with severe systemic disease or debilitation, initial IV:** 0.15–0.25 mg/kg given over 20–30 sec. **Pediatric:** 0.05–0.2 mg/kg IV.

*Induction of general anesthesia, before use of other general anesthetics, in medicated clients.*

**Adults, premedicated clients up to 55 years of age, IV, initial:** 0.15–0.35 mg/kg. If less than 55 years of age, 0.25 mg/kg may be given over 20–30 sec, allowing 2 min for effect. **Adults, premedicated clients over 55 years of age who are good risk surgical clients, initial, IV:** 0.2 mg/kg. **Adults, premedicated clients over 55 years of age with severe systemic disease or debilitation, initial, IV:** 0.15 mg/kg may be sufficient.

*Maintenance of balanced anesthesia for short surgical procedures.*

**IV:** Incremental injections about 25% of the dose used for induction when signs indicate anesthesia is lightening.

*NOTE:* Narcotic preanesthetic medication may include fentanyl, 1.5–2 mcg/kg IV 5 min before induction; morphine, up to 0.15 mg/kg IM; meperidine, up to 1 mg/kg IM; or, Innovar, 0.02 mL/kg IM. Sedative

**M**

preanesthetic medication may include secobarbital sodium, 200 mg PO or hydroxyzine pamoate, 100 mg PO. Except for fentanyl, all preanesthetic medications should be given 1 hr prior to midazolam. Doses should always be individualized.

## DENTAL CONCERNS
### General
1. Check vital signs every 5 min during general anesthesia because of cardiovascular and respiratory side effects.
2. Monitor vital signs at regular intervals during recovery.
3. Titrate all doses. Extent of CNS depression is dependent on dose.
4. This drug causes amnesia, especially in the elderly.
5. Obese patients may have a longer recovery period because of an increased half-life.
6. Patients may require assistance with ambulation until drowsiness has subsided.
### Client/Family Teaching
1. Drug may cause dizziness and drowsiness. Avoid alcohol, CNS depressants, and activities that require mental alertness (i.e., driving) for 24 hr following drug administration.
2. Repeat postprocedure instructions and obtain in writing as may not fully recall instructions; transient amnesia is normal and memory of procedure may be minimal.

# Miglitol
(**MIG**-lih-tohl)
**Pregnancy Category:** B
Glyset **(Rx)**
**Classification:** Antidiabetic, oral

See also *Antidiabetic Agents.*
**Action/Kinetics:** Acts by delaying digestion of ingested carbohydrates resulting in smaller rise in blood glucose levels after meals. Does not enhance insulin secretion or increase insulin sensitivity. Does not cause hypoglycemia when given in fasted state. Absorption is saturable at high doses (i.e., only 50% to 70% of 100 mg dose is absorbed while 25 mg dose is

100% absorbed). **Peak levels:** 2–3 hr. Drug is not metabolized and is eliminated unchanged in urine. Dose must be reduced in those with impaired renal function.
**Uses:** Alone as adjunct to diet to treat non-insulin-dependent diabetes. With sulfonylurea when diet plus either miglitol or a sulfonylurea alone do not result in adequate control (effects of sulfonylurea and miglitol are additive).
**Contraindications:** Lactation, diabetic ketoacidosis, inflammatory bowel disease, colonic ulceration, partial intestinal obstruction, those predisposed to intestinal obstruction, chronic intestinal diseases associated with marked disorders of digestion or absorption, conditions that may deteriorate due to increased gas formation in the intestine, hypersensitivity to drug.
**Special Concerns:** When given with sulfonylurea or insulin, miglitol causes further decrease in blood sugar and increased risk of hypoglycemia. Safety and efficacy have not been determined in children.
**Side Effects:** *GI:* Flatulence, diarrhea, abdominal pain, soft stools, abdominal discomfort. *Dermatologic:* Skin rash (transient).
**Drug Interactions:** No drug interactions reported that would impact on dental health or the dental process.
**How Supplied:** *Tablets:* 25 mg, 50 mg, 100 mg

## Dosage
- **Tablets**
*Type II diabetes.*
**Individualize dosage. Initial:** 25 mg t.i.d. with first bite of each main meal (some may benefit from starting with 25 mg once daily to minimize GI side effects). After 4 to 8 weeks of 25 mg t.i.d. dose, increase dosage to 50 mg t.i.d. for about 3 months. Measure glycosylated hemoglobin; if not satisfactory, increase dose to 100 mg t.i.d. **Maintenance:** 50 mg t.i.d., up to 100 mg t.i.d. (maximum).

## DENTAL CONCERNS

See also *Dental Concerns* for *Antidiabetic Agents*.

**General**

1. Place dental chair in semisupine position to help eliminate or minimize GI adverse effects of the drug.

---

# Minocycline hydrochloride

(mih-no-**SYE**-kleen)

**Pregnancy Category:** D

Alti-Minocycline ✦, Apo-Minocycline ✦, Dynacin, Minocin, Novo-Minocycline ✦, Vectrin **(Rx)**

**Classification:** Antibiotic, tetracycline

See also *Anti-Infectives* and *Tetracyclines*.

**Action/Kinetics:** In fasting adults, 90% to 100% of an oral dose is absorbed. **Peak plasma levels:** 1–4 hr. Absorption is less affected by milk or food than for other tetracyclines. **t½, elimination:** 11–26 hr. Metabolized in the liver.

**Uses:** See also *Tetracyclines*. To eliminate meningococci from the nasopharynx of asymptomatic *Neisseria meningitidis* carriers in which the risk of meningococcal meningitis is high. *Note:* Due to adverse CNS effects, it is now recommended that rifampin be used in treating meningococcus carriers when the drug susceptibility is not known or when the organism is sulfa-resistant. Minocycline is indicated only when rifampin is contraindicated.

Granulomas of the skin caused by *Mycobacterium marinum*. In combination with gonococcal regimens for presumptive treatment of coexisting chlamydial infections. Uncomplicated gonogoccal urethritis in adult males. Treatment of uncomplicated urethral, endocervical, or rectal infections caused by *Chlamydia trachomatis* or *Ureaplasma urealyticum* in adults. Intrapleurally as a sclerosing agent to control pleural effusions associated with metastatic tumors. Treatment of cholera and nocar-

diosis. Adjunctive treatment of inflammatory acne unresponsive to oral tetracycline HCl or oral erythromycin.

**Contraindications:** See also *Tetracyclines*.

**Special Concerns:** See also *Tetracyclines*.

**Side Effects:** See also *Tetracyclines*.

**Additional Side Effects:** Blue-gray pigmentation areas of cutaneous inflammation, vertigo, ataxia, drowsiness, ***Stevens-Johnson syndrome*** (rare).

**Drug Interactions:** See also *Tetracyclines*.

**How Supplied:** *Capsules:* 50 mg, 100 mg; *Powder for injection:* 100 mg; *Syrup:* 50 mg/5 mL; *Tablets:* 100 mg.

## Dosage

• **Capsules, Injection, Suspension, Tablets**

*Infections against which effective, including asymptomatic meningococcus carriers.*

**Adults, initial:** 200 mg; **then,** 100 mg q 12 hr. An alternative regimen is 100–200 mg initially followed by 50 mg q 6 hr. The length of treatment is 5 days for meningococcus carriers.

**Children over 8 years of age, initial:** 4 mg/kg; **then,** 2 mg/kg q 12 hr.

*Mycobacterial infections.*

100 mg PO b.i.d. for 6–8 weeks.

*Uncomplicated gonococcal urethritis in adult males.*

100 mg b.i.d. for 5 days.

*Uncomplicated urethral, endocervical, or rectal infections due to* Chlamydia trachomatis *or* Ureaplasma urealyticum.

100 mg PO b.i.d. for at least 7 days.

*Nongonococcal urethritis caused by* C. trachomatis *or* Mycoplasma.

100/day PO in 1 or 2 divided doses for 1 to 3 weeks.

*Sclerosing agent to control pleural effusions associated with metastatic cancer.*

300 mg diluted with 40–50 mL of 0.9% NaCl injection and instilled into

**M**

---

✦ = Available in Canada                    ***bold italic*** = life-threatening side effect

the pleural space through a thoracostomy tube.

*Cholera in conjunction with fluid and electrolyte replacement.*
**Initial:** 200 mg PO; **then,** 100 mg PO 12 hr for 48–72 hr.

*Adjunct to treat inflammatory acne unresponsive to PO tetracycline HCl or erythromycin.*
50 mg PO 1–3 times/day.

## DENTAL CONCERNS

See also *Dental Concerns* for *Anti-Infectives* and *Tetracyclines*.
**General**
1. Has been reported to cause intrinsic staining in erupted permanent teeth which is not associated with the calcification stage.
2. Minocycline HCl readily distributes to gingival crevicular fluid.
3. Minocycline HCl may cause drowsiness. Caution patients about driving or performing tasks that require much thought or concentration.

# Minoxidil, oral
(mih-**NOX**-ih-dil)
**Pregnancy Category:** C
Loniten **(Rx)**
**Classification:** Antihypertensive, depresses sympathetic nervous system

See also *Antihypertensive Agents.*
**Action/Kinetics:** Decreases elevated BP by decreasing peripheral resistance by a direct effect. Causes increase in renin secretion, increase in cardiac rate and output, and salt/water retention. Does not cause orthostatic hypotension. **Onset:** 30 min. **Peak plasma levels:** reached within 60 min; **plasma t½:** 4.2 hr. **Duration:** 24–48 hr. Ninety percent absorbed from GI tract; excretion: renal (90% metabolites). The time needed to reach the maximum effect is inversely related to the dose.
**Uses:** Severe hypertension not controllable by the use of a diuretic plus two other antihypertensive drugs. Usually taken with at least two other antihypertensive drugs (a diuretic and a drug to minimize tachycardia such as a beta-adrenergic blocking agent). Minoxidil can produce severe side effects; it should be reserved for resistant cases of hypertension. Close medical supervision required, including possible hospitalization during initial administration. Topically to promote hair growth in balding men.
**Contraindications:** Pheochromocytoma. Within 1 month after a MI. Dissecting aortic aneurysm.
**Special Concerns:** Safe use during lactation not established. Use with caution and at reduced dosage in impaired renal function. Geriatric clients may be more sensitive to the hypotensive and hypothermic effects of minoxidil; also, it may be necessary to decrease the dose in these clients due to age-related decreases in renal function. BP controlled too rapidly may cause syncope, stroke, MI, and ischemia of affected organs. Experience with use in children is limited.
**Side Effects:** *CV:* Edema, ***pericardial effusion that may progress to tamponade*** (acute compression of heart caused by fluid or blood in pericardium), CHF, angina pectoris, changes in direction of T waves, increased HR. In children, rebound hypertension following slow withdrawal. *GI:* N&V. *CNS:* Headache, fatigue. *Hypersensitivity:* Rashes, including bullous eruptions and **Stevens-Johnson syndrome.** *Hematologic:* Initially, decrease in hematocrit, hemoglobin, and erythrocyte count but all return to normal. Rarely, thrombocytopenia and leukopenia. *Other:* Hypertrichosis (enhanced hair growth, pigmentation and thickening of fine body hair 3–6 weeks after initiation of therapy), breast tenderness, darkening of skin.
**Drug Interactions**
*CNS depressant drugs, especially those used in conscious sedation* / ↑ Hypotension
*Indomethacin* / ↓ Effects
*NSAIDS* / ↓ Effects
*Sympathomimetics* / ↓ Effects
**How Supplied:** *Tablet:* 2.5 mg, 10 mg

**Dosage**
• **Tablets**
  *Hypertension.*
**Adults and children over 12 years: Initial,** 5 mg/day. For optimum control, dose can be increased to 10, 20, and then 40 mg in single or divided doses/day. Daily dosage should not exceed 100 mg. **Children under 12 years: Initial,** 0.2 mg/kg/day. Effective dose range: 0.25–1.0 mg/kg/day. Dosage must be titrated to individual response. Daily dosage should not exceed 50 mg.

## DENTAL CONCERNS

See also *Dental Concerns* for *Antihypertensive Agents.*
**General**
1. Patients on chronic drug therapy may develop blood dyscrasias. Symptoms include fever, sore throat, and bleeding, and poor wound healing.
**Consultation with Primary Care Provider**
1. Patients with symptoms of blood dyscrasias should be referred to their primary care provider for complete blood counts. Treatment should be postponed until the results are known.

# Mirtazapine
(mir-**TAZ**-ah-peen)
**Pregnancy Category:** C
Remeron **(Rx)**
**Classification:** Noradrenergic and specific serotonergic antagonist

See also *Antidepressants, Tricyclic.*
**Action/Kinetics:** Enhances central noradrenergic and serotonergic activity, perhaps by antagonism at central presynaptic alpha-2 adrenergic inhibitory autoreceptors and heteroreceptors. Also a potent antagonist of 5-HT$_2$, 5-HT$_3$ and histamine H$_1$ receptors. Moderate antagonist of peripheral alpha-1 adrenergic receptors and muscarinic receptors. Rapidly and completely absorbed from the GI tract. **Peak plasma levels:** Within 2 hr. **t½:** 20–40 hr. Extensively metabolized in the liver and excreted in both the urine (75%) and feces (15%). Females exhibit significantly longer elimination half-lives than males.
**Uses:** Treatment of depression.
**Contraindications:** Use in combination with an MAO inhibitor or within 14 days of initiating or discontinuing therapy with an MAO inhibitor.
**Special Concerns:** Use with caution in those with impaired renal or hepatic disease, in geriatric clients, during lactation, in CV or cerebrovascular disease that can be exacerbated by hypotension (e.g., history of MI, angina, ischemic stroke), and in conditions that would predispose to hypotension (e.g., dehydration, hypovolemia, treatment with antihypertensive medications). The effect of mirtazapine for longer than 6 weeks has not been evaluated, although treatment is indicated for 6 months or longer. Safety and efficacy have not been determined in children.
**Side Effects:** Side effects with an incidence of 0.1% or greater are listed. *CNS:* Somnolence, dizziness, activation of mania or hypomania, suicidal ideation, sedation, drowsiness, abnormal dreams, abnormal thinking, tremor, confusion, hypesthesia, apathy, depression, hypokinesia, vertigo, twitching, agitation, anxiety, amnesia, hyperkinesia, paresthesia, ataxia, delirium, delusions, depersonalization, dyskinesia, extrapyramidal syndrome, increased libido, abnormal coordination, dysarthria, hallucinations, neurosis, dystonia, hostility, increased reflexes, emotional lability, euphoria, paranoid reaction. *Oral:* Dry mouth, glossitis, gum hemorrhage, stomatitis. *GI:* N&V, anorexia, constipation, ulcer, eructation, cholecystitis, colitis, abnormal liver function tests. *CV:* Hypertension, vasodilation, angina pectoris, *MI,* bradycardia, ventricular ex-

**M**

trasystoles, syncope, migraine, hypotension. *Hematologic:* Agranulocytosis. *Body as a whole:* Asthenia, flu syndrome, back pain, malaise, abdominal pain, acute abdominal syndrome, chills, fever, facial edema, photosensitivity reaction, neck rigidity, neck pain, enlarged abdomen. *Respiratory:* Dyspnea, increased cough, sinusitis, epistaxis, bronchitis, asthma, pneumonia. *GU:* Urinary frequency, UTI, kidney calculus, cystitis, dysuria, urinary incontinence, urinary retention, vaginitis, hematuria, breast pain, amenorrhea, dysmenorrhea, leukorrhea, impotence. *Musculoskeletal:* Myalgia, myasthenia, arthralgia, arthritis, tenosynovitis. *Dermatologic:* Pruritus, rash, acne, exfoliative dermatitis, dry skin, herpes simplex, alopecia. *Metabolic/nutritional:* Increased appetite, weight gain, peripheral edema, edema, thirst, dehydration, weight loss. *Ophthalmic:* Eye pain, abnormal accommodation, conjunctivitis, keratoconjunctivitis, lacrimation disorder, glaucoma. *Miscellaneous:* Deafness, hyperacusis, ear pain.

**Drug Interactions**
*Alcohol* / Additive impairment of motor skills
*Diazepam* / Additive impairment of motor skills

**How Supplied:** *Tablet:* 15 mg, 30 mg

### Dosage
• **Tablets**
*Treatment of depression.*
**Initial:** 15 mg/day given as a single dose, preferably in the evening before sleep. Those not responding to the 15-mg dose may respond to doses up to a maximum of 45 mg/day. Do not make dose changes at intervals of less than 1 to 2 weeks. Consider treatment for up to 6 months.

### DENTAL CONCERNS

See also *Dental Concerns* for *Antidepressants, Tricyclic.*
**General**
1. Risk of hypotensive episode if sedation or general anesthesia is necessary. Consult with the appropriate health care provider.

# Misoprostol
(my-soh-**PROST**-ohl)
**Pregnancy Category:** X
Cytotec **(Rx)**
**Classification:** Prostaglandin

**Action/Kinetics:** Synthetic prostaglandin $E_1$ analog that inhibits gastric acid secretion, protects the gastric mucosa by increasing bicarbonate and mucous production, and decreases pepsin levels during basal conditions. Rapidly converted to the active misoprostol acid. **Time for peak levels of misoprostol acid:** 12 min. **$t^{1/2}$, misoprostol acid:** 20–40 min. Misoprostol acid is less than 90% bound to plasma protein. *NOTE:* Misoprostol does not prevent development of duodenal ulcers in clients on NSAIDs.

**Uses:** Prevention of aspirin and other nonsteroidal anti-inflammatory-induced gastric ulcers in clients with a high risk of gastric ulcer complications (e.g., geriatric clients with debilitating disease) or in those with a history of ulcer. *Non-FDA Approved Uses:* Treat duodenal ulcers including those unresponsive to histamine $H_2$ antagonists. With cyclosporine and prednisone to decrease the incidence of acute graft rejection in renal transplant clients (the drug improves renal function).

**Contraindications:** Allergy to prostaglandins, pregnancy, during lactation (may cause diarrhea in nursing infants).

**Special Concerns:** Use with caution in clients with renal impairment and in clients older than 64 years of age. Safety and efficacy have not been established in children less than 18 years of age. Misoprostol may cause miscarriage with potentially serious bleeding.

**Side Effects:** *GI:* Diarrhea, abdominal pain, nausea, dyspepsia, flatulence, vomiting, constipation. *Gynecologic:* Spotting, cramps, dysmenorrhea, hypermenorrhea, menstrual disorders, postmenopausal vaginal bleeding. *Miscellaneous:* Headache.

**How Supplied:** *Tablet:* 100 mcg, 200 mcg

**Dosage**
• **Tablets**
**Adults:** 200 mcg q.i.d. with food. Dose can be reduced to 100 mcg if the larger dose cannot be tolerated. In renal impairment, the 200-mcg dose can be reduced if necessary.

## DENTAL CONCERNS
**General**
1. Avoid NSAIDs and aspirin-containing products in patients taking this drug with active peptic ulcer disease.
**Consultation with Primary Care Provider**
1. Consultation with the appropriate health care provider may be necessary in order to assess level of disease control.

## Montelukast sodium
(mon-teh-**LOO**-kast)
**Pregnancy Category:** B
Singulair **(Rx)**
**Classification:** Antiasthmatic

**Action/Kinetics:** Cysteinyl leukotrienes and leukotriene receptor occupation are associated with symptoms of asthma, including airway edema, smooth muscle contraction, and inflammation. Montelukast binds with cysteinyl leukotriene receptors thus preventing the action of cysteinyl leukotrienes. Rapidly absorbed after PO use. **Time to peak levels:** 3–4 hr for 10 mg tablet and 2–2.5 hr for 5 mg tablet. Metabolized in liver and mainly excreted in feces. **t½:** 2.7–5.5 hr.
**Uses:** Prophylaxis and chronic treatment of asthma in adults and children aged 6 years of age and older.
**Contraindications:** Use to reverse bronchospasm in acute asthma attacks, including status asthmaticus. Use to abruptly substitute for inhaled or oral corticosteroids. Use as monotherapy to treat and manage exercise-induced bronchospasm. Use with known aspirin or NSAID sensitivity.
**Special Concerns:** Use with caution during lactation. Safety and efficacy have not been determined for children less than 6 years of age.
**Side Effects:** *Adolescents and adults aged 15 and older. GI:* Dyspepsia, infectious gastroenteritis, abdominal pain, dental pain. *CNS:* Headache, dizziness. *Body as a whole:* Asthenia, fatigue, trauma. *Respiratory:* Influenza, cough, nasal congestion. *Dermatologic:* Rash. *Miscellaneous:* Pyuria.
*Children, aged 6 to 14 years. GI:* Nausea, diarrhea. *Respiratory:* Pharyngitis, laryngitis, otitis, sinusitis. *Miscellaneous:* Viral infection.
**How Supplied:** *Tablets:* 10 mg. *Chewable tablets:* 5 mg.

**Dosage**
• **Tablets**
*Asthma.*
**Adolescents and adults age 15 years and older:** 10 mg daily taken in evening.
• **Chewable tablets**
*Asthma.*
**Pediatric clients aged 6 to 14 years:** 5 mg chewable tablet daily taken in evening.

## DENTAL CONCERNS
See also *Dental Concerns* for *Theophylline Derivatives.*
**Client/Family Teaching**
1. Remember to provide your dental health professional with updated information regarding your breathing status and medications.

## Moricizine hydrochloride
(mor-**IS**-ih-zeen)
**Pregnancy Category:** B
Ethmozine **(Rx)**
**Classification:** Antiarrhythmic, class I

See also *Antiarrhythmic Drugs.*
**Action/Kinetics:** Causes a stabilizing effect on the myocardial membranes as well as local anesthetic activity.

Shortens phase II and III repolarization leading to a decreased duration of the action potential and an effective refractory period. Also, there is a decrease in the maximum rate of phase zero depolarization and a prolongation of AV conduction in clients with ventricular tachycardia. **Onset:** 2 hr. **Peak plasma levels:** 30–120 min. **t½:** 1.5–3.5 hr (reduced after multiple dosing). **Duration:** 10–24 hr. 95% is protein bound. Significant first-pass effect. Metabolized almost completely by the liver with metabolites excreted through both the urine and feces; the drug induces its own metabolism. Food delays the rate of absorption resulting in lower peak plasma levels; however, the total amount absorbed is not changed.

**Uses:** Documented life-threatening ventricular arrhythmias (e.g., sustained ventricular tachycardia) where benefits of the drug are determined to outweigh the risks. *Non-FDA Approved Uses:* Ventricular premature contractions, couplets, and nonsustained ventricular tachycardia.

**Contraindications:** Preexisting second- or third-degree block, right bundle branch block when associated with bifascicular block (unless the client has a pacemaker), cardiogenic shock. Use during lactation.

**Special Concerns:** There is the possibility of increased risk of death when used in clients with non-life-threatening cardiac arrhythmias. Safety and effectiveness in children less than 18 years of age have not been determined. Geriatric clients have a higher rate of side effects. Increased survival rates following use of antiarrhythmic drugs have not been proven in clients with ventricular arrhythmias. Use with caution in clients with sick sinus syndrome due to the possibility of sinus bradycardia, sinus pause, or sinus arrest. Use with caution in clients with CHF.

**Side Effects:** *CV: Proarrhythmias, including new rhythm disturbances or worsening of existing arrhythmias;* ECG abnormalities, including conduction defects, sinus pause, junctional rhythm, AV block; palpitations, *sustained ventricular tachycardia,* cardiac chest pain, CHF, *cardiac death,* hypotension, hypertension, atrial fibrillation, atrial flutter, syncope, bradycardia, *cardiac arrest, MI, pulmonary embolism,* vasodilation, thrombophlebitis, *cerebrovascular events. CNS:* Dizziness (common), anxiety, headache, fatigue, nervousness, paresthesias, sleep disorders, tremor, anxiety, hypoesthesias, depression, euphoria, somnolence, agitation, confusion, *seizures,* hallucinations, loss of memory, vertigo, coma. *Oral:* Dry mouth, bitter taste. *GI:* Nausea, abdominal pain, vomiting, diarrhea, dyspepsia, anorexia, ileus, flatulence, dysphagia. *Musculoskeletal:* Asthenia, abnormal gait, akathisia, ataxia, abnormal coordination, dyskinesia, pain. *GU:* Urinary retention, dysuria, urinary incontinence, urinary frequency, impotence, kidney pain, decreased libido. *Respiratory:* Dyspnea, apnea, asthma, hyperventilation, pharyngitis, cough, sinusitis. *Opthalmologic:* Nystagmus, diplopia, blurred vision, eye pain, periorbital edema. *Dermatologic:* Rash, pruritus, dry skin, urticaria. *Miscellaneous:* Sweating, drug fever, hypothermia, temperature intolerance, swelling of the lips and tongue, speech disorder, tinnitus, jaundice.

**Drug Interactions:** No specific interactions have been reported with drugs that are used in dentistry. However, lowest effective dose should be used, such as a local anesthetic, vasoconstrictor, or anticholinergic, if required.

**How Supplied:** *Tablet:* 200 mg, 250 mg, 300 mg

## Dosage

• **Tablets**

*Antiarrhythmic.*

**Adults:** 600–900 mg/day in equally divided doses q 8 hr. If needed, the dose can be increased in increments of 150 mg/day at 3-day intervals until the desired effect is obtained. In clients with hepatic or renal impairment, the initial dose should be 600 mg or less with close monitoring and dosage adjustment.

## DENTAL CONCERNS

See also *Dental Concerns* for *Antiarrhythmic Drugs*.

## Morphine hydrochloride
(**MOR**-feen)
Pregnancy Category: C
Morphitec-1, -5, -10, -20 ✿, M.O.S. ✿, M.O.S.-S.R. ✿ (Rx)

## Morphine sulfate
(**MOR**-feen **SUL**-fayt)
Pregnancy Category: C
Astramorph PF, Duramorph, Infumorph, Kadian, M-Eslon ✿, Morphine HP ✿, M.O.S.-Sulfate ✿, MS Contin, MS-IR, MSIR Capsules, Oramorph SR, RMS, RMS Rectal Suppositories, Roxanol, Roxanol 100, Roxanol Rescudose, Roxanol UD, Statex ✿ (C-II) (Rx)
Classification: Opioid analgesic, morphine type

See also *Opioid Analgesics*.
**Action/Kinetics:** Morphine is the prototype for opiate analgesics. **Onset:** approximately 15–60 min, based on epidural or intrathecal use. **Peak effect:** 30–60 min. **Duration:** 3–7 hr. **t½:** 1.5–2 hr. Oral morphine is only one-third to one-sixth as effective as parenteral products.
**Uses:** Intrathecally, epidurally, PO (including sustained-release products), or by continuous IV infusion for acute or chronic pain. In low doses, morphine is more effective against dull, continuous pain than against intermittent, sharp pain. Large doses, however, will dull almost any kind of pain. Preoperative medication. To facilitate induction of anesthesia and reduce dose of anesthetic. *Non-FDA Approved Uses:* Acute LV failure (for dyspneic seizures) and pulmonary edema. Morphine should not be used with papaverine for analgesia in biliary spasms but may be used with papaverine in acute vascular occlusions.

**Additional Contraindications:** Epidural or intrathecal morphine if infection is present at injection site, in clients on anticoagulant therapy, bleeding diathesis, if client has received parenteral corticosteroids within the past 2 weeks.
**Special Concerns:** May increase the length of labor. Clients with known seizure disorders may be at greater risk for morphine-induced seizure activity.
**How Supplied:** Morphine hydrochloride: *Syrup:* 1 mg/mL, 5 mg/mL, 10 mg/mL, 20 mg/mL; *Concentrate:* 20 mg/mL, 50 mg/mL; *Suppository:* 10 mg, 20 mg, 30 mg; *Tablets:* 10 mg, 20 mg, 40 mg, 60 mg; *Slow-release tablets:* 30 mg, 60 mg. Morphine sulfate: *Capsule:* 15 mg, 30 mg; *Capsule, extended release:* 20 mg, 50 mg, 100 mg; *Concentrate:* 20 mg/mL; *Injection:* 0.5 mg/mL, 1 mg/mL, 2 mg/mL, 4 mg/mL, 5 mg/mL, 8 mg/mL, 10 mg/mL, 15 mg/mL, 25 mg/mL, 50 mg/mL; *Solution:* 10 mg/5 mL, 20 mg/5 mL; *Suppository:* 5 mg, 10 mg, 20 mg, 30 mg; *Tablet:* 10 mg, 15 mg, 30 mg; *Tablet, extended release:* 15 mg, 30 mg, 60 mg, 100 mg, 200 mg

### Dosage

- **Capsules, Tablets, Oral Solution, Soluble Tablets, Syrup**
  *Analgesia.*
  10–30 mg q 4 hr.
- **Sustained-Release Tablets**
  *Analgesia.*
  30 mg q 8–12 hr, depending on client needs and response. Kadian is indicated for once-daily dosing at doses of 20, 50, or 100 mg where analgesia is indicated for just a few days.
- **IM, SC**
  *Analgesia.*
  **Adults:** 5–20 mg/70 kg q 4 hr as needed; **pediatric:** 100–200 mcg/kg up to a maximum of 15 mg.
- **IV Infusion**
  *Analgesia.*
  **Adults:** 2.5–15 mg/70 kg in 4–5 mL of water for injection (should be administered slowly over 4–5 min).

M

- **IV Infusion, Continuous**
  *Analgesia.*
  **Adults:** 0.1–1 mg/mL in D5W by a controlled-infusion pump.
- **Rectal Suppositories**
  **Adults:** 10–20 mg q 4 hr.
- **Intrathecal**
  **Adults:** 0.2–1 mg as a single daily injection.
- **Epidural**

**Initial:** 5 mg/day in the lumbar region; if analgesia is not manifested in 1 hr, increasing doses of 1–2 mg can be given, not to exceed 10 mg/day. For continuous infusion, 2–4 mg/day with additional doses of 1–2 mg if analgesia is not satisfactory.

## DENTAL CONCERNS

See also *Dental Concerns* for *Opioid Analgesics.*

# Nabumetone
(nah-**BYOU**-meh-tohn)
**Pregnancy Category:** B
Relafen **(Rx)**
**Classification:** Nonsteroidal anti-inflammatory agent

See also *Nonsteroidal Anti-Inflammatory Drugs.*
**Action/Kinetics: Time to peak plasma levels:** 2.5–4 hr. **t½ of active metabolite:** 22.5–30 hr.
**Uses:** Acute and chronic treatment of osteoarthritis and rheumatoid arthritis. Has also been used to treat mild to moderate pain including postextraction dental pain, postsurgical episiotomy pain, and soft tissue athletic injuries.
**Contraindications:** Lactation.
**Special Concerns:** Safety and efficacy have not been determined in children.
**How Supplied:** *Tablet:* 500 mg, 750 mg

### Dosage
- **Tablets**
  *Osteoarthritis, rheumatoid arthritis.*
  **Adults, initial:** 1,000 mg as a single dose; **maintenance:** 1,500–2,000 mg/day. Doses greater than 2,000 mg/day have not been studied.

## DENTAL CONCERNS

See also *Dental Concerns* for *Nonsteroidal Anti-Inflammatory Drugs.*

# Nadolol
(**NAY**-doh-lohl)
**Pregnancy Category:** C
Alti-Nadolol ✢, Apo-Nadol ✢, Corgard, Novo-Nadolol ✢ **(Rx)**
**Classification:** Beta-adrenergic blocking agent

See also *Beta-Adrenergic Blocking Agents.*
**Action/Kinetics:** Manifests both beta-1- and beta-2-adrenergic blocking activity. Has no membrane stabilizing or intrinsic sympathomimetic activity. Low lipid solubility. **Peak serum concentration:** 3–4 hr. **t½:** 20–24 hr (permits once-daily dosage). **Duration:** 17–24 hr. Absorption variable, averaging 30%; steady plasma level achieved after 6–9 days of administration. Excreted unchanged by the kidney.
**Uses:** Hypertension, either alone or with other drugs (e.g., thiazide diuretic). Angina pectoris. *Non-FDA Approved Uses:* Prophylaxis of migraine, ventricular arrhythmias, aggressive behavior, essential tremor, tremors associated with lithium or parkinsonism, antipsychotic-induced akathisia, rebleeding of esophageal varices, situational anxiety, reduce intraocular pressure.
**Contraindications:** Hypersensitivity to nadolol, cardiogenic shock, 2nd or 3rd degree heart block, sinus bradycardia, CHF, cardiac failure. Bronchial asthma or bronchospasm, including severe COPD.

**Special Concerns:** Diabetes mellitus, hyperthyroidism, lactation, myasthenia gravis, peripheral vascular disease, renal disease.
**Side Effects:** *Oral:* Dry mouth, taste disturbances. *CV:* AV block, bradycardia, **CHF,** hypotension, palpitations. *CNS:* Depression, dizziness, drowsiness, fatigue, hallucinations, headache, lethargy, paresthesias. *GI:* Colitis, constipation, cramps, diarrhea, flatulence, hepatomegaly, nausea, vomiting. *Hematologic:* **Agranulocytosis, thrombocytopenia.** *Allergic:* fever, sore throat, respiratory distress, rash, pharyngitis, **laryngospasm, anaphylaxis.** *Skin:* pruritus, rash, fever. *Ophthalmic:* Dry, burning eyes. *GU:* Dysuria, impotence, nocturia. *Other:* Hypoglycemia or hyperglycemia. *Respiratory:* **Bronchospasm,** cough, dyspnea, **laryngospasm,** nasal stuffiness, pharyngitis, respiratory dysfunction, wheezing.
**Drug Interactions:** See also *Drug Interactions* for *Beta-Adrenergic Blocking Agents* and *Antihypertensive Agents.*
**How Supplied:** *Tablet:* 20 mg, 40 mg, 80 mg, 120 mg, 160 mg

**Dosage** ————————————
• **Tablets**
*Hypertension.*
**Initial:** 40 mg/day; **then,** may be increased in 40- to 80-mg increments until optimum response obtained.
**Maintenance:** 40–80 mg/day although up to 240–320 mg/day may be needed.
*Angina.*
**Initial:** 40 mg/day; **then,** increase dose in 40- to 80-mg increments q 3–7 days until optimum response obtained. **Maintenance:** 40–80 mg/day, although up to 160–240 mg/day may be needed.
*Aggressive behavior.*
40–160 mg/day.
*Antipsychotic-induced akathisia.*
40–80 mg/day.
*Essential tremor.*
120–240 mg/day.
*Lithium-induced tremors.*
20–40 mg/day.
*Tremors associated with parkinsonism.*
80–320 mg/day.
*Prophylaxis of migraine.*
40–80 mg/day.
*Rebleeding from esophageal varices.*
40–160 mg/day.
*Situational anxiety.*
20 mg.
*Ventricular arrhythmias.*
10–640 mg/day.
*Reduction of intraocular pressure.*
10–20 mg b.i.d.
*NOTE:* Dosage for all uses should be decreased in clients with renal failure.

## DENTAL CONCERNS

See also *Dental Concerns* for *Beta-Adrenergic Blocking Agents* and *Antihypertensive Agents.*
**Client/Family Teaching**
1. Review the importance of good oral hygiene in order to prevent soft tissue inflammation.
2. Review the proper use of oral hygiene aids in order to prevent injury.
3. Daily home fluoride treatments for persistent dry mouth.
4. Avoid mouth rinses with alcohol because alcohol can exacerbate dry mouth.
5. Dry mouth can be treated with tart, sugarless gum or candy, water, or with saliva substitutes if dry mouth persists.

# Naloxone hydrochloride
(nal-**OX**-ohn)
**Pregnancy Category:** B
Narcan **(Rx)**
**Classification:** Opioid antagonist

See also *Opioid Antagonists.*
**Action/Kinetics:** Combines competitively with opiate receptors and blocks or reverses the action of narcotic analgesics. Since the duration of action of naloxone is shorter than that of the narcotic analgesics, the respiratory depression may return

---

when the narcotic antagonist has worn off. **Onset: IV,** 2 min; **SC, IM: <5 min. Time to peak effect: 5–15 min. Duration:** Dependent on dose and route of administration but may be as short as 45 min. **t½:** 60–100 min. Metabolized in the liver to inactive products; eliminated through the kidneys.

**Uses:** Respiratory depression induced by natural and synthetic narcotics, including butorphanol, methadone, nalbuphine, pentazocine, and propoxyphene. Drug of choice when nature of depressant drug is not known. Diagnosis of acute opiate overdosage. Not effective when respiratory depression is induced by hypnotics, sedatives, or anesthetics and other nonopioid CNS depressants. Adjunct to increase BP in septic shock. *Non-FDA Approved Uses:* Treatment of Alzheimer's dementia, alcoholic coma, and schizophrenia.

**Contraindications:** Sensitivity to drug. Opioid addicts (drug may cause severe withdrawal symptoms). Not recommended for use in neonates.

**Special Concerns:** Safe use during lactation and in children is not established.

**Side Effects:** N&V, sweating, hypertension, tremors, sweating due to reversal of opioid depression. If used postoperatively, excessive doses may cause *ventricular tachycardia and fibrillation,* hypo- or hypertension, pulmonary edema, and *seizures (infrequent).*

**Drug Interactions:** No drug interactions of concern to dental health have been reported.

**How Supplied:** *Injection:* 0.02 mg/mL, 0.4 mg/mL, 1 mg/mL

**Dosage** ————————
• **IV, IM, SC**
  *Narcotic overdose.*
**Initial:** 0.4–2 mg IV; if necessary, additional IV doses may be repeated at 2- to 3-min intervals. If no response after 10 mg, reevaluate diagnosis. **Pediatric, initial:** 0.01 mg/kg IV; **then,** 0.1 mg/kg IV, if needed. The

SC or IM route may be used if an IV route is not available.

*To reverse postoperative narcotic depression.*

**Adults: IV, initial,** 0.1- to 0.2-mg increments at 2- to 3-min intervals; **then,** repeat at 1- to 2-hr intervals if necessary. Supplemental IM dosage increases the duration of reversal. **Children: Initial,** 0.005–0.01 mg IV at 2- to 3-min intervals until desired response is obtained.

*Reverse narcotic-induced depression in neonates.*

**Initial:** 0.01 mg/kg IV, IM, or SC. May be repeated using adult administration guidelines.

## DENTAL CONCERNS

See also *Dental Concerns* for *Opioid Antagonists.*

# Naltrexone
(nal-**TREX**-ohn)
**Pregnancy Category:** C
ReVia **(Rx)**
**Classification:** Opioid antagonist

See also *Opioid Antagonists.*

**Action/Kinetics:** Competitively binds to opiate receptors, thereby reversing or preventing the effects of narcotics. **Peak plasma levels:** 1 hr. **Duration:** 24–72 hr. Metabolized in the liver; a major metabolite—6-beta-naltrexol—is active. **Peak serum levels, after 50 mg: naltrexone,** 8.6 ng/mL; **6-beta-naltrexol,** 99.3 ng/mL. **t½: naltrexone,** approximately 4 hr; **6-beta-naltrexol,** 13 hr. Naltrexone and its metabolites are excreted in the urine.

**Uses:** To prevent opioid use in former narcotic addicts. Adjunct to the psychosocial treatment for alcoholism. *Non-FDA Approved Uses:* To treat eating disorders and postconcussional syndrome not responding to other approaches.

**Contraindications:** Clients taking opioid analgesics, those dependent on opioids, those in acute withdrawal from opioids. Liver failure, acute hepatitis.

**Special Concerns:** Use with caution during lactation. Safety during lactation and in children under 18 years of age has not been established.

**Side Effects:** *CNS:* Headache, anxiety, nervousness, sleep disorders, dizziness, change in energy level, depression, confusion, restlessness, disorientation, hallucinations, nightmares, bad dreams, paranoia, fatigue, drowsiness. *Oral:* Xerostomia. *GI:* N&V, diarrhea, constipation, anorexia, abdominal pain or cramps, flatulence, ulcers, increased appetite, weight gain or loss, increased thirst, hemorrhoids. *CV:* Phlebitis, edema, increased BP, changes in ECG, palpitations, epistaxis, tachycardia. *GU:* Delayed ejaculation, increased urinary frequency or urinary discomfort, increased or decreased interest in sex. *Respiratory:* Cough, sore throat, nasal congestion, rhinorrhea, sneezing, excess secretions, hoarseness, SOB, heaving breathing, sinus trouble. *Dermatologic:* Rash, oily skin, itching, pruritus, acne, cold sores, alopecia, athlete's foot. *Musculoskeletal:* Joint/muscle pain, muscle twitches, tremors, pain in legs, knees, or shoulders. *Ophthalmologic:* Blurred vision, aching or strained eyes, burning eyes, light-sensitive eyes, swollen eyes. *Other:* Hepatotoxicity, tinnitus, painful or clogged ears, chills, swollen glands, inguinal pain, cold feet, "hot" spells, "pounding" head, fever, yawning, side pains.

A severe narcotic withdrawal syndrome may be precipitated if naltrexone is administered to a dependent individual. The syndrome may begin within 5 min and may last for up to 2 days.

**How Supplied:** *Tablet:* 50 mg

**Dosage** ————————
• **Tablets**
    *To produce blockade of opiate actions.*

**Initial:** 25 mg followed by an additional 25 mg in 1 hr if no withdrawal symptoms occur. **Maintenance:** 50 mg/day.

*Alternate dosing schedule for blockade of opiate actions.*
The weekly dose of 350 mg may be given as: (a) 50 mg/day on weekdays and 100 mg on Saturday; (b) 100 mg/48 hr; (c) 100 mg every Monday and Wednesday and 150 mg on Friday; or, (d) 150 mg q 72 hr.
    *Alcoholism.*
50 mg once daily for up to 12 weeks. Treatment for longer than 12 weeks has not been studied.

## DENTAL CONCERNS

See also *Dental Concerns* for *Opioid Antagonists.*

# Naproxen
(nah-**PROX**-en)
**Pregnancy Category:** B
Apo-Naproxen ✿, EC-Naprosyn, Naprosyn, Napron X, Naxen ✿, Novo–Naprox ✿, Nu-Naprox ✿, PMS-Naproxen ✿ **(Rx)**

# Naproxen sodium
(nah-**PROX**-en)
**Pregnancy Category:** B
Anaprox, Anaprox DS, Apo-Napro-Na ✿, Apo-Napro-Na DS ✿, Naprelan, Novo–Naprox Sodium ✿, Novo-Naprox Sodium DS ✿, Synflex ✿, Synflex DS ✿ **(Rx)**, Aleve **(OTC)**
**Classification:** Nonsteroidal, anti-inflammatory analgesic

See also *Nonsteroidal Anti-Inflammatory Drugs.*
**Action/Kinetics: Peak serum levels of naproxen:** 2–4 hr; **for sodium salt:** 1–2 hr. **t½ for naproxen:** 12–15 hr; **for sodium salt:** 12–13 hr. **Onset, immediate release for analgesia:** 1–2 hr. **Duration, analgesia:** Approximately 7 hr. **Onset, 24 hr (both immediate and delayed release):** 30 min; **duration:** 24 hr. The onset of anti-inflammatory effects may take up to 2 weeks and may last 2–4 weeks. More than 90% bound to plasma protein. Food delays

**N**

the rate but not the amount of drug absorbed.

**Uses: Rx.** Mild to moderate pain. Musculoskeletal and soft tissue inflammation including rheumatoid arthritis, osteoarthritis, bursitis, tendinitis, ankylosing spondylitis. Primary dysmenorrhea, acute gout. Juvenile rheumatoid arthritis (naproxen only). *NOTE:* The delayed-release or enteric-coated products are not recommended for initial treatment of pain because, compared to other naproxen products, absorption is delayed. *Non-FDA Approved Uses:* Antipyretic in cancer clients, sunburn, acute migraine (sodium salt only), prophylaxis of migraine, migraine due to menses, PMS (sodium salt only). **OTC.** Relief of minor aches and pains due to the common cold, headache, toothache, muscular aches, backache, minor arthritis pain, pain due to menstrual cramps. Decrease fever.

**Contraindications:** Use of naproxen and naproxen sodium simultaneously. Lactation. Use of delayed-release product for initial treatment of acute pain.

**Special Concerns:** Safety and effectiveness of naproxen have not been determined in children less than 2 years of age; the safety and effectiveness of naproxen sodium have not been established in children. Geriatric clients may manifest increased total plasma levels of naproxen.

**Drug Interactions**
*Methotrexate* / Possibility of a fatal interaction
*Probenecid* / ↓ Plasma clearance of naproxen

**How Supplied:** Naproxen: *Enteric coated tablet:* 375 mg, 500 mg; *Suspension:* 25 mg/mL; *Tablet:* 250 mg, 375 mg, 500 mg. Naproxen sodium: *Tablet:* 220 mg, 275 mg, 550 mg; *Tablet, extended release:* 375 mg, 500 mg

**Dosage** ─────────────

NAPROXEN
• **Oral Suspension, Tablets**
*Rheumatoid arthritis, osteoarthritis, ankylosing spondylitis, pain, dys-menorrhea, acute tendinitis, bursitis.*

**Adults, individualized, usual:** 250–500 mg b.i.d. May increase to 1.5 g for short periods of time. Improvement should be observed within 2 weeks; if no improvement is seen, an additional 2-week course of therapy should be considered.
*Acute gout.*

**Adults, initial:** 750 mg; **then,** 250 mg naproxen q 8 hr until symptoms subside.
*Juvenile rheumatoid arthritis.*
Naproxen only, 10 mg/kg/day in two divided doses. If the suspension is used, the following dosage can be used: **13 kg:** 2.5 mL b.i.d.; **25 kg:** 5 mL b.i.d.; **38 kg:** 7.5 mL b.i.d.

• **Delayed Release Tablets**
*Rheumatoid arthritis, osteoarthritis, ankylosing spondylitis, pain, dys-menorrhea, acute tendinitis, bursitis.*
375–500 mg b.i.d.

NAPROXEN SODIUM
• **Tablets (Rx)**
*Rheumatoid arthritis, osteoarthritis, ankylosing spondylitis, pain, dys-menorrhea, acute tendinitis, bursitis.*

**Adults:** 275–550 mg b.i.d. in the morning and evening. May be increased to 1.65 g for short periods of time.
*Acute gout.*

**Adults, initial:** 825 mg; **then,** 275 mg q 8 hr until symptoms subside.
*Mild to moderate pain, primary dysmenorrhea, acute bursitis and tendinitis.*

**Adults, initial:** 550 mg; **then,** 275 mg q 6–8 hr as needed. Total daily dose should not exceed 1,375 mg.

• **Controlled Release Tablets**
*Rheumatoid arthritis, osteoarthritis, ankylosing spondylitis, pain, dys-menorrhea, acute tendinitis, bursitis.*

**Adults:** 750 mg or 1,000 mg once daily, not to exceed 1,000 mg/day.
*Acute gout.*

**Adults:** 1,000 mg once daily. For short periods of time, 1,500 mg may be given.

- **Tablets (OTC)**
**Adults:** 200 mg q 8–12 hr with a full glass of liquid. For some clients, 400 mg initially followed by 200 mg 12 hr later will provide better relief. Dose should not exceed 600 mg in a 24-hr period. Geriatric clients should not take more than 200 mg q 12 hr. Not for use in children less than 12 years of age unless directed by a physician.

## DENTAL CONCERNS

See also *Dental Concerns* for *Nonsteroidal Anti-Inflammatory Drugs.*

# Nedocromil sodium
(neh-**DAH**-kroh-mill)
**Pregnancy Category:** B
Tilade **(Rx)**
**Classification:** Antiasthmatic

**Action/Kinetics:** Inhibits the release of various mediators, such as histamine, leukotriene $C_4$, and prostaglandin $D_2$, from a variety of cell types associated with asthma. Has no intrinsic bronchodilator, antihistamine, or glucocorticoid activity; also, systemic bioavailability is low. **t½:** 3.3 hr. About 89% bound to plasma protein; excreted unchanged.

**Uses:** Maintenance therapy in adults and children (age six and older) with mild to moderate bronchial asthma.

**Contraindications:** Use for the reversal of acute bronchospasms, especially status asthmaticus.

**Special Concerns:** Use with caution during lactation. Safety and efficacy have not been established in children less than 12 years of age. Nedocromil has not been shown to be able to substitute for the total dose of corticosteroids.

**Side Effects:** *Respiratory:* Coughing, pharyngitis, rhinitis, upper respiratory tract infection, increased sputum, bronchitis, dyspnea, ***bronchospasm.*** *Oral:* Dry mouth, unpleasant taste. *GI tract:* N&V, dyspepsia, abdominal pain, diarrhea. *CNS:* Dizziness, dysphonia. *Skin:* Rash, sensation of warmth. *Body as a whole:* Headache, chest pain, fatigue, arthritis. *Miscellaneous:* Viral infection.

**How Supplied:** *Metered dose inhaler:* 1.75 mg/inh

## Dosage
- **Metered Dose Inhaler**
  *Bronchial asthma.*
**Adults and children over 12 years of age:** Two inhalations q.i.d. at regular intervals in order to provide 14 mg/day. If the client is under good control on q.i.d. dosing (i.e., requiring inhaled or oral beta agonist no more than twice a week or no worsening of symptoms occur with respiratory infections), a lower dose can be tried. In such instances, the dose should first be reduced to 10.5 mg/day (i.e., used t.i.d.); then, after several weeks with good control, the dose can be reduced to 7 mg/day (i.e., used b.i.d.).

## DENTAL CONCERNS
**General**
1. The patient may require a semisupine position for the dental chair to help with breathing.
2. Dental procedures may cause the patient anxiety which could result in an asthma attack. Make sure that the patient has his/her sympathomimetic inhaler present or have the inhaler from the office emergency kit present.
3. Morning and shorter appointments as well as methods for addressing anxiety levels in the patient can help to reduce the amount of stress that the patient is experiencing.
4. Sulfites present in vasoconstrictors can precipitate an asthma attack.
5. Decreased saliva flow can put the patient at risk for dental caries, periodontal disease, and candidiasis.
**Consultation with Primary Care Provider**
1. Consultation may be necessary in order to evaluate the patient's level of disease control.

**N**

---

***bold italic*** = life-threatening side effect

2. Consultation may be necessary in order to determine the patient's ability to tolerate stress.

**Client/Family Teaching**

1. Daily home fluoride treatments for persistent dry mouth.

2. Avoid alcohol-containing mouth rinses.

3. Dry mouth can be treated with tart, sugarless gum or candy, water, or with saliva substitutes if dry mouth persists. Review technique for use and care of prescribed inhalers and respiratory equipment. Rinsing of equipment and of mouth after use is imperative in preventing oral fungal infections.

# Nefazodone hydrochloride
(nih-**FAY**-zoh-dohn)
**Pregnancy Category:** C
Serzone **(Rx)**
**Classification:** Antidepressant

**Action/Kinetics:** Exact antidepressant mechanism not known. Inhibits neuronal uptake of serotonin and norepinephrine and antagonizes central 5-HT$_2$ receptors and alpha-1-adrenergic receptors (which may cause postural hypotension). Produces none to slight anticholinergic effects, moderate sedation, and slight orthostatic hypotension. **Peak plasma levels:** 1 hr. t½: 2–4 hr. **Time to reach steady state:** 4–5 days. Extensively metabolized by the liver with less than 1% excreted unchanged in the urine. Food delays the absorption of nefazodone and decreases the bioavailability by approximately 20%.

**Uses:** Treatment of depression.

**Contraindications:** Use with terfenadine or astemizole; in combination with an MAO inhibitor or within 14 days of discontinuing MAO inhibitor therapy. Clients hypersensitive to nefazodone or other phenylpiperazine antidepressants.

**Special Concerns:** Use with caution in clients with a recent history of MI, unstable heart disease and taking digoxin, or a history of mania. Use with caution during lactation. Safety and efficacy have not been determined in individuals below 18 years of age. There is a possibility of a suicide attempt in depression that may persist until significant remission occurs.

**Side Effects:** *CNS:* Dizziness, insomnia, agitation, somnolence, lightheadedness, activation of mania or hypomania, confusion, memory impairment, paresthesia, abnormal dreams, decreased concentration, ataxia, incoordination, psychomotor retardation, tremor, hypertonia, decreased libido, vertigo, twitching, depersonalization, hallucinations, *suicide thoughts/attempt,* apathy, euphoria, hostility, abnormal gait, abnormal thinking, derealization, paranoid reaction, dysarthria, myoclonus, *neuroleptic malignant syndrome (rare).* *CV:* Postural hypotension, hypotension, sinus bradycardia, tachycardia, hypertension, syncope, ventricular extrasystoles, angina pectoris, *CVA (rare).* *Oral:* Dry mouth, periodontal abscess, gingivitis, mouth ulceration, stomatitis. *GI:* Nausea, constipation, dyspepsia, diarrhea, increased appetite, vomiting, eructation, colitis, gastritis, esophagitis, peptic ulcer, rectal hemorrhage. *Dermatologic:* Pruritus, dry skin, acne, alopecia, urticaria, maculopapular rash, vesiculobullous rash, eczema. *Musculoskeletal:* Asthenia, arthralgia, arthritis, tenosynovitis, muscle stiffness, bursitis. *Respiratory:* Pharyngitis, increased cough, dyspnea, bronchitis, asthma, pneumonia, laryngitis, voice alteration, epistaxis, hiccups. *Hematologic:* Ecchymosis, anemia, leukopenia, lymphadenopathy. *Ophthalmologic:* Blurred vision, abnormal vision, visual field defect, dry eye, eye pain, abnormal accommodation, diplopia, conjunctivitis, mydriasis, keratoconjunctivitis, photophobia, night blindness. *Body as a whole:* Headache, infection, flu syndrome, chills, fever, neck rigidity, allergic reaction, malaise, photosensitivity, facial edema, hangover effect, enlarged abdomen, hernia, pelvic pain, halitosis, cellulitis, weight loss, gout, dehydration. *GU:*

Urinary frequency, UTI, urinary retention, vaginitis, breast pain, cystitis, urinary urgency, metrorrhagia, amenorrhea, polyuria, vaginal hemorrhage, breast enlargement, menorrhagia, urinary incontinence, abnormal ejaculation, hematuria, nocturia, kidney calculus. *Miscellaneous:* Peripheral edema, thirst, abnormal LFTs, ear pain, hyperacusis, deafness, taste loss.

**Drug Interactions**

*Alprazolam* / ↑ Plasma levels of alprazolam

*Astemizole* / ↑ Plasma levels of astemizole resulting in QT prolongation and possible serious CV events, including death due to ventricular tachycardia of the torsades de pointes type

*MAO inhibitors* / Serious and possibly fatal reactions including symptoms of hyperthermia, rigidity, myoclonus, autonomic instability with possible rigid fluctuations of VS, and mental status changes that may include extreme agitation progressing to delirium and coma

*Terfenadine* / ↑ Plasma levels of terfenadine resulting in QT prolongation and possible serious CV events, including death due to ventricular tachycardia of the torsades de pointes type

*Triazolam* / ↑ Plasma levels of triazolam

**How Supplied:** *Tablet:* 100 mg, 150 mg, 200 mg, 250 mg

**Dosage** ——————————

• **Tablets**

*Antidepressant.*

**Adults, initial:** 200 mg/day given in two divided doses. Increase dose in increments of 100–200 mg/day at intervals of no less than 1 week. The effective dose range is 300–600 mg/day. The initial dose for elderly or debilitated clients is 100 mg/day given in two divided doses.

**DENTAL CONCERNS**

See also *Dental Concerns* for *Antidepressants, Tricyclic.*

1. There is no information available regarding the use of this drug with vasoconstrictors.

# Nelfinavir mesylate

(nel-**FIN**-ah-veer)
**Pregnancy Category:** B
Viracept **(Rx)**
**Classification:** Antiviral, protease inhibitor

See also *Antiviral Drugs.*

**Action/Kinetics:** HIV-1 protease inhibitor which results in the production of immature, non-infectious viruses. Activity is increased when used with didanosine, lamivudine, stavudine, zalcitabine, or zidovudine. **Peak plasma levels:** 2–4 hr. **Steady-state plasma levels:** 3–4 mcg/mL. Food increases plasma levels 2–3 fold. **t½, terminal:** 3.5–5 hr. Metabolites (one of which is as active as parent compound) and unchanged drug excreted mainly in feces.

**Uses:** Treat HIV infection when antiretroviral therapy is required.

**Contraindications:** Administration with astemizole, cisapride, midazolam, rifampin, terfenadine, or triazolam. Hypersensitivity.

**Special Concerns:** Use with caution with hepatic impairment. Safety and efficacy have not been determined in children less than 2 years of age.

**Side Effects:** Side effects were determined when used in combination with other antiviral drugs. *Oral:* Mouth ulcers. *GI:* N&V, diarrhea, flatulence, abdominal pain, anorexia, dyspepsia, epigastric pain, GI bleeding, hepatitis, pancreatitis. *CNS:* Anxiety, depression, dizziness, emotional lability, hyperkinesia, insomnia, migraine, paresthesia, *seizures,* sleep disorder, somnolence, *suicide ideation.* *Hematologic:* Anemia, leukopenia, thrombocytopenia. *Respiratory:* Dyspnea, rhinitis, sinusitis, pharyngitis. *GU:* Kidney calculus, sexual dysfunction, urine abnormality. *Ophthalmic:* Eye disorder, acute ir-

**N**

itis. *Musculoskeletal:* Arthralgia, arthritis, cramps, myalgia, myasthenia, myopathy. *Dermatologic:* Dermatitis, folliculitis, fungal dermatitis, maculopapular rash, pruritus, urticaria, sweating. *Miscellaneous:* Asthenia, dehydration, allergic reaction, back pain, fever, headache, malaise, pain, accidental injury.

**Drug Interactions**

*Anticonvulsants* / Possible ↓ plasma levels of nelfinavir

*Astemizole* / Potential for serious and life-threatening cardiac arrhythmias

*Terfenadine* / Potential for serious and life-threatening cardiac arrhythmias

**Dosage**

• **Powder, Tablets**

*HIV.*

**Adults:** 750 mg (i.e., 3 250-mg tablets) t.i.d. in combination with nucleoside analogs. **Children, 2 to 13 years:** 20-30 mg/kg/dose t.i.d.

## DENTAL CONCERNS

See also *General Dental Concerns* for *All Anti-Infectives* and *Antiviral Drugs.*

**General**

1. Examine patients for oral signs and symptoms of opportunistic infection.
2. Patients on chronic drug therapy may develop blood dyscrasias. Symptoms include fever, sore throat, and bleeding, and poor wound healing.
3. Palliative therapy may be required for patients with oral adverse effects.

**Consultation with Primary Care Provider**

1. Patients with symptoms of blood dyscrasias should be referred to their primary care provider for complete blood counts. Treatment should be postponed until the results are known.
2. Medical consultation may be necessary in order to assess patient's level of disease control.

**Client/Family Teaching**

1. Review the importance of good oral hygiene in order to prevent soft tissue inflammation.
2. Review the proper use of oral hygiene aids in order to prevent injury.
3. Report oral sores, lesions, or bleeding to the dentist.
4. Update patient's dental record (medication/health history) as needed.

# Nevirapine

(neh-**VYE**-rah-peen)

**Pregnancy Category:** C

Viramune **(Rx)**

**Classification:** Antiviral

See also *Antiviral Drugs.*

**Action/Kinetics:** By binding tightly to reverse transcriptase, nevirapine prevents viral RNA from being converted into DNA. In combination with a nucleoside analogue, it reduces the amount of virus circulating in the body and increases CD4+ cell counts. Readily absorbed, with peak plasma levels occurring 4 hr after a 200-mg dose. Extensively metabolized in the liver. Excreted through both the urine (about 90%) and the feces (about 10%). Induces its own metabolism such that following chronic use the half-life decreases from about 45 hr following a single dose to 25 to 30 hr following multiple dosing with 200 or 400 mg daily.

**Uses:** In combination with nucleoside analogues (e.g., AZT, lamivudine, didanosine, zalcitabine) for the treatment of HIV-1 infections in adults who have experienced clinical and immunologic deterioration. Always use in combination with at least one other antiretroviral agent, as resistant viruses emerge rapidly when nevirapine is used alone. The use of nevirapine with protease inhibitors (e.g., saquinavir, indinavir, ritonavir) is not recommended.

**Contraindications:** Lactation.

**Special Concerns:** The duration of benefit from therapy may be limited. Nevirapine is not a cure for HIV infections; clients may continue to experience illnesses associated with HIV infections, including opportunistic infections. Nevirapine has not been shown to reduce the risk of transmitting HIV to others through sexual contact or blood contamination. Use with caution in impaired renal or hepatic function. Safety and efficacy have not been determined in children.

**Side Effects:** *Oral:* Ulcerative stomatits. *GI:* Nausea, abnormal LFTs, diarrhea, abdominal pain, hepatitis. *CNS:* Headache, fatigue, paresthesia. *Hematologic:* Decreased hemoglobin, decreased platelets, decreased neutrophils. *Miscellaneous:* ***Rash (may be severe and life-threatening),*** fever, peripheral neuropathy, myalgia.

**Drug Interactions:** None reported that may have potential dental concerns. However, nevirapine can induce cytochrome P450 enzymes.

**How Supplied:** *Tablet:* 200 mg

**Dosage**
• **Tablets**
    *HIV-1 infections.*
**Initial:** 200 mg/day for 14 days.
**Maintenance:** 200 mg b.i.d. (e.g., 7:00 a.m. and 7:00 p.m.) in combination with a nucleoside analogue antiretroviral agent.

## DENTAL CONCERNS

See also *Dental Concerns* for *Antiviral Drugs* and *Anti-Infectives.*
**General**
1. Examine patient for oral signs and symptoms of opportunistic infection.
**Consultation with Primary Care Provider**
1. Medical consultation may be necessary in order to assess patient's level of disease control.
**Client/Family Teaching**
1. Review the importance of good oral hygiene in order to prevent soft tissue inflammation.
2. Review the proper use of oral hygiene aids in order to prevent injury.
3. Secondary oral infection may occur. Seek dental treatment immediately if this happens.

# Niacin (Nicotinic acid)
(NYE-ah-sin, nih-koh-**TIN**-ick **AH**-sid)
**Pregnancy Category:** C
Nia-Bid, Niaspan, Nico-400, Nicobid, Nicolar, Nicotinex, Slo-Niacin, Span-Niacin, Tega-Span (Rx and OTC)

# Niacinamide
(nye-ah-**SIN**-ah-myd)
**Pregnancy Category:** C
Papulex ✦ (Rx: Injection; OTC: Tablets)
**Classification:** Vitamin B complex

**Action/Kinetics:** Niacin (nicotinic acid) and niacinamide are water-soluble, heat-resistant vitamins prepared synthetically. Niacin (after conversion to the active niacinamide) is a component of the coenzymes nicotinamide-adenine dinucleotide and nicotinamide-adenine dinucleotide phosphate, which are essential for oxidation-reduction reactions involved in lipid metabolism, glycogenolysis, and tissue respiration. Deficiency of niacin results in pellagra, the most common symptoms of which are dermatitis, diarrhea, and dementia. In high doses niacin also produces vasodilation. Reduces serum cholesterol and triglycerides in types II, III, IV, and V hyperlipoproteinemia (mechanism unknown). **Peak serum levels:** 45 min; **t½:** 45 min.

**Uses:** Prophylaxis and treatment of pellagra; niacin deficiency. Treat hyperlipidemia in clients not responding to either diet or weight loss. Reduce the risk of recurrent nonfatal MI and promote regression of atherosclerosis when combined with bile-binding resins.

**Contraindications:** Severe hypotension, hemorrhage, arterial bleeding, liver dysfunction, peptic ulcer. Use of the extended-release tablets and capsules in children.

**Special Concerns:** Extended-release niacin may be hepatotoxic. Use with caution in diabetics, gall bladder disease, and clients with gout.

**N**

---

**Side Effects:** *GI:* N&V, diarrhea, peptic ulcer activation, abdominal pain. *Dermatologic:* Flushing, warm feeling, skin rash, pruritus, dry skin, itching and tingling feeling, keratosis nigricans. *Other:* Hypotension, headache, macular cystoid edema, amblyopia. *NOTE:* Megadoses are accompanied by serious toxicity including the symptoms listed in the preceding as well as liver damage, hyperglycemia, hyperuricemia, arrhythmias, tachycardia, and dermatoses.

**Drug Interactions:** No drug interactions reported of concern to dentistry.

**How Supplied:** Niacin: *Capsule:* 100 mg; *Capsule, extended release:* 125 mg, 250 mg, 400 mg, 500 mg, 750 mg; *Elixir:* 50 mg/5 mL; *Tablet:* 50 mg, 100 mg, 250 mg, 500 mg; *Tablet, extended release:* 250 mg, 500 mg, 750 mg, 1,000 mg. Niacinamide: *Tablet:* 50 mg, 100 mg, 500 mg

**Dosage** ―――――――
NIACIN

• **Extended-Release Capsules, Tablets, Extended-Release Tablets, Capsules, Elixir**
*Vitamin.*
**Adults:** Up to 500 mg/day; **pediatric:** Up to 300 mg/day.
*Antihyperlipidemic.*
**Adults, initial:** 1 g t.i.d.; **then:** increase dose in increments of 500 mg/day q 2–4 weeks as needed. **Maintenance:** 1–2 g t.i.d. (up to a maximum of 8 g/day).
• **IM, IV**
*Pellagra.*
**Adults, IM:** 50–100 mg 5 or more times/day. **IV, slow:** 25–100 mg 2 or more times/day. **Pediatric, IV slow:** Up to 300 mg/day.
NIACINAMIDE
• **Tablets**
*Vitamin.*
**Adults:** Up to 500 mg/day. **Pediatric:** Up to 300 mg/day. Capsules not recommended for use in children.

## DENTAL CONCERNS
**General**
1. Monitor vital signs at every appointment because of cardiovascular and respiratory side effects.
2. Have the patient sit up slowly and remain seated for at least two minutes after being supine in order to minimize the risk of orthostatic hypotension.
3. Decreased saliva flow can put the patient at risk for dental caries, periodontal disease, and candidiasis.
4. Consider repositioning dental chair to semisupine condition for patient discomfort because of GI side effects.

**Client/Family Teaching**
1. Daily home fluoride treatments for persistent dry mouth.
2. Avoid alcohol-containing mouth rinses.
3. Dry mouth can be treated with tart, sugarless gum or candy, water, or with saliva substitutes if dry mouth persists.

# Nicardipine hydrochloride
(nye-**KAR**-dih-peen)
**Pregnancy Category:** C
Cardene, Cardene IV, Cardene SR **(Rx)**
**Classification:** Calcium channel blocking agent (antianginal, antihypertensive)

See also *Calcium Channel Blocking Agents.*

**Action/Kinetics:** Moderately decreases CO and significantly decreases peripheral vascular resistance. **Onset of action:** 20 min. **Maximum plasma levels:** 30–120 min. Significant first-pass metabolism. Food (especially fats) will decrease the amount of drug absorbed from the GI tract. Steady-state plasma levels are reached after 2–3 days of therapy. **Therapeutic serum levels:** 0.028–0.050 mcg/mL. $t\frac{1}{2}$, **at steady state:** 8.6 hr. **Maximum BP-lowering effects, immediate release:** 1–2 hr; **maximum BP-lowering effects, sustained release:** 2–6 hr. **Duration:** 8 hr. Highly bound to plasma protein (> 95%) and metabolized by the liver with excretion through both the urine and feces.

**Uses: Immediate release:** Chronic stable angina (effort-associated angina) alone or in combination with beta-adrenergic blocking agents.

**Immediate and sustained released:** Hypertension alone or in combination with other antihypertensive drugs.

**IV:** Short-term treatment of hypertension when PO therapy is not desired or possible.

*Non-FDA Approved Uses:* CHF.

**Contraindications:** Clients with advanced aortic stenosis due to the effect on reducing afterload. During lactation. Hypersensitivity, hypotension < 90 mm Hg, 2nd or 3rd degree heart block, sick sinus syndrome.

**Special Concerns:** Safety and efficacy in children less than 18 years of age have not been established. Use with caution in clients with CHF, especially in combination with a beta blocker due to the possibility of a negative inotropic effect. Use with caution in clients with impaired liver function, reduced hepatic blood flow, or impaired renal function. Initial increase in frequency, duration, or severity of angina.

**Side Effects:** *CV:* Pedal edema, flushing, increased angina, palpitations, tachycardia, other edema, abnormal ECG, hypotension, postural hypotension, syncope, *MI, AV block,* ventricular extrasystoles, peripheral vascular disease. *CNS:* Dizziness, headache, somnolence, malaise, nervousness, insomnia, abnormal dreams, vertigo, depression, confusion, amnesia, anxiety, weakness, psychoses, hallucinations, paranoia. *Oral:* Dry mouth, sore throat, gingival hyperplasia. *GI:* N&V, dyspepsia, constipation. *Neuromuscular:* Asthenia, myalgia, paresthesia, hyperkinesia, arthralgia. *Miscellaneous:* Rash, dyspnea, SOB, nocturia, polyuria, allergic reactions, abnormal liver chemistries, hot flashes, impotence, rhinitis, sinusitis, nasal congestion, chest congestion, tinnitus, equilibrium disturbances, abnormal or blurred vision, infection, atypical chest pain.

**Drug Interactions**

*Anesthetics* / ↑ Effect of nicardipine

*Barbiturates* / ↓ Effect of nicardipine

*Carbamazepine* / ↑ Effect of nicardipine due to ↓ breakdown by liver

*Fentanyl* / Possible severe hypotension or ↑ fluid volume

*Indomethacin* / ↓ Effect of nicardipine

*NSAIDs* / ↓ Possible effect of nicardipine

*Phenobarbital* / ↓ Effect of nicardipine

*Other drugs with hypotensive effects* / ↑ Effect of nicardipine

**How Supplied:** *Capsule:* 20 mg, 30 mg; *Capsule, extended release:* 30 mg, 45 mg, 60 mg; *Injection:* 2.5 mg/mL

## Dosage

- **Capsules, Immediate Release**
  *Angina, hypertension.*
**Initial, usual:** 20 mg t.i.d. (range: 20–40 mg t.i.d.). Wait 3 days before increasing dose to ensure steady-state plasma levels.

- **Capsules, Sustained Release**
  *Hypertension.*
**Initial:** 30 mg b.i.d. (range: 30–60 mg b.i.d.).

*NOTE:* In renal impairment, the initial dose should be 20 mg t.i.d. In hepatic impairment, the initial dose should be 20 mg b.i.d.

- **IV**
  *Hypertension.*
**Individualize dose. Initial:** 5 mg/hr; the infusion rate may be increased to a maximum of 15 mg/hr (by 2.5-mg/hr increments q 15 min). For a more rapid reduction in BP, initiate at 5 mg/hr but increase the rate q 5 min in 2.5-mg/hr increments until a maximum of 15 mg/hr is reached. **Maintenance:** 3 mg/hr. The IV infusion rate to produce an average plasma level similar to a particular PO dose is as follows: 20 mg q 8 hr is equivalent to 0.5 mg/hr; 30 mg q 8 hr is equivalent to 1.2 mg/hr;

**N**

and 40 mg q 8 hr is equivalent to 2.2 mg/hr.

## DENTAL CONCERNS

See also *Dental Concerns* for *Calcium Channel Blocking Agents*.
**General**
1. Quarterly visits to assess for gingival hyperplasia.
2. Vasoconstrictors should be used with caution, in low doses, and with careful aspiration. Epinephrine-impregnated gingival retraction cords should be avoided
**Client/Family Teaching**
1. Practice frequent careful oral hygiene to minimize the incidence and severity of drug-induced gingival hyperplasia.
2. Need for frequent visits with a dental health professional if hyperplasia occurs

# Nicotine polacrilex (Nicotine Resin Complex)

(**NIK**-oh-teen)
**Pregnancy Category:** X
Nicorette, Nicorette DS, Nicorette Plus ✹ (OTC)
**Classification:** Smoking deterrent

**Action/Kinetics:** Following chewing, nicotine is released from an ion exchange resin in the gum product, providing blood nicotine levels approximating those produced by smoking cigarettes. The amount of nicotine released depends on the rate and duration of chewing. Following repeated administration q 30 min, nicotine blood levels reach 25–50 ng/mL. If the gum is swallowed, only a minimum amount of nicotine is released. Metabolized mainly by the liver, with about 10%–20% excreted unchanged in the urine.

**Uses:** Adjunct with behavioral modification in smokers wishing to give up the smoking habit. Is considered only as an initial aid, with the ultimate goal being abstention from all forms of nicotine. Most likely to benefit are individuals with the following characteristics:
a. smoke brands of cigarettes containing more than 0.9 mg nicotine;
b. smoke more than 15 cigarettes daily;
c. inhale cigarette smoke deeply and frequently;
d. smoke most frequently during the morning;
e. smoke the first cigarette of the day within 30 min of arising;
f. indicate cigarettes smoked in the morning are the most difficult to give up;
g. smoke even if the individual is ill and confined to bed;
h. find it necessary to smoke in places where smoking is not allowed. *NOTE:* Nicotine may be effective in improving the course of difficult-to-treat ulcerative colitis.

**Contraindications:** Pregnancy, lactation, nonsmokers, serious arrhythmias, angina, vasospastic disease, active temporomandibular joint disease. Use in individuals less than 18 years of age.

**Special Concerns:** Safety and effectiveness in children and adolescents who smoke have not been determined. Use with caution in hypertension, PUD, oral or pharyngeal inflammation, gastritis, stomatitis, hyperthyroidism, insulin-dependent diabetes, and pheochromocytoma.

**Side Effects:** *CNS:* Dizziness, irritability, headache. *Oral:* Dry mouth, sore mouth or throat, salivation. *GI:* N&V, indigestion, GI upset, eructation. *Other:* Hiccoughs, sore jaw muscles.

**Drug Interactions**
*Caffeine* / Possibly ↓ blood levels of caffeine due to ↑ rate of breakdown by liver
*Imipramine* / Possibly ↓ blood levels of imipramine due to ↑ rate of breakdown by liver
*Pentazocine* / Possibly ↓ blood levels of pentazocine due to ↑ rate of breakdown by liver
*Propoxyphene* / ↑ of propoxyphene
**How Supplied:** *Gum:* 2 mg, 4 mg

## Dosage
• **Gum**

**Initial:** One piece of gum chewed whenever the urge to smoke occurs; best results are obtained when the gum is chewed on a fixed schedule, at intervals of 1 to 2 hr, with at least 9 pieces chewed per day. **Maintenance:** 9–12 pieces of gum daily during the first month, not to exceed 30 pieces daily of the 2-mg strength and 20 pieces daily of the 4-mg strength.

## DENTAL CONCERNS

### General

1. Assess vital signs at every appointment because of cardiovascular side effects.
2. Chewing the nicotine polacrilex dose form may aggravate TMJ.

### Client/Family Teaching

1. Review the importance of good oral hygiene in order to prevent periodontal inflammation.
2. Review the proper use of oral hygiene aids in order to prevent injury.
3. Daily home fluoride treatments for persistent dry mouth.
4. Avoid alcohol-containing mouth rinses.
5. Dry mouth can be treated with tart, sugarless gum or candy, water, or with saliva substitutes if dry mouth persists.

When used in conjunction with a smoking cessation program in the dental office:

1. Must want to stop smoking and should do so immediately.
2. Use gum only as directed. When client has the urge to smoke, chew one piece slowly for about 30 min. If a slight tingling becomes evident, stop chewing until sensation subsides.
3. Acidic beverages, such as coffee, juices, soft drinks, and wine, interfere with buccal absorption of nicotine from the gum; thus, avoid eating and drinking 15 min before and during chewing as effects may be diminished.
4. Gum will not stick to dentures or appliances.
5. Identify individuals and local support groups that can help with smoking cessation and provide emotional and psychologic support throughout the endeavor. Participate in a formal smoking cessation program.

# Nicotine transdermal system

(**NIK**-oh-teen)
**Pregnancy Category:** D
Habitrol, Prostep **(Rx)**, Nicoderm CQ Step 1, Step 2, or Step 3, Nicotrol **(OTC)**
**Classification:** Smoking deterrent

**Action/Kinetics:** Nicotine transdermal system is a multilayered film that provides systemic delivery of varying amounts of nicotine over a 24-hr period after applying to the skin. The nicotine transdermal system produces an initial (first day of use) increase in BP, an increase in HR (3%–7%), and a decrease in SV after 10 days. Metabolized in the liver to a large number of metabolites, all of which are less active than nicotine. **t½, following removal of the system from the skin:** 3–4 hr.

**Uses:** As an aid to stopping smoking for the relief of nicotine withdrawal symptoms. Should be used in conjunction with a comprehensive behavioral smoking cessation program.

**Contraindications:** Hypersensitivity or allergy to nicotine or any components of the therapeutic system. Use in children and during pregnancy, labor, and delivery. Lactation. Use in those with heart disease, hypertension, a recent MI, severe or worsening angina pectoris, and those taking certain antidepressants or antiasthmatic drugs. Use in severe renal impairment.

**Special Concerns:** Pregnant smokers should be encouraged to try to stop smoking using educational and behavioral interventions before using the nicotine transdermal system. The product should only be used during pregnancy if the potential benefit outweighs the potential risk of nico-

**N**

*bold italic* = life-threatening side effect

tine to the fetus. The use of nicotine transdermal systems for longer than 3 months has not been studied. Clients with coronary heart disease (history of MI and/or angina pectoris), serious cardiac arrhythmias, or vasospastic diseases (e.g., Buerger's disease, Prinzmetal's variant angina) should be screened carefully before using the transdermal system. Use with caution in clients with hyperthyroidism, pheochromocytoma, insulin-dependent diabetes (nicotine causes the release of catecholamines), in active peptic ulcers, in accelerated hypertension, and during lactation.

**Side Effects:** *NOTE:* The incidence of side effects is complicated by the fact that clients manifest effects of nicotine withdrawal or by concurrent smoking.

*Dermatologic:* Erythema, pruritus, or burning at the site of application; cutaneous hypersensitivity, sweating, rash at application site. *Body as a whole:* Allergy, back pain. *Oral:* Dry mouth. *GI:* Diarrhea, dyspepsia, abdominal pain, constipation, N&V. *Musculoskeletal:* Arthralgia, myalgia. *CNS:* Abnormal dreams, somnolence, dizziness, impaired concentration, headache, insomnia. *CV:* Tachycardia, hypertension. *Respiratory:* Increased cough, pharyngitis, sinusitis. *GU:* Dysmenorrhea.

**Drug Interactions**
*Propoxyphene* / ↓ Metabolism of propoxyphene

**How Supplied:** *Film, extended release:* 7 mg/24 hr, 11 mg/24 hr, 14 mg/24 hr, 15 mg/16 hr, 21 mg/24 hr, 22 mg/24 hr

**Dosage** ⎯⎯⎯⎯⎯⎯⎯⎯
• **Transdermal System**
HABITROL (Rx)
**Healthy clients, initial:** 21 mg/day for 4–8 weeks; **then,** 14 mg/day for 2–4 weeks and 7 mg/day for 2–4 weeks. **Light smokers, those who weigh less than 100 lb or who have CV disease:** 14 mg/day for 4–8 weeks; **then,** 7 mg/day for 2–4 weeks.
PROSTEP (Rx)

**Clients weighing 100 lb or more:** 22 mg/day for 4–8 weeks; **then,** 11 mg/day for 2–4 weeks. **Clients weighing less than 100 lb:** 11 mg/day for 4–8 weeks.
NICODERM CQ (OTC)
**Light smokers (10 or less cigarettes/day):** One 14-mg/24-hr patch for 16 or 24 hr/day for 6 weeks; **then,** one 7-mg/24-hr patch for 16 or 24 hr/day for 2 weeks. **Heavy smokers (>10 cigarettes/day):** One 21-mg/24-hr patch for 16 or 24 hr/day for 6 weeks; **then,** one 14-mg/24-hr patch for 16 or 24 hr/day for 2 weeks, followed by one 7-mg/24-hr patch for 16 or 24 hr for 2 weeks.
NICOTROL (OTC)
**Those who smoke > 10 cigarettes/day:** 15 mg/day for 6 weeks. The patch is to be worn for 16 hr and removed at bedtime.

## DENTAL CONCERNS

1. Decreased saliva flow can put the patient at risk for dental caries, periodontal disease, and candidiasis.
**Client/Family Teaching**
1. Daily home fluoride treatments for persistent dry mouth.
2. Avoid alcohol-containing mouth rinses.
3. Dry mouth can be treated with tart, sugarless gum or candy, water, or with saliva substitutes if dry mouth persists.

When used in conjunction with a smoking cessation program in the dental office:
1. Use extreme caution during application; avoid contact with active systems. If contact occurs, wash area with water only. The eyes should not be touched. These systems can be a dermal irritant and cause contact dermatitis.
2. Any persistent skin irritations such as erythema, edema, or pruritus at the application site as well as any generalized skin reactions such as hives, urticaria, or a generalized rash should be reported and the system removed.
3. Follow manufacturer's guidelines for proper system application. Re-

view information sheet that comes with the product which contains instructions on how to use and dispose of the transdermal systems properly.

4. Stop smoking completely. If smoking continues, may experience adverse side effects due to higher nicotine levels in the body.

5. Participate in a formal smoking cessation program. The success or failure of smoking cessation depends on the quality, intensity, and frequency of supportive care.

6. Nicotine in any form can be toxic and addictive; nicotine transdermal systems may lead to dependence. To minimize this risk, withdraw use of the transdermal system gradually after 4–8 weeks of use.

7. Symptoms of nicotine withdrawal include craving, nervousness, restlessness, irritability, mood lability, anxiety, drowsiness, sleep disturbances, impaired concentration, increased appetite, headache, myalgia, constipation, fatigue, and weight gain; report if evident as dosage may require adjustment.

8. Change site of application daily; do not reuse for 1 week.

9. With Nicotrol, remove patch at bedtime and apply upon arising.

10. Keep all products used and unused away from children and pets; sufficient nicotine is still present in used systems to cause toxicity.

11. If therapy is unsuccessful after 4 weeks, discontinue and identify reasons for failure so that a later attempt may be more successful.

# Nifedipine

(nye-**FED**-ih-peen)
**Pregnancy Category:** C
Adalat, Adalat CC, Adalat P.A. 10 and 20 ✤, Adalat XL ✤, Apo-Nifed ✤, Apo-Nifed PA ✤, Gen-Nifedipine ✤, Novo-Nifedin ✤, Nu-Nifed ✤, Procardia, Procardia XL, Taro-Nifedipine ✤ **(Rx)**
**Classification:** Calcium channel blocking agent (antianginal, antihypertensive)

See also *Calcium Channel Blocking Agents.*

**Action/Kinetics:** Variable effects on AV node effective and functional refractory periods. CO is moderately increased while peripheral vascular resistance is significantly decreased. **Onset:** 20 min. **Peak plasma levels:** 30 min (up to 4 hr for extended-release). **t½:** 2–5 hr. **Therapeutic serum levels:** 0.025–0.1 mcg/mL. **Duration:** 4–8 hr (12 hr for extended-release). Low-fat meals may slow the rate but not the extent of absorption. Metabolized in the liver to inactive metabolites.

**Uses:** Vasospastic (Prinzmetal's or variant) angina. Chronic stable angina without vasospasm, including angina due to increased effort (especially in clients who cannot take beta blockers or nitrates or who remain symptomatic following clinical doses of these drugs). Essential hypertension (sustained-release only). *Non-FDA Approved Uses:* PO, sublingually, or chewed in hypertensive emergencies. Also prophylaxis of migraine headaches, primary pulmonary hypertension, severe pregnancy-associated hypertension, esophageal diseases, Raynaud's phenomenon, CHF, asthma, premature labor, biliary and renal colic, and cardiomyopathy. To prevent strokes and to decrease the risk of CHF in geriatric hypertensives.

**Contraindications:** Hypersensitivity. Lactation.

**Special Concerns:** Use with caution in impaired hepatic or renal function and in elderly clients. Initial increase in frequency, duration, or severity of angina (may also be seen in clients being withdrawn from beta blockers and who begin taking nifedipine).

**Side Effects:** *CV:* Peripheral and pulmonary edema, MI, hypotension, palpitations, syncope, CHF (especially if used with a beta blocker), decreased platelet aggregation, arrhythmias, tachycardia. Increased frequency, length, and duration of

**N**

angina when beginning nifedipine therapy. *Oral:* Dry mouth, gingival hyperplasia. *GI:* Nausea, diarrhea, constipation, flatulence, abdominal cramps, dysgeusia, vomiting, eructation, gastroesophageal reflux, melena. *CNS:* Dizziness, lightheadedness, giddiness, nervousness, sleep disturbances, headache, weakness, depression, migraine, psychoses, hallucinations, disturbances in equilibrium, somnolence, insomnia, abnormal dreams, malaise, anxiety. *Dermatologic:* Rash, dermatitis, urticaria, pruritus, photosensitivity, erythema multiforme, ***Stevens-Johnson syndrome.*** *Respiratory:* Dyspnea, cough, wheezing, SOB, respiratory infection, throat, nasal, or chest congestion. *Musculoskeletal:* Muscle cramps or inflammation, joint pain or stiffness, arthritis, ataxia, myoclonic dystonia, hypertonia, asthenia. *Hematologic:* Thrombocytopenia, leukopenia, purpura, anemia. *Other:* Fever, chills, sweating, blurred vision, sexual difficulties, flushing, transient blindness, hyperglycemia, hypokalemia, allergic hepatitis, hepatitis, tinnitus, gynecomastia, polyuria, nocturia, erythromelalgia, weight gain, epistaxis, facial and periorbital edema, hypoesthesia, gout, abnormal lacrimation, breast pain, dysuria, hematuria.

**Drug Interactions**
*Anesthetics* / ↑ Effect of nifedipine
*Barbiturates* / ↓ Effect of nifedipine
*Carbamazepine* / ↑ Effect of nifedipine due to ↓ breakdown by liver
*Fentanyl* / Possible severe hypotension or ↑ fluid volume
*Indomethacin* / ↓ Effect of nifedipine
*NSAIDs* / ↓ Possible effect of nifedipine
*Phenobarbital* / ↓ Effect of nifedipine
*Other drugs with hypotensive effects* / ↑ Effect of nifedipine

**How Supplied:** *Capsule:* 10 mg, 20 mg; *Tablet, extended release:* 30 mg, 60 mg, 90 mg

**Dosage** ⎯⎯⎯⎯⎯⎯⎯⎯⎯⎯
• **Capsules**

**Individualized. Initial:** 10 mg t.i.d. (range: 10–20 mg t.i.d.); **maintenance:** 10–30 mg t.i.d.–q.i.d. Clients with coronary artery spasm may respond better to 20–30 mg t.i.d.–q.i.d. Doses greater than 120 mg/day are rarely needed while doses greater than 180 mg/day are not recommended.
• **Sustained-Release Tablets**
**Initial:** 30 or 60 mg once daily for Procardia XL and 30 mg once daily for Adalat CC. Titrate over a 7- to 14-day period. Dosage can be increased as required and as tolerated, to a maximum of 120 mg/day for Procardia XL and 90 mg/day for Adalat CC.

*Investigational, hypertensive emergencies.*
10–20 mg given PO, sublingually (by puncturing capsule and squeezing contents under the tongue), or chewed (capsule is punctured several times and then chewed).

## DENTAL CONCERNS

See also *Dental Concerns* for *Calcium Channel Blocking Agents.*
**General**
1. Frequent visits to assess for gingival hyperplasia.
2. Vasoconstrictors should be used with caution, in low doses, and with careful aspiration. Epinephrine-impregnated gingival retraction cords should be avoided.
3. Keep nitroglycerin avaliable during dental visit in case dental visits precipitate angina attacks.
**Client/Family Teaching**
1. Practice frequent careful oral hygiene to minimize the incidence and severity of drug-induced gingival hyperplasia.
2. Need for frequent visits with a dental health professional if hyperplasia occurs.

# Nimodipine
(nye-**MOH**-dih-peen)
**Pregnancy Category:** C
Nimotop, Nimotop I.V. ✿ **(Rx)**
**Classification:** Calcium channel blocking agent

See also *Calcium Channel Blocking Agents*.
**Action/Kinetics:** Has a greater effect on cerebral arteries than arteries elsewhere in the body (probably due to its highly lipophilic properties). Mechanism to reduce neurologic deficits following subarachnoid hemorrhage not known. **Peak plasma levels:** 1 hr. **t½:** 1–2 hr. Significantly bound (over 95%) to plasma protein. Undergoes first-pass metabolism in the liver; metabolites excreted through the urine.

**Uses:** Improvement of neurologic deficits due to spasm following subarachnoid hemorrhage from ruptured congenital intracranial aneurysms; clients should have Hunt and Hess grades of I–III. *Non-FDA Approved Uses:* Migraine headaches and cluster headaches.

**Contraindications:** Lactation.

**Special Concerns:** Safety and efficacy have not been established in children. Use with caution in clients with impaired hepatic function and reduced hepatic blood flow. The half-life may be increased in geriatric clients.

**Side Effects:** *CV:* Hypotension, peripheral edema, CHF, ECG abnormalities, tachycardia, bradycardia, palpitations, rebound vasospasm, hypertension, hematoma, ***DIC, DVT.*** *Oral:* Dry mouth, gingival hyperplasia. *GI:* Nausea, dyspepsia, diarrhea, abdominal discomfort, cramps, ***GI hemorrhage,*** vomiting. *CNS:* Headache, depression, lightheadedness, dizziness. *Hepatic:* Abnormal liver function test, hepatitis, jaundice. *Hematologic:* Thrombocytopenia, anemia, purpura, ecchymosis. *Dermatologic:* Rash, dermatitis, pruritus, urticaria. *Miscellaneous:* Dyspnea, muscle pain or cramps, acne, itching, flushing, diaphoresis, wheezing, hyponatremia.

**Drug Interactions**
*Anesthetics* / ↑ Effect of nimodipine
*Barbiturates* / ↓ Effect of nimodipine
*Carbamazepine* / ↑ Effect of nimodipine due to ↓ breakdown by liver
*Fentanyl* / Possible severe hypotension or ↑ fluid volume
*Indomethacin* / ↓ Effect of nimodipine
*NSAIDs* / ↓ Possible effect of nimodipine
*Phenobarbital* / ↓ Effect of nimodipine
*Other drugs with hypotensive effects* / ↑ Effect of nimodipine

**How Supplied:** *Capsule:* 30 mg

**Dosage** ─────────────
• **Capsules**
**Adults:** 60 mg q 4 hr beginning within 96 hr after subarachnoid hemorrhage and continuing for 21 consecutive days. The dosage should be reduced to 30 mg q 4 hr in clients with hepatic impairment.

## DENTAL CONCERNS

See also *Dental Concerns* for *Calcium Channel Blocking Agents*.
**Client/Family Teaching**
1. Practice frequent careful oral hygiene to minimize the incidence and severity of drug-induced gingival hyperplasia.
2. Need for frequent visits with a dental health professional if hyperplasia occurs.

# Nitroglycerin IV
(nye-troh-**GLIH**-sir-in)
**Pregnancy Category:** C
Nitro-Bid IV, Nitroglycerin in 5% Dextrose, Tridil **(Rx)**
**Classification:** Antianginal agent (coronary vasodilator)

See also *Antianginal Drugs—Nitrates/Nitrites*.
**Action/Kinetics: Onset:** 1–2 min; **duration:** 3–5 min (dose-dependent).
**Uses:** Hypertension associated with surgery (e.g., associated with ET intubation, skin incision, sternotomy, anesthesia, cardiac bypass, immediate postsurgical period). CHF associated

with acute MI. Angina unresponsive to usual doses of organic nitrate or beta-adrenergic blocking agents. Cardiac-load reducing agent. Produce controlled hypotension during surgical procedures.

**Special Concerns:** Dosage has not been established in children.

**How Supplied:** *Injection:* 0.5 mg/mL, 5 mg/mL

**Dosage** ⸻

• **IV Infusion Only**

**Initial:** 5 mcg/min delivered by precise infusion pump. May be increased by 5 mcg/min q 3–5 min until response is seen. If no response seen at 20 mcg/min, dose can be increased by 10–20 mcg/min until response noted. Monitor titration continuously until client reaches desired level of response.

## DENTAL CONCERNS

See also *Dental Concerns* for *Antianginal Drugs—Nitrates/Nitrites.*

# Nitroglycerin sublingual
(nye-troh-**GLIH**-sir-in)
**Pregnancy Category:** C
Nitrostat **(Rx)**
**Classification:** Antianginal agent (coronary vasodilator)

See also *Antianginal Drugs—Nitrates/Nitrites.*

**Action/Kinetics: Sublingual. Onset:** 1–3 min; **duration:** 30–60 min.

**Uses:** Agents of choice for prophylaxis and treatment of angina pectoris.

**Special Concerns:** Dosage has not been established in children.

**How Supplied:** *Tablet:* 0.3 mg, 0.4 mg, 0.6 mg

**Dosage** ⸻

• **Sublingual Tablets**

150–600 mcg under the tongue or in the buccal pouch at first sign of attack; may be repeated in 5 min if necessary (no more than 3 tablets should be taken within 15 min). For prophylaxis, tablets may be taken 5–10 min prior to activities that may precipitate an attack.

## DENTAL CONCERNS

See also *Dental Concerns* for *Antianginal Drugs—Nitrates/Nitrites.*

# Nitroglycerin sustained-release capsules
(nye-troh-**GLIH**-sir-in)
**Pregnancy Category:** C
Nitroglyn **(Rx)**

# Nitroglycerin sustained-release tablets
(nye-troh-**GLIH**-sir-in)
**Pregnancy Category:** C
Nitrogard-SR ✹, Nitrong, Nitrong SR ✹ **(Rx)**
**Classification:** Antianginal agent (coronary vasodilator)

See also *Antianginal Drugs—Nitrates/Nitrites.*

**Action/Kinetics: Sustained-release. Onset:** 20–45 min; **duration:** 3–8 hr.

**Uses:** To prevent anginal attacks. "Possibly effective" for the prophylaxis or treatment of anginal attacks.

**Special Concerns:** Dosage has not been established in children.

**How Supplied:** Nitroclycerin sustained-release capsules: *Capsule, extended release:* 2.5 mg, 6.5 mg, 9 mg. Nitroglycerin sustained-release tablets: *Tablet, extended release:* 2.6 mg, 6.5 mg

**Dosage** ⸻

• **Sustained-Release Capsules**

2.5, 6.5, or 9 mg q 8–12 hr.

• **Sustained-Release Tablets**

1.3, 2.6, or 6.5 mg q 8–12 hr.

## DENTAL CONCERNS

See also *Dental Concerns* for *Antianginal Drugs—Nitrates/Nitrites.*

# Nitroglycerin transdermal system
(nye-troh-**GLIH**-sir-in)
**Pregnancy Category:** C
Deponit 0.2 mg/hr and 0.4 mg/hr, Minitran 0.1 mg/hr, 0.2 mg/hr, 0.4 mg/hr, and 0.6 mg/hr, Nitrek 0.2 mg/hr, 0.4 mg/hr, and 0.6 mg/hr, Ni-

trodisc 0.2 mg/hr, 0.3 mg/hr, and 0.4 mg/hr, Nitro-Dur 0.1 mg/hr, 0.2 mg/hr, 0.3 mg/hr, 0.4 mg/hr, 0.6 mg/hr, and 0.8 mg/hr, Transderm-Nitro 0.1 mg/hr, 0.2 mg/hr, 0.4 mg/hr, and 0.6 mg/hr **(Rx)**
**Classification:** Antianginal agent (coronary vasodilator)

See also *Antianginal Drugs—Nitrates/Nitrites.*
**Action/Kinetics: Onset:** 30–60 min; **duration:** 8–24 hr. The amount released each hour is indicated in the name.
**Uses:** Prophylaxis of angina pectoris due to CAD. *NOTE:* There is some evidence that nitroglycerin patches stop preterm labor.
**Special Concerns:** Dosage has not been established in children.
**How Supplied:** *Film, extended release:* 0.1 mg/hr, 0.2 mg/hr, 0.3 mg/hr, 0.4 mg/hr, 0.6 mg/hr, 0.8 mg/hr

**Dosage** ⸻
• **Topical Patch**
**Initial:** 0.2–0.4 mg/hr (initially the smallest available dose in the dosage series) applied each day to skin site free of hair and free of excessive movement (e.g., chest, upper arm).
**Maintenance:** Additional systems or strengths may be added depending on the clinical response.

## DENTAL CONCERNS

See also *Dental Concerns* for *Antianginal Drugs—Nitrates/Nitrites.*

# Nitroglycerin translingual spray
(nye-troh-**GLIH**-sir-in)
**Pregnancy Category:** C
Nitrolingual **(Rx)**
**Classification:** Antianginal agent (coronary vasodilator)

See also *Antianginal Drugs—Nitrates/Nitrites.*
**Action/Kinetics: Onset:** 2 min; **duration:** 30–60 min.

**Uses:** Coronary artery disease to relieve an acute attack or used prophylactically 10–15 min before beginning activities that can cause an acute anginal attack.
**Special Concerns:** Dosage has not been established in children.
**How Supplied:** *Spray:* 0.4 mg/spray

**Dosage** ⸻
• **Spray**
*Termination of acute attack.*
One to two metered doses (400–800 mcg) on or under the tongue q 5 min as needed; no more than three metered doses should be administered within a 15-min period.
*Prophylaxis.*
One to two metered doses 5–10 min before beginning activities that might precipitate an acute attack.

## DENTAL CONCERNS

See also *Dental Concerns* for *Antianginal Drugs—Nitrates/Nitrites.*
**Client/Family Teaching**
1. Do *not* inhale the spray. Spray under the tongue.
2. Seek immediate medical attention if chest pain persists.

# Nizatidine
(nye-**ZAY**-tih-deen)
**Pregnancy Category:** C
Axid **(Rx)**, Axid AR **(OTC)**
**Classification:** Histamine H₂ receptor antagonist

See also *Histamine H₂ Antagonists.*
**Action/Kinetics:** Decreases gastric acid secretion by blocking the effect of histamine on histamine $H_2$ receptors. Does not affect the P-450 and P-448 drug metabolizing enzymes. **Onset:** 30 min. **Peak plasma levels:** 0.5–3 hr after a PO dose. **Time to peak effect:** 0.5–3 hr. **Duration, nocturnal:** Up to 12 hr; **basal:** Up to 8 hr. **t½:** 1–2 hr. Approximately 60% of a PO dose is excreted unchanged in the urine. Clients with moderate to severe renal impairment manifest a significant prolongation of t½ with decreased clearance.

**Uses:** Treatment of acute duodenal ulcer and maintenance following healing of a duodenal ulcer. GERD, including erosive and ulcerative esophagitis. Short-term treatment of benign gastric ulcer. OTC use to prevent meal-induced heartburn.

**Contraindications:** Hypersensitivity to $H_2$ receptor antagonists. Cirrhosis of the liver, impaired renal or hepatic function. Lactation.

**Special Concerns:** Safety and efficacy have not been determined in children.

**Side Effects:** *CNS:* Headache, fatigue, somnolence, insomnia, dizziness, abnormal dreams, anxiety, nervousness, confusion (rare). *Oral:* Dry mouth. *GI:* N&V, diarrhea, pancreatitis, constipation, abdominal discomfort, flatulence, dyspepsia, anorexia. *Dermatologic:* Exfoliative dermatitis, erythroderma, pruritus, urticaria, erythema multiforme. *CV:* Asymptomatic ventricular tachycardia; *rarely, cardiac arrhythmias or arrest following rapid IV use. Respiratory:* Rhinitis, pharyngitis, sinusitis, cough. *Body as a whole:* Asthenia, back pain, chest pain, infection, fever, myalgia. *Miscellaneous:* Impotence, loss of libido, thrombocytopenia, sweating, gynecomastia, hyperuricemia, eosinophilia, gout, and cholestatic or hepatocellular effects (resulting in increased AST, ALT, or alkaline phosphatase).

**Drug Interactions**
*Antacids containing Al and Mg hydroxides* / ↓ Nizatidine absorption by about 10%
*Aspirin, high doses* / ↑ Salicylate serum levels
*Simethicone* / ↓ Nizatidine absorption by about 10%

**How Supplied:** *Capsule:* 150 mg, 300 mg; *Tablet:* 75 mg

**Dosage** —————
AXID
• **Capsules**
*Active duodenal ulcer.*
**Adults:** Either 300 mg once daily at bedtime or 150 mg b.i.d. The dose should be 150 mg/day if the $C_{CR}$ is 20–50 mL/min and 150 mg every

other day if $C_{CR}$ is less than 20 mL/min.
*Prophylaxis following healing of duodenal ulcer.*
**Adults:** 150 mg/day at bedtime. The dose should be 150 mg every other day if $C_{CR}$ is 20–50 mL/min and 150 mg every 3 days if $C_{CR}$ is less than 20 mL/min.
*Treatment of benign gastric ulcer.*
**Adults:** 150 mg b.i.d. or 300 mg at bedtime.
*Gastroesophageal reflux disease, including erosive and ulcerative esophagitis.*
**Adults:** 150 mg b.i.d.
AXID AR
• **Tablets**
*Heartburn.*
1 tablet b.i.d.

---

## DENTAL CONCERNS
**General**
1. Avoid alcohol, caffeine, and aspirin-containing prescription and nonprescription drugs.
**Client/Family Teaching**
1. Avoid alcohol-containing mouth rinses and beverages.

# Norfloxacin
(nor-**FLOX**-ah-sin)
**Pregnancy Category:** C
Chibroxin Ophthalmic Solution, Noroxin, Noroxin Ophthalmic Solution ✲ **(Rx)**
**Classification:** Fluoroquinolone anti-infective

---

See also *Anti-Infectives* and *Fluoroquinolones.*

**Action/Kinetics:** Active against gram-positive and gram-negative organisms by inhibiting bacterial DNA synthesis. Not effective against obligate anaerobes. **Peak plasma levels:** 1.4–1.6 mcg/mL after 1–2 hr following a dose of 400 mg and 2.5 mcg/mL 1–2 hr after a dose of 800 mg. **t½:** 3–4.5 hr. Food decreases the absorption of norfloxacin. Approximately 30% excreted unchanged in the urine and 30% through the feces.
**Uses: Systemic:** Uncomplicated UTIs caused by *Escherichia coli, Klebsiella pneumoniae, Enterobacter*

cloacae, *Proteus mirabilis, P. vulgaris, Pseudomonas aeruginosa, Citrobacter freundii, Staphylococcus aureus, S. epidermidis, Enterococcus faecalis, Enterobacter aerogenes, S. saprophyticus,* and *S. agalactiae.* Complicated UTIs caused by *E. faecalis, E. coli, K. pneumoniae, P. mirabilis, P. aeruginosa,* or *Serratia marcescens.* Urethral gonorrhea and endocervical gonococcal infections due to penicillinase- or non-penicillinase-producing *Neisseria gonorrhoeae.* Prostatitis due to *E. coli.*

**Ophthalmic:** Superficial ocular infections involving the cornea or conjunctiva due to *Staphylococcus, S. aureus, Streptococcus pneumoniae, E. coli, Haemophilus aegyptius, H. influenzae, K. pneumoniae, N. gonorrhoeae, Proteus* species, *Enterobacter aerogenes, Serratia marcescens, Pseudomonas aeruginosa,* and *Vibrio* species.

**Contraindications:** Hypersensitivity to nalidixic acid, cinoxacin, or norfloxacin. Lactation, infants, and children. Ophthalmic use for dendritic keratitis, vaccinia, varicella, mycobacterial infections of the eye, fungal disease of the eye, and use with steroid combinations after uncomplicated removal of a corneal foreign body.

**Special Concerns:** Use with caution in clients with a history of seizures and in impaired renal function. Geriatric clients eliminate norfloxacin more slowly.

**Side Effects:** See also *Side Effects* for *Fluoroquinolones.*

*Oral:* Dry/painful mouth, stomatitis. *GI:* Nausea, vomiting, diarrhea, abdominal pain or discomfort, dyspepsia, flatulence, constipation, pseudomembranous colitis. *CNS:* Headache, dizziness, fatigue, malaise, drowsiness, depression, insomnia, confusion, psychoses. *Hematologic:* Decreased hematocrit, eosinophilia, leukopenia, neutropenia, either increased or decreased platelets. *Dermatologic:* Photosensitivity, rash, pruritus, exfoliative dermatitis, ***toxic***

***epidermal necrolysis,*** erythema, erythema multiforme, ***Stevens-Johnson syndrome.*** *Other:* Paresthesia, hypersensitivity, fever, visual disturbances, hearing loss, crystalluria, cylindruria, candiduria, myoclonus (rare), hepatitis, pancreatitis, arthralgia.

*Following ophthalmic use:* Conjunctival hyperemia, photophobia, chemosis, bitter taste in mouth.

**Additional Drug Interactions**
*Sodium bicarbonate* / ↓ Absorption of sodium bicarbonate.

**How Supplied:** *Ophthalmic solution:* 0.3%; *Tablet:* 400 mg

## Dosage
- **Tablets**
  *Uncomplicated UTIs due to* E. coli, K. pneumoniae, *or* P. mirabilis.
  400 mg q 12 hr for 3 days.
  *Uncomplicated UTIs due to other organisms.*
  400 mg q 12 hr for 7–10 days.
  *Complicated UTIs.*
  400 mg q 12 hr for 10–21 days. Maximum dose for UTIs should not exceed 800 mg/day.
  *Uncomplicated gonorrhea.*
  800 mg as a single dose.
  *Impaired renal function, with* $C_{CR}$ *equal to or less than 30 mL/min/1.73 m².*
  400 mg/day for 7–10 days.
  *Prostatis due to* E. coli.
  400 mg q 12 hr for 28 days.
- **Ophthalmic Solution**
  *Acute infections.*
  **Initially,** 1–2 gtt q 15–30 min; **then,** reduce frequency as infection is controlled.
  *Moderate infections.*
  1–2 gtt 4–6 times/day.

## DENTAL CONCERNS

See also *General Dental Concerns for All Anti-Infectives* and for *Fluoroquinolones.*

### General
1. Ingestible sodium bicarbonate products (i.e., air polishing systems) can only be used 2 hours after taking enoxacin.

N

---

2. Determine why the patient is taking the medication.

3. Decreased saliva flow can put the patient at risk for dental caries, periodontal disease, and candidiasis.

**Consultation with Primary Care Provider**

1. Consult with the patient's health care provider if an acute dental infection occurs and the patient requires another anti-infective.

**Client/Family Teaching**

1. Review the importance of good oral hygiene in order to prevent soft tissue inflammation.

2. Daily home fluoride treatments for persistent dry mouth.

3. Avoid alcohol-containing mouth rinses and beverages.

4. Avoid caffeine-containing beverages.

5. Dry mouth can be treated with tart, sugarless gum or candy, water, sugar-free beverages, or with saliva substitutes if dry mouth persists.

6. Patient may want to wear dark glasses in order to avoid photophobia, which can occur with the dental light.

7. Discontinue treatment and inform dentist immediately if the patient experiences pain or inflammation in his or her tendons. Rest and avoid exercise.

# Nortriptyline hydrochloride
(nor-**TRIP**-tih-leen)
**Pregnancy Category:** C

Aventyl, Pamelor **(Rx)**
**Classification:** Antidepressant, tricyclic

See also *Antidepressants, Tricyclic.*

**Action/Kinetics:** Manifests moderate anticholinergic and sedative effects but slight orthostatic hypotensive effects. **Effective plasma levels:** 50–150 ng/mL. **t½:** 18–44 hr. **Time to reach steady state:** 4–19 days.

**Uses:** Treatment of symptoms of depression. Chronic, severe neurogenic pain. Dermatologic disorders including chronic urticaria, angioedema, and nocturnal pruritus in atopic eczema.

**Contraindications:** Use in children.

**Special Concerns:** Safety and efficacy have not been determined in children.

**How Supplied:** *Capsule:* 10 mg, 25 mg, 50 mg, 75 mg; *Solution:* 10 mg/5 mL

**Dosage**

• **Capsules, Oral Solution**
*Depression.*
**Adults:** 25 mg t.i.d.–q.i.d. Dose individualized; begin at a low dosage and increase as needed. **Doses above 150 mg/day are not recommended. Elderly clients:** 30–50 mg/day in divided doses.
*Dermatologic disorders.*
75 mg/day.

## DENTAL CONCERNS

See also *Dental Concerns* for *Antidepressants, Tricyclic.*

# Ofloxacin
(oh-**FLOX**-ah-zeen)
**Pregnancy Category:** C
Floxin, Floxin I.V., Floxin Otic, Ocuflox **(Rx)**
**Classification:** Antibacterial, fluoroquinolone

See also *Anti-Infectives.*

**Action/Kinetics:** Effective against a wide range of gram-positive and gram-negative aerobic and anaerobic bacteria. Penicillinase has no effect on the activity of ofloxacin. Widely distributed to body fluids.

**Maximum serum levels:** 1–2 hr. **t½, first phase:** 5–7 hr; **second phase:** 20–25 hr. **Peak serum levels at steady state, after PO doses:** 1.5 mcg/mL after 200-mg doses, 2.4 mcg/mL after 300-mg doses, and 2.9 mcg/mL after 400-mg doses. **Peak serum levels after IV doses:** 2.7 mcg/mL after 200-mg dose and 4 mcg/mL after 400-mg dose. Between 70% and 80% is excreted unchanged in the urine.

**Uses: Systemic:** Pneumonia or acute bacterial exacerbations of chronic bronchitis or community-acquired pneumonia due to *Haemophilus influenzae* or *Streptococcus pneumoniae*. Not a drug of first choice in the treatment of presumed or confirmed pneumococcal pneumonia. Not effective for syphilis.

Acute, uncomplicated urethral and cervical gonorrhea due to *Neisseria gonorrhoeae;* nongonococcal urethritis, and cervicitis due to *Chlamydia trachomatis*. Mixed infections of the urethra and cervix due to *N. gonorrhoeae* and *C. trachomatis*.

Mild to moderate skin and skin structure infections due to *Staphylococcus aureus, Streptococcus pyogenes,* or *Proteus mirabilis*.

Uncomplicated cystitis due to *Citrobacter diversus, Enterobacter aerogenes, Escherichia coli, Klebsiella pneumoniae, P. mirabilis,* or *Pseudomonas aeruginosa*. Complicated UTIs due to *E. coli, K. pneumoniae, P. mirabilis, C. diversus,* or *P. aeruginosa*. Prostatitis due to *E. coli*. Monotherapy for pelvic inflammatory disease.

IV therapy is indicated when the client is unable to take PO medication.

**Ophthalmic:** Treatment of conjunctivitis caused by *S. aureus, Staphylococcus epidermidis, S. pneumoniae, Enterobacter cloacae, H. influenzae, P. mirabilis,* and *P. aeruginosa*. Corneal ulcers caused by susceptible organisms.

**Otic:** Otitis externa in clients one year of age and older. Acute otitis media from age one to twelve with tympanostomy tubes. Chronic suppurative otitis media in those twelve years and older who have perforated tympanic membranes.

**Contraindications:** Hypersensitivity to quinolone antibacterial agents. Use during lactation. Use for syphilis (ineffective). Ophthalmic use in dendritic keratitis, vaccinia, varicella, mycobacterial infections of the eye, fungal diseases of the eye, and with steroid combinations after uncomplicated removal of a corneal foreign body.

**Special Concerns:** Safety and effectiveness of the systemic forms have not been established in children, adolescents under the age of 18 years, pregnant women, and lactating women. Safety and effectiveness of the ophthalmic form have not been established in children less than 1 year of age. Use with caution in clients with known or suspected CNS disorders such as severe cerebral atherosclerosis, epilepsy, or factors that predispose to seizures. The effectiveness of the IV dosage form in treating severe infections has not been determined.

**Side Effects:** See also *Side Effects* for *Fluroquinolones*.

*Oral:* Dry or painful mouth, canidiasis, dysgeusia. *GI:* Nausea, diarrhea, vomiting, abdominal pain or discomfort, dyspepsia, flatulence, constipation, pseudomembranous colitis, decreased appetite. *CNS:* Headache, dizziness, fatigue, malaise, somnolence, depression, insomnia, seizures, sleep disorders, nervousness, anxiety, cognitive change, dream abnormality, euphoria, hallucinations, vertigo. *CV:* Chest pain, edema, hypertension, palpitations, vasodilation. *Hypersensitivity reactions:* Dyspnea, ***anaphylaxis***. *GU:* External genital pruritus in women, vaginitis, vaginal discharge; burning, irritation, pain, and rash of the female genitalia; glucosuria, proteinuria, hematuria, pyuria, dysmenorrhea, menorrhagia, metrorrhagia, urinary frequency or pain. *Respiratory:* Cough, rhinorrhea. *Dermatolog-*

*ic:* Diaphoresis, vasculitis, photosensitivity, rash, pruritus. *Hematologic:* Leukocytosis, lymphocytopenia, eosinophilia. *Musculoskeletal:* Asthenia, extremity pain, arthralgia, myalgia, possibility of osteochondrosis. *Miscellaneous:* Chills, malaise, syncope, hyperglycemia or hypoglycemia, whole body pain, thirst, weight loss, photophobia, trunk pain, paresthesia, visual disturbances, hypersensitivity, hearing loss, fever.

*After ophthalmic use:* Transient ocular burning or discomfort, stinging, redness, itching, photophobia, tearing, and dryness.

**Drug Interactions**
*Antacids* / ↓ Effects of antacids

**How Supplied:** *Injection:* 4 mg/mL, 20 mg/mL, 40 mg/mL; *Ophthalmic solution:* 0.3%; *Tablet:* 200 mg, 300 mg, 400 mg

**Dosage** ———————————
• **Tablets, IV**
*Pneumonia, exacerbation of chronic bronchitis.*
400 mg q 12 hr for 10 days.
*Acute uncomplicated gonorrhea.*
One 400-mg dose. The Centers for Disease Control also recommend adding doxycycline.
*Cervicitis/urethritis due to* C. trachomatis *or* N. gonorrhoeae.
300 mg q 12 hr for 7 days.
*Mild to moderate skin and skin structure infections.*
400 mg q 12 hr for 10 days.
*Cystitis due to* E. coli *or* K. pneumoniae.
200 mg q 12 hr for 3 days.
*Cystitis due to other organisms.*
200 mg q 12 hr for 7 days.
*Complicated UTIs.*
200 mg q 12 hr for 10 days.
*Prostatitis.*
300 mg q 12 hr for 6 weeks.
*Chlamydia.*
300 mg PO b.i.d. for 7 days.
*Epididymitis.*
300 mg PO b.i.d. for 10 days.
*Pelvic inflammatory disease, outpatient.*
400 mg PO b.i.d. for 14 days.
*NOTE:* The dose should be adjusted in clients with a $C_{CR}$ of 50 mL/min

or less. If the $C_{CR}$ is 10–50 mL/min, the dosage interval should be q 24 hr, and if $C_{CR}$ is less than 10 mL/min, the dose should be half the recommended dose given q 24 hr.
• **Ophthalmic Solution (0.3%)**
*Conjunctivitis.*
**Initial:** 1–2 gtt in the affected eye(s) q 2–4 hr for the first 2 days; **then,** 1–2 gtt q.i.d. for five additional days.
• **Otic Solution (0.3%)**
*Otitis externa, otitis media.*
Apply b.i.d.

## DENTAL CONCERNS

See also *General Dental Concerns for All Anti-Infectives* and for *Fluoroquinolones.*
**General**
1. Ingestible sodium bicarbonate products (i.e., air polishing systems) can only be used 2 hours after taking ofloxacin.
2. Examine for signs and symptoms of oral fungal infections.
3. Determine why the patient is taking the medication.
4. Decreased saliva flow can put the patient at risk for dental caries, periodontal disease, and candidiasis.
**Consultation with Primary Care Provider**
1. Consult with the patient's health care provider if an acute dental infection occurs and the patient requires another anti-infective.
**Client/Family Teaching**
1. Review the importance of good oral hygiene in order to prevent soft tissue inflammation.
2. Daily home fluoride treatments for persistent dry mouth.
3. Avoid alcohol-containing mouth rinses and beverages.
4. Avoid caffeine-containing beverages.
5. Dry mouth can be treated with tart, sugarless gum or candy, water, sugar-free beverages, or with saliva substitutes if dry mouth persists.
6. Patient may want to wear dark glasses in order to avoid photophobia, which can occur with the dental light.
7. Avoid direct sunlight, as a photo-

sensitivity reaction may occur. If exposed, wear sunglasses, protective clothing, and sunscreen.

8. Discontinue treatment and inform dentist immediately if the patient experiences pain or inflammation in his or her tendons. Rest and avoid exercise.

# Olanzapine
(oh-**LAN**-zah-peen)
**Pregnancy Category:** C
Zyprexa **(Rx)**
**Classification:** Antipsychotic agent, miscellaneous

**Action/Kinetics:** A thienobenzodiazepine antipsychotic believed to act by antagonizing dopamine $D_{1-4}$ and serotonin ($5HT_2$) receptors. Also binds to muscarinic, histamine $H_{1,}$ and alpha-1 adrenergic receptors, which can explain many of the side effects. Well absorbed from the GI tract. **Peak plasma levels:** 6 hr after PO dosing. Undergoes significant first-pass metabolism with about 40% metabolized before it reaches the systemic circulation. Food does not affect the rate or extent of absorption. Significantly bound to plasma proteins. Unchanged drug and metabolites are excreted through both the urine and feces.

**Uses:** Management of psychotic disorders.

**Contraindications:** Lactation.

**Special Concerns:** Use with caution in geriatric clients, as the drug may be excreted more slowly in this population. Use with caution in impaired hepatic function. Use care in giving olanzapine to those where there is a chance of increased core body temperature (e.g., strenuous exercise, exposure to extreme heat, concomitant anticholinergic drug administration, dehydration). Due to anticholinergic side effects, use with caution in clients with significant prostatic hypertrophy, narrow-angle glaucoma, or a history of paralytic ileus. Safety and efficacy have not

been determined in children less than 18 years of age.

**Side Effects:** *Neuroleptic malignant syndrome:* Hyperpyrexia, muscle rigidity, altered mental status, irregular pulse or BP, tachycardia, diaphoresis, cardiac dysrhythmia, rhabdomyolysis, *acute renal failure, death. Oral:* Dry mouth, increased salivation, aphthous stomatitis, gingivitis, glossitis, mouth ulceration, oral moniliasis, periodontal abscess, tongue edema. *GI:* Dysphagia, constipation, increased appetite, N&V, thirst, eructation, esophagitis, rectal incontinence, flatulence, gastritis, gastroenteritis, hepatitis, melena, *rectal hemorrhage,. CNS:* Tardive dyskinesia, seizures, somnolence, agitation, insomnia, nervousness, hostility, dizziness, anxiety, personality disorder, akathisia, hypertonia, tremor, amnesia, impaired articulation, euphoria, stuttering, *suicide,* abnormal gait, alcohol misuse, antisocial reaction, ataxia, CNS stimulation, coma, delirium, depersonalization, hypesthesia, hypotonia, incoordination, decreased libido, obsessive-compulsive symptoms, phobias, somatization, stimulant misuse, stupor, vertigo, withdrawal syndrome. *CV:* Tachycardia, orthostatic/postural hypotension, hypotension, *CVA, hemorrhage, heart arrest,* migraine, palpitation, vasodilation, ventricular extrasystoles. *Body as a whole:* Headache, fever, abdominal pain, chest pain, neck rigidity, intentional injury, flu syndrome, chills, facial edema, hangover effect, malaise, moniliasis, neck pain, pelvic pain, photosensitivity. *Respiratory:* Rhinitis, increased cough, pharyngitis, dyspnea, apnea, asthma, epistaxis, hemoptysis, hyperventilation, voice alteration. *GU:* Premenstrual syndrome, hematuria, metrorrhagia, urinary incontinence, UTI, abnormal ejaculation, amenorrhea, breast pain, cystitis, decreased or increased menstruation, dysuria, female lactation, impotence, menorrhagia, polyuria, pyuria, urinary retention, urinary frequency, impaired urination, enlarged uterine fibroids. *Hematologic:* Leukocytosis, lymphadenopathy, thrombocytopenia. *Metabolic/nutritional:* Weight gain or loss, peripheral edema, lower extremity edema, dehydration, hyperglycemia, hyperkalemia, hyperuricemia, hypoglycemia, hypokalemia, hyponatremia, ketosis, water intoxication. *Musculoskeletal:* Joint pain, extremity pain, twitching, arthritis, back and hip pain, bursitis, leg cramps, myasthenia, rheumatoid arthritis. *Dermatologic:* Vesiculobullous rash, alopecia, contact dermatitis, dry skin, eczema, hirsutism, seborrhea, skin ulcer, urticaria. *Ophthalmic:* Amblyopia, blepharitis, corneal lesion, cataract, diplopia, dry eyes, eye hemorrhage, eye inflammation, eye pain, ocular muscle abnormality. *Otic:* Deafness, ear pain, tinnitus. *Miscellaneous:* Diabetes mellitus, goiter, cyanosis, taste perversion.

**Drug Interactions**
*Carbamazepine* / ↑ Clearance of olanzepine due to ↑ rate of metabolism
*CNS depressants* / ↑ Effect of CNS depressants
**How Supplied:** *Tablet:* 5 mg, 7.5 mg, 10 mg

**Dosage** ————————
• **Tablets**
  *Psychoses.*
**Adults, initial:** 5–10 mg once daily without regard to meals. Goal is 10 mg daily; increments to reach 10 mg can be in 5-mg amounts but at an interval of 1 week. Doses higher than 10 mg daily are recommended only after clinical assessment and should not be greater than 20 mg/day. The recommended initial dose is 5 mg in those who are debilitated, who have a predisposition to hypotensive reactions, who may have factors that cause a slower metabolism of olanzapine (e.g., nonsmoking female clients over 65 years of age), or who may be more sensitive to the drug. It is recommended that clients who respond to the drug be continued on it at the lowest possible dose to maintain remission

with periodic evaluation to determine continued need for the drug.

**DENTAL CONCERNS**

See also *Dental Concerns* for *Antipsychotic Agents, Phenothiazines.*

# Olopatadine hydrochloride
(oh-loh-pah-**TIH**-deen)
**Pregnancy Category:** C
Patanol **(Rx)**
**Classification:** Antihistamine, ophthalmic

See also *Antihistamines.*
**Action/Kinetics:** Selective histamine H-1 receptor antagonist. Little is absorbed into the systemic circulation.
**Uses:** Prevention of itching in allergic conjunctivitis.
**Contraindications:** Not to be injected. Not to be instilled while the client is wearing contact lenses.
**Special Concerns:** Use with caution during lactation. Safety and efficacy have not been determined for children less than 3 years of age.
**Side Effects:** *Ophthalmic:* Burning or stinging, dry eye, foreign body sensation, hyperemia, keratitis, lid edema, pruritus. *Nose/throat:* Pharyngitis, rhinitis, sinusitis. *Oral:* Taste perversion. *Miscellaneous:* Headache, asthenia, cold syndrome.
**Drug Interactions:** None reported.
**How Supplied:** *Solution:* 0.1% Solution in a 5–mL drop dispenser

**Dosage** ————————
• **Solution (0.1%)**
  *Allergic conjunctivitis.*
**Adults and children over 3 years of age:** 1–2 gtt in each affected eye b.i.d. at an interval of 6–8 hr.

**DENTAL CONCERNS**
1. Protective eye coverings may be necessary during dental treatment.

# Omeprazole
(oh-**MEH**-prah-zohl)
**Pregnancy Category:** C

Losec ✿, Prilosec **(Rx)**
**Classification:** Agent to suppress gastric acid secretion

**Action/Kinetics:** Thought to be a gastric pump inhibitor in that it blocks the final step of acid production by inhibiting the $H^+$–$K^+$ proton ATPase system at the secretory surface of the gastric parietal cell. Both basal and stimulated acid secretions are inhibited. Serum gastrin levels are increased during the first 1 or 2 weeks of therapy and are maintained at such levels during the course of therapy. Because omeprazole is acid-labile, the product contains an enteric-coated granule formulation; however, absorption is rapid. **Peak plasma levels:** 0.5–3.5 hr. **Onset:** Within 1 hr. **t½:** 0.5–1 hr. **Duration:** Up to 72 hr (due to prolonged binding of the drug to the parietal $II^+$–$K^+$; ATPase enzyme). Significantly bound (95%) to plasma protein. Metabolized in the liver and inactive metabolites are excreted through the urine. Consider dosage adjustment in Asians.

**Uses:** Short-term (4- to 8-week) treatment of active duodenal ulcer, active benign gastric ulcer, erosive esophagitis (all grades), and heartburn and other symptoms associated with GERD. In combination with clarithromycin for eradication of *Helicobacter pylori* and active duodenal ulcer. Long-term maintenance therapy for healed erosive esophagitis. Long-term treatment of pathologic hypersecretory conditions such as Zollinger-Ellison syndrome, multiple endocrine adenomas, and systemic mastocytosis. *Non-FDA Approved Uses:* In combination with amoxicillin for eradication of *H.* pylori.

**Contraindications:** Lactation. Use as maintenance therapy for duodenal ulcer disease.

**Special Concerns:** Bioavailability may be increased in geriatric clients. Use with caution during lactation. Symptomatic effects with omeprazole do not preclude gastric malignan-cy. Safety and effectiveness have not been determined in children.

**Side Effects:** *CNS:* Headache, dizziness. Possibly, anxiety disorders, abnormal dreams, vertigo, insomnia, nervousness, apathy, paresthesia, somnolence, depression, aggression, hallucinations, hemifacial dysesthesia, tremors, confusion. *Oral:* Dry mouth, mucosal atrophy of the tongue, taste perversion, candidiasis. *GI:* Diarrhea, N&V, abdominal pain, abdominal swelling, constipation, flatulence, anorexia, fecal discoloration, esophageal candidiasis, irritable colon, gastric fundic gland polyps, gastroduodenal carcinoids. *Hepatic:* **Pancreatitis.** Overt liver disease, including hepatocellular, cholestatic, or mixed hepatitis; *liver necrosis, hepatic failure,* hepatic encephalopathy. *CV:* Angina, chest pain, tachycardia, bradycardia, palpitation, peripheral edema, elevated BP. *Respiratory:* Upper respiratory infection, pharyngeal pain, bronchospasms, cough, epistaxis. *Dermatologic:* Rash, severe generalized skin reaction including *toxic epidermal necrolysis, Stevens-Johnson syndrome;* erythema multiforme, skin inflammation, urticaria, pruritus, alopecia, dry skin, hyperhidrosis. *GU:* UTI, acute interstitial nephritis, urinary frequency, hematuria, proteinuria, glycosuria, testicular pain, microscopic pyuria, gynecomastia. *Hematologic:* Pancytopenia, thrombocytopenia, anemia, leukocytosis, neutropenia, hemolytic anemia, *agranulocytosis. Musculoskeletal:* Asthenia, back pain, myalgia, joint pain, muscle cramps, muscle weakness, leg pain. *Miscellaneous:* Rash, angioedema, fever, pain, gout, fatigue, malaise, weight gain, tinnitus, alteration in taste.

When used with clarithromycin the following *additional* side effects were noted: Tongue discoloration, rhinitis, pharyngitis, and flu syndrome.

*NOTE:* Data are lacking on the effect of long-term hypochlorhydria and hypergastrinemia on the risk of developing tumors.

**Drug Interactions**

*Ampicillin (esters)* / Possible ↓ absorption of ampicillin esters due to ↑ pH of stomach

*Diazepam* / ↑ Plasma levels of diazepam due to ↓ rate of metabolism by the liver

*Ketoconazole* / Possible ↓ absorption of ketoconazole due to ↑ pH of stomach

*Phenytoin* / ↑ Plasma levels of phenytoin due to ↓ rate of metabolism of the liver

**How Supplied:** *Enteric coated capsule:* 10 mg, 20 mg

**Dosage** ─────────────
• **Capsules, Eneric-Coated**
*Active duodenal ulcer.*
**Adults,** 20 mg/day for 4–8 weeks.
*Erosive esophagitis, heartburn, symptoms associated with GERD.*
**Adults:** 20 mg/day for 4–8 weeks.
**Maintenance of healing erosive esophagitis:** 20 mg daily.
*Treatment of* H. pylori, *reduction of risk of duodenal ulcer recurrence.*
**Days 1–14:** Omeprazole, 40 mg daily in the morning, plus clarithromycin, 500 mg t.i.d. Days **15–28:** Omeprazole, 20 mg daily.
*Pathologic hypersecretory conditions.*
**Adults, initial**: 60 mg/day; **then,** dose individualized although doses up to 120 mg t.i.d. have been used. Daily doses > 80 mg should be divided.
*Gastric ulcers.*
**Adults:** 40 mg once daily for 4–8 weeks.

## DENTAL CONCERNS
**General**
1. A semisupine position for the dental chair may be necessary to help minimize or avoid GI effects of the disease.
2. Determine the patient's ability to tolerate aspirin or NSAID-related products.
3. Decreased saliva flow can put the patient at risk for dental caries, periodontal disease, and candidiasis.

**Client/Family Teaching**
1. Review the importance of good oral hygiene in order to prevent soft tissue inflammation.
2. Review the proper use of oral hygiene aids in order to prevent injury.
3. Daily home fluoride treatments for persistent dry mouth.
4. Avoid alcohol-containing mouth rinses and beverages.
5. Avoid caffeine-containing beverages.
6. Dry mouth can be treated with tart, sugarless gum or candy, water, sugar-free beverages, or with saliva substitutes if dry mouth persists.

# Oxaprozin
(**ox**-ah-**PROH**-zin)
**Pregnancy Category:** C
Daypro **(Rx)**
**Classification:** Nonsteroidal anti-inflammatory drug

See also *Nonsteroidal Anti-Inflammatory Drugs.*

**Uses:** Acute and chronic use to manage rheumatoid arthritis and osteoarthritis.

**How Supplied:** *Tablet:* 600 mg

**Dosage** ─────────────
• **Tablets**
*Rheumatoid arthritis.*
**Adults:** 1,200 mg once daily. Lower and higher doses may be required in certain clients.
*Osteoarthritis.*
**Adults:** 1,200 mg once daily. For clients with a lower body weight or with a milder disease, 600 mg/day may be appropriate.
The maximum daily use for either rheumatoid arthritis or osteoarthritis is 1,800 mg (or 26 mg/kg, whichever is lower) given in divided doses.

## DENTAL CONCERNS

See also *Dental Concerns* for *Nonsteroidal Anti-Inflammatory Drugs.*

─────COMBINATION DRUG─────

# Oxycodone and Acetaminophen
(ox-ee-**KOH**-dohn, ah-**SEAT**-ah-**MIN**-oh-fen)

**Pregnancy Category:** C
Endocet, Oxycocet ✹, Percocet ✹,
Percocet-Demi ✹, Roxicet **(C-II) (Rx)**
**Classification:** Analgesic

See also *Acetaminophen* and *Opioid Analgesics*.
**Content: Endocet and Roxicet Tablets:** *Opioid analgesic:* Oxycodone hydrochloride, 5 mg. *Analgesic:* Acetaminophen, 325 mg. **Roxicet Oral Solution:** *Opioid analgesic:* Oxycodone hydrochloride, 5 mg/5 mL. *Analgesic:* Acetaminophen, 325 mg/5 mL.
**Uses:** Relief of moderate to moderately severe pain.
**Contraindications:** Hypersensitivity to either oxycodone or acetaminophen.
**Special Concerns:** Can produce drug dependence and has abuse potential. The respiratory depressant effects of oxycodone can be exaggerated in clients with head injury, other intracranial lesions, or a preexisting increase in intracranial pressure. Use with caution in clients who are elderly, are debilitated, have severely impaired hepatic or renal function, are hyperthyroid, have Addison's disease, have prostatic hypertrophy, or have urethral stricture. Use for acute abdominal conditions may obscure the diagnosis or clinical course. Use with caution during lactation. Safety and efficacy in children have not been established.
**Side Effects:** Commonly, dizziness, lightheadedness, N&V, and sedation; these effects are more common in ambulatory clients than nonambulatory clients. Other side effects include euphoria, dysphoria, constipation, skin rash, and pruritus. See also individual components.
**Drug Interactions**
*Anticholinergic drugs* / Production of paralytic ileus
*Antidepressants, tricyclic* / ↑ Effect of either the tricyclic antidepressant or oxycodone
*CNS depressants (including other opioid analgesics, phenothiazines, antianxiety drugs, sedative-hypnotics, anesthetics, alcohol)* / Additive CNS depression
*MAO inhibitors* / ↑ Effect of either the MAO inhibitor or oxycodone

**Dosage**
• **Oral Solution, Tablets**
    *Analgesic.*
**Adults:** 5 mL of the oral solution q 6 hr or 1 tablet q 6 hr as needed for pain.

**DENTAL CONCERNS**

See also *Dental Concerns* for *Opioid Analgesics* and *Acetaminophen*.

**P**

# Paclitaxel
(**PACK**-lih-**tax**-el)
**Pregnancy Category:** D
Taxol **(Rx)**
**Classification:** Antineoplastic, miscellaneous

See also *Antineoplastic Agents*.
**Action/Kinetics:** Naturally occurring antineoplastic agent that promotes the assembly of microtubules from tubulin dimers and stabilizes microtubules by preventing depolymerization. The stabilization results in the inhibition of the normal dynamic reorganization of the microtubule network that is required for vital interphase and mitotic cellular functions. Also induces abnormal "bundles" of microtubules throughout the cell cycle and multiple esters of microtubules during mitosis. Following IV administration, there is a biphasic decline in plasma levels. The

initial rapid decline is due to distribution to the peripheral compartment and significant elimination, whereas the second phase is due, in part, to a slow efflux of the drug from the peripheral compartment. Metabolized by the liver with small amounts of unchanged drug excreted in the urine.

**Uses:** Metastatic carcinoma of the ovary after failure of first-line or subsequent chemotherapy. Breast cancer after combination chemotherapy has failed or there has been relapse within 6 months of adjuvant chemotherapy (prior therapy must have included an anthracycline unless contraindicated). Second-line treatment of AIDS-related Kaposi's sarcoma. *Non-FDA Approved Uses:* Alone or in combination with other chemotherapeutic drugs for advanced head and neck cancer, previously untreated extensive-stage small-cell lung cancer, adenocarcinoma of the upper GI tract, hormone-refractory prostate cancer, advanced non-small-cell lung cancer, and leukemias.

**Contraindications:** Hypersensitivity to paclitaxel, in those with a hypersensitivity to products containing polyoxyethylated castor oil (Cremophor EL), clients with a baseline neutropenia below 1,500 cells/mm³, and those with AIDS-related Kaposi's sarcoma with baseline neutrophil counts below 1,000 cells/mm³. Lactation.

**Special Concerns:** Use with caution in clients with impaired hepatic function. Safety and efficacy have not been determined in children.

**Side Effects:** *Hypersensitivity reactions:* Severe symptoms usually occur during the first hour of therapy and occur during both the first or second course of therapy despite premedication. Severe symptoms include *dyspnea, angioedema,* hypotension, or generalized urticaria all of which require immediate cessation of the drug and aggressive treatment therapy. Symptoms not requiring treatment include milder dyspnea, flushing, skin reactions, hypotension, or tachycardia. *Hematologic:* Neutropenia and leukopenia (common),

thrombocytopenia, anemia, infections, bleeding, packed cell transfusions, platelet transfusions. *CV:* Bradycardia and hypotension (including during the infusion), hypertension, *severe CV events (including asymptomatic ventricular tachycardia, bigeminy, syncope, complete AV block),* abnormal ECG (including nonspecific repolarization abnormalities, sinus tachycardia, premature beats). *Musculoskeletal:* Peripheral neuropathy (including mild paresthesia), myalgia, arthralgia. *Oral:* Mucositis. *GI:* N&V, diarrhea. *Miscellaneous:* Alopecia, fever associated with severe neutropenia; infections of the urinary tract and upper respiratory tract as well as *sepsis due to neutropenia.*

**Drug Interactions**
*Ketoconazole* / Inhibition of metabolism of paclitaxel by ketoconazole

**How Supplied:** *Injection:* 6 mg/mL

**Dosage** ─────────────
• **IV Infusion**
*Metastatic carcinoma of the ovary.*
**Adults:** 135 mg/m² given IV over 3 hr q 3 weeks after failure of first-line or subsequent chemotherapy.
*Metastatic breast cancer.*
**Adults:** 175 mg/m² given IV over 3 hr q 3 weeks after failure of chemotherapy for metastatic disease or relapse within 6 months of adjuvant chemotherapy.
*AIDS-related Kaposi's sarcoma.*
135 mg/m² given IV over 3 hr q 3 weeks or 100 mg/m² given IV over 3 hr q 2 weeks.

## DENTAL CONCERNS

See also *Dental Concerns* for *Antineoplastic Agents.*

# Paroxetine hydrochloride
(pah-**ROX**-eh-teen)
**Pregnancy Category:** B
Paxil **(Rx)**
**Classification:** Antidepressant, selective serotonin reuptake inhibitor

**Action/Kinetics:** Inhibits neuronal reuptake of serotonin in the CNS resulting in potentiation of serotonergic activity in the CNS. It appears to have weak effects on neuronal uptake of norepinephrine and dopamine. Has no anticholinergic effects, does not cause orthostatic hypotension, produces a slight sedative effect. Completely absorbed from the GI tract. **Time to peak plasma levels:** 5.2 hr. **Peak plasma levels:** 61.7 ng/mL. **t½:** 21 hr. **Time to reach steady state:** About 10 days. Plasma levels are increased in impaired renal and hepatic function as well as in geriatric clients. Extensively metabolized in the liver to inactive metabolites. Approximately two-thirds of the drug is excreted through the urine and one-third is excreted in the feces.

**Uses:** Treatment of major depressive episodes, panic disorder with or without agoraphobia (as defined in DSM-IV), and obsessive-compulsive disorders (as defined in DSM-III-R). *Non-FDA Approved Uses:* Headaches, diabetic neuropathy, premature ejaculation.

**Contraindications:** Use in clients taking MAO inhibitors. Use of alcohol.

**Special Concerns:** Use with caution and initially at reduced dosage in elderly clients as well as in those with impaired hepatic or renal function, with a history of mania, with a history of seizures, in clients with diseases or conditions that could affect metabolism or hemodynamic responses, and during lactation. Concurrent administration of paroxetine with lithium or digoxin should be undertaken with caution. Safety and efficacy have not been determined in children.

**Side Effects:** The side effects listed were observed with a frequency up to 1 in 1,000 clients.

*CNS:* Headache, somnolence, insomnia, agitation, **seizures,** tremor, anxiety, activation of mania or hypomania, dizziness, nervousness, paresthesia, drugged feeling, myoclonus, CNS stimulation, confusion, amnesia, impaired concentration, depression, emotional lability, vertigo, abnormal thinking, akinesia, alcohol abuse, ataxia, **convulsions, possibility of a suicide attempt** depersonalization, hallucinations, hyperkinesia, hypertonia, incoordination, lack of emotion, manic reaction, paranoid reaction. *Oral:* Dry mouth, dysphagia, glossitis, increased salivation, mouth ulceration. *GI:* Nausea, abdominal pain, diarrhea, vomiting, constipation, decreased appetite, flatulence, oropharynx disorder ("lump" in throat, tightness in throat), dyspepsia, increased appetite, bruxism, eructation, gastritis, **rectal hemorrhage,** abnormal LFTs. *Hematologic:* Anemia, leukopenia, lymphadenopathy, purpura. *CV:* Palpitation, vasodilation, postural hypotension, hypertension, syncope, tachycardia, bradycardia, conduction abnormalities, abnormal ECG, hypotension, migraine, peripheral vascular disorder. *Dermatologic:* Sweating, rash, pruritus, acne, alopecia, dry skin, ecchymosis, eczema, furunculosis, urticaria. *Metabolic/Nutritional:* Edema, weight gain, weight loss, hyperglycemia, peripheral edema, thirst. *Respiratory:* Respiratory disorder (cold symptoms or upper respiratory infection), pharyngitis, yawn, increased cough, rhinitis, asthma, bronchitis, dyspnea, epistaxis, hyperventilation, pneumonia, respiratory flu, sinusitis. *GU:* Abnormal ejaculation (usually delay), erectile difficulties, sexual dysfunction, impotence, urinary frequency, urinary difficulty or hesitancy, decreased libido, anorgasmia in women, difficulty in reaching climax/orgasm in women, abortion, amenorrhea, breast pain, cystitis, dysmenorrhea, dysuria, menorrhagia, nocturia, polyuria, urethritis, urinary incontinence, urinary retention, vaginitis. *Musculoskeletal:* Asthenia, back pain, myopathy, myalgia, myasthenia, neck pain, arthralgia, arthritis. *Ophthalmologic:* Blurred vision, abnormality of accommodation, eye pain, mydriasis. *Otic:* Ear pain, otitis media, tinnitus. *Miscellaneous:* Fever, chest pain, trauma, taste perver-

**P**

sion or loss, chills, malaise, allergic re-action, **carcinoma,** face edema, mon-iliasis, anorexia.

*NOTE:* Over 4- to 6-week period, there was evidence of adaptation to side effects such as nausea and dizzi-ness but less adaptation to dry mouth, somnolence, and asthenia.

**Drug Interactions**

*Cimetidine* / ↑ Effect of paroxetine due to ↓ breakdown by the liver

*Diazepam* / ↑ Half-life of diazepam

*MAO inhibitors* / Possibility of seri-ous, and sometimes fatal, reactions including hyperthermia, rigidity, myoclonus, autonomic instability with possible rapid fluctuations in VS, and mental status changes in-cluding extreme agitation progress-ing to delirium and coma

*Phenobarbital* / Possible ↓ effect of paroxetine due to ↑ breakdown by the liver

*Phenytoin* / Possible ↓ effect of pa-roxetine due to ↑ breakdown by the liver; also, paroxetine ↓ levels of phenytoin

**How Supplied:** *Tablet:* 10 mg, 20 mg, 30 mg, 40 mg

**Dosage** ────────────
• **Tablets**
  *Depression.*
**Adults:** 20 mg/day, usually given as a single dose in the morning. Some clients not responding to the 20-mg dose may benefit from increasing the dose in 10-mg/day increments, up to a maximum of 50 mg/day. Dose changes should be made at intervals of at least 1 week.
  *Panic disorders.*
**Adults, initial:** 10 mg/day usually given in the morning; **then,** increase by 10-mg increments each week un-til a dose of 40 mg/day is reached. Maximum daily dose: 60 mg.
  *Obsessive-compulsive disorders.*
**Adults, initial:** 20 mg/kg; **then,** in-crease by 10-mg increments a day in intervals of at least 1 week until a dose of 40 mg/kg is reached. Maxi-mum daily dose: 60 mg.
  *Headaches.*
10–50 mg/day.
  *Diabetic neuropathy.*
10–60 mg/day.

*Premature ejaculation in men.*
20 mg/day.
*NOTE:* Geriatric or debilitated cli-ents, those with severe hepatic or re-nal impairment, **initial:** 10 mg/day, up to a maximum of 40 mg/day for all uses.

**DENTAL CONCERNS**

See also *Dental Concerns* for *Antide-pressants, Tricylic* and *Selective Se-rotonin Reuptake Inhibitors.*

# Penciclovir
(pen-**SIGH**-kloh-veer)
**Pregnancy Category:** B
Denavir **(Rx)**
**Classification:** Antiviral drug

See also *Antiviral Drugs.*
**Action/Kinetics:** Active against herpes simplex viruses (HSVs), in-cluding HSV-1 and HSV-2. In infect-ed cells penciclovir is converted to penciclovir triphosphate by cellular kinases. Penciclovir triphosphate in-hibits HSV polymerase competitively with deoxyguanosine triphosphate which inhibits herpes viral DNA syn-thesis and replication. Not absorbed through the skin.
**Uses:** Treatment of recurrent herpes labialis (cold sores) in adults.
**Contraindications:** Lactation. Ap-plication of the drug to mucous membranes.
**Special Concerns:** Use with cau-tion if applied around the eyes due to the possibility of irritation. The effect of the drug in immunocompromised clients has not been determined. Safety and efficacy have not been determined in children.
**Side Effects:** *Oral:* Taste perversion. *Dermatologic:* Reaction at the site of application, hypesthesia, local anes-thesia, erythematous rash, mild erythe-ma. *Miscellaneous:* Headache.
**How Supplied:** *Cream:* 10 mg/g.

**Dosage** ────────────
• **Cream (10 mg/g)**
  *Cold sores.*
Apply q 2 hr while awake for 4 days.

## DENTAL CONCERNS

See also *Dental Concerns* for *Antiviral Drugs.*

**General**

1. Document onset, location, description, and extent of lesions. Note frequency of occurrence and any triggers or prodrome.

2. Postpone dental treatment when active oral herpetic lesion is present.

**Client/Family Teaching**

1. Discard toothbrush or other oral hygiene products during period of infection in order to prevent reinoculation.

2. Avoid contact with mucous membranes; apply to lips and face only. Use finger cot or latex glove to help prevent herpes infection on fingers.

3. Use sunscreens and lip balms with a sunscreen when sun exposed to prevent recurrence and to diminish intensity of outbreaks.

4. Report if lesions do not improve or if a foul odor or purulent drainage appears.

# Penicillin G benzathine, parenteral

(pen-ih-**SILL**-in, **BEN**-zah-theen)

**Pregnancy Category:** B

Bicillin 1200 L-A ✦, Bicillin L-A, Megacillin Suspension ✦, Permapen **(Rx)**

**Classification:** Antibiotic, penicillin

See also *Anti-Infectives* and *Penicillins.*

**Action/Kinetics:** Penicillin G is neither penicillinase resistant nor acid stable. The product is a long-acting (repository) form of penicillin in an aqueous vehicle; it is administered as a sterile suspension. **Peak plasma levels: IM** 0.03–0.05 unit/mL.

**Uses:** Most gram-positive (streptococci, staphylococci, pneumococci) and some gram-negative (gonococci, meningococci) organisms. Syphilis. Prophylaxis of glomerulonephritis and rheumatic fever. Surgical infec-

tions, secondary infections following tooth extraction, tonsillectomy.

**Contraindications:** Hypersensitivity to penicillins.

**Special Concerns:** Hypersensitivity to cephalosporins.

**Side Effects:** See also *Anti-Infectives* and *Penicillins.*

**Drug Interactions:** See also *Anti-Infectives* and *Penicillins.*

*Aspirin* / ↑ Penicillin concentrations

*Probenecid* / ↑ Penicillin concentrations

**How Supplied:** *Injection:* 300,000 U/mL, 600,000 U/mL

## Dosage

• **Parenteral Suspension (IM Only)**

*Upper respiratory tract infections, erysipeloid, yaws.*

**Adults:** 1,200,000 units as a single dose; **older children:** 900,000 units as a single dose; **children under 27 kg:** 300,000–600,000 units as a single dose; **neonates:** 50,000 units/kg as a single dose.

*Early syphilis.*

**Adults:** 2,400,000 units as a single dose.

*Late syphilis.*

**Adults:** 2,400,000 units q 7 days for 3 weeks.

*Neurosyphilis.*

**Adults:** Penicillin G, 12,000,000–24,000,000 units IV/day for 10–14 days followed by penicillin G benzathine, 2,400,000 units IM q week for 3 weeks.

*Congenital syphilis, older children.*

50,000 units/kg IM (up to adult dose of 2,400,000 units).

*Prophylaxis of rheumatic fever.*

**Adults and children over 27.3 kg:** 1,200,000 units/ q 4 weeks; **children and infants less than 27.3 kg:** 50,000 units/kg as a single dose.

## DENTAL CONCERNS

See also *Dental Concerns* for *Penicillins.*

**P**

# Penicillin V potassium (Phenoxymethyl-penicillin potassium)

(pen-ih-**SILL**-in )
**Pregnancy Category:** B
Apo-Pen-VK ✿, Beepen-VK, Betapen-VK, Ledercillin VK, Nadopen-V ✿, Novo–Pen-VK ✿, Nu-Pen-VK ✿, Penicillin VK, Pen-V, Pen-Vee K, PVF K ✿, Robicillin VK, V-Cillin K, Veetids 125, 250, and 500 **(Rx)**
**Classification:** Antibiotic, penicillin

See also *Anti-Infectives* and *Penicillins.*

**Action/Kinetics:** Related closely to penicillin G. Products are not penicillinase resistant but are acid stable and resist inactivation by gastric secretions. Well absorbed from the GI tract and not affected by foods. **Peak plasma levels:** Penicillin V, **PO:** 2.7 mcg/mL after 30–60 min; penicillin V potassium, **PO:** 1–9 mcg/mL after 30–60 min. **t½:** 30 min. Periodic blood counts and renal function tests are indicated during long-term usage.

**Uses:** Penicillin-sensitive staphylococci, pneumococci, streptococci, gonococci. Vincent's infection of the oropharynx. Lyme disease. **Prophylaxis:** Rheumatic fever, chorea, bacterial endocarditis, pre- and postsurgery. Should *not* be used as prophylaxis for GU instrumentation or surgery, sigmoidoscopy, or childbirth or during the acute stage of severe pneumonia, bacteremia, arthritis, empyema, pericarditis, and meningitis. Penicillin G, IV, should be used for treating neurologic complications due to Lyme disease.

**Contraindications:** Hypersensitivity to penicillins.

**Special Concerns:** More and more strains of staphylococci are resistant to penicillin V, necessitating culture and sensitivity studies. Hypersensitivity to cephalosporins.

**Side Effects:** See also *Anti-Infectives* and *Penicillins.*

**Drug Interactions:** See also *Anti-Infectives* and *Penicillins.*

*Probenecid* / ↑ Penicillin concentrations

**Additional Drug Interactions**
*Contraceptives, oral* / ↓ Effectiveness of oral contraceptives
*Neomycin, oral* / ↓ Absorption of penicillin V

**How Supplied:** *Powder for reconstitution:* 125 mg/5 mL, 250 mg/5 mL; *Tablet:* 250 mg, 500 mg

## Dosage

• **Oral Solution, Tablets**
*Streptococcal infections.*
**Adults and children over 12 years:** 125–250 mg q 6–8 hr for 10 days. **Children, usual:** 25–50 mg/kg/day in divided doses q 6–8 hr.

*Pneumococcal or staphylococcal infections, fusospirochetosis of oropharynx.*
**Adults and children over 12 years:** 250–500 mg q 6–8 hr.

*Prophylaxis of rheumatic fever/chorea.*
125–250 mg b.i.d.

*Prophylaxis of bacterial endocarditis.*
**Adults and children over 27 kg:** 2 g 30–60 min prior to procedure; **then,** 1 g q 6 hr. **Pediatric:** 1 g 30–60 min prior to procedure; **then,** 500 mg/ q 6 hr.

*Anaerobic infections.*
250 mg q.i.d. See also *Penicillin G, Procaine, Aqueous, Sterile.*

*Prophylaxis of septicemia caused by* Staphylococcus pneumoniae *in children with sickle cell anemia.*
125 mg b.i.d.

*Streptococcal pharyngitis in children.*
250 mg b.i.d. for 10 days.

*Streptococcal otitis media and sinusitis.*
250–500 mg q 6 hr for 14 days.

*Lyme disease.*
250–500 mg q.i.d. for 10–20 days (for children less than 2 years of age, 50 mg/kg/day in four divided doses for 10–20 days).

*NOTE:* 250 mg penicillin V is equivalent to 400,000 units.

*Vincent's infection of the oropharynx.*
250 mg to 500 mg q 6 to 8 hr.

## DENTAL CONCERNS

See also *Dental Concerns* for *Penicillins.*

### Client/Family Teaching

1. Clients with a history of rheumatic fever or congenital heart disease need to use and understand the importance of antibiotic prophylaxis prior to any invasive medical or dental procedure.
2. Report if throat and/or ear symptoms do not improve after 48 hr of therapy; may need to reevaluate and alter therapy.
3. With oral administration, if a reaction is going to occur, you usually see it after the second dose. Seek medical intervention immediately if respiratory distress or skin wheals appear.
4. Use an additional nonhormonal form of birth control if taking oral contraceptives because their effectiveness may be diminished.

---

# Pentobarbital

(pen-toe-**BAR**-bih-tal)
**Pregnancy Category:** D
Nembutal **(C-II) (Rx)**

# Pentobarbital sodium

(pen-toe-**BAR**-bih-tal)
**Pregnancy Category:** D
Nembutal Sodium, Nova-Rectal ✦,
Novo-Pentobarb ✦ **(C-II) (Rx)**
**Classification:** Sedative-hypnotic,
barbiturate type

---

See also *Barbiturates.*
**Action/Kinetics:** Short-acting. **t½:**
19–34 hr. Is 60%–70% protein bound.
**Uses: PO:** Sedative. Short-term treatment of insomnia (no more than 2 weeks). Preanesthetic. **Rectal:** Sedation, short-term treatment of insomnia (no more than 2 weeks). **Parenteral:** Short-term treatment of insomnia (no more than 2 weeks). Preanes-

thetic. Anticonvulsant in anesthetic doses for emergency treatment of acute convulsive states (e.g., status epilepticus, eclampsia, meningitis, tetanus, and toxic reactions to strychnine or local anesthetics). *Non-FDA Approved Uses:* Parenterally to induce coma to protect the brain from ischemia and increased ICP following stroke and head trauma.
**Special Concerns:** Dosage should be reduced in geriatric and debilitated clients and in those with impaired hepatic or renal function.
**How Supplied:** Pentobarbital: *Elixir:* 18.2 mg/5 mL. Pentobarbital sodium: *Capsule:* 50 mg, 100 mg; *Injection:* 50 mg/mL; *Suppository:* 30 mg, 60 mg, 120 mg, 200 mg

### Dosage

- **Capsules**
  *Sedation.*
  **Adults:** 20 mg t.i.d.–q.i.d. **Pediatric:** 2–6 mg/kg/day, depending on age, weight, and degree of sedation desired.
  *Preoperative sedation.*
  **Adults:** 100 mg. **Pediatric:** 2–6 mg/kg/day (maximum of 100 mg), depending on age, weight, and degree of sedation desired.
  *Hypnotic.*
  **Adults:** 100 mg at bedtime.
- **Suppositories, Rectal**
  *Hypnotic.*
  **Adults:** 120–200 mg at bedtime; **infants, 2–12 months (4.5–9 kg):** 30 mg; **1–4 years (9–18.2 kg):** 30 or 60 mg; **5–12 years (18.2–36.4 kg):** 60 mg; **12–14 years (36.4–50 kg):** 60 or 120 mg.
- **IM**
  *Hypnotic/preoperative sedation.*
  **Adults:** 150–200 mg; **pediatric:** 2–6 mg/kg (not to exceed 100 mg).
  *Anticonvulsant.*
  **Pediatric, initially:** 50 mg; **then,** after 1 min, additional small doses may be given, if needed, until the desired effect is achieved.
- **IV**
  *Sedative/hypnotic.*

**P**

---

**Adults:** 100 mg followed in 1 min by additional small doses, if required, up to a total of 500 mg.
*Anticonvulsant.*
**Adults, initial:** 100 mg; **then,** after 1 min, additional small doses may be given, if needed, up to a total of 500 mg. **Pediatric, initially:** 50 mg; **then,** after 1 min, additional small doses may be given, if needed, until the desired effect is achieved.

## DENTAL CONCERNS

See also *Dental Concerns* for *Barbiturates.*
**Client/Family Teaching**
1. Drug may cause drowsiness and morning-after "hangover."
2. Avoid alcohol or any other CNS depressants.
3. With insomnia, drug is for short-term use only; with long-term use one can experience rebound insomnia.

# Pergolide mesylate

(**PER**-go-lyd)
**Pregnancy Category:** B
Permax **(Rx)**
**Classification:** Antiparkinson agent

See also *Antiparkinson Agents.*
**Action/Kinetics:** Potent dopamine receptor (both $D_1$ and $D_2$) agonist. About 90% of the drug is bound to plasma proteins. Metabolized in the liver and excreted through the urine.
**Uses:** Adjunctive treatment to levodopa/carbidopa in Parkinson's disease.
**Contraindications:** Hypersensitivity to pergolide or ergot derivatives.
**Special Concerns:** Use with caution during lactation and in clients prone to cardiac dysrhythmias, preexisting dyskinesia, and preexisting states of confusion or hallucinations. Safety and efficacy have not been determined in children.
**Side Effects:** The most common side effects are listed. *CV:* Postural hypotension, palpitation, vasodilation, syncope, hypotension, hypertension, **arrhythmias, MI.** *Oral:* Dry mouth, sialadenitis, aphthous stomatitis, taste alteration. *GI:* Nausea (common), vomiting, diarrhea, constipation, dyspepsia, anorexia. *CNS:* Dyskinesia (common), dizziness, dystonia, hallucinations, confusion, insomnia, somnolence, anxiety, tremor, depression, abnormal dreams, psychosis, personality disorder, extrapyramidal syndrome, akathisia, paresthesia, incoordination, akinesia, neuralgia, hypertonia, speech disorders. *Musculoskeletal:* Arthralgia, bursitis, twitching, myalgia. *Respiratory:* Rhinitis, dyspnea, hiccup, epistaxis. *Dermatologic:* Sweating, rash. *Ophthalmologic:* Abnormal vision, double vision, eye disorders. *GU:* UTI, urinary frequency, hematuria. *Whole body:* Pain in chest, abdomen, neck, or back; headache, asthenia, flu syndrome, chills, facial edema, infection. *Miscellaneous:* Peripheral edema, anemia, weight gain.
**Drug Interactions**
*Butyrophenones* / ↓ Effect of pergolide due to dopamine antagonist effect
*Metoclopramide* / ↓ Effect of pergolide due to dopamine antagonist effect
*Phenothiazines* / ↓ Effect of pergolide due to dopamine antagonist effect
*Thioxanthines* / ↓ Effect of pergolide due to dopamine antagonist effect
**How Supplied:** *Tablet:* 0.05 mg, 0.25 mg, 1 mg

## Dosage

• **Tablets**
*Parkinsonism.*
**Adults, initial:** 0.05 mg/day for the first 2 days; **then,** increase dose gradually by 0.1 or 0.15 mg/day every third day over the next 12 days. The dosage may then be increased by 0.25 mg/day every third day until the therapeutic dosage level is reached. The mean therapeutic daily dosage is 3 mg used concurrently with levodopa/carbidopa (expressed as levodopa) at a dose of 650 mg/day. The effectiveness of doses of pergolide greater than 5 mg/day has not been evaluated.

## DENTAL CONCERNS
### General
1. Monitor vital signs at every appointment because of cardiovascular side effects.
2. Have the patient sit up slowly and remain seated for at least two minutes after being supine in order to minimize the risk of orthostatic hypotension.
3. Decreased saliva flow can put the patient at risk for dental caries, periodontal disease, and candidiasis.
4. Shorter appointments may be necessary because of the effects of Parkinson's disease on muscle.
5. Determine the presence of movement disorders such as extrapyramidal symptoms, tardive dyskinesia, or akathesia. They may interfere with the ability of the patient to perform oral health care or they can complicate dental treatment.
6. A semisupine position for the dental chair may be necessary to help minimize or avoid GI adverse effects.

### Consultation with Primary Care Provider
1. Consultation may be required in order to assess the extent of disease control.

### Client/Family Teaching
1. Daily home fluoride treatments for persistent dry mouth.
2. Avoid alcohol-containing mouth rinses and beverages.
3. Avoid caffeine-containing beverages.
4. Dry mouth can be treated with tart, sugarless gum or candy, water, sugar-free beverages, or with saliva substitutes if dry mouth persists.

# Phenelzine sulfate
(FEN-ell-zeen)
**Pregnancy Category: C**
Nardil **(Rx)**
Classification: Antidepressant, monoamine oxidase inhibitor

**Action/Kinetics:** MAO inhibitor that prevents the enzyme from metabolizing biogenic amines. Antidepressant effect of phenelzine believed to be due to accumulation of biogenic amines in presynaptic granules, increasing the concentration of neurotransmitter released upon nerve stimulation. **Onset:** Few days to several months. Beneficial effects at doses of 60 mg/day may not be seen for at least 4 weeks. Clinical effects of the drug may be observed for up to 2 weeks after termination of therapy.

**Uses:** Depression characterized as atypical, nonendogenous, or neurotic; most often used in those clients who have mixed anxiety and depression and phobic or hypochondriacal symptoms. Not usually first-line therapy; reserve for those who have failed to respond to drugs more commonly used. *Non-FDA Approved Uses:* Alone or as an adjunct to treat bulimia nervosa, agoraphobia with panic attcks, globus hystericus syndrome, and chronic headache. Also for orthostatic hypotension, refractory migraine headaches, narcolepsy, obsessive-compulsive disorder, panic attacks, posttraumatic stress disorder, and social phobia.

**Contraindications:** Pheochromocytoma, CHF, history of liver disease, abnormal liver function tests. Use with other sympathomimetic drugs due to the possibility of hypertensive crisis. Phenelzine is also contraindicated with the use of many other drugs (see *Drug Interactions*). Use in children under the age of 16 years.

**Special Concerns:** Use with caution in combination with antihypertensive drugs, including thiazide diuretics and β-blockers, due to the possibility of severe hypotensive effects. The safe use during pregnancy or lactation has not been determined. Use with caution in geriatric clients.

**Side Effects:** *CNS:* Dizziness, headache, drowsiness, sleep disturbances (insomnia, hypersomnia), fatigue, weakness, tremors, twitching, myoclonic movements, hyperreflexia, jitteriness, palilalia, euphoria, nystag-

P

mus, paresthesias, ataxia, *shock-like coma,* toxic delirium, manic reaction, *convulsions,* acute anxiety reaction, precipitation of schizophrenia. *Oral:* Dry mouth. *GI:* Constipation, GI disturbances, reversible jaundice. Rarely, *fatal necrotizing hepatocellular damage. CV:* Postural hypotension, edema. *GU:* Anorgasmia, ejaculatory disturbances, urinary retention. *Metabolic:* Weight gain, hypernatremia, hypermetabolic syndrome. *Dermatologic:* Skin rash, sweating. *Ophthalmic:* Blurred vision, glaucoma. *Miscellaneous:* Leukopenia, edema of the glottis, fever associated with increased muscle tone.

**Drug Interactions**
*Alcohol* / Possibility of excitation, seizures, delirium, hyperpyrexia, circulatory collapse, coma, death
*Anesthetics, general* / ↑ Hypotensive effect; use together with caution. Phenelzine should be discontinued at least 10 days before elective surgery
*Anticholinergic drugs, atropine* / MAO inhibitors ↑ effect of anticholinergic drugs
*Antidepressants, tricyclic* / Comcomitant use may result in excitation, sweating, tachycardia, tachypnea, hyperpyrexia, disseminated intravascular coagulation, delirium, tremors, convulsions, death. At least 7–10 days should elapse between discontinuing an MAO inhibitor and initiating a new drug. However, such combinations have been used together successfully
*Fluoxetine* / Possibility of hyperthermia, rigidity, myoclonic movements, death. At least 10 days should elapse between discontinuation of phenelzine and initiation of fluoxetine; and, at least 5 weeks should elapse between discontinuing fluoxetine and beginning phenelzine
*Opioid analgesics (especially meperidine)* / Possibility of excitation, seizures, delirium, hyperpyrexia, circulatory collapse, coma, death
*Phenothiazines* / ↑ Effect of phenothizines due to ↓ breakdown by the liver; also, ↑ chance of severe extrapyramidal effects and hypertensive crisis
*Succinylcholine* / ↑ Effect of succinylcholine due to ↓ breakdown in the plasma by pseudocholinesterase
*Sympathomimetic drugs—amphetamine, cocaine, dopa, ephedrine, epinephrine, metaraminol, methyldopa, methylphenidate, norepinephrine, phenylephrine, phenylpropanolamine. Many OTC cold products, hay fever medications, and nasal decongestants contain one or more of these drugs* / All peripheral, metabolic, cardiac, and central effects are potentiated for up to 2 weeks after termination of MAO inhibitor therapy. Symptoms include acute hypertensive crisis with possible intracranial hemorrhage, hyperthermia, coma, and possibly death

**How Supplied:** *Tablets:* 15 mg.

**Dosage** ————————————
• **Tablets**
  *Treatment of depression.*
**Adults, initial:** 15 mg t.i.d.; **then,** increase the dose to 60 mg/day at a fairly rapid pace (some may require 90 mg/day). **Maintenance:** After the maximum beneficial effect has been observed, the dose should be reduced slowly over several weeks to a range of 15 mg/day or every other day to as high as 45 mg/day or every other day. **Geriatric, initial:** 0.8–1 mg/kg daily in divided doses; **then,** increase as needed to a maximum of 60 mg/day.

## DENTAL CONCERNS

See also *Dental Concerns* for *Antidepressants, Tricyclic.*
**General**
1. Possibility of hypertensive episode with vasoconstrictors.
2. Patient should not be prescribed prescription or over-the-counter products that contain aspirin.

# Phenobarbital
(fee-no-**BAR**-bih-tal)
**Pregnancy Category:** D
Barbilixir ✦, Solfoton **(C-IV) (Rx)**

# Phenobarbital sodium

(fee-no-**BAR**-bih-tal)
**Pregnancy Category:** D
Luminal Sodium **(C-IV) (Rx)**
**Classification:** Sedative, anticonvulsant, barbiturate type

See also *Barbiturates.*
**Action/Kinetics:** Long-acting. **t½:** 53–140 hr. **Onset:** 30 to more than 60 min. **Duration:** 10–16 hr. **Anticonvulsant therapeutic serum levels:** 15–40 mcg/mL. **Time for peak effect, after IV:** up to 15 min. Distributed more slowly than other barbiturates due to lower lipid solubility. Is 50%–60% protein bound. Twenty-five percent eliminated unchanged in the urine.

**Uses: PO:** Sedative, hypnotic (short-term), anticonvulsant (partial and generalized tonic-clonic or cortical focal seizures); emergency control of acute seizure disorders such as status epilepticus, meningitis, tetanus, eclampsia, toxicity of local anesthetics. **Parenteral:** Sedative, hypnotic (short-term), preanesthetic, anticonvulsant, emergency control of acute seizure disorders.

**Special Concerns:** The dose should be reduced in geriatric and debilitated clients as well as those with impaired hepatic or renal function.

**Additional Side Effects:** Chronic use may result in headache, fever, and megaloblastic anemia.

**How Supplied:** Phenobarbital: *Capsule:* 16 mg; *Elixir:* 20 mg/5 mL; *Tablet:* 15 mg, 16 mg, 16.2 mg, 30 mg, 60 mg, 100 mg. Phenobarbital sodium: *Injection:* 30 mg/mL, 60 mg/mL, 65 mg/mL, 130 mg/mL

## Dosage

PHENOBARBITAL, PHENOBARBITAL SODIUM

• **Capsules, Elixir, Tablets**
*Sedation.*
**Adults:** 30–120 mg/day in two to three divided doses. **Pediatric:** 2 mg/kg (60 mg/m²) t.i.d.
*Hypnotic.*
**Adults:** 100–200 mg at bedtime. **Pediatric:** Dose should be determined by provider, based on age and weight.
*Anticonvulsant.*
**Adults:** 60–100 mg/day in single or divided doses. **Pediatric:** 3–6 mg/kg/day in single or divided doses.

• **IM, IV**
*Sedation.*
**Adults:** 30–120 mg/day in two to three divided doses.
*Preoperative sedation.*
**Adults:** 100–200 mg IM only, 60–90 min before surgery. **Pediatric:** 1–3 mg/kg IM or IV 60–90 min prior to surgery.
*Hypnotic.*
**Adults:** 100–320 mg IM or IV.
*Acute convulsions.*
**Adults:** 200–320 mg IM or IV; may be repeated in 6 hr if needed. **Pediatric:** 4–6 mg/kg/day for 7–10 days to achieve a blood level of 10 15 mcg/mL (or 15 mg/kg/day, IV or IM).
*Status epilepticus.*
**Adults:** 15–20 mg/kg IV (given over 10–15 min); may be repeated if needed. **Pediatric:** 15–20 mg/kg given over a 10- to 15-min period.

## DENTAL CONCERNS

See also *Dental Concerns* for *Barbiturates.*

# Phenylephrine hydrochloride

(fen-ill-**EF**-rin)
**Pregnancy Category:** C
**Nasal:** Alconefrin 12, 25, and 50, Children's Nostril, Doktors, Duration, Neo-Synephrine Solution, Nostril, Rhinall, Vicks Sinex. **Ophthalmic:** AK-Dilate, Dionephrine ✦, Mydfrin 2.5%, Neo-Synephrine, Neo-Synephrine Viscous, Phenoptic, Prefrin Liquifilm, Relief. **Parenteral:** Neo-Synephrine. (Rx: Parenteral and Ophthalmic Solutions 2.5% or greater; OTC: Nasal products and ophthalmic solutions 0.12% or less)
**Classification:** Alpha-adrenergic agent (sympathomimetic)

See also *Sympathomimetic Drugs* and *Nasal Decongestants.*

**Action/Kinetics:** Stimulates alpha-adrenergic receptors, producing pronounced vasoconstriction and hence an increase in both SBP and DBP; reflex bradycardia results from increased vagal activity. Also acts on alpha receptors producing vasoconstriction in the skin, mucous membranes, and the mucosa as well as mydriasis by contracting the dilator muscle of the pupil. **IV: Onset,** immediate; **duration,** 15–20 min. **IM, SC: Onset,** 10–15 min; **duration:** 0.5–2 hr for IM and 50–60 min for SC. *Nasal decongestion (topical):* **Onset:** 15–20 min; **duration,** 30 min–4 hr. *Ophthalmic:* **Time to peak effect for mydriasis,** 15–60 min for 2.5% solution and 10–90 min for 10% solution. **Duration:** 0.5–1.5 hr for 0.12%, 3 hr for 2.5%, and 5–7 hr with 10% (when used for mydriasis). Excreted in urine.

**Uses: Systemic:** Vascular failure in shock, shock-like states, drug-induced hypotension or hypersensitivity. To maintain BP during spinal and inhalation anesthesia; to prolong spinal anesthesia. As a vasoconstrictor in regional analgesia. Paroxysmal SVT. **Nasal:** Nasal congestion due to allergies, sinusitis, common cold, or hay fever. **Ophthalmologic: 0.12%:** Temporary relief of redness of the eye associated with colds, hay fever, wind, dust, sun, smog, smoke, contact lens. **2.5% and 10%:** Decongestant and vasoconstrictor, treatment of uveitis with posterior synechiae, open-angle glaucoma, refraction without cycloplegia, ophthalmoscopic examination, funduscopy, prior to surgery.

**Contraindications:** Severe hypertension, ventricular tachycardia.

**Special Concerns:** Use with extreme caution in geriatric clients, severe arteriosclerosis, bradycardia, partial heart block, myocardial disease, hyperthyroidism and during pregnancy and lactation. Nasal and ophthalmic use of phenylephrine may be systemically absorbed. Use of the 2.5% or 10% ophthalmic solutions in children may cause hypertension and irregular heart beat. In geriatric clients, chronic use of the 2.5% or 10% ophthalmic solutions may cause rebound miosis and a decreased mydriatic effect.

**Side Effects:** *CV:* Reflex bradycardia, arrhythmias (rare). *CNS:* Headache, excitability, restlessness. *Ophthalmologic:* Rebound miosis and decreased mydriatic response in geriatric clients, blurred vision.

**Additional Drug Interactions**
*Anesthetics, halogenated hydrocarbon* / May sensitize myocardium → serious arrhythmias

**How Supplied:** *Injection:* 10 mg/mL; *Liquid:* 5 mg/5 mL; *Nasal solution:* 0.125%, 0.25%, 0.5%, 1%; *Ophthalmic solution:* 0.12%, 2.5%, 10%; *Nasal spray:* 0.25%, 0.5%, 1%

**Dosage** ————————————
- **IM, IV, SC**
  *Vasopressor, mild to moderate hypotension.*
  **Adults:** 2–5 mg (range: 1–10 mg), not to exceed an initial dose of 5 mg IM or SC repeated no more often than q 10–15 min; or, 0.2 mg (range: 0.1–0.5 mg), not to exceed an initial dose of 0.5 mg IV repeated no more often than q 10–15 min. **Pediatric:** 0.1 mg/kg (3 mg/m²) IM or SC repeated in 1–2 hr if needed.
  *Vasopressor, severe hypotension and shock.*
  **Adults:** 10 mg by continuous IV infusion using 250–500 mL 5% dextrose injection or 0.9% sodium chloride injection given at a rate of 0.1–0.18 mg/min initial; **then,** give at a rate of 0.04–0.06 mg/min.
  *Prophylaxis of hypotension during spinal anesthesia.*
  **Adults:** 2–3 mg IM or SC 3–4 min before anesthetic given; subsequent doses should not exceed the previous dose by more than 0.1–0.2 mg. No more than 0.5 mg should be given in a single dose. **Pediatric:** 0.044–0.088 mg/kg IM or SC.
  *Hypotensive emergencies during spinal anesthesia.*
  **Adults, initial:** 0.2 mg IV; dose can be increased by no more than 0.2

mg for each subsequent dose not to exceed 0.5 mg/dose.

*Prolongation of spinal anesthesia.*
2–5 mg added to the anesthetic solution increases the duration of action up to 50% without increasing side effects or complications.

*Vasoconstrictor for regional anesthesia.*
Add 1 mg to every 20 mL of local anesthetic solution. If more than 2 mg phenylephrine is used, pressor reactions can be expected.

*Paroxysmal SVT.*
**Initial:** 0.5 mg (maximum) given by rapid IV injection (over 20–30 seconds). Subsequent doses are determined by BP and should not exceed the previous dose by more than 0.1–0.2 mg and should never be more than 1 mg.

• **Nasal Solution, Nasal Spray**
**Adults and children over 12 years of age:** 2–3 gtt of the 0.25% or 0.5% solution into each nostril q 3–4 hr as needed. In resistant cases, the 1% solution can be used but no more often than q 4 hr. **Children, 6–12 years of age:** 2–3 gtt of the 0.25% solution q 3–4 hr as needed. **Infants, greater than 6 months of age:** 1–2 gtt of the 0.16% solution into each nostril q 3–4 hr.

• **Ophthalmic Solution, 0.12%, 2.5%, 10%**

*Vasoconstriction, pupillary dilation.*
1 gtt of the 2.5% or 10% solution on the upper limbus a few minutes following 1 gtt of topical anesthetic (prevents stinging and dilution of solution by lacrimation). An additional drop may be needed after 1 hr.

*Uveitis.*
1 gtt of the 2.5% or 10% solution with atropine. To free recently formed posterior synechiae, 1 gtt of the 2.5% or 10% solution to the upper surface of the cornea. Treatment should be continued the following day, if needed. In the interim, hot compresses should be applied for 5–10 min t.i.d. using 1 gtt of 1% or 2%

atropine sulfate before and after each series of compresses.

*Glaucoma.*
1 gtt of 10% solution on the upper surface of the cornea as needed. Both the 2.5% and 10% solutions may be used with miotics in clients with open-angle glaucoma.

*Surgery.*
2.5% or 10% solution 30–60 min before surgery for wide dilation of the pupil.

*Refraction.*
**Adults:** 1 gtt of a cycloplegic (homatropine HBr, atropine sulfate, cyclopentolate, tropicamide HCl, or a combination of homatropine and cocaine HCl) in each eye followed in 5 min with 1 gtt of 2.5% phenylephrine solution and in 10 min with another drop of cycloplegic. The eyes are ready for refraction in 50–60 min. **Children:** 1 gtt of atropine sulfate, 1%, in each eye followed in 10–15 min with 1 gtt of phenylephrine solution, 2.5%, and in 5–10 min with a second drop of atropine sulfate, 1%. The eyes are ready for refraction in 1–2 hr.

*Ophthalmoscopic examination.*
1 gtt of 2.5% solution in each eye. The eyes are ready for examination in 15–30 min and the effect lasts for 1–3 hr.

*Minor eye irritations.*
1–2 gtt of the 0.12% solution in the eye(s) up to q.i.d. as needed.

## DENTAL CONCERNS

See also *Dental Concerns* for *Sympathomimetic Drugs* and *Nasal Decongestants*.

# Phenytoin (Diphenylhydantoin)
(**FEN**-ih-toyn, dye-**fen**-ill-hy-**DAN**-toyn)
**Pregnancy Category:** C
Dilantin Infatab, Dilantin-125, Novo-Phenytoin ✹ **(Rx)**

# Phenytoin sodium, extended
(**FEN**-ih-toyn)
**Pregnancy Category:** C
Dilantin Kapseals **(Rx)**

# Phenytoin sodium, parenteral
(**FEN**-ih-toyn)
**Pregnancy Category:** C
Dilantin Sodium **(Rx)**

# Phenytoin sodium prompt
(**FEN**-ih-toyn)
**Pregnancy Category:** C
Diphenylan Sodium **(Rx)**
**Classification:** Anticonvulsant, hydantoin type; antiarrhythmic (type I)

See also *Anticonvulsants.*
**Action/Kinetics:** Acts in the motor cortex of the brain to reduce the spread of electrical discharges from the rapidly firing epileptic foci in this area. Phenytoin extended is designed for once-a-day dosage. It has a slow dissolution rate—no more than 35% in 30 min, 30%–70% in 60 min, and less than 85% in 120 min. Absorption is variable following PO dosage. **Peak serum levels: PO,** 4–8 hr. Since the rate and extent of absorption depend on the particular preparation, the same product should be used for a particular client. **Peak serum levels (following IM):** 24 hr (wide variation). **Therapeutic serum levels:** 5–20 mcg/mL. t½: 8–60 hr (average: 20–30 hr). **Steady state:** 7–10 days after initiation. Biotransformed in the liver. Both inactive metabolites and unchanged drug are excreted in the urine.

As an antiarrhythmic, phenytoin increases the electrical stimulation threshold of heart muscle, although it is less effective than quinidine, procainamide, or lidocaine. **Onset:** 30–60 min. **Duration:** 24 hr or more. t½: 22–36 hr. **Therapeutic serum level:** 10–20 mcg/mL.
**Uses:** Chronic epilepsy, especially of the tonic-clonic, psychomotor type. Not effective against absence

seizures and may even increase the frequency of seizures in this disorder. Parenteral phenytoin is sometimes used to treat status epilepticus and to control seizures during neurosurgery.

PO for certain PVCs and IV for PVCs and tachycardia. Particularly useful for arrhythmias produced by digitalis overdosage.

*Non-FDA Approved Uses:* Paroxysmal choreoathetosis; to treat blistering and erosions in clients with recessive dystrophic epidermolysis bullosa; episodic dyscontrol; trigeminal neuralgia; as a muscle relaxant in neuromyotonia, myotonia congenita, or myotonic muscular dystrophy; to treat cardiac symptoms in overdosage of tricyclic antidepressants. Severe preeclampsia.

**Contraindications:** Hypersensitivity to hydantoins, exfoliative dermatitis, sinus bradycardia, second- and third-degree AV block, clients with Adams-Stokes syndrome, SA block. Lactation.
**Special Concerns:** Use with caution in acute, intermittent porphyria. Administer with extreme caution to clients with a history of asthma or other allergies, impaired renal or hepatic function, and heart disease (hypotension, severe myocardial insufficiency). Abrupt withdrawal may cause status epilepticus. Combined drug therapy is required if petit mal seizures are also present.
**Side Effects:** *CNS:* Most commonly, drowsiness, ataxia, dysarthria, confusion, insomnia, nervousness, irritability, depression, tremor, numbness, headache, psychoses, *increased seizures.* Choreoathetosis following IV use. *Oral:* Gingival hyperplasia, oral ulceration, loss of taste. *GI:* N&V, either diarrhea or constipation. *Dermatologic:* Various dermatoses including a measles-like rash (common), scarlatiniform, maculopapular, and urticarial rashes. Rarely, drug-induced lupus erythematosus, *Stevens-Johnson syndrome,* exfoliative or purpuric dermatitis, and *toxic epidermal necrolysis.* Alopecia, hirsutism. Skin reactions may necessitate

withdrawal of therapy. *Hematopoietic:* Leukopenia, granulocytopenia, thrombocytopenia, pancytopenia, **agranulocytosis,** macrocytosis, megaloblastic anemia, leukocytosis, monocytosis, eosinophilia, simple anemia, **aplastic anemia, hemolytic anemia.** *Hepatic:* Liver damage, toxic hepatitis, hypersensitivity reactions involving the liver including hepatocellular degeneration and **fatal hepatocellular necrosis.** *Ophthalmic:* Diplopia, nystagmus, conjunctivitis. *Miscellaneous:* Hyperglycemia, chest pain, edema, fever, photophobia, weight gain, **pulmonary fibrosis,** lymph node hyperplasia, gynecomastia, periarteritis nodosa, depression of IgA, soft tissue injury at injection site, coarsening of facial features, Peyronie's disease, enlarged lips.

*Rapid parenteral administration may cause serious CV effects, including hypotension, arrhythmias, CV collapse, and heart block, as well as CNS depression.*

Many clients have a partial deficiency in the ability of the liver to degrade phenytoin, and as a result, toxicity may develop after a small PO dose. Liver and kidney function tests and hematopoietic studies are indicated prior to and periodically during drug therapy.

**Drug Interactions**

*Acetaminophen* / ↓ Effect of acetaminophen due to ↑ breakdown by liver; however, hepatotoxicity may be ↑

*Alcohol, ethyl* / In alcoholics, ↓ effect of phenytoin due to ↑ breakdown by liver

*Antacids* / ↓ Effect of phenytoin due to ↓ GI absorption

*Antidepressants, tricyclic* / May ↑ incidence of epileptic seizures or ↑ effect of phenytoin by ↓ plasma protein binding

*Barbiturates* / Effect of phenytoin may be ↑, ↓, or not changed; possible ↑ effect of barbiturates

*Benzodiazepines* / ↑ Effect of phenytoin due to ↓ breakdown by liver

*Carbamazepine* / ↓ Effect of phenytoin or carbamazepine due to ↑ breakdown by liver

*Cimetidine* / ↑ Effect of phenytoin due to ↓ breakdown by liver

*Clonazepam* / ↓ Plasma levels of clonazepam or phenytoin; or, ↑ risk of phenytoin toxicity

*Corticosteroids* / Effect of corticosteroids ↓ due to ↑ breakdown by liver; also, corticosteroids may mask hypersensitivity reactions due to phenytoin

*Doxycycline* / ↓ Effect of doxycycline due to ↑ breakdown by liver

*Fluconazole* / ↑ Effect of phenytoin due to ↓ breakdown by liver

*Ibuprofen* / ↑ Effect of phenytoin

*Meperidine* / ↓ Effect of meperidine due to ↑ breakdown by liver; toxic effects of meperidine may ↑ due to accumulation of active metabolite (normeperidine)

*Metronidazole* / ↑ Effect of phenytoin due to ↓ breakdown by liver

*Miconazole* / ↑ Effect of phenytoin due to ↓ breakdown by liver

*Phenothiazines* / ↑ Effect of phenytoin due to ↓ breakdown by liver

*Phenylbutazone* / ↑ Effect of phenytoin due to ↓ breakdown by liver and ↓ plasma protein binding

*Salicylates* / ↑ Effect of phenytoin by ↓ plasma protein binding

*Sucralfate* / ↓ Effect of phenytoin due to ↓ absorption from GI tract

*Sulfonamides* / ↑ Effect of phenytoin due to ↓ breakdown in liver

*Trimethoprim* / ↑ Effect of phenytoin due to ↓ breakdown by liver

**How Supplied:** Phenytoin: *Chew tablet:* 50 mg; *Suspension:* 100 mg/4 mL, 125 mg/5 mL. Phenytoin sodium, extended: *Capsule, extended release:* 30 mg, 100 mg. Phenytoin sodium, parenteral: *Injection:* 50 mg/mL. Phenytoin sodium prompt: *Capsule:* 100 mg

**Dosage**

• **Oral Suspension, Chewable Tablets**
   *Seizures.*

**Adults, initial:** 100 mg (125 mg of the suspension) t.i.d.; adjust dosage at 7- to 10-day intervals until seizures are controlled; **usual, maintenance:** 300–400 mg/day, although 600 mg/day (625 mg of the suspension) may be required in some. **Pediatric, initial:** 5 mg/kg/day in two to three divided doses; **maintenance,** 4–8 mg/kg (up to maximum of 300 mg/day). Children over 6 years may require up to 300 mg/day. **Geriatric:** 3 mg/kg initially in divided doses; **then,** adjust dosage according to serum levels and response. Once dosage level has been established, the extended capsules may be used for once-a-day dosage.

• **Capsules, Extended-Release Capsules**

*Seizures.*

**Adults, initial:** 100 mg t.i.d.; adjust dose at 7- to 10-day intervals until control is achieved. An initial loading dose of 12–15 mg/kg divided into two to three doses over 6 hr followed by 100 mg t.i.d. on subsequent days may be preferred if seizures are frequent. **Pediatric:** See dose for Oral Suspension and Chewable Tablets.

*Arrhythmias.*

**Adults:** 200–400 mg/day.

• **IV**

*Status epilepticus.*

**Adults, loading dose:** 10–15 mg/kg at a rate not to exceed 50 mg/min; **then,** 100 mg PO or IV q 6–8 hr. **Pediatric, loading dose:** 15–20 mg/kg in divided doses of 5–10 mg/kg given at a rate of 1–3 mg/kg/min.

*Arrhythmias.*

**Adults:** 100 mg q 5 min up to maximum of 1 g.

• **IM**

Dose should be 50% greater than the PO dose.

*Neurosurgery.*

100–200 mg q 4 hr during and after surgery (during first 24 hr, no more than 1,000 mg should be administered; after first day, give maintenance dosage).

## DENTAL CONCERNS

See also *Dental Concerns* for *Anticonvulsants.*

**Client/Family Teaching**

1. To minimize bleeding from the gums and prevent gingival hyperplasia, practice good oral hygiene. Brush teeth with a soft toothbrush, massage the gums, and floss every day.

# Pirbuterol acetate
(peer-**BYOU**-ter-ohl)
**Pregnancy Category:** C
Maxair Autohaler **(Rx)**
**Classification:** Sympathomimetic, bronchodilator

See also *Sympathomimetic Drugs.*

**Action/Kinetics:** Causes bronchodilation by stimulating beta-2-adrenergic receptors. Has minimal effects on beta-1 receptors. Also inhibits histamine release from mast cells, causes vasodilation, and increases ciliary motility. **Onset, inhalation:** Approximately 5 min. **Time to peak effect:** 30–60 min. **Duration:** 5 hr.

**Uses:** Alone or with theophylline or steroids, for prophylaxis and treatment of bronchospasm in asthma and other conditions with reversible bronchospasms, including bronchitis, emphysema, bronchiectasis, obstructive pulmonary disease. May be used with or without theophylline or steroids.

**Contraindications:** Cardiac arrhythmias due to tachycardia; tachycardia caused by digitalis toxicity.

**Special Concerns:** Safety and efficacy have not been determined in children less than 12 years of age.

**Additional Side Effects:** *CV:* PVCs, hypotension. *CNS:* Hyperactivity, hyperkinesia, anxiety, confusion, depression, fatigue, syncope. *Oral:* Bad taste or taste change, stomatitis, glossitis, dry mouth. *GI:* Diarrhea, anorexia, loss of appetite, abdominal pain, abdominal cramps. *Dermatologic:* Rash, edema, pruritus, alopecia. *Miscellaneous:* Flushing, numbness in extremities, weight gain.

**How Supplied:** *Aerosol solid w/adapter:* 0.2 mg/inh

**Dosage** ———————————
• **Inhalation Aerosol**
**Adults and children over 12 years:** 0.2–0.4 mg (1–2 inhalations) q 4–6 hr, not to exceed 12 inhalations (2.4 mg) daily.

## DENTAL CONCERNS

See also *Dental Concerns* for *Sympathomimetic Drugs.*

# Piroxicam
(peer-**OX**-ih-kam)
Alti-Piroxicam ✿, Apo-Piroxicam ✿, Dom-Piroxicam ✿, Feldene, Gen-Piroxicam ✿, Novo-Pirocam ✿, Nu-Pirox ✿, PMS-Piroxicam ✿, Pro-Piroxicam ✿, Rho-Piroxicam ✿ **(Rx)**
**Classification:** Nonsteroidal anti-inflammatory drug

See also *Nonsteroidal Anti-Inflammatory Drugs.*
**Action/Kinetics:** May inhibit prostaglandin synthesis. Effect is comparable to that of aspirin, but with fewer GI side effects and less tinnitus. May be used with gold, corticosteroids, and antacids. **Peak plasma levels:** 1.5–2 mcg/mL after 3–5 hr (single dose). **Steady-state plasma levels** (after 7–12 days): 3–8 mcg/mL. **t½:** 50 hr. **Analgesia, onset:** 1 hr; **duration:** 2–3 days. **Anti-inflammatory activity, onset:** 7–12 days; **duration:** 2–3 weeks. Metabolites and unchanged drug excreted in urine and feces.
**Uses:** Acute and chronic treatment of rheumatoid arthritis and osteoarthritis. *Non-FDA Approved Uses:* Juvenile rheumatoid arthritis, primary dysmenorrhea, sunburn.
**Contraindications:** Safe use during pregnancy has not been determined. Lactation.
**Special Concerns:** Safety and efficacy have not been established in children. Increased plasma levels and

elimination half-life may be observed in geriatric clients (especially women).

**How Supplied:** *Capsule:* 10 mg, 20 mg

**Dosage** ———————————
• **Capsules**
   *Anti-inflammatory, antirheumatic.*
**Adults:** 20 mg/day in one or more divided doses. Effect of therapy should not be assessed for 2 weeks.

## DENTAL CONCERNS

See also *Dental Concerns* for *Nonsteroidal Anti-Inflammatory Drugs.*

# Pramipexole
(prah-mih-**PEX**-ohl)
**Pregnancy Category:** C
Mirapex **(Rx)**
**Classification:** Antiparkinson drug

See also *Antiparkinson Agents.*
**Action/Kinetics:** Thought to act by stimulating dopamine (especially $D_3$) receptors in striatum. Rapidly absorbed. **Peak levels:** 2 hr. Food increases time for maximum levels to occur. **t½, terminal:** About 8 hr (12 hr in geriatric clients). Excreted mainly unchanged in urine. Clearance decreases with age.
**Uses:** Idiopathic Parkinson's disease.
**Contraindications:** Lactation.
**Special Concerns:** Safety and efficacy have not been determined in children.
**Side Effects:** *CNS:* Hallucinations (especially in elderly), dizziness, somnolence, insomnia, confusion, amnesia, hypesthesia, dystonia, akathisia, abnormal thinking, decreased libido, myoclonus. *CV:* Orthostatic hypotension. *Body as a whole:* Asthenia, general edema, malaise, fever. *Oral:* Dry mouth, taste perversion. *GI:* Nausea, constipation, anorexia, dysphagia. *Miscellaneous:* Vision abnormalities, impotence, peripheral edema, decreased weight.

**P**

---

**Drug Interactions**

*Butyrophenones* / Possible ↓ effect of pramipexole

*Cimetidine* / ↑ Levodopa levels and half-life

*CNS Depressants* / Additive CNS depression

*Metoclopramide* / Possible ↓ effect of pramipexole

*Phenothiazines* / Possible ↓ effect of pramipexole

*Thioxanthines* / Possible ↓ effect of pramipexole

**How Supplied:** *Tablets:* 0.125 mg, 0.25 mg, 1 mg, 1.5 mg

**Dosage** ————————

• **Tablets**

*Parkinsonism.*

**Initial:** Start with 0.125 mg t.i.d.; **then,** increase dose by 0.125 mg t.i.d. weekly for 7 weeks (i.e., dose at week 7 is 1.5 mg t.i.d.). **Maintenance:** 1.5–4.5 mg/day in equally divided doses t.i.d. with or without comcomitant levodopa (about 800 mg/day).

Impaired renal function, $C_{CR}$, over 60 mL/min: Start with 0.125 mg t.i.d., up to maximum of 1.5 mg t.i.d. $C_{CR}$, 25–59 mL/min: Start with 0.125 mg b.i.d., up to maximum of 1.5 mg b.i.d. $C_{CR}$, 15–24 mL/min: Start with 0.125 mg once daily, up to maximum of 1.5 mg once daily.

**DENTAL CONCERNS**

**General**

1. Monitor vital signs at every appointment because of cardiovascular side effects.

2. Have the patient sit up slowly and remain seated for at least two minutes after being supine in order to minimize the risk of orthostatic hypotension.

3. Decreased saliva flow can put the patient at risk for dental caries, periodontal disease, and candidiasis.

4. A semisupine position for the dental chair may be necessary to help minimize or avoid GI adverse effects.

**Consultation with Primary Care Provider**

1. Consultation may be required in order to assess extent of disease control and patient's ability to tolerate stress.

**Client/Family Teaching**

1. Review the importance of good oral hygiene in order to prevent soft tissue inflammation.

2. Review the proper use of oral hygiene aids in order to prevent injury.

3. Daily home fluoride treatments for persistent dry mouth.

4. Avoid alcohol-containing mouth rinses and beverages.

5. Avoid caffeine-containing beverages.

6. Dry mouth can be treated with tart, sugarless gum or candy, water, sugar-free beverages, or with saliva substitutes if dry mouth persists.

—————————————

# Pravastatin sodium

(prah-vah-**STAH**-tin)

**Pregnancy Category:** X

Pravachol **(Rx)**

**Classification:** Antihyperlipidemic agent

—————————————

See also *Antihyperlipidemic Agents—HMG-CoA Reductase Inhibitors.*

**Action/Kinetics:** Competitively inhibits HMG-CoA reductase enzyme, which reduces cholesterol synthesis. Drug increases survival in heart transplant recipients. Rapidly absorbed from the GI tract. **Peak plasma levels:** 1–1.5 hr. Significant first-pass extraction and metabolism in the liver, which is the site of action of the drug; thus, plasma levels may not correlate well with lipid-lowering effectiveness. **t½, elimination:** 77 hr. Metabolized in the liver; approximately 20% of a PO dose is excreted through the urine and 70% in the feces.

**Uses:** Adjunct to diet for reducing elevated total and LDL cholesterol levels in clients with primary hypercholesterolemia (type IIa and IIb) when the response to a diet with restricted saturated fat and cholesterol has not been effective. Reduce the risk of heart attack and slow progression of coronary atherosclerosis in those with hypercholesterolemia and heart disease. *Non-FDA Approved Uses:* To lower cholesterol levels in those with heterozygous familial hypercholesterolemia, familial combined hyperlipidemia, diabetic dyslipidemia in non-insulin-dependent diabetics, hypercholesterolemia secondary to nephrotic syndrome, homozygous familial hypercholesterolemia in those not completely devoid of LDL receptors but who have a decreased level of LDL receptor activity.

**Contraindications:** To treat hypercholesterolemia due to hyperalphaproteinemia. Active liver disease; unexplained, persistent elevations in liver function tests. Use during pregnancy and lactation and in children less than 18 years of age.

**Special Concerns:** Use with caution in clients with a history of liver disease, renal insufficiency, or heavy alcohol use.

**Side Effects:** *Musculoskeletal:* Rhabdomyolysis with renal dysfunction secondary to myoglobinuria, myalgia, myopathy, arthralgias, localized pain. *CNS:* CNS vascular lesions characterized by ***perivascular hemorrhage,*** edema, and mononuclear cell infiltration of perivascular spaces; headache, dizziness, psychic disturbances. Dizziness, vertigo, memory loss, anxiety, insomnia, depression. *GI:* N&V, diarrhea, abdominal pain, cramps, constipation, flatulence, heartburn, anorexia. *Hepatic:* Hepatitis (including chronic active hepatitis), fatty change in liver, cirrhosis, ***fulminant hepatic necrosis, hepatoma,*** pancreatitis, cholestatic jaundice. *GU:* Gynecomastia, erectile dysfunction, loss of libido. *Ophthalmic:* Progression of cataracts, lens opacities, ophthalmoplegia. *Hypersensitivity reaction:* Vasculitis, purpura, polymyalgia rheumatica, ***angioedema,*** lupus erythematosus–like syndrome, thrombocytopenia, ***hemolytic anemia,*** leukopenia, positive ANA, arthritis, arthralgia, urticaria, asthenia, ESR increase, fever, chills, photosensitivity, malaise, dyspnea, ***toxic epidermal ne-***

***crolysis, Stevens-Johnson syndrome.*** *Dermatologic:* Alopecia, pruritus, skin nodules, discoloration of skin, dryness of skin and mucous membranes, changes in hair and nails. *Neurologic:* Dysfunction of certain cranial nerves resulting in alteration of taste, impairment of extraocular movement, and facial paresis; paresthesia, peripheral neuropathy, tremor, vertigo, memory loss peripheral nerve palsy. *Respiratory:* Common cold, rhinitis, cough. *Hematologic:* Anemia, transient asymptomatic eosinophilia, thrombocytopenia, leukopenia. *Miscellaneous:* Rash, pruritus, cardiac chest pain, fatigue, influenza.

**Drug Interactions**
*Cyclosporine* / ↑ Risk of myopathy or rhabdomyolysis
*Erythromycin* / ↑ Risk of myopathy or rhabdomyolysis

**How Supplied:** *Tablet:* 10 mg, 20 mg, 40 mg

**Dosage**
• **Tablets**
**Initial:** 10–20 mg once daily at bedtime (geriatric clients should take 10 mg once daily at bedtime). **Maintenance dose:** 10–40 mg once daily at bedtime (maximum dose for geriatric clients is 20 mg/day).

**DENTAL CONCERNS**

See also *Dental Concerns* for *Antihyperlipidemic Agents.*

# Prazosin hydrochloride
(**PRAY**-zoh-sin)
**Pregnancy Category:** C
Alti-Prazosin ✿, Apo-Prazo ✿, Minipress, Novo-Prazin ✿, Nu-Prazo ✿, Rho-Prazosin ✿ **(Rx)**
**Classification:** Antihypertensive, alpha-1-adrenergic blocking agent

See also *Alpha-1-Adrenergic Blocking Agents* and *Antihypertensive Agents.*

**Action/Kinetics:** Produces selective blockade of postsynaptic alpha-1-adrenergic receptors. Dilates arterioles and veins, thereby decreasing total peripheral resistance and decreasing DBP more than SBP. CO, HR, and renal blood flow are not affected. Can be used to initiate antihypertensive therapy; most effective when used with other agents (e.g., diuretics, beta-adrenergic blocking agents). **Onset:** 2 hr. Absorption not affected by food. **Maximum effect:** 2–3 hr; **duration:** 6–12 hr. **t½:** 2–3 hr. Full therapeutic effect: 4–6 weeks. Metabolized extensively; excreted primarily in feces.

**Uses:** Mild to moderate hypertension alone or in combination with other antihypertensive drugs. *Non-FDA Approved Uses:* CHF refractory to other treatment. Raynaud's disease, benign prostatic hypertrophy.

**Contraindications:** Hypersensitivity to prazosin, doxazosin, or terazosin. Severe CHF.

**Special Concerns:** Safe use in children has not been established. Use with caution during lactation. Geriatric clients may be more sensitive to the hypotensive and hypothermic effects of prazosin; also, it may be necessary to decrease the dose in these clients due to age-related decreases in renal function.

**Side Effects: First-dose effect:** *Marked hypotension* and syncope 30–90 min after administration of initial dose (usually 2 or more mg), increase of dosage, or addition of other antihypertensive agent. *CNS:* Dizziness, drowsiness, headache, fatigue, paresthesias, depression, vertigo, nervousness, hallucinations. *CV:* Palpitations, syncope, tachycardia, orthostatic hypotension, aggravation of angina. *Oral:* Dry mouth. *GI:* N&V, diarrhea or constipation, abdominal pain, pancreatitis. *GU:* Urinary frequency or incontinence, impotence, priapism. *Respiratory:* Dyspnea, nasal congestion, epistaxis. *Dermatologic:* Pruritus, rash, sweating, alopecia, lichen planus. *Miscellaneous:* Asthenia, edema, symptoms of lupus erythematosus, blurred vision, tinnitus, arthralgia, myalgia, reddening of sclera, eye pain, conjunctivitis, edema, fever.

**Drug Interactions**
*Epinephrine* / ↑ Antihypertensive effect
*Indomethacin* / ↓ Effect of prazosin
*NSAIDs* / ↓ Effect of prazosin

**How Supplied:** *Capsule:* 1 mg, 2 mg, 5 mg

**Dosage** ———
• **Capsules**
*Hypertension.*
**Individualized: Initial,** 1 mg b.i.d.–t.i.d.; **maintenance:** if necessary, increase gradually to 6–15 mg/day in two to three divided doses. Daily dose should not exceed 20 mg, although some clients have benefitted from doses of 40 mg daily. If used with diuretics or other antihypertensives, reduce dose to 1–2 mg t.i.d. **Pediatric, less than 7 years of age, initial:** 0.25 mg b.i.d.–t.i.d. adjusted according to response. **Pediatric, 7–12 years of age, initial:** 0.5 mg b.i.d.–t.i.d. adjusted according to response.

## DENTAL CONCERNS

See also *Dental Concerns* for *Antihypertensive Agents* and *Alpha-1-Adrenergic Blocking Agents.*
**General**
1. Restrict use of sodium-containing agents such as saline IV fluids for patients with sodium restrictions.
2. Dental procedures may cause the patient anxiety or place stress on the heart. Assess cardiovascular patient for this risk.
3. Early morning and shorter appointments, as well as methods for addressing anxiety levels in the patient, can help reduce the amount of stress the patient is experiencing.

# Prednisone
(**PRED**-nih-sohn)
**Pregnancy Category:** C
**Oral Solution:** Prednisone Intensol Concentrate **(Rx). Syrup:** Liquid Pred **(Rx). Tablets:** Alti-Prednisone ✿, Apo-Prednisone ✿, Deltasone, Jaa Prednisone ✿, Meticorten, Novo-Prednisone ✿, Orasone 1, 5, 10, 20, and

50, Panasol-S, Sterapred DS, Winpred
★ **(Rx)**
**Classification:** Corticosteroid, synthetic

See also *Corticosteroids.*
**Action/Kinetics:** Three to five times as potent as cortisone or hydrocortisone. May cause moderate fluid retention. Metabolized in the liver to prednisolone, the active form.
**Special Concerns:** Use during pregnancy only if benefits outweigh risks. Dose must be highly individualized.
**How Supplied:** *Concentrate:* 5 mg/mL; *Solution:* 5 mg/5 mL; *Syrup:* 5 mg/5 mL; *Tablet:* 1 mg, 2.5 mg, 5 mg, 10 mg, 20 mg, 50 mg

**Dosage**
• **Oral Concentrate, Syrup, Tablets**
*Acute, severe conditions.*
**Initial:** 5–60 mg/day in four equally divided doses after meals and at bedtime. Decrease gradually by 5–10 mg q 4–5 days to establish minimum maintenance dosage (5–10 mg) or discontinue altogether until symptoms recur.
*Replacement.*
**Pediatric:** 0.1–0.15 mg/kg/day.
*COPD.*
30–60 mg/day for 1–2 weeks; then taper.
*Ophthalmopathy due to Graves' disease.*
60 mg/day; **then,** taper to 20 mg/day.
*Duchenne's muscular dystrophy.*
0.75–1.5 mg/kg/day (used to improve strength).

**DENTAL CONCERNS**

See also *Dental Concerns* for *Corticosteroids.*

# Prilocaine hydrochloride
(**PRY**-loh-kayn)
**Pregnancy Category:** B
Citanest, Citanest Forte with epinephrine

**Classification:** Amide local anesthetic

See also *Amide Local Anesthetic Agents.*
**Action/Kinetics:** Blocks nerve action potential by inhibiting ion fluxes across the cell membrane. **Onset:** 2–10 min. **Duration:** 2–4 hr. Renally excreted and metabolized in the liver.
**Uses:** Local dental anesthesia.
**Contraindications:** See also *Amide Local Anesthetic Agents.*
**Special Concerns:** Elderly, large doses of prilocaine HCl in patients with myasthenia gravis, risk of methemoglobinemia.
**Side Effects:** See also *Amide Local Anesthetic Agents.*
**Drug Interactions:** See also *Amide Local Anesthetic Agents.*
**How Supplied:** *Injection without vasoconstrictor:* 4%; *Injection with vasoconstrictor:* 4% solution with 1:200,000 epinephrine

**Dosage**
• **Injection without Vasoconstrictor**
*Dental anesthesia.*
40–80 mg not to exceed 400 mg over a 2-hr dental appointment. Dose should be adjusted down for medically compromised, debilitated, or elderly patients. (See also *Appendix 9.*)
• **Injection with Vasoconstrictor**
*Dental anesthesia.*
40–80 mg not to exceed 400 mg over a 2-hr dental appointment. Dose should be adjusted down for medically compromised, debilitated, or elderly patients. (See also *Appendix 9.*)

**DENTAL CONCERNS**

See also *Dental Concerns* for *Amide Local Anesthetic Agents.*

# Procainamide hydrochloride
(proh-**KAYN**-ah-myd)

**Pregnancy Category:** C
Apo-Procainamide ✷, Procan SR ✷,
Procanbid, Pronestyl, Pronestyl-SR
**(Rx)**
**Classification:** Antiarrhythmic, class
IA

See also *Antiarrhythmic Agents.*

**Action/Kinetics:** Produces a direct cardiac effect to prolong the refractory period of the atria and to a lesser extent the bundle of His-Purkinje system and ventricles. Large doses may cause AV block. Some anticholinergic and local anesthetic effects. **Onset: PO,** 30 min; **IV,** 1–5 min. **Time to peak effect, PO:** 90–120 min; **IM,** 15–60 min; **IV,** immediate. **Duration:** 3 hr. **t½:** 2.5–4.7 hr. **Therapeutic serum level:** 4–8 mcg/mL. **Protein binding:** 15%. From 40% to 70% excreted unchanged. Metabolized in the liver (16%–21% by slow acetylators and 24%–33% by fast acetylators) to the active N-acetylprocainamide (NAPA); has antiarrhythmic properties with a longer half-life than procainamide.

**Uses:** Documented ventricular arrhythmias (e.g., sustained ventricular tachycardia) that may be life threatening in clients where benefits of treatment clearly outweigh risks. Antiarrhythmic drugs have not been shown to improve survival in clients with ventricular arrhythmias.

**Contraindications:** Hypersensitivity to drug, complete AV heart block, lupus erythematosus, torsades de pointes, asymptomatic ventricular premature contractions. Lactation.

**Special Concerns:** There is an increased risk of death in those with non-life-threatening arrhythmias. Although used in children, safety and efficacy have not been established. Use with extreme caution in clients for whom a sudden drop in BP could be detrimental, in CHF, acute ischemic heart disease, or cardiomyopathy. Also, use with caution in clients with liver or kidney dysfunction, preexisting bone marrow failure or cytopenia of any type, development of first-degree heart block while on

procainamide, myasthenia gravis, and those with bronchial asthma or other respiratory disorders. May cause more hypotension in geriatric clients; also, in this population, the dose may have to be decreased due to age-related decreases in renal function.

**Side Effects:** *Body as a whole:* Lupus erythematosus–like syndrome especially in those on maintenance therapy and who are slow acetylators. Symptoms include arthralgia, pleural or abdominal pain, arthritis, pleural effusion, pericarditis, fever, chills, myalgia, skin lesions, hematologic changes. *CV:* Following IV use: Hypotension, ***ventricular asystole or fibrillation, partial or complete heart block.*** Rarely, second-degree heart block after PO use. *Oral:* Dry mouth, bitter taste. *GI:* N&V, diarrhea, anorexia, abdominal pain. *Hematologic:* Thrombocytopenia, ***agranulocytosis,*** neutropenia. ***Rarely, hemolytic anemia.*** *Dermatologic:* Urticaria, pruritus, angioneurotic edema, flushing, maculopapular rash. *CNS:* Depression, dizziness, weakness, giddiness, psychoses, hallucinations. *Other:* Granulomatous hepatitis, weakness, fever, chills.

**Drug Interactions**
*Anticholinergic agents, atropine* /
Additive anticholinergic effects
*Barbiturates* / ↓ Effects
*Cholinergic agents* / Anticholinergic activity of procainamide antagonizes effect of cholinergic drugs
*Ethanol* / Effect of procainamide may be altered, but because the main metabolite is active as an antiarrhythmic, specific outcome not clear
*Lidocaine* / Additive cardiodepressant effects
*Sodium bicarbonate* / ↑ Effect of procainamide due to ↓ excretion by the kidney
*Succinylcholine* / Procainamide ↑ muscle relaxation produced by succinylcholine
*Trimethoprim* / ↑ Effect of procainamide due to ↑ serum levels
**How Supplied:** *Capsule:* 250 mg, 375 mg, 500 mg; *Injection:* 100

mg/mL, 500 mg/mL; *Tablet:* 250 mg, 375 mg, 500 mg; *Tablet, extended release:* 250 mg, 500 mg, 750 mg, 1000 mg

**Dosage** ———————————
• **Capsules, Extended-Release Tablets, Tablets**
**Adults, initial:** 50 mg/kg/day in divided doses q 3 hr. **Usual, 40–50 kg:** 250 mg q 3 hr of standard formulation or 500 mg q 6 hr of sustained-release; **60–70 kg:** 375 mg q 3 hr of standard formulation or 750 mg q 6 hr of sustained-release; **80–90 kg:** 500 mg q 3 hr of standard formulation or 1 g q 6 hr of sustained-release; **over 100 kg:** 625 mg q 3 hr of standard formulation or 1.25 g q 6 hr of sustained-release. **Pediatric:** 15–50 mg/kg/day divided q 3–6 hr (up to a maximum of 4 g/day).
• **Procanbid Extended-Release Tablets**
*Life-threatening arrhythmias.*
500 or 1,000 mg b.i.d.
• **IM**
*Ventricular arrhythmias.*
**Adults, initial:** 50 mg/kg/day divided into fractional doses of ⅛–¼ given q 3–6 hr until PO therapy is possible. **Pediatric:** 20–30 mg/kg/day divided q 4–6 hr (up to a maximum of 4 g/day).
*Arrhythmias associated with surgery or anesthesia.*
**Adults:** 100–500 mg.
• **IV**
**Initial loading infusion:** 20 mg/min (for up to 25–30 min). **Maintenance infusion:** 2–6 mg/min. **Pediatric, initial loading dose:** 3–5 mg/kg/dose over 5 min (maximum of 100 mg); **maintenance:** 20–80 mcg/kg/min continuous infusion (maximum of 2 g/day).

## DENTAL CONCERNS

See also *Dental Concerns* for *Antiarrhythmic Agents.*
**General**
1. Have the patient sit up slowly and remain seated for at least two minutes after being supine in order to minimize the risk of orthostatic hypotension.
2. Patients on chronic drug therapy may develop blood dyscrasias. Symptoms include fever, sore throat, bleeding, and poor wound healing.
**Consultation with Primary Care Provider**
1. Patients with symptoms of blood dyscrasias should be referred to their primary care provider for complete blood counts. Treatment should be postponed until the results are known.
**Client/Family Teaching**
1. Review the proper use of oral hygiene aids in order to prevent injury.
2. Daily home fluoride treatments for persistent dry mouth.

---

# Propranolol hydrochloride
(proh-**PRAN**-oh-lohl)
**Pregnancy Category:** C
Apo-Propranolol ✤, Detensol ✤, Dom-Propranolol ✤, Inderal, Inderal 10, 20, 40, 60, 80, and 90, Inderal LA, Novo-Pranol ✤, Nu-Propranolol ✤, PMS Propranolol ✤, Propranolol Intensol **(Rx)**
**Classification:** Beta-adrenergic blocking agent; antiarrhythmic (type II)

P

See also *Beta-Adrenergic Blocking Agents.*
**Action/Kinetics:** Manifests both beta-1- and beta-2-adrenergic blocking activity. Antiarrhythmic action is due to both beta-adrenergic receptor blockade and a direct membrane-stabilizing action on the cardiac cell. Has no intrinsic sympathomimetic activity and has high lipid solubility. **Onset, PO:** 30 min; **IV:** immediate. **Maximum effect:** 1–1.5 hr. **Duration:** 3–5 hr. **t½:** 2–3 hr (8–11 hr for long-acting). **Therapeutic serum level, antiarrhythmic:** 0.05–0.1 mcg/mL. Completely metabolized by liver and excreted in urine. Although food increases bioavailability, absorption may be decreased.

372 PROPRANOLOL HYDROCHLORIDE

**Uses:** Hypertension (alone or in combination with other antihypertensive agents). Angina pectoris, hypertrophic subaortic stenosis, prophylaxis of MI, pheochromocytoma, prophylaxis of migraine, essential tremor. Cardiac arrhythmias. Anxiety, aggressive behavior.

**Contraindications:** Hypersensitivity to propranolol, cardiogenic shock, 2nd or 3rd degree heart block, sinus bradycardia, congestive heart failure, cardiac failure. Bronchial asthma, bronchospasms including severe COPD.

**Special Concerns:** Children, diabetes mellitus, hepatic disease, hyperthyroidism, hypotension, lactation, myasthenia gravis, peripheral vascular disease, renal disease. It is dangerous to use propranolol for pheochromocytoma unless an alpha-adrenergic blocking agent is already in use.

**Side Effects:** *Oral:* Dry mouth. *CV:* AV block, bradycardia, *CHF,* hypotension, peripheral vascular insufficiency, vasodilation. *CNS:* Bizarre dreams, depression, disorientation, fatigue, hallucinations, lethargy, paresthesias. *GI:* Acute pancreatitis, colitis, constipation, cramps, diarrhea, hepatomegaly, nausea, vomiting. *Hematologic: Agranulocytosis, thrombocytopenia. Allergic:* Fever, sore throat, respiratory distress, rash, pharyngitis, *laryngospasm, anaphylaxis. Skin:* Fever, pruritus, rash. *Ophthalmic:* Dry eyes. *GU:* Decreased libido, impotence, urinary tract infection. *Other:* Hypoglycemia. *Respiratory: Bronchospasm,* dyspnea, wheezing.

**Additional Side Effects:** Psoriasis-like eruptions, skin necrosis, SLE (rare).

**Drug Interactions:** See also *Drug Interactions* for *Beta-Adrenergic Blocking Agents* and *Antihypertensive Agents.*

**How Supplied:** *Capsule, extended release:* 60 mg, 80 mg, 120 mg, 160 mg; *Concentrate:* 80 mg/mL; *Injection:* 1 mg/mL; *Solution:* 20 mg/5 mL, 40 mg/5 mL; *Tablet:* 10 mg, 20 mg, 40 mg, 60 mg, 80 mg

**Dosage** ————
• **Tablets, Sustained-Release Capsules, Oral Solution, Concentrate**
*Hypertension.*
**Initial:** 40 mg b.i.d. or 80 mg of sustained-release/day; **then,** increase dose to maintenance level of 120–240 mg/day given in two to three divided doses or 120–160 mg of sustained-release medication once daily. Maximum daily dose should not exceed 640 mg. **Pediatric, initial:** 0.5 mg/kg b.i.d.; dose may be increased at 3- to 5-day intervals to a maximum of 1 mg/kg b.i.d. The dosage range should be calculated by weight and not by body surface area.
*Angina.*
**Initial:** 80–320 mg b.i.d., t.i.d., or q.i.d.; or, 80 mg of sustained-release once daily; **then,** increase dose gradually to maintenance level of 160 mg/day of sustained-release capsule. The maximum daily dose should not exceed 320 mg.
*Arrhythmias.*
10–30 mg t.i.d.–q.i.d. given after meals and at bedtime.
*Hypertrophic subaortic stenosis.*
20–40 mg t.i.d.–q.i.d. before meals and at bedtime or 80–160 mg of sustained-release medication given once daily.
*MI prophylaxis.*
180–240 mg/day given in three to four divided doses. Total daily dose should not exceed 240 mg.
*Pheochromocytoma, preoperatively.*
60 mg/day for 3 days before surgery, given concomitantly with an alpha-adrenergic blocking agent.
*Inoperable tumors.*
30 mg/day in divided doses.
*Migraine.*
**Initial:** 80 mg sustained-release medication given once daily; **then,** increase dose gradually to maintenance of 160–240 mg/day in divided doses. If a satisfactory response has not been observed after 4–6 weeks, the drug should be discontinued and withdrawn gradually.
*Essential tremor.*

**Initial:** 40 mg b.i.d.; **then,** 120 mg/day up to a maximum of 320 mg/day.

*Aggressive behavior.*
80–300 mg/day.

*Anxiety.*
80–320 mg/day.

## DENTAL CONCERNS

See also *Dental Concerns* for *Beta-Adrenergic Blocking Agents* and *Antihypertensive Agents.*

**Client/Family Teaching**

1. Review the importance of good oral hygiene in order to prevent soft tissue inflammation.
2. Review the proper use of oral hygiene aids in order to prevent injury.
3. Daily home fluoride treatments for persistent dry mouth.
4. Avoid alcohol-containing mouth rinses and beverages.
5. Avoid caffeine-containing beverages.
6. Dry mouth can be treated with tart, sugarless gum or candy, water, sugar-free beverages, or with saliva substitutes if dry mouth persists.

# Pseudoephedrine hydrochloride

(soo-doh-eh-**FED**-rin)
**Pregnancy Category:** B
Allermed, Balminil Decongestant Syrup ✦, Cenafed, Children's Congestion Relief, Children's Sudafed Liquid, Congestion Relief, Decofed Syrup, DeFed-60, Dorcol Children's Decongestant Liquid, Efidac/24, Eltor 120 ✦, Genaphed, Halofed, PediaCare Infants' Oral Decongestant Drops, PMS-Pseudoephedrine ✦, Pseudo, Pseudo-Gest, Seudotabs, Sinustop Pro, Sudafed, Sudafed 12 Hour **(OTC)**

# Pseudoephedrine sulfate

(soo-doh-eh-**FED**-rin)
**Pregnancy Category:** B
Afrin Extended-Release Tablets, Drixoral Day ✦, Drixoral N.D. ✦, Drixoral Non-Drowsy Formula **(OTC)**
**Classification:** Direct- and indirect-acting sympathomimetic, nasal decongestant

See also *Sympathomimetic Drugs.*

**Action/Kinetics:** Produces direct stimulation of both alpha-(pronounced) and beta-adrenergic receptors, as well as indirect stimulation through release of norepinephrine from storage sites. Results in decongestant effect on the nasal mucosa. Systemic administration eliminates possible damage to the nasal mucosa. **Onset:** 15–30 min. **Time to peak effect:** 30–60 min. **Duration:** 3–4 hr. **Extended-release: duration,** 8–12 hr. Urinary excretion slowed by alkalinization, causing reabsorption of drug.

**Uses:** Nasal congestion associated with sinus conditions, otitis, allergies. Relief of eustachian tube congestion.

**Additional Contraindications:** Lactation. Use of sustained-release products in children less than 12 years of age.

**Special Concerns:** Use with caution in newborn and premature infants due to a higher risk of side effects. Geriatric clients may be more prone to age-related prostatic hypertrophy.

**How Supplied:** Pseudoephedrine hydrochloride: *Liquid:* 7.5 mg/0.8 mL, 30 mg/5 mL; *Syrup:* 15 mg/5 mL, 30 mg/5 mL; *Tablet:* 30 mg, 60 mg; *Tablet, extended release:* 120 mg, 240 mg. Pseudoephedrine sulfate: *Tablet:* 60 mg

## Dosage

HYDROCHLORIDE

• **Oral Solution, Syrup, Tablets**
*Decongestant.*
**Adults:** 60 mg q 4–6 hr, not to exceed 240 mg in 24 hr. **Pediatric, 6–12 years:** 30 mg using the oral solution or syrup q 4–6 hr, not to exceed 120 mg in 24 hr; **2–6 years:** 15 mg using the oral solution or syrup q 4–6 hr, not to exceed 60 mg in 24 hr. For children less than 2 years of age, the dose must be individualized.

• **Extended-Release Capsules, Tablets**
*Decongestant.*

**Adults and children over 12 years:** 120 mg q 12 hr or 240 mg q 24 hr. Use is not recommended for children less than 12 years of age.

SULFATE

- **Extended-Release Tablets**
  *Decongestant.*

**Adults and children over 12 years:** 120 mg q 12 hr. Use is not rec-ommended for children less than 12 years of age.

## DENTAL CONCERNS

See also *Dental Concerns* for *Sympathomimetic Drugs* and *Nasal Decongestants.*

## Quetiapine fumarate

(kweh-**TYE**-ah-peen)
**Pregnancy Category:** C
Seroquel **(Rx)**
**Classification:** Antipsychotic drug

**Action/Kinetics:** Mechanism unknown but may act as an antagonist at dopamine $D_2$ and serotonin $5HT_2$ receptors. Side effects may be due to antagonism of other receptors (e.g., histamine $H_1$, dopamine $D_1$, adrenergic alpha-1 and alpha-2, serotonin $5HT_{1A}$). Rapidly absorbed. **Peak plasma levels:** 1.5 hr. Metabolized by liver and excreted through urine and feces. **t½, terminal:** About 6 hr.

**Uses:** Management of psychoses.

**Contraindications:** Lactation.

**Special Concerns:** Use with caution in liver disease, in those at risk for aspiration pneumonia, and in those with history of seizures or conditions that lower seizure threshold (e.g., Alzheimer's). Safety and efficacy have not been determined in children.

**Side Effects:** Side effects with incidence of 1% or more are listed. Incidence of extrapyramidal and anticholinergic side effects are much lower than conventional antipsychotics. *Body as a whole:* Asthenia, rash, fever, weight gain, back pain, flu syndrome. *CNS:* Headache, somnolence, dizziness, hypertonia, dysarthria. *Oral:* Dry mouth. *GI:* Constipation, dyspepsia, anorexia, abdominal pain. *CV:* Orthostatic hypotension, syncope, tachycardia, palpitation. *Respiratory:* Pharyngitis, rhinitis, increased cough, dyspnea. *Miscellaneous:* Peripheral edema, sweating, leukopenia, ear pain. *Note:* **Neuroleptic malignant syndrome** and **seizures,** although rare, may occur.

**Drug Interactions**

*Barbiturates* / ↓ Effect of quetiapine due to ↑ breakdown by liver

*Carbamazepine* / ↓ Effect of quetiapine due to ↑ breakdown by liver

*Glucocorticoids* / ↓ Effect of quetiapine due to ↑ breakdown by liver

*Phenytoin* / ↓ Effect of quetiapine due to ↑ breakdown by liver

*Thioridazine* / ↑ Clearance of quetiapine

**How Supplied:** *Tablets:* 25 mg, 100 mg, 200 mg

**Dosage**

- **Tablets**
  *Psychoses.*

**Initial:** 25 mg b.i.d., with increases of 25 to 50 mg b.i.d. or t.i.d. on second and third day, as tolerated. Target dose range, by fourth day, is 300 to 400 mg daily. Further dosage adjustments can occur at intervals of 2 or more days. The antipsychotic dose range is 150–750 mg/day.

## DENTAL CONCERNS

See also *Dental Concerns* for *Antipsychotic Agents, Phenothiazines.*

# Quinapril hydrochloride

(**KWIN**-ah-prill)
**Pregnancy Category:** D
Accupril **(Rx)**
**Classification:** Angiotensin-converting enzyme inhibitor

See also *Angiotensin-Converting Enzyme Inhibitors.*
**Action/Kinetics: Onset:** 1 hr.
**Time to peak serum levels:** 1 hr.
**Peak decrease in BP:** 2–4 hr. Metabolized to quinaprilat, the active metabolite. **t½, quinaprilat:** 2 hr. **Duration:** 24 hr. Significantly bound to plasma proteins. Metabolized with approximately 60% excreted through the urine and 37% excreted in the feces. Also appears to improve endothelial function, an early marker of coronary atherosclerosis.
**Uses:** Alone or in combination with a thiazide diuretic for the treatment of hypertension. Adjunct with a diuretic or digitalis to treat CHF in those not responding adequately to diuretics or digitalis.
**Special Concerns:** Use with caution during lactation. Safety and effectiveness have not been determined in children. Geriatric clients may be more sensitive to the effects of quinapril and manifest higher peak quinaprilat blood levels.
**Side Effects:** *CV:* Vasodilation, tachycardia, ***heart failure,*** palpitations, ***MI, CVA, hypertensive crisis,*** angina pectoris, orthostatic hypotension, ***cardiac rhythm disturbances, cardiogenic shock.*** *Oral:* Dry mouth or throat. *GI:* Constipation, N&V, abdominal pain, ***GI hemorrhage.*** *CNS:* Somnolence, vertigo, nervousness, depression, headache, dizziness, fatigue. *Hematologic:* ***Agranulocytosis,*** bone marrow depression, thrombocytopenia. *Dermatologic:* ***Angioedema of the lips, tongue, glottis, and larynx;*** sweating, pruritus, exfoliative dermatitis, photosensitivity, dermatopolymyositis. *Body as a whole:* Malaise, back pain. *GU:* Oliguria and/or progressive azotemia and rarely ***acute renal failure and/or death in severe***

***heart failure.*** Worsening renal failure. *Respiratory:* Pharyngitis, cough, asthma, bronchospasm. *Miscellaneous:* Oligohydramnios in fetuses exposed to the drug in utero. Abnormal liver function tests, pancreatitis, syncope, hyperkalemia, amblyopia, viral infections.
**Drug Interactions**
See also *Angiotensin-Converting Enzyme Inhibitors.*
*Tetracyclines* / ↓ Absorption of tetracycline due to high magnesium content of quinapril tablets
**How Supplied:** *Tablet:* 5 mg, 10 mg, 20 mg, 40 mg

**Dosage**
• **Tablets**
*Hypertension.*
**Initial:** 10 mg/day; **then,** adjust dosage based on BP response at peak (2–6 hr) and trough (predose) blood levels. The dose should be adjusted at 2-week intervals. **Maintenance:** 20, 40, or 80 mg daily as a single dose or in two equally divided doses. With impaired renal function, the initial dose should be 10 mg if the $C_{CR}$ is greater than 60 mL/min, 5 mg if the $C_{CR}$ is between 30 and 60 mL/min, and 2.5 mg if the $C_{CR}$ is between 10 and 30 mL/min. If the initial dose is well tolerated, the drug may be given the following day as a b.i.d. regimen.
*CHF.*
**Initial:** 5 mg b.i.d. If this dose is well tolerated, titrate clients at weekly intervals until an effective dose, usually 20–40 mg daily in two equally divided doses, is attained. Undesirable hypotension, orthostasis, or azotemia may prevent this dosage level from being reached.

## DENTAL CONCERNS

See also *Dental Concerns* for *Angiotensin-Converting Enzyme Inhibitors* and *Antihypertensive Agents.*

# Quinidine bisulfate

(**KWIN**-ih-deen)

Pregnancy Category: D
Biquin Durules ✦ (Rx)

# Quinidine gluconate
(**KWIN**-ih-deen)
Pregnancy Category: C
Quinaglute Dura-Tabs, Quinalan, Quinate ✦ (Rx)

# Quinidine polygalacturonate
(**KWIN**-ih-deen)
Pregnancy Category: C
Cardioquin (Rx)

# Quinidine sulfate
(**KWIN**-ih-deen)
Pregnancy Category: C
Apo-Quinidine ✦, Quinidex Extentabs, Quinora (Rx)
**Classification:** Antiarrhythmic, class IA

See also *Antiarrhythmic Agents.*
**Action/Kinetics:** Reduces the excitability of the heart and depresses conduction velocity and contractility. Prolongs the refractory period and increases conduction time. It also decreases CO and possesses anticholinergic, antimalarial, antipyretic, and oxytocic properties. **PO: Onset:** 0.5–3 hr. **Maximum effects, after IM:** 30–90 min. **t½:** 6–7 hr. **Time to peak levels, PO:** 3–5 hr for gluconate salt, 1–1.5 hr for sulfate salt, and 6 hr for polygalacturonate salt; **IM:** 1 hr. **Therapeutic serum levels:** 2–6 mcg/mL. **Protein binding:** 60%–80%. **Duration:** 6–8 hr for tablets/capsules and 12 hr for extended-release tablets. Metabolized by liver. Urine pH affects rate of urinary excretion (10%–50% excreted unchanged).
**Uses:** Premature atrial, AV junctional, and ventricular contractions. Treatment and control of atrial flutter, established atrial fibrillation, paroxysmal atrial tachycardia, paroxysmal AV junctional rhythm, paroxysmal and chronic atrial fibrillation, paroxysmal ventricular tachycardia not associated with complete heart block, maintenance therapy after electrical conversion of atrial flutter or fibrilla-

tion. The parenteral route is indicated when PO therapy is not feasible or immediate effects are required. *Non-FDA Approved Uses:* Gluconate salt for life-threatening *Plasmodium falciparum* malaria.
**Contraindications:** Hypersensitivity to drug or other cinchona drugs. Myasthenia gravis, history of thrombocytopenic purpura associated with quinidine use, digitalis intoxication evidenced by arrhythmias or AV conduction disorders. Also, complete heart block, left bundle branch block, or other intraventricular conduction defects manifested by marked QRS widening or bizarre complexes. Complete AV block with an AV nodal or idioventricular pacemaker, aberrant ectopic impulses and abnormal rhythms due to escape mechanisms. History of drug-induced torsades de pointes or long QT syndrome.
**Special Concerns:** Safety in children and during lactation has not been established. Quinidine should be used with extreme caution in clients in whom a sudden change in BP might be detrimental or in those suffering from extensive myocardial damage, subacute endocarditis, bradycardia, coronary occlusion, disturbances in impulse conduction, chronic valvular disease, considerable cardiac enlargement, frank CHF, and renal or hepatic disease. Cautious use is also recommended in clients with acute infections, hyperthyroidism, muscular weakness, respiratory distress, and bronchial asthma. The dose in geriatric clients may have to be reduced due to age-related changes in renal function.
**Side Effects:** *CV:* Widening of QRS complex, hypotension, *cardiac asystole,* ectopic ventricular beats, *ventricular tachycardia or fibrillation, torsades de pointes,* paradoxical tachycardia, *arterial embolism,* ventricular extrasystoles (one or more every 6 beats), prolonged QT interval, *complete AV block, ventricular flutter.* GI: N&V, abdominal pain, anorexia, diarrhea, urge to defecate as well as urinate, esophagitis (rare). *CNS:* Syn-

cope, headache, confusion, excitement, vertigo, apprehension, delirium, dementia, ataxia, depression. *Dermatologic:* Rash, urticaria, exfoliative dermatitis, photosensitivity, flushing with intense pruritus, eczema, psoriasis, pigmentation abnormalities. *Allergic:* Acute asthma, angioneurotic edema, ***respiratory arrest,*** dyspnea, fever, ***vascular collapse,*** purpura, vasculitis, hepatic dysfunction (including granulomatous hepatitis), ***hepatic toxicity.*** *Hematologic:* Hypoprothrombinemia, ***acute hemolytic anemia,*** thrombocytopenic purpura, ***agranulocytosis,*** thrombocytopenia, leukocytosis, neutropenia, shift to left in WBC differential. *Ophthalmologic:* Blurred vision, mydriasis, alterations in color perception, decreased field of vision, double vision, photophobia, optic neuritis, night blindness, scotomata. *Other:* Liver toxicity including hepatitis, lupus nephritis, tinnitus, decreased hearing acuity, arthritis, myalgia, increase in serum skeletal muscle CPK, lupus erythematosus.

**Drug Interactions**
*Anticholinergic agents, Atropine /* Additive effect on blockade of vagus nerve action
*Barbiturates /* ↓ Effect of quinidine due to ↑ breakdown by liver
*Cholinergic agents /* Quinidine antagonizes effect of cholinergic drugs
*Neuromuscular blocking agents /* ↑ Respiratory depression
*Skeletal muscle relaxants /* ↑ Skeletal muscle relaxation
*Sodium bicarbonate /* ↑ Effect of quinidine due to ↓ renal excretion
*Tricyclic antidepressants /* ↑ Effect of antidepressant due to ↓ clearance
**How Supplied:** Quinidine bisulfate: *Sustained-release tablet:* 250 mg. Quinidine gluconate: *Injection:* 80 mg/mL; *Tablet, extended release:* 324 mg. Quinidine polygalacturonate: *Tablet:* 275 mg. Quinidine sulfate: *Tablet:* 200 mg, 300 mg; *Tablet, extended release:* 300 mg

**Dosage** —————————————
• **Quinidine    Bisulfate    Controlled-Release Tablets**
*Antiarrhythmic.*
**Initial:** Test dose of 200 mg in the morning (to ascertain hypersensitivity). In the evening, administer 500 mg. **Then,** beginning the next day, 500–750 mg/12 hr. **Maintenance:** 0.5–1.25 g morning and evening.
• **Quinidine    Polygalacturonate Tablets, Quinidine Sulfate Tablets**
*Premature atrial and ventricular contractions.*
**Adults:** 200–300 mg t.i.d.–q.i.d.
*Paroxysmal SVTs.*
**Adults:** 400–600 mg q 2–3 hr until the paroxysm is terminated.
*Conversion of atrial flutter.*
**Adults:** 200 mg q 2–3 hr for five to eight doses; daily doses can be increased until rhythm is restored or toxic effects occur.
*Conversion of atrial flutter, maintenance therapy.*
**Adults:** 200–300 mg t.i.d.–q.i.d. Large doses or more frequent administration may be required in some clients.
• **Quinidine    Gluconate    Sustained-Release Tablets, Quinidine Sulfate Sustained-Release Tablets**
*All uses.*
**Adults:** 300–600 mg q 8–12 hr.
• **Quinidine Gluconate Injection (IM or IV)**
*Acute tachycardia.*
**Adults, initial:** 600 mg IM; **then,** 400 mg IM repeated as often as q 2 hr.
*Arrhythmias.*
**Adults:** 330 mg IM or less IV (as much as 500–750 mg may be required).
*P. falciparum malaria.*
Two regimens may be used. (1) *Loading dose:* 15 mg/kg in 250 mL NSS given over 4 hr; **then,** 24 hr after beginning the loading dose, institute 7.5 mg/kg infused over 4 hr and given q 8 hr for 7 days or until PO therapy can be started. (2) *Loading dose:* 10 mg/kg in 250 mL NSS infused over 1–2 hr followed immediately by 0.02 mg/kg/min for up to

**Q**

———————————————————————

72 hr or until parasitemia decreases to less than 1% or PO therapy can be started.

## DENTAL CONCERNS

See also *Dental Concerns* for *Antiarrhythmic Agents*.

**General**

1. Have the patient sit up slowly and remain seated for at least two minutes after being supine in order to minimize the risk of orthostatic hypotension.
2. Patients on chronic drug therapy may develop blood dyscrasias.

Symptoms include fever, sore throat, bleeding, and poor wound healing.

**Consultation with Primary Care Provider**

1. Patients with symptoms of blood dyscrasias should be referred to their primary care provider for complete blood counts. Treatment should be postponed until the results are known.

**Client/Family Teaching**

1. Review the proper use of oral hygiene aids in order to prevent injury.
2. Daily home fluoride treatments for persistent dry mouth.

---

# R

## Raloxifene hydrochloride

(ral-**OX**-ih-feen)

**Pregnancy Category:** X

Evista **(Rx)**

**Classification:** Estrogen receptor modulator

---

**Action/Kinetics:** Selective estrogen receptor modulator that reduces bone resorption and decreases overall bone turnover. Considered an estrogen antagonist that acts by combining with estrogen receptors. Has not been associated with endometrial proliferation, breast enlargement, breast pain, or increased risk of breast cancer. Also decreases total and LDL cholesterol levels. Absorbed rapidly after PO; significant first-pass effect. Excreted primarily in feces with small amounts excreted in urine.

**Uses:** Prevention of osteoporosis in postmenopausal women. Not effective in reducing hot flashes or flushes associated with estrogen deficiency.

**Contraindications:** In women who are or who might become pregnant, active or history of venous thromboembolic events (e.g., DVT, pulmonary embolism, retinal vein thrombosis). Use in premenopausal women, during lactation, or in pediatric clients. Concurrent use with systemic estrogen or hormone replacement therapy.

**Special Concerns:** Use with caution with highly protein-bound drugs, including clofibrate, diazepam, diazoxide, ibuprofen, indomethacin, and naproxen. Effect on bone mass density beyond 2 years of treatment is not known.

**Side Effects:** *CV:* Hot flashes, migraine. *Body as a whole:* Infection, flu syndrome, chest pain, fever, weight gain, peripheral edema. *CNS:* Depression, insomnia. *GI:* Nausea, dyspepsia, vomiting, flatulence, GI disorder, gastroenteritis. *GU:* Vaginitis, urinary tract infection, cystitis, leukorrhea, endometrial disorder. *Respiratory:* Sinusitis, pharyngitis, increased cough, pneumonia, laryngitis. *Musculoskeletal:* Arthralgia, myalgia, leg cramps, arthritis. *Dermatologic:* Rash, sweating.

**Drug Interactions**

*Ampicillin* / ↓ Absorption of ampicillin

**How Supplied:** *Tablets:* 60 mg

---

**Dosage**

• **Tablets**

*Prevention of osteoporosis in post-menopausal women.*
**Adults:** 60 mg once daily.

## DENTAL CONCERNS
### General
1. Avoid prolonged immobilization and restrictions of movement as with travel due to increased risk of venous thromboembolic events. Stop 3 days prior to and during prolonged immobilization such as with surgery or prolonged bedrest.
2. It may be necessary to give the patient breaks during longer appointments to stretch or move the legs.
3. Shorter appointments may be necessary if procedure does not allow for breaks.
### Consultation with Primary Care Provider
1. Consultation with the appropriate health care provider may be necessary in order to evaluate the patient's ability to tolerate stress and the level of disease control.

# Ramipril
(**RAM**-ih-prill)
**Pregnancy Category:** D
Altace **(Rx)**
**Classification:** Angiotensin-converting enzyme inhibitor

See also *Angiotensin-Converting Enzyme Inhibitors.*
**Action/Kinetics: Onset:** 1–2 hr. **Time to peak serum levels:** 1 hr (1–2 hr for ramiprilat, the active metabolite). Ramiprilat has approximately six times the ACE inhibitory activity than ramipril. **t½:** 1–2 hr (13–17 hr for ramiprilat); prolonged in impaired renal function. **Duration:** 24 hr. Metabolized in the liver with 60% excreted through the urine and 40% in the feces. Food decreases the rate, but not the extent, of absorption of ramipril.
**Uses:** Alone or in combination with other antihypertensive agents (especially thiazide diuretics) for the treatment of hypertension. Treatment of

CHF following MI to decrease risk of CV death and decrease the risk of failure-related hospitalization and progression to severe or resistant heart failure.
**Contraindications:** Hypersensitivity to ACE inhibitors. Use during lactation.
**Special Concerns:** Geriatric clients may manifest higher peak blood levels of ramiprilat.
**Side Effects:** *CV:* Hypotension, chest pain, palpitations, angina pectoris, *MI, arrhythmias. Oral:* Dry mouth. *GI:* N&V, abdominal pain, diarrhea, dysgeusia, anorexia, constipation, dyspepsia, enzyme changes suggesting pancreatitis, dysphagia, gastroenteritis, increased salivation. *CNS:* Headache, dizziness, fatigue, insomnia, sleep disturbances, somnolence, depression, nervousness, malaise, vertigo, anxiety, amnesia, *convulsions,* tremor. *Respiratory:* Cough, dyspnea, upper respiratory tract infection, asthma, *bronchospasm. Hematologic:* Leukopenia, eosinophilia. Rarely, decreases in hemoglobin or hematocrit. *Dermatologic:* Diaphoresis, photosensitivity, pruritus, rash, dermatitis, purpura. *Body as a whole:* Paresthesias, angioedema, asthenia, syncope, fever, muscle cramps, myalgia, arthralgia, arthritis, neuralgia, neuropathy, influenza, edema. *Miscellaneous:* Impotence, tinnitus, hearing loss, vision disturbances, epistaxis, weight gain, proteinuria.
**Drug Interactions:** See also *Angiotensin-Converting Enzyme Inhibitors.*
**How Supplied:** *Capsule:* 1.25 mg, 2.5 mg, 5 mg, 10 mg

## Dosage
- **Capsules**
  *Hypertension.*
**Initial:** 2.5 mg once daily in clients not taking a diuretic; **maintenance:** 2.5–20 mg/day as a single dose or two equally divided doses. *Clients taking diuretics or who have a $C_{CR}$*

R

*less than 40 mL/min/1.73 m²:* initially 1.25 mg/day; dose may then be increased to a maximum of 5 mg/day.

*CHF following MI.*

**Initial:** 2.5 mg b.i.d. Clients intolerant of this dose may be started on 1.25 mg b.i.d. The target maintenance dose is 5 mg b.i.d.

## DENTAL CONCERNS

See also *Dental Concerns* for *Angiotensin-Converting Enzyme Inhibitors* and *Antihypertensive Agents.*

# Ranitidine hydrochloride
(rah-**NIH**-tih-deen)
**Pregnancy Category:** B
Alti-Ranitidine HCl ✸, Apo-Ranitidine ✸, Novo-Ranidine ✸, Nu-Ranit ✸, Zantac, Zantac-C ✸, Zantac Efferdose, Zantac GELdose Capsules **(Rx)**, Zantac 75 **(OTC)**
**Classification:** H₂ receptor antagonist

See also *Histamine H₂ Antagonists.*
**Action/Kinetics:** Competitively inhibits gastric acid secretion by blocking the effect of histamine on histamine H₂ receptors. Weak inhibitor of cytochrome P-450 (drug-metabolizing enzymes); thus, drug interactions involving inhibition of hepatic metabolism are not expected to occur. Food increases the bioavailability. **Peak effect: PO,** 1–3 hr; **IM, IV,** 15 min. **t½:** 2.5–3 hr. **Duration, nocturnal:** 13 hr; **basal:** 4 hr. **Serum level to inhibit 50% stimulated gastric acid secretion:** 36–94 ng/mL. From 30% to 35% of a PO dose and from 68% to 79% of an IV dose excreted unchanged in urine.
**Uses:** Short-term (4–8 weeks) and maintenance treatment of duodenal ulcer. Pathologic hypersecretory conditions such as Zollinger-Ellison syndrome and systemic mastocytosis. Short-term treatment of active, benign gastric ulcers. Maintenance of healing of gastric ulcers. Gastroesophageal reflux disease, including erosive esophagitis. Maintenance of healing of erosive esophagitis. *Non-FDA Approved Uses:* Prophylaxis of pulmonary aspiration of acid during anesthesia, prevent gastric damage from NSAIDs, prevent stress ulcers, prevent acute upper GI bleeding, as part of multidrug regimen to eradicate *Helicobacter pylori.*
**Contraindications:** Cirrhosis of the liver, impaired renal or hepatic function.
**Special Concerns:** Use with caution during lactation and in clients with decreased hepatic or renal function. Safety and efficacy not established in children.
**Side Effects:** *GI:* Constipation, N&V, diarrhea, abdominal pain, pancreatitis (rare). *CNS:* Headache, dizziness, malaise, insomnia, vertigo, confusion, anxiety, agitation, depression, fatigue, somnolence, hallucinations. *CV:* Bradycardia or tachycardia, premature ventricular beats following rapid IV use (especially in clients predisposed to cardiac rhythm disturbances), ***cardiac arrest.*** *Hematologic:* Thrombocytopenia, granulocytopenia, leukopenia, pancytopenia (sometimes with marrow hypoplasia), ***agranulocytosis, autoimmune hemolytic or aplastic anemia.*** *Hepatic:* Hepatotoxicity, jaundice, hepatitis, increase in ALT. *Dermatologic:* Erythema multiforme, rash, alopecia. *Allergic:* ***Bronchospasm, anaphylaxis,*** angioneurotic edema (rare), rashes, fever, eosinophilia. *Other:* Arthralgia, gynecomastia, impotence, loss of libido, blurred vision, pain at injection site, local burning or itching following IV use.
**Drug Interactions**
*Antacids* / Antacids may ↓ the absorption of ranitidine
*Diazepam* / ↓ Effect of diazepam due to ↓ absorption from GI tract
**How Supplied:** *Capsule:* 150 mg, 300 mg; *Granule for reconstitution:* 150 mg; *Injection:* 1 mg/mL, 25 mg/mL; *Syrup:* 15 mg/mL; *Tablet:* 75 mg, 150 mg, 300 mg; *Tablet, effervescent:* 150 mg

## Dosage ─────────

• **Capsules (Soft Gelatin), Effervescent Tablets and Granules, Syrup, Tablets**

*Duodenal ulcer, short-term.*
**Adults:** 150 mg b.i.d. or 300 mg at bedtime to heal ulcer, although 100 mg b.i.d. will inhibit acid secretion and may be as effective as the higher dose. **Maintenance:** 150 mg at bedtime.

*Pathologic hypersecretory conditions.*
**Adults:** 150 mg b.i.d. (up to 6 g/day has been used in severe cases).

*Benign gastric ulcer.*
**Adults:** 150 mg b.i.d. for active ulcer.
**Maintenance:** 150 mg at bedtime

*Gastroesophageal reflux disease.*
**Adults:** 150 mg b.i.d.

*Erosive esophagitis.*
**Adults:** 150 mg q.i.d.

*Maintenenace of healing of erosive esophagitis.*
**Adults:** 150 mg b.i.d.

• **IM, IV**

*Treatment and maintenance for duodenal ulcer, hypersecretory conditions, gastroesophageal reflux.*
**Adults, IM:** 50 mg q 6–8 hr. **Intermittent IV injection or infusion:** 50 mg q 6–8 hr, not to exceed 400 mg/day. **Continuous IV infusion:** 6.25 mg/hr.

*Zollinger-Ellison clients.*
**Continuous IV infusion:** Dilute ranitidine in 5% dextrose injection to a concentration no greater than 2.5 mg/mL with an initial infusion rate of 1 mg/kg/hr. If after 4 hr the client shows a gastric acid output of greater than 10 mEq/hr or if symptoms appear, the dose should be increased by 0.5-mg/kg/hr increments and the acid output measured. Doses up to 2.5 mg/kg/hr may be necessary.

## DENTAL CONCERNS
### General
1. A semisupine position for the dental chair may be necessary to help minimize or avoid GI adverse effects.
2. Avoid alcohol, caffeine, and aspirin-containing prescription and nonprescription drugs.

# Repaglinide
(re-**PAY**-glin-eyed)
**Pregnancy Category:** C
Prandin **(Rx)**
**Classification:** Oral antidiabetic

See also *Antidiabetic Agents: Hypoglycemic Agents.*

**Action/Kinetics:** Lowers blood glucose by stimulating release of insulin from pancreas. Action depends on functioning beta cells in pancreatic islets. Rapidly and completely absorbed from GI tract. **Peak plasma levels:** 1 hr. Completely metabolized in liver with most excreted in feces.

**Uses:** Adjunct to diet and exercise in type 2 diabetes mellitus. In combination with metformin to lower blood glucose where hyperglycemia can not be controlled by exercise, diet, or either drug alone.

**Contraindications:** Lactation. Diabetic ketoacidosis, with or without coma. Type 1 diabetes.

**Special Concerns:** Use with caution in impaired hepatic function. Safety and efficacy have not been determined in children.

**Side Effects:** *CV:* Chest pain, angina, ischemia. *GI:* Nausea, diarrhea, constipation, vomiting, dyspepsia. *Respiratory:* URI, sinusitis, rhinitis, bronchitis. *Musculoskeletal:* Arthralgia, back pain. *Miscellaneous:* Hypoglycemia, headache, paresthesia, chest pain, urinary tract infection, tooth disorder, allergy.

**Drug Interactions:** See *Antidiabetic Agents, Hypoglycemic Agents.*

**How Supplied:** *Tablets:* 0.5 mg, 1 mg, 2 mg

## Dosage
• **Tablets**
*Type 2 diabetes mellitus.*
Individualize dosage. **Initial:** In those not previously treated or whose HbA1-C is less than 8%, give 0.5 mg. For those previously treated or whose HbA1-C is 8% or more, give 1 or 2 mg before each meal. **Dose range:** 0.5–4 mg taken with

meals. **Maximum daily dose:** 16 mg.

## DENTAL CONCERNS

See also *Dental Concerns* for *Antidiabetic Agents: Hypoglycemic Agents.*

---

# Rifabutin
(**rif**-ah-**BYOU**-tin)
**Pregnancy Category:** B
Mycobutin **(Rx)**
**Classification:** Antitubercular drug

**Action/Kinetics:** Inhibits DNA-dependent RNA polymerase in susceptible strains of *Escherichia coli* and *Bacillus subtilis.* Rapidly absorbed from the GI tract. **Peak plasma levels after a single dose:** 3.3 hr. **Mean terminal t½:** 45 hr. About 85% is bound to plasma proteins. High-fat meals slow the rate, but not the extent, of absorption. About 30% of a dose is excreted in the feces and 53% in the urine, primarily as metabolites. The 25-O-desacetyl metabolite is equal in activity to rifabutin.

**Uses:** Prevention of disseminated *Mycobacterium avium* complex (MAC) disease in clients with advanced HIV infection.

**Contraindications:** Hypersensitivity to rifabutin or other rifamycins (e.g., rifampin). Use in clients with active tuberculosis. Lactation.

**Special Concerns:** Safety and efficacy have not been determined in children, although the drug has been used in HIV-positive children.

**Side Effects:** *Oral:* Taste perversion, discolored saliva (brownish-orange). *GI:* Anorexia, abdominal pain, diarrhea, dyspepsia, eructation, flatulence, N&V. *Respiratory:* Chest pain, chest pressure or pain with dyspnea. *CNS:* Insomnia, *seizures,* paresthesia, aphasia, confusion. *Musculoskeletal:* Asthenia, myalgia, arthralgia, myositis. *Body as a whole:* Fever, headache, generalized pain, flu-like syndrome. *Dermatologic:* Rash, skin discoloration. *Hematologic:* Neutropenia, leukopenia, anemia, eosinophilia, thrombocytopenia. *Miscella-*

*neous:* Discolored urine, nonspecific T wave changes on ECG, hepatitis, hemolysis, uveitis.

**Drug Interactions:** Rifabutin has liver enzyme-inducing properties and may be expected to have similar interactions as does rifampin. However, rifabutin is a less potent enzyme inducer than rifampin.

**How Supplied:** *Capsule:* 150 mg

## Dosage

- **Capsules**

  *Prophylaxis of MAC disease in clients with advanced HIV infection.*
  **Adults:** 300 mg/day.

## DENTAL CONCERNS

See also *General Dental Concerns for All Anti-Infectives.*
**General**
1. Examine patient for oral signs and symptoms of opportunistic infection.
2. Determine why the patient is taking the drug.
3. Patients on chronic drug therapy may develop blood dyscrasias. Symptoms include fever, sore throat, bleeding, and poor wound healing.
**Consultation with Primary Care Provider**
1. Medical consultation may be necessary in order to assess patient's ability to tolerate stress.
2. Patients with symptoms of blood dyscrasias should be referred to their primary care provider for complete blood counts. Treatment should be postponed until the results are known.
**Client/Family Teaching**
1. Review the importance of good oral hygiene in order to prevent soft tissue inflammation.
2. Avoid alcohol-containing mouth rinses and beverages.

---

# Rifampin
(rih-**FAM**-pin)
**Pregnancy Category:** C
Rifadin, Rimactane, Rofact ✶ **(Rx)**
**Classification:** Primary antitubercular agent

**Action/Kinetics:** Semisynthetic antibiotic derived from *Streptomyces mediterranei*. Suppresses RNA synthesis by binding to the beta subunit of DNA-dependent RNA polymerase. This prevents attachment of the enzyme to DNA and blockade of RNA transcription. Both bacteriostatic and bactericidal; most active against rapidly replicating organisms. Well absorbed from the GI tract; widely distributed in body tissues. **Peak plasma concentration:** 4–32 mcg/mL after 2–4 hr. **t½:** 1.5–5 hr (higher in clients with hepatic impairment). In normal clients t½ decreases with usage. Metabolized in liver; 60% is excreted in feces.

**Uses:** All types of tuberculosis. Must be used in conjunction with at least one other tuberculostatic drug (such as isoniazid, ethambutol, pyrazinamide) but is the drug of choice for retreatment. Also for treatment of asymptomatic meningococcal carriers to eliminate *Neisseria meningitidis*. *Investigational:* Used in combination for infections due to *Staphylococcus aureus* and *S. epidermidis* (endocarditis, osteomyelitis, prostatitis); Legionnaire's disease; in combination with dapsone for leprosy; prophylaxis of meningitis due to *Haemophilus influenzae* and gram-negative bacteremia in infants.

**Contraindications:** Hypersensitivity; not recommended for intermittent therapy.

**Special Concerns:** Safe use during lactation has not been established. Safety and effectiveness not determined in children less than 5 years of age. Use with extreme caution in clients with hepatic dysfunction.

**Side Effects:** *Oral:* Sore mouth and tongue, red-orange saliva, stomatitis, glossitis, candidiasis, bleeding. *GI:* N&V, diarrhea, anorexia, gas, pseudomembranous colitis, pancreatitis, cramps, heartburn, flatulence. *CNS:* Headache, drowsiness, fatigue, ataxia, dizziness, confusion, generalized numbness, fever, difficulty in concentrating. *Hepatic:* Jaundice, hepatitis.

Increases in AST, ALT, bilirubin, alkaline phosphatase. *Hematologic:* Thrombocytopenia, eosinophilia, hemolysis, leukopenia, **hemolytic anemia.** *Allergic:* Flu-like symptoms, dyspnea, wheezing, SOB, purpura, pruritus, urticaria, skin rashes, sore mouth and tongue, conjunctivitis. *Renal:* Hematuria, hemoglobinuria, renal insufficiency, acute renal failure. *Miscellaneous:* Visual disturbances, muscle weakness or pain, arthralgia, decreased BP, osteomalacia, menstrual disturbances, edema of face and extremities, adrenocortical insufficiency, increases in BUN and serum uric acid. *NOTE:* Body fluids and feces may be red-orange.

**Drug Interactions**

*Acetaminophen* / ↓ Effect of acetaminophen due to ↑ breakdown by liver

*Barbiturates* / ↓ Effect of barbiturates due to ↑ breakdown by liver

*Benzodiazepines* / ↓ Effect of benzodiazepines due to ↑ breakdown by liver

*Corticosteroids* / ↓ Effect of corticosteroids due to ↑ breakdown by liver

*Halothane* / ↑ Risk of hepatotoxicity and hepatic encephalopathy

*Ketoconazole* / ↓ Effect of either ketoconazole or rifampin

*Sulfones* / ↓ Effect of sulfones due to ↑ breakdown by liver

**How Supplied:** *Capsule:* 150 mg, 300 mg; *Powder for injection:* 600 mg

**Dosage** ———————

• **Capsules, IV**
  *Pulmonary tuberculosis.*
  **Adults:** Single dose of 600 mg/day; **children over 5 years:** 10–20 mg/kg/day, not to exceed 600 mg/day.
  *Meningococcal carriers.*
  **Adults:** 600 mg b.i.d. for 2 days; **children:** 10–20 mg/kg q 12 hr for four doses. Dosage should not exceed 600 mg/day.

---

## DENTAL CONCERNS

See also *General Dental Concerns for All Anti-Infectives.*

**General**

1. Examine patient for oral signs and symptoms of opportunistic infection.
2. Determine why the patient is taking the drug.
3. Patients on chronic drug therapy may develop blood dyscrasias. Symptoms include fever, sore throat, bleeding, and poor wound healing.

**Consultation with Primary Care Provider**

1. Medical consultation may be necessary in order to assess patient's ability to tolerate stress.
2. Patients with symptoms of blood dyscrasias should be referred to their primary care provider for complete blood counts. Treatment should be postponed until the results are known.

**Client/Family Teaching**

1. Review the importance of good oral hygiene in order to prevent soft tissue inflammation.
2. Avoid alcohol-containing mouth rinses and beverages.
3. Must take daily for months to effectively treat tuberculosis. Do not stop taking or skip doses of medication.
4. Rifampin may impart a red-orange color to urine, feces, saliva, sputum, and tears; contact lenses may become *permanently* discolored.

---

# Risperidone
(ris-**PAIR**-ih-dohn)
**Pregnancy Category:** C
Risperdal **(Rx)**
**Classification:** Antipsychotic

**Action/Kinetics:** Mechanism may be due to a combination of antagonism of dopamine ($D_2$) and serotonin ($5\text{-}HT_2$) receptors. Also has high affinity for the alpha-1, alpha-2, and histamine-1 receptors. Metabolized significantly in the liver to the active metabolite 9-hydroxyrisperidone, which has equal receptor-binding activity as risperidone. Thus, the effect is likely due to both the parent compound and the metabolite. Food does not affect either the rate or extent of absorption. **Peak plasma levels, risperidone:** 1 hr; **peak plasma levels, 9-hydroxyrisperidone:** 3 hr for extensive metabolizers and 17 hr for poor metabolizers. **$t\frac{1}{2}$, risperidone and 9-methylrisperidone:** 3 and 21 hr, respectively, for extensive metabolizers and 20 and 30 hr, respectively, for poor metabolizers. The clearance of the drug is decreased in geriatric clients and in clients with hepatic and renal impairment.

**Uses:** Treatment of psychotic disorders.

**Contraindications:** Lactation.

**Special Concerns:** Use with caution in clients with known CV disease (including history of MI or ischemia, heart failure, conduction abnormalities), cerebrovascular disease, and conditions that predispose the client to hypotension (e.g., dehydration, hypovolemia, use of antihypertensive drugs). Use with caution in clients who will be exposed to extreme heat or when taken with other CNS drugs or alcohol. The effectiveness of risperidone for more than 6–8 weeks has not been studied. Safety and effectiveness have not been established for children.

**Side Effects:** *Neuroleptic malignant syndrome:* Hyperpyrexia, muscle rigidity, altered mental status, autonomic instability (i.e., irregular pulse or BP, tachycardia, diaphoresis, cardiac dysrhythmia), elevated CPK, rhabdomyolysis, *acute renal failure, death. CNS:* Tardive dyskinesia (especially in geriatric clients), somnolence, insomnia, agitation, anxiety, aggressive reaction, extrapyramidal symptoms, headache, dizziness, increased dream activity, decreased sexual desire, nervousness, impaired concentration, depression, apathy, catatonia, euphoria, increased libido, amnesia, increased duration of sleep, dysarthria, vertigo, stupor, paresthesia, confusion. *Oral:* Increased or decreased salivation, toothache, stomatitis, dry mouth. *GI:* Constipation, nausea, dyspepsia, vomiting, abdominal pain, anorexia, flatulence, diarrhea, increased appetite, melena, dysphagia, hemorrhoids, gastritis. *CV:* Prolongation of the QT interval that might lead to ***torsades de pointes,***. Orthostatic hypotension, tachycardia, palpitation, hypertension or hypotension, ***AV block, MI.*** *Respiratory:* Rhinitis, coughing, upper respiratory infection, sinusitis, pharyngitis, dyspnea. *Body as a whole:* Arthralgia, back pain, chest pain, fever, fatigue, rigors, malaise, edema, flu-like symptoms, increase or decrease in weight. *Hematologic:* Purpura, anemia, hypochromic anemia. *GU:* Polyuria, polydipsia, urinary incontinence, hematuria, dysuria, menorrhagia, orgastic dysfunction, dry vagina, erectile dysfunction, nonpuerperal lactation, amenorrhea, female breast pain, leukorrhea, mastitis, dysmenorrhea, female perineal pain, intermenstrual bleeding, ***vaginal hemorrhage,*** failure to ejaculate. *Dermatologic:* Rash, dry skin, seborrhea, increased pigmentation, increased or decreased sweating, acne, alopecia, hyperkeratosis, pruritus, skin exfoliation. *Ophthalmic:* Abnormal vision, abnormal accommodation, xerophthalmia. *Miscellaneous:* Increased prolactin, photosensitivity, diabetes mellitus, thirst, myalgia, epistaxis.

**Drug Interactions:** See also *Antipsychotic Agents, Phenothiazines.* *Carbamazepine* / ↑ Clearance of risperidone following chronic use of carbamazepine

**How Supplied:** *Solution:* 1 mg/mL; *Tablet:* 1 mg, 2 mg, 3 mg, 4 mg

## Dosage

- **Oral Solution, Tablets**
  *Antipsychotic.*

**Adults, initial:** 1 mg b.i.d. Once daily dosing can also be used. Can be increased by 1 mg b.i.d. on the second and third days, as tolerated, to reach a dose of 3 mg b.i.d. by the third day. Further increases in dose should occur at intervals of about 1 week. **Maximal effect:** 4–6 mg/day. Doses greater than 6 mg/day were not shown to be more effective and were associated with greater incidence of side effects. Safety of doses greater than 16 mg/day have not been studied. The initial dose is 0.5 mg b.i.d. for clients who are elderly or debilitated, those with severe renal or hepatic impairment, and those predisposed to hypotension or in whom hypotension would pose a risk. Dosage increases in these clients should be in increments of 0.5 mg b.i.d. Dosage increases above 1.5 mg b.i.d. should occur at intervals of about 1 week.

## DENTAL CONCERNS

See also *Dental Concerns* for *Antipsychotic Agents, Phenothiazines.*
**General**
1. Vasoconstrictors should be used with caution and in low doses. Avoid epinephrine-containing gingival retraction cords.

# Ritonavir
(rih-**TOH**-nah-veer)
**Pregnancy Category:** B
Norvir **(Rx)**
**Classification:** Antiviral drug, protease inhibitor

See also *Anitiviral Drugs.*
**Action/Kinetics:** Ritonavir is a peptidomimetic inhibitor of both the HIV-1 and HIV-2 proteases. Inhibition of HIV protease results in the enzyme incapable of processing the "gag-pool" polyprotein precursor that leads to production of noninfectious immature HIV particles. **Peak concentrations after 600 mg of the solution:** 2 hr after fasting and 4 hr after nonfasting. **t½:** 3–5 hr. The drug is metabolized by the cytochrome P450 system. Metabolites and unchanged drug are excreted through both the feces and urine.
**Uses:** Alone or in combination with nucleoside analogues (ddC or AZT) for the treatment of HIV infection.

R

---

Use of ritonavir may result in a reduction in both mortality and AIDS-defining clinical events. Clinical benefit has not been determined for periods longer than 6 months.

**Contraindications:** Hypersensitivity.

**Special Concerns:** Ritonavir is not considered a cure for HIV infection; clients may continue to manifest illnesses associated with advanced HIV infection, including opportunistic infections. Also, therapy with ritonavir has not been shown to decrease the risk of transmitting HIV to others through sexual contact or blood contamination. Use with caution in those with impaired hepatic function and during lactation. Hemophiliacs treated with protease inhibitors may manifest spontaneous bleeding episodes. Safety and efficacy have not been determined in children less than 12 years of age.

**Side Effects:** Side effects listed are those with a frequency of 2% or greater. *Oral:* Circumoral paresthesia, taste perversion, local throat irritation, dry mouth. *GI:* N&V, diarrhea, anorexia, flatulence, constipation, abdominal pain, dyspepsia. *Nervous:* Peripheral paresthesia, dizziness, insomnia, paresthesia, somnolence, abnormal thinking. *Body as a whole:* Asthenia, headache, malaise, fever. *Dermatologic:* Sweating, rash. *Miscellaneous:* Vasodilation, hyperlipidemia, myalgia, pharyngitis.

**Drug Interactions:** Ritonavir is expected to produce large increases in the plasma levels of a number of drugs, including astemizole, buproprion, cisapride, erythromycin, meperidine, phenothiazines, piroxicam, propoxyphene, tefenadine. This may lead to an increased risk of arrhythmias, hematologic complications, seizures, or other serious adverse effects.

Ritonavir may produce a decrease in the plasma levels of the following drugs: sedative/hypnotics.

Ritonavir may produce an increase in the plasma levels of the following drugs: clarithromycin, fluconazole, fluoxetine, desipramine, theophylline.

Coadministration of ritonavir with the following drugs may cause extreme sedation and respiratory depression and thus should not be combined: alprazolam, clorazepate, diazepam, estazolam, flurazepam, midazolam, triazolam, and zolpidem.

*Metronidazole* / Possible disulfiram-like reaction.

**How Supplied:** *Capsules:* 100 mg; *Oral solution:* 600 mg/7.5 mL

## Dosage

- **Capsules, Oral Solution**
  *Treatment of HIV infection.*
  600 mg b.i.d. If nausea is experienced upon initiation of therapy, dose escalation may be tried as follows: 300 mg b.i.d. for 1 day, 400 mg b.i.d. for 2 days, 500 mg b.i.d. for 1 day, and then 600 mg b.i.d. thereafter.

## DENTAL CONCERNS

See also *Dental Concerns* for *Antiviral Drugs.*

**General**

1. Semisupine position for dental chair in order to help alleviate or minimize GI discomfort from the drug.
2. Examine patient for oral signs and symptoms of opportunistic infection.
3. Decreased saliva flow can put the patient at risk for dental caries, periodontal disease, and candidiasis.
4. Frequent recall in order to evaluate healing of infection.

**Consultation with Primary Care Provider**

1. Medical consultation may be necessary in order to assess patient's ability to tolerate stress.
2. Medical consultation may be necessary in order to assess patient's level of disease control.

**Client/Family Teaching**

1. Review the importance of good oral hygiene in order to prevent soft tissue inflammation.
2. Review the proper use of oral hygiene aids in order to prevent injury.

3. Secondary oral infection may occur. Seek dental treatment immediately if this happens.

4. Daily home fluoride treatments for persistent dry mouth.

5. Avoid alcohol-containing mouth rinses and beverages.

6. Avoid caffeine-containing beverages.

7. Dry mouth can be treated with tart, sugarless gum or candy, water, sugar-free beverages, or with saliva substitutes if dry mouth persists.

---

# Ropinirole hydrochloride
(roh-**PIN**-ih-roll)
**Pregnancy Category:** C
Requip **(Rx)**
**Classification:** Antiparkinson agent

See also *Antiparkinson Agents*.

**Action/Kinetics:** Mechanism is not known but believed to involve stimulation of postsynaptic $D_2$ dopamine receptors in caudate-putamen in brain. Causes decreases in both systolic and diastolic BP at doses above 0.25 mg. Rapidly absorbed. **Peak plasma levels:** 1–2 hr. Food reduces maximum concentration. **t½, elimination:** 6 hr. First pass effect; extensively metabolized in liver.

**Uses:** Treat signs and symptoms of idiopathic Parkinson's disease.

**Contraindications:** Lactation.

**Special Concerns:** Safety and efficacy have not been determined in children.

**Side Effects:** *Oral:* Dry mouth. *CNS:* Hallucinations, cause and/or exacerbate pre-existing dyskinesia. *CV:* Syncope (sometimes with bradycardia), postural hypotension.

**Drug Interactions**
*Ciprofloxacin* / Significant ↑ in ropinirole plasma levels
*Estrogens* / ↓ Oral clearance of ropinirole

**How Supplied:** *Tablets:* 0.25 mg, 0.5 mg, 1 mg, 2 mg, 5 mg

## Dosage
• **Tablets**
  *Parkinson's disease.*

**Week 1:** 0.25 mg t.i.d. **Week 2:** 0.5 mg t.i.d. **Week 3:** 0.75 mg t.i.d. **Week 4:** 1 mg t.i.d. After week 4, daily dose, if necessary, may be increased by 1.5 mg/day on weekly basis up to dose of 9 mg/day. This may be followed by increase of up to 3 mg/day weekly to total dose of 24 mg/day.

## DENTAL CONCERNS
**General**
1. Monitor vital signs at every appointment because of cardiovascular side effects.

2. Have the patient sit up slowly and remain seated for at least two minutes after being supine in order to minimize the risk of orthostatic hypotension.

3. Decreased saliva flow can put the patient at risk for dental caries, periodontal disease, and candidiasis.

4. Patients on chronic drug therapy may develop blood dyscrasias. Symptoms include fever, sore throat, bleeding, and poor wound healing.

**Consultation with Primary Care Provider**
1. Patients with symptoms of blood dyscrasias should be referred to their primary care provider for complete blood counts. Treatment should be postponed until the results are known.

2. Consultation may be required in order to assess extent of disease control and patient's ability to tolerate stress.

**Client/Family Teaching**
1. Review the importance of good oral hygiene in order to prevent soft tissue inflammation.

2. Review the proper use of oral hygiene aids in order to prevent injury.

3. Daily home fluoride treatments for persistent dry mouth.

4. Avoid alcohol-containing mouth rinses and beverages.

5. Avoid caffeine-containing beverages.

6. Dry mouth can be treated with tart, sugarless gum or candy, water, sugar-free beverages, or with saliva substitutes if dry mouth persists.

R

---

# Salmeterol xinafoate

(sal-**MET**-er-ole)
**Pregnancy Category:** C
Serevent **(Rx)**
**Classification:** Beta-2 adrenergic agonist

See also *Sympathomimetic Drugs.*

**Action/Kinetics:** Selective for beta-2 adrenergic receptors which are located in the bronchi and heart causing relaxation of bronchial smooth muscle and inhibition of release of mediators of immediate hypersensitivity, especially from mast cells. Significantly bound to plasma proteins. Cleared by hepatic metabolism.

**Uses:** Long-term maintenance treatment of asthma. Prevention of bronchospasms in clients over 12 years of age with reversible obstructive airway disease, including nocturnal asthma. Prevention of exercise-induced bronchospasms. Inhalation powder for long-term maintenance treatment of asthma in clients aged 12 years or older.

**Contraindications:** Use in clients who can be controlled by short-acting, inhaled beta-2 agonists. Use to treat acute symptoms of asthma or in those who have worsening or deteriorating asthma. Lactation.

**Special Concerns:** The drug is not a substitute for PO or inhaled corticosteroids. The safety and efficacy of using salmeterol with a spacer or other devices has not been studied adequately. Use with caution in impaired hepatic function; with cardiovascular disorders, including coronary insufficiency, cardiac arrhythmias, and hypertension; with convulsive disorders or thyrotoxicosis; and in clients who respond unusually to sympathomimetic amines. Because of the potential of the drug interfering with uterine contractility, use of salmeterol during labor should be restricted to those in whom benefits clearly outweigh risks. Safety and efficacy have not

been determined in children less than 12 years of age.

**Side Effects:** *Respiratory:* Paradoxical bronchospasms, upper or lower respiratory tract infection, nasopharyngitis, disease of nasal cavity/sinus, cough, pharyngitis, allergic rhinitis, laryngitis, tracheitis, bronchitis. *Allergic: **Immediate hypersensitivity reactions,*** including urticaria, rash, and **bronchospasm.** *CV:* Palpitations, chest pain, increased BP, tachycardia. *CNS:* Headache, sinus headache, tremors, nervousness, malaise, fatigue, dizziness, giddiness. *Oral:* Dry mouth, dental pain. *GI:* Stomachache. *Musculoskeletal:* Joint pain, back pain, muscle cramps, muscle contractions, myalgia, myositis, muscle soreness. *Miscellaneous:* Flu, dental pain, rash, skin eruption, dysmenorrhea.

**Drug Interactions**
*Tricyclic antidepressants* / Potentiation of the effect of salmeterol

**How Supplied:** *Metered dose inhaler:* 21 mcg/inh

**Dosage**
- **Metered Dose Inhaler**
*Maintenance of bronchodilation, prevention of symptoms of asthma, including nocturnal asthma.*
**Adults and children over 12 years of age:** Two inhalations (42 mcg) b.i.d. (morning and evening, approximately 12 hr apart).
*Prevention of exercise-induced bronchospasms.*
**Adults and children over 12 years of age:** Two inhalations (42 mcg) at least 30–60 min before exercise. Additional doses should not be used for 12 hr.
- **Inhalation Powder (Diskus)**
*Maintenance treatment of asthma.*
**Adults and children over 12 years of age:** 50 mcg (one inhalation) b.i.d. in the morning and evening.
*NOTE:* Even though the metered dose inhaler and the inhalation

powder are used for the same conditions, they are not interchangeable.

## DENTAL CONCERNS

See also *Dental Concerns* for *Sympathomimetic Drugs.*
1. Do not use this drug during an acute asthma attack.

## Saquinavir mesylate
(sah-**KWIN**-ah-veer)
**Pregnancy Category:** B
Fortovase, Invirase **(Rx)**
**Classification:** Antiviral drug, protease inhibitor

See also *Antiviral Drugs.*

**Action/Kinetics:** Saquinavir inhibits the activity of HIV protease and prevents the cleavage of viral polyproteins. Has a low bioavailability after PO use, probably due to incomplete absorption and first-pass metabolism. A high-fat meal or high-calorie meal increases the amount of drug absorbed. Over 98% bound to plasma protein. About 87% metabolized in the liver by the cytochrome P450 system. Both metabolites and unchanged drug are excreted mainly through the feces. It is believed the bioavailability of Fortovase is greater than Invirase.

**Uses:** Combined with AZT or zalcitabine (ddC) for treatment of advanced HIV infection in selected clients. No data are available regarding the benefit of combination therapy of saquinavir with AZT or ddC on HIV disease progression or survival.

**Contraindications:** Lactation.

**Special Concerns:** Photoallergy or phototoxicity may occur; thus, clients should take protective measures against exposure to ultraviolet or sunlight until tolerance is assessed. Use with caution in those with hepatic insufficiency. Hemophiliacs treated with protease inhibitors for HIV infections may manifest spontaneous bleeding episodes. Safety and efficacy have not been determined in HIV-infected children or adolescents less than 16 years of age.

**Side Effects:** Side effects listed are for saquinavir combined with either AZT or ddC. *Oral:* Ulceration of buccal mucosa, cheilitis, gingivitis, glossitis, stomatitis, tooth disorder, dry mouth, alteration in taste. *GI:* Diarrhea, abdominal discomfort, nausea, dyspepsia, abdominal pain, constipation, dysphagia, eructation, blood-stained or discolored feces, gastralgia, gastritis, GI inflammation, *rectal hemorrhage,* hemorrhoids, hepatomegaly, hepatosplenomegaly, melena, pain, painful defecation, pancreatitis, parotid disorder, pelvic salivary glands disorder, vomiting, frequent bowel movements. *CNS:* Headache, paresthesia, numbness of extremity, dizziness, peripheral neuropathy, ataxia, confusion, *convulsions,* dysarthria, dysesthesia, hyperesthesia, hyperreflexia, hyporeflexia, face numbness, facial pain, paresis, poliomyelitis, progressive multifocal leukoencephalopathy, spasms, tremor, agitation, amnesia, anxiety, depression, excessive dreaming, euphoria, hallucinations, insomnia, reduced intellectual ability, irritability, lethargy, libido disorder, overdose effect, psychic disorder, somnolence, speech disorder. *Musculoskeletal:* Musculoskeletal pain, myalgia, arthralgia, arthritis, back pain, muscle cramps, musculoskeletal disorder, stiffness, tissue changes, trauma. *Body as a whole:* Allergic reaction, chest pain, edema, fever, intoxication, external parasites, retrosternal pain, shivering, wasting syndrome, weight decrease, abscess, angina tonsillaris, candidiasis, hepatitis, herpes simplex, herpes zoster, infections (bacterial, mycotic, staphylococcal), influenza, lymphadenopathy, tumor. *CV:* Cyanosis, heart murmur, heart valve disorder, hypertension, hypotension, syncope, distended vein, HR disorder. *Metabolic:* Dehydration, hyperglycemia, weight decrease. *Hematologic:* Anemia, microhemorrhages, pancytope-

**S**

nia, splenomegaly, thrombocytopenia. *Respiratory:* Bronchitis, cough, dyspnea, epistaxis, hemoptysis, laryngitis, pharyngitis, pneumonia, respiratory disorder rhinitis, sinusitis, URTI. *GU:* Enlarged prostate, vaginal discharge, micturition disorder, UTI. *Dermatologic:* Acne, dermatitis, seborrheic dermatitis, eczema, erythema, folliculitis, furunculosis, hair changes, hot flushes, photosensitivity reaction, changes in skin pigment, maculopapular rash, skin disorder, skin nodules, skin ulceration, increased sweating, urticaria, verruca, xeroderma. *Ophthalmic:* Dry eye syndrome, xerophthalmia, blepharitis, eye irritation, visual disturbance. *Otic:* Earache, ear pressure, decreased hearing, otitis, tinnitus.

**Drug Interactions**
*Astemizole* / Possibility of prolongation of QT intervals → serious CV adverse effects
*Carbamazepine* / ↓ Blood levels of saquinavir
*Clindamycin* / ↑ Blood levels of clindamycin
*Dexamethasone* / ↓ Blood levels of saquinavir
*Itraconazole* / ↑ Blood levels of itraconazole
*Ketoconazole* / ↑ Blood levels of ketoconazole
*Phenobarbital* / ↓ Blood levels of saquinavir
*Terfenadine* / Possibility of prolongation of QT intervals → serious CV adverse effects
**How Supplied:** *Capsules:* 200 mg

**Dosage** ⎯⎯⎯⎯⎯⎯⎯⎯⎯⎯
• **Fortovase Capsules**
*HIV infections in combination with AZT or ddC.*
Six 200-mg capsules (i.e., 1,200 mg) taken t.i.d. with meals or up to 2 hr after meals.
• **Invirase Capsules**
*HIV infections in combination with AZT or ddC.*
Three 200-mg capsules of saquinavir t.i.d. taken within 2 hr of a full meal. The recommended doses of AZT or ddC as part of combination therapy are: AZT, 200 mg t.i.d., or ddC, 0.75

mg t.i.d. However, base dosage adjustments of AZT or ddC on the known toxicity profile of the individual drug. This form of the drug will be phased out.

## DENTAL CONCERNS

See also *Dental Concerns* for *Antiviral Drugs.*
**General**
1. Examine patient for oral signs and symptoms of opportunistic infection.
2. Patients on chronic drug therapy may develop blood dyscrasias. Symptoms include fever, sore throat, and bleeding, and poor wound healing.
3. Palliative therapy may be required for patients with oral adverse effects.
**Consultation with Primary Care Provider**
1. Medical consultation may be necessary in order to assess patient's level of disease control.
2. Patients with symptoms of blood dyscrasias should be referred to their primary care provider for complete blood counts. Treatment should be postponed until the results are known.
**Client/Family Teaching**
1. Review the importance of good oral hygiene in order to prevent soft tissue inflammation.
2. Review the proper use of oral hygiene aids in order to prevent injury.
3. Report oral sores, lesions, or bleeding to the dentist.
4. Update patient's dental record (medication/health history) as needed.

# Secobarbital sodium
(see-koh-**BAR**-bih-tal)
**Pregnancy Category:** D
Novo-Secobarb ✽, Seconal Sodium
**(C-II) (Rx)**
**Classification:** Barbiturate sedative-hypnotic

See also *Barbiturates.*
**Action/Kinetics:** Short-acting. Distributed quickly due to high lipid

solubility. **Onset:** 10–15 min. **t½:** 15–40 hr. **Duration:** 3–4 hr. Is 46%–70% protein bound.

**Uses: Parenteral:** Intermittent use as a sedative, hypnotic, or preanesthetic.

**Special Concerns:** Elderly or debilitated clients may be more sensitive to the drug and require reduced dosage.

**How Supplied:** *Injection:* 50 mg/mL

**Dosage** ————————————

• **IM, IV**
*Hypnotic.*
**Adults:** 100–200 mg IM or 50–250 mg IV.
*Preoperative sedative.*
**Adults:** 1 mg/kg IM 10–15 min before procedure. **Children:** 4–5 mg/kg IM.
*Dentistry in clients who will receive nerve block.*
100–150 mg IV.
*Status epilepticus.*
**Children:** 15–20 mg/kg IV over 10–15 min.

## DENTAL CONCERNS

See also *Dental Concerns* for *Barbiturates.*

# Selegiline hydrochloride (Deprenyl)
(seh-**LEH**-jih-leen)
**Pregnancy Category:** C
Carbex, Eldepryl, Novo-Selegiline ✦ **(Rx)**
**Classification:** Antiparkinson agent

See also *Antiparkinson Agents.*

**Action/Kinetics:** Precise mechanism of action is not known; does inhibit MAO, type B. May act through other mechanisms to increase dopaminergic activity, including interference with dopamine uptake at the synapse. Metabolites include amphetamine and methamphetamine, which may contribute to the effects of the drug. Rapidly absorbed and metabolized. **Maximum plasma levels:** 0.5–2 hr.

**Uses:** Adjunct in the treatment of Parkinson's disease in clients being treated with levodopa/carbidopa who have manifested a decreased response to this therapy. *NOTE:* No evidence that selegiline is effective in clients not taking levodopa.

**Contraindications:** Hypersensitivity to the drug. Doses greater than 10 mg/day. Use with meperidine (and usually other opiates).

**Special Concerns:** Use with caution during lactation. Safety and efficacy in children have not been established.

**Side Effects:** *CNS:* Dizziness, lightheadedness, fainting, confusion, hallucinations, vivid dreams/nightmares, headache, anxiety, drowsiness, depression, mood changes, delusions, fatigue, disorientation, apathy, malaise, vertigo, overstimulation, sleep disturbance, transient irritability, weakness, lethargy, personality change. *Skeletal Muscle:* Tremor, chorea, loss of balance, blepharospasm, restlessness, increased bradykinesia, facial grimace, dystonic symptoms, tardive dyskinesia, dyskinesia, involuntary movements, muscle cramps, heavy leg, falling down, stiff neck, freezing, festination, increased apraxia. *Altered Sensations/pain:* Headache, tinnitus, migraine, back or leg pain, supraorbital pain, burning throat, chills, numbness of fingers/toes, taste disturbance, generalized aches. *CV:* Orthostatic hypotension, hypertension, arrhythmia, angina pectoris, palpitations, hypotension, tachycardia, syncope, peripheral edema, sinus bradycardia. *Oral:* Dry mouth. *GI:* N&V, constipation, anorexia, weight loss, poor appetite, dysphagia, diarrhea, rectal bleeding, **GI bleeding (worsening of pre-existing ulcer disease),** heartburn. *GU:* Nocturia, slow urination, urinary hesitancy or retention, prostatic hypertrophy, urinary frequency, sexual dysfunction. *Miscellaneous:* Blurred vision, increased sweating, diaphore-

**S**

sis, facial hair, hair loss, rash, photosensitivity, hematoma, asthma, diplopia, SOB, speech affected.

**Drug Interactions**

*Fluoxetine (Prozac)* / Possibility of death—five weeks should elapse between discontinuing fluoxetine and beginning selegiline and 14 days between discontinuing selegiline and initiation of fluoxetine

*Meperidine and other opioid analgesics* / Symptoms include stupor, muscle rigidity, severe agitation, hyperthermia, hallucinations, death.

**How Supplied:** *Capsule:* 5 mg; *Tablet:* 5 mg

**Dosage** ─────────────

• **Capsules, Tablets**

*Parkinsonism in those receiving levodopa/carbidopa.*

**Adults:** 5 mg taken at breakfast and lunch, not to exceed 10 mg/day.

## DENTAL CONCERNS

**General**

1. Monitor vital signs at every appointment because of cardiovascular side effects.

2. Have the patient sit up slowly and remain seated for at least two minutes after being supine in order to minimize the risk of orthostatic hypotension.

3. Decreased saliva flow can put the patient at risk for dental caries, periodontal disease, and candidiasis.

4. Determine the presence of movement disorders such as extrapyramidal symptoms, tardive dyskinesia, or akathisia. They may interfere with the ability of the patient to perform oral health care or they can complicate dental treatment.

**Consultation with Primary Care Provider**

1. Consultation may be required in order to assess extent of disease control and the patient's ability to tolerate stress.

2. If patient demonstrates signs and symptoms of tardive dyskinesia or akathisia refer him back to the appropriate health care provider.

**Client/Family Teaching**

1. Daily home fluoride treatments for persistent dry mouth.

2. Avoid alcohol-containing mouth rinses and beverages.

3. Avoid caffeine-containing beverages.

4. Dry mouth can be treated with tart, sugarless gum or candy, water, sugar-free beverages, or with saliva substitutes if dry mouth persists.

# Sertraline hydrochloride

(**SIR**-trah-leen)

**Pregnancy Category:** B

Zoloft **(Rx)**

**Classification:** Antidepressant, selective serotonin reuptake inhibitor

───────────────

See also *Selective Serotonin Reuptake Inhibitors.*

**Action/Kinetics:** Believed to act by inhibiting CNS neuronal uptake of serotonin. No significant affinity for adrenergic, cholinergic, dopaminergic, histaminergic, serotonergic, GABA, or benzodiazepine receptors. Steady-state plasma levels are usually reached after 1 week of once daily dosing but is increased to 2–3 weeks in older clients. **Time to peak plasma levels:** 4.5–8.4 hr. **Peak plasma levels:** 20–55 ng/mL. **Time to reach steady state:** 7 days. **Terminal elimination t½:** 1–4 days (including active metabolite). Washout period is 7 days. Food decreases the time to reach peak plasma levels. Undergoes significant first-pass metabolism, significant (98%) binding to serum proteins. Excreted through the urine (40%–45%) and feces (40%–45%). Metabolized to N-desmethyl-sertraline, which has minimal antidepressant activity.

**Uses:** Treatment of depression with reduced psychomotor agitation, anxiety, and insomnia. Obsessive-compulsive disorders in adults and children as defined in DSM-III-R. Treatment of panic disorder, with or without agoraphobia.

**Contraindications:** Use in combination with an MAO inhibitor or within 14 days of discontinuing treatment with an MAO inhibitor.

**Special Concerns:** Use with caution in hepatic or renal dysfunction, with seizure disorders, during lactation, and in diseases or conditions that may affect hemodynamic responses or metabolism. Safety and efficacy have not been determined in children. The plasma clearance may be lower in elderly clients. The possibility of a suicide attempt is possible in depression and may persist until significant remission occurs.

**Side Effects:** A large number of side effects is possible; listed are those side effects with a frequency of 0.1% or greater. *Oral:* Dry mouth, increased salivation, teeth grinding, taste perversion or change, aphthous stomatitis. *GI:* Nausea and diarrhea (common), constipation, dyspepsia, vomiting, flatulence, anorexia, abdominal pain, thirst, increased appetite, gastroenteritis, dysphagia, eructation. *CV:* Palpitations, hot flushes, edema, hypertension, hypotension, peripheral ischemia, postural hypotension or dizziness, syncope, tachycardia. *CNS:* Headache (common), insomnia (common), somnolence, agitation, nervousness, anxiety, dizziness, tremor, fatigue, impaired concentration, yawning, paresthesia, hypoesthesia, twitching, hypertonia, confusion, ataxia or abnormal coordination, abnormal gait, hyperesthesia, hyperkinesia, abnormal dreams, aggressive reaction, amnesia, apathy, delusion, depersonalization, depression, aggravated depression, emotional lability, euphoria, hallucinations, neurosis, paranoid reaction, *suicide ideation or attempt,* abnormal thinking, hypokinesia, migraine, nystagmus, vertigo. *Dermatologic:* Rash, acne, excessive sweating, alopecia, pruritus, cold and clammy skin, facial edema, erythematous rash, maculopapular rash, dry skin. *Musculoskeletal:* Myalgia, arthralgia, arthrosis, dystonia, muscle cramps or weakness. *GU:* Urinary frequency, micturition disorders, menstrual disorders, dysmenorrhea, dysuria, painful menstruation, intermenstrual bleeding, sexual dysfunction and decreased libido, nocturia, polyuria, dysuria, urinary incontinence. *Respiratory:* Rhinitis, pharyngitis, yawning, bronchospasm, coughing, dyspnea, epistaxis. *Ophthalmologic:* Blurred vision, abnormal vision, abnormal accommodation, conjunctivitis, diplopia, eye pain, xerophthalmia. *Otic:* Tinnitus, earache. *Body as a whole:* Asthenia, fever, chest pain, chills, back pain, weight loss or weight gain, generalized edema, malaise, flushing, hot flashes, rigors, lymphadenopathy, purpura.

**Drug Interactions:** Because sertraline is highly bound to plasma proteins, its use with other drugs that are also highly protein bound may lead to displacement, resulting in higher plasma levels of the drug and possibly increased side effects.

*Alcohol* / Concurrent use is not recommended in depressed clients

*Benzodiazepines* / ↓ Clearance of benzodiazepines metabolized by hepatic oxidation

*Cimetidine* / ↑ Half-life and blood levels of sertraline

*Diazepam* / ↑ Plasma levels of desmethyldiazepam (significance not known)

*MAO inhibitors* / Serious and possibly fatal reactions including hyperthermia, rigidity, autonomic instability with possible rapid fluctuation of VS, myoclonus, changes in mental status (e.g., extreme agitation, delirium, coma)

**How Supplied:** *Tablet:* 50 mg, 100 mg

## Dosage
- **Tablets**

  *Depression.*

**Adults, initial:** 50 mg once daily either in the morning or evening. Clients not responding to a 50-mg dose may benefit from doses up to a maximum of 200 mg/day.

---

*Obsessive-compulsive disorder.*
**Adults:** 50–200 mg/day. **Children, 6 to 12 years:** 25 mg once a day; **adolescents, 13 to 17 years:** 50 mg once a day.

*Panic attacks.*
**Adults, initial:** 25 mg/day for the first week; **then,** dosage ranges from 50–200 mg/day, based on response and tolerance.

## DENTAL CONCERNS

See also *Dental Concerns* for *Antidepressants, Tricyclic* and *Selective Serotonin Reuptake Inhibitors.*

# Sibutramine hydrochloride monohydrate

(sih-**BYOU**-trah-meen)
**Pregnancy Category:** C
Meridia **(Rx) (C-IV)**
**Classification:** Anti-obesity drug

**Action/Kinetics:** Main effect is likely due to primary and secondary amine metabolites of sibutramine. Inhibits reuptake of norepinephrine (NE) and serotonin (5HT), resulting in enhanced NE and 5HT activity and reduced food intake. Significant improvement in serum uric acid. Rapidly absorbed from GI tract. Extensive first-pass metabolism in liver. **Peak plasma levels of active metabolites:** 3–4 hr. **t½, sibutramine:** 1.1 hr; **t½, active metabolites:** 14–16 hr. Excreted in urine and feces.

**Uses:** Management of obesity, including weight loss and maintenance of weight loss. Recommended for obese clients with initial body mass index of 30 kg/m² or more or 27 kg/m² in presence of hypertension, diabetes, or dyslipidemia. Use in conjunction with reduced calorie diet. Safety and efficacy have not been determined for more than 1 year.

**Contraindications:** Lactation. Use in clients receiving MAO inhibitors, who have anorexia nervosa, those taking centrally-acting appetite suppressant drugs, those with history of coronary artery disease, CHF, arrhythmias, or stroke. Use in severe renal impairment or hepatic dysfunction. Use with serotonergic drugs, such as fluoxetine, fluvoxamine, paroxetine, sertraline, venlafaxine, sumatriptan, and dihydroergotamine; also, use with dextromethorphan, meperidine, pentazocine, fentanyl, lithium, or tryptophan.

**Special Concerns:** Use with caution in geriatric clients. Safety and efficacy have not been determined in children less than 16 years of age. Use with caution in narrow angle glaucoma, history of seizures, or with drugs that may raise BP (e.g., phenylpropanolamine, ephedrine, pseudoephedrine). Exclude organic causes (e.g., untreated hypothyroidism) before use.

**Side Effects:** *Body as a whole:* Headache, back pain, flu syndrome, injury/accident, asthenia, chest pain, neck pain, allergic reaction. *Oral:* Dry mouth, aphthous stomatitis, taste perversion. *GI:* Anorexia, abdominal pain, constipation, N&V, rectal disorder, increased appetite, dyspepsia, gastritis. *CNS:* Insomnia, dizziness, paresthesia, nervousness, anxiety, depression, somnolence, CNS stimulation, emotional lability. *CV:* Increased blood pressure, tachycardia, vasodilation, migraine, palpitation. *Dermatologic:* Sweating, rash, herpes simplex, acne. *Musculoskeletal:* Arthralgia, myalgia, tenosynovitis, joint disorder. *Respiratory:* Rhinitis, pharyngitis, sinusitis, increase cough, laryngitis. *GU:* Dysmenorrhea, UTI, vaginal monilia, metrorrhagia. *Otic:* Ear disorder, ear pain. *Miscellaneous:* Thirst, generalized edema.

**How Supplied:** *Capsules:* 5 mg, 10 mg, 15 mg

## Dosage
- **Capsules**
  *Obesity.*

**Adults, initial:** 10 mg once daily (usually in morning) with or without food. If there is adequate weight loss, dose may be titrated after 4 weeks to total of 15 mg once daily.

Daily dose should not exceed 15 mg.

## DENTAL CONCERNS

1. Monitor vital signs at every appointment because of cardiovascular side effects.
2. Decreased saliva flow can put the patient at risk for dental caries, periodontal disease, and candidiasis.

**Client/Family Teaching**

1. Daily home fluoride treatments for persistent dry mouth.
2. Avoid alcohol-containing mouth rinses and beverages.
3. Avoid caffeine-containing beverages.
4. Dry mouth can be treated with tart, sugarless gum or candy, water, sugar-free beverages, or with saliva substitutes if dry mouth persists.

# Sildenafil citrate

(sill-**DEN**-ah-fill)
**Pregnancy Category:** B
Viagra **(Rx)**
**Classification:** Drug for erectile dysfunction

**Action/Kinetics:** Nitric oxide activates the enzyme guanylate cyclase, which causes increased levels of guanosine monophosphate (cGMP) and subsequently smooth muscle relaxation in the corpus cavernosum and allowing inflow of blood. Sildenafil enhances effect of nitric oxide by inhibiting phosphodiesterase type 5 which is responsible for degradation of cGMP in the corpus cavernosum. When sexual stimulation causes local release of nitric oxide, inhibition of phosphodiesterse type 5 by sildenafil causes increased levels of cGMP in the corpus cavernosum and thus smooth muscle relaxation and inflow of blood resulting in an erection. Drug has no effect in absence of sexual stimulation. Rapidly absorbed after PO use. Absorption is decreased when taken with high fat meal. Metabolized in liver where it is converted to active metabolite (N-desmethyl sildenafil). **t½, sildenafil**

**and metabolite:** 4 hr. Excreted mainly in feces (80%) with about 13% excreted in urine. Reduced clearance is seen in geriatric clients.
**Uses:** Treatment of erectile dysfunction.
**Contraindications:** Concomitant use with organic nitrates in any form or with other treatments for erectile dysfunction. Use in newborns, children, or women.
**Special Concerns:** Use with caution in clients with anatomical deformation of penis, in those with predisposition to priapism (e.g., sickle cell anemia, multiple myeloma, leukemia), in bleeding disorders or active peptic ulceration, and in those with genetic disorders of retinal phosphodiesterases.
**Side Effects:** Listed are side effects with incidence of 2% or greater. *CNS:* Headache, dizziness. *Oral:* Dry mouth, glossitis. *GI:* Dyspepsia, diarrhea. *Dermatologic:* Flushing, rash. *Ophthalmic:* Mild and transient predominantly color tinge to vision, increased sensitivity to light, blurred vision. *Respiratory:* Nasal congestion, respiratory tract infection. *Miscellaneous:* UTI, back pain, flu syndrome, arthralgia.
**Drug Interactions**
*Cimetadine* / ↑ Plasma levels of sildenafil
*Erythromycin* / ↑ Plasma levels of sildenafil
*Itraconazole* / ↑ Plasma levels of sildenafil
*Ketoconazole* / ↑ Plasma levels of sildenafil
*Nitrates* / ↑ Risk for adverse cardiovascular events
*Rifampin* / ↓ Plasma levels of sildenafil
**How Supplied:** *Tablets:* 25 mg, 50 mg, 100 mg

## Dosage

• **Tablets**
  *Treat erectile dysfunction.*
For most clients, 50 mg no more than once daily, as needed, about 1 hr before sexual activity. May be taken

anywhere from 0.5 hr to 4 hr before sexual activity. Depending on tolerance and effectiveness, dose may be increased to maximum of 100 mg or decreased to 25 mg. Starting dose of 25 mg should be considered in those with hepatic or renal impairment or if taken with erythromycin, itraconzole, or ketoconazole.

## DENTAL CONCERNS
### General
1. Avoid potentially interacting drugs.

# Simvastatin
(**sim**-vah-**STAH**-tin)
**Pregnancy Category:** X
Zocor **(Rx)**
**Classification:** Antihyperlipidemic

See also *Antihyperlipidemic Agents— HMG-CoA Reductase Inhibitors.*

**Action/Kinetics:** Inhibits HMG-CoA reductase enzyme, which reduces cholesterol synthesis. **Peak therapeutic response:** 4–6 weeks. Approximately 85% absorbed; significant first-pass effect with less than 5% of a PO dose reaching the general circulation. Metabolites excreted in the feces (60%) and urine (13%).

**Uses:** Adjunct to diet for the reduction of elevated total and LDL cholesterol levels in types IIa and IIb hypercholesterolemia when the response to diet and other approaches have been inadequate. Prophylaxis of heart attack and decrease in incidence of cardiac death in those with CHD and elevated cholesterol levels. *Non-FDA Approved Uses:* Heterozygous familial hypercholesterolemia, familial combined hyperlipidemia, diabetic dyslipidemia in non-insulin-dependent diabetes, hyperlipidemia secondary to the nephrotic syndrome, and homozygous familial hypercholesterolemia in clients with defective LDL receptors.

**Contraindications:** Active liver disease or unexplained persistent increases in liver function tests. Use in pregnancy, during lactation, or in children.

**Special Concerns:** Use with caution in clients who have a history of liver disease/consume large quantities of alcohol or with drugs that affect steroid levels or activity. Higher plasma levels may be observed in clients with severe renal insufficiency. Safety and efficacy have not been determined in children less than 18 years of age.

**Side Effects:** *Oral:* stomatitis. *Musculoskeletal:* Rhabdomyolysis with renal dysfunction secondary to myoglobinuria, myopathy, arthralgias. *GI:* N&V, diarrhea, abdominal pain, constipation, flatulence, dyspepsia, pancreatitis, anorexia. *Hepatic:* Hepatitis (including chronic active hepatitis), cholestatic jaundice, cirrhosis, fatty change in liver, *fulminant hepatic necrosis, hepatoma. Neurologic:* Dysfunction of certain cranial nerves resulting in alteration of taste, impairment of extraocular movement, and facial paresis. Paresthesia, peripheral neuropathy, peripheral nerve palsy. *CNS:* Headache, tremor, vertigo, memory loss, anxiety, insomnia, depression. *Hypersensitivity Reactions:* Although rare, the following symptoms have been noted. *An-gioedema, anaphylaxis,* lupus erythematous–like syndrome, vasculitis, purpura, thrombocytopenia, leukopenia, *hemolytic anemia,* polymyalgia rheumatica, positive ANA, ESR increase, arthritis, arthralgia, asthenia, urticaria, photosensitivity, chills, fever, flushing, malaise, dyspnea, *toxic epidermal necrolysis, erythema multiforme (including Stevens-Johnson syndrome). GU:* Gynecomastia, loss of libido, erectile dysfunction. *Ophthalmologic:* Lens opacities, ophthalmoplegia. *Hematologic:* Transient asymptomatic eosinophilia, anemia, thrombocytopenia, leukopenia. *Miscellaneous:* Upper respiratory infection, asthenia, alopecia, edema.

**Drug Interactions**
*Cyclosporine /* ↑ Risk of myopathy or rhabdomyolysis
*Erythromycin /* ↑ Risk of myopathy or rhabdomyolysis

**How Supplied:** *Tablet:* 5 mg, 10 mg, 20 mg, 40 mg

**Dosage** ──────────────
* **Tablets**

**Adults, initially:** 5–10 mg once daily in the evening; **maintenance:** 5–40 mg/day as a single dose in the evening. Consider a starting dose of 5 mg/day for clients with LDL less than 190 mg/dL and 10 mg/day for clients with LDL greater than 190 mg/dL. For geriatric clients, the starting dose should be 5 mg/day with maximum LDL reductions seen with 20 mg or less daily.

## DENTAL CONCERNS

See also *Dental Concerns* for *Antihyperlipidemic Agents—HMG-CoA Reductase Inhibitors.*

# Sparfloxacin

(spar-**FLOX**-ah-sin)
**Pregnancy Category:** C
Zagam **(Rx)**
**Classification:** Fluoroquinolone antibiotic

See also *Fluoroquinolones.*
**Action/Kinetics:** Well absorbed. **Peak serum levels:** 4–5 hr. 50% excreted in the urine.
**Uses:** Community acquired pneumonia due to *Chlamydia pneumoniae, Haemophilus influenzae, Haemophilus parainfluenzae, Moraxella catarrhalis, Mycoplasma pneumoniae,* or *Streptococcus pneumoniae.* Acute bacterial exacerbations of chronic bronchitis caused by *C. pneumoniae, Enterobacter cloacae, H. influenzae, H. parainfluenzae, Klebsiella pneumoniae, M. catarrhalis, Staphylococcus aureus,* or *S. pneumoniae.*
**Contraindications:** Hypersensitivity, photosensitivity, disopyramide, amiodarone, and class Ia and III antiarrhythmics, terfenadine, bepridil; patients with prolonged Qtc intervals, hypokalemia, significant bradycardia

**Special Concerns:** Safety and efficacy have not been determined in children less than 18 years of age.
**Side Effects:** See also *Fluoroquinolones.*
**Drug Interactions:** Avoid concurrent use with erythromycin, terfenadine, tricyclic antidepressants, phenothiazines.
*Antacids* / ↓ Absorption of antacids
**How Supplied:** *Tablets:* 200 mg

**Dosage** ──────────────
* **Tablets**
  *Community-acquired pneumonia, acute bacterial exacerbations of chronic bronchitis.*

**Adults over 18 years of age:** Two 200-mg tablets taken on the first day as a loading dose. Then, one 200-mg tablet q 24 hr for a total of 10 days of therapy (i.e., a total of 11 tablets). For clients with a $C_{CR}$ less than 50 mL/min, the loading dose is two 200-mg tablets taken on the first day. Then, one 200-mg tablet q 48 hr for a total of 9 days (i.e., a total of 6 tablets).

## DENTAL CONCERNS

See also *General Dental Concerns for All Anti-Infectives* and for *Fluoroquinolones.*
**General**
1. Determine why the patient is taking the medication.
2. Decreased saliva flow can put the patient at risk for dental caries, periodontal disease, and candidiasis.
3. Place dental chair in semisupine position due to the GI adverse effects of the drug.
**Consultation with Primary Care Provider**
1. Consult with the patient's health care provider if an acute dental infection occurs and the patient requires another anti-infective.
**Client/Family Teaching**
1. You may want to wear dark glasses in order to avoid photophobia, which can occur with the dental light.
2. Avoid direct sunlight, as a photo-

sensitivity reaction may occur. If exposed, wear sunglasses, protective clothing, and sunscreen.

# Sucralfate
(sue-**KRAL**-fayt)
**Pregnancy Category: B**
Apo-Sucralfate ✤, Carafate, Novo-Sucralate ✤, Nu-Sucralfate ✤, Sulcrate ✤, Sulcrate Suspension Plus ✤ **(Rx)**
**Classification:** Antiulcer drug

**Action/Kinetics:** Thought to form an ulcer-adherent complex with albumin and fibrinogen at the site of the ulcer, protecting it from further damage by gastric acid. May also form a viscous, adhesive barrier on the surface of the gastric mucosa and duodenum. It adsorbs pepsin, thus inhibiting its activity. May be used in conjunction with antacids. Approximately 90% excreted in the feces. **Duration:** 5 hr.

**Uses:** Short-term treatment (up to 8 weeks) of active duodenal ulcers. Maintenance for duodenal ulcer at decreased dosage after healing of acute ulcers. *Non-FDA Approved Uses:* Hasten healing of gastric ulcers, chronic treatment of gastric ulcers. Treatment of reflux and peptic esophagitis. Treatment of aspirin- and NSAID-induced GI symptoms; prevention of stress ulcers and GI bleeding in critically ill clients. The suspension has been used to treat oral and esophageal ulcers due to chemotherapy, radiation, or sclerotherapy.
*Note:* Even though healing of ulcers may result, the frequency or severity of subsequent attacks is not áltered.

**Special Concerns:** Safety for use in children and during lactation has not been fully established. A successful course resulting in healing of ulcers will not alter posthealing frequency or severity of duodenal ulceration.

**Side Effects:** *Oral:* Dry mouth. *GI:* Constipation (most common); also, N&V, diarrhea, indigestion, flatulence, gastric discomfort. *Hypersensitivity:* Urticaria, *angioedema, respiratory difficulty,* rhinitis. *Miscellaneous:*

Back pain, dizziness, sleepiness, vertigo, rash, pruritus, facial swelling, *laryngospasm.*

**Drug Interactions**
*Antacids containing aluminum /* ↑ Total body burden of aluminum
*Cimetidine /* ↓ Absorption of cimetidine due to binding to sucralfate
*Ciprofloxacin /* ↓ Absorption of ciprofloxacin due to binding to sucralfate
*Ketoconazole /* ↓ Bioavailability of ketoconazole
*Norfloxacin /* ↓ Absorption of norfloxacin due to binding to sucralfate
*Ranitidine /* ↓ Absorption of ranitidine due to binding to sucralfate
*Tetracycline /* ↓ Absorption of tetracycline due to binding to sucralfate
*Theophylline /* ↓ Absorption of theophylline due to binding to sucralfate

**How Supplied:** *Suspension:* 1 g/10 mL; *Tablet:* 1 g

**Dosage** —————————
• **Suspension, Tablets**
**Adults: usual:** 1 g q.i.d. (10 mL of the suspension) 1 hr before meals and at bedtime (it may also be taken 2 hr after meals). The drug should be taken for 4–8 weeks unless X-ray films or endoscopy have indicated significant healing. **Maintenance (tablets only):** 1 g b.i.d.

## DENTAL CONCERNS
**General**
1. A semisupine position for the dental chair may be necessary to help minimize or avoid GI adverse effects.
2. Avoid alcohol, caffeine, and aspirin-containing prescription and nonprescription drugs.

**Client/Family Teaching**
1. Review the importance of good oral hygiene in order to prevent soft tissue inflammation.
2. Review the proper use of oral hygiene aids in order to prevent injury.

# Sulfacetamide sodium
(sul-fah-**SEAT**-ah-myd)

AK-Sulf, Balsulph ♣, Bleph-10, Bleph-10 Liquifilm ♣, Cetamide, Diosulf ♣, Isopto-Cetamide, I-Sulfacet, Ocu-Sul-10, Ocu-Sul-15, Ocu-Sul-30, Ocusulf-10, Ophthacet, Ophtho-Sulf ♣, PMS-Sulfacetamide Sodium ♣, Sebizon, Sodium Sulamyd, Spectro-Sulf, Steri-Units Sulfacetamide, Sulf-10, Sulfair, Sulfair 10, Sulfair 15, Sulfair Forte, Sulfamide, Sulfex 10% ♣, Sulten-10 **(Rx)**
**Classification:** Sulfonamide, topical

See also *Sulfonamides*.
**Uses:** Topically for conjunctivitis, corneal ulcer, and other superficial ocular infections. As an adjunct to systemic sulfonamides to treat trachoma.
**Contraindications:** In infants less than 2 months of age. Use in the presence of epithelial herpes simplex keratitis, vaccinia, varicella, and other viral diseases of the cornea and conjunctiva. Mycobacterial or fungal infections of the ocular structures. After uncomplicated removal of a corneal foreign body.
**Special Concerns:** Safe use during pregnancy and lactation or in children less than 12 years of age has not been established. Use with caution in clients with dry eye syndrome. Ophthalmic ointments may retard corneal wound healing.
**Side Effects:** *When used topically:* Itching, local irritation, periorbital edema, burning and transient stinging, headache, bacterial or fungal corneal ulcers. *NOTE:* Sulfonamides may cause serious systemic side effects, including severe hypersensitivity reactions. Symptoms include fever, skin rash, GI disturbances, bone marrow depression, ***Stevens-Johnson syndrome, toxic epidermal necrolysis,*** exfoliative dermatitis, photosensitivity. Fatalities have occurred.
**Drug Interactions:** Preparations containing silver are incompatible with sulfacetamide sodium.
**How Supplied:** *Lotion:* 10%; *Ophthalmic ointment:* 10%; *Ophthalmic solution:* 10%, 15%, 30%

**Dosage** ————————
• **Ophthalmic Solution, 10%,**

**15%, 20%**
   *Conjunctivitis or other superficial ocular infections.*
1–2 gtt in the conjunctival sac q 1–4 hr. Doses may be tapered by increasing the time interval between doses as the condition improves.
   *Trachoma.*
2 gtt q 2 hr with concomitant systemic sulfonamide therapy.
• **Ophthalmic Ointment (10%)**
Apply approximately ¼ in. into the lower conjunctival sac 3–4 times/day and at bedtime. Alternatively, 0.5–1 in. is placed in the conjunctival sac at bedtime along with use of drops during the day.
   *For cutaneous infections.*
Apply locally (10%) to affected area b.i.d.–q.i.d.
• **Lotion**
   *Seborrheic dermatitis.*
Apply 1–2 times/day (for mild cases, apply overnight).
   *Cutaneous bacterial infections.*
Apply b.i.d.–q.i.d. until infection clears.

## DENTAL CONCERNS
### General
1. Patients on chronic drug therapy may develop blood dyscrasias. Symptoms include fever, sore throat, bleeding, and poor wound healing.
2. It may be necessary to position the dental chair in a semisupine position in order to minimize the GI effects of the drug.
### Consultation with Primary Care Provider
1. Patients with symptoms of blood dyscrasias should be referred to their primary care provider for complete blood counts. Treatment should be postponed until the results are known.
2. Consultation may be required in order to assess extent of disease control.

# Sulindac
(sul-**IN**-dak)
Apo-Sulin ♣, Clinoril, Novo–Sundac ♣, Nu-Sulindac ♣ **(Rx)**

**Classification:** Nonsteroidal anti-inflammatory drug

See also *Nonsteroidal Anti-Inflammatory Drugs.*

**Action/Kinetics:** Biotransformed in the liver to a sulfide, the active metabolite. **Peak plasma levels of sulfide:** after fasting, 2 hr; after food, 3–4 hr. **Onset, anti-inflammatory effect:** within 1 week; **duration, anti-inflammatory effect:** 1–2 weeks. **t½,** of sulindac: 7.8 hr; of metabolite: 16.4 hr. Excreted in both urine and feces.

**Uses:** Acute and chronic treatment of rheumatoid arthritis, osteoarthritis, ankylosing spondylitis, acute gouty arthritis; acute, painful shoulder; tendinitis, bursitis. *Non-FDA Approved Uses:* Juvenile rheumatoid arthritis, sunburn.

**Contraindications:** Use with active GI lesions or a history of recurrent GI lesions.

**Special Concerns:** Safety and efficacy have not been established for children. Safe use during pregnancy has not been established. Use with caution during lactation.

**Additional Side Effects:** Hypersensitivity, pancreatitis, GI pain (common), maculopapular rash. Stupor, *coma,* hypotension, and diminished urine output.

**Additional Drug Interactions:** *Sulindac* ↑ Effect of warfarin due to ↓ plasma protein binding.

**How Supplied:** *Tablet:* 150 mg, 200 mg

**Dosage**

• **Tablets**
*Osteoarthritis, rheumatoid arthritis, ankylosing spondylitis.*
**Adults:** 150 mg b.i.d.
*Acute painful shoulder, acute gouty arthritis.*
**Adults:** 200 mg b.i.d. for 7–14 days.
*Antigout.*
**Adults:** 200 mg b.i.d. for 7 days.

## DENTAL CONCERNS

See also *Dental Concerns* for *Nonsteroidal Anti-Inflammatory Drugs.*

**T**

# Tamoxifen
(tah-**MOX**-ih-fen)
**Pregnancy Category:** D
Apo-Tamox ✦, Gen-Tamoxifen, Nolvadex, Nolvadex-D ✦, Novo–Tamoxifen ✦, Tamofen ✦, Tamone ✦, Tamoplex ✦ **(Rx)**
**Classification:** Antiestrogen

See also *Antineoplastic Agents.*
**Action/Kinetics:** Antiestrogen believed to compete with estrogen for estrogen-binding sites in target tissue (breast); also blocks uptake of estradiol. **Steady-state plasma levels (after 10 mg b.i.d. for 3 months):** 120 ng/mL for tamoxifen and 336 ng/mL for N-desmethyl tamoxifen. **Steady-state levels, tamoxifen:** About 4 weeks; **for N-desmethylta-** moxifen: About 8 weeks (**t½ for metabolite:** about 14 days). Metabolized to the equally active N-desmethyltamoxifen. Tamoxifen and metabolites are excreted mainly through the feces. Objective response may be delayed 4–10 weeks with bone metastases.

**Uses:** Adjuvant treatment of axillary node-negative or node-positive breast cancer in women following total or segmental mastectomy, axillary dissection, and breast irradiation. Metastatic breast cancer in premenopausal women as an alternative to oophorectomy or ovarian irradiation (especially in wowen with estrogen-positive tumors). Advanced metastatic breast cancer in men. *Non-FDA Approved Uses:* Mastalgia, gynecomastia (to treat pain and size), prophylaxis of breast cancer in high-risk women, pancreatic carcinoma, advanced or recurrent endometrial and hepatocellular carcinoma.

**Contraindications:** Lactation.

**Special Concerns:** Use with caution in clients with leukopenia or thrombocytopenia. Women should not become pregnant while taking tamoxifen.

**Side Effects:** *Oral:* Altered sense of taste. *GI:* N&V, distaste for food, anorexia, diarrhea, abdominal cramps. *CV:* Peripheral edema, superficial phlebitis, deep vein thrombosis, ***pulmonary embolism, thromboembolic disorders (especially when tamoxifen is combined with other cytotoxic agents).*** *CNS:* Depression, dizziness, lightheadedness, headache, fatigue. *Hepatic:* Rarely, fatty liver, cholestasis, hepatitis, ***hepatic necrosis.*** *GU:* Hot flashes, vaginal bleeding and discharge, menstrual irregularities, pruritus vulvae, ovarian cysts, hyperplasia of the uterus, polyps, uterine carcinoma. *Other:* Skin rash, skin changes, hypercalcemia, musculoskeletal pain, hyperlipidemias, weight gain or loss, increased bone and tumor pain, mild to moderate thrombocytopenia and leukopenia, retinopathy, hair thinning or partial loss, fluid retention, coughing. In men, may be loss of libido and impotency. Impotence and loss of libido in males after discontinuing therapy.

**Drug Interactions**

*Anticoagulants* / ↑ Hypoprothrombinemic effect

*Bromocriptine* / ↑ Serum levels of tamoxifen and N-desmethyl tamoxifen

**How Supplied:** *Tablet:* 10 mg, 20 mg

**Dosage** ———————

• **Tablets**

*Breast cancer.*

10–20 mg b.i.d. (morning and evening) or 20 mg daily. Doses of 10 mg b.i.d.–t.i.d. for 2 years and 10 mg b.i.d. for 5 years have been used.

There is no evidence that doses greater than 20 mg daily are more effective.

*Mastalgia.*

10 mg/day for 4 months.

## DENTAL CONCERNS

See also *Dental Concerns* for *Antineoplastic Agents.*

# Tamsulosin hydrochloride

(tam-**SOO**-loh-sin)

**Pregnancy Category:** B

Flomax **(Rx)**

**Classification:** Alpha-1 adrenergic blocking agent

**Action/Kinetics:** Blockade of alpha-1 receptors (probably alpha$_{1A}$) in prostate results in relaxation of smooth muscles in bladder neck and prostate; thus, urine flow rate is improved and there is a decrease in symptoms of BPH. Food interferes with the rate of absorption. **t½, elimination:** 5–7 hr. Significantly bound to plasma proteins. Extensively metabolized in liver; excreted through urine and feces.

**Uses:** Treatment of signs and symptoms of BPH. Rule out prostatic carcinoma before using tamsulosin.

**Contraindications:** Use to treat hypertension, with other alpha-adrenergic blocking agents, or in women or children.

**Special Concerns:** Use with caution with concurrent administration of warfarin.

**Side Effects:** *Body as a whole:* Headache, infection, asthenia, back pain, chest pain. *CV:* Postural hypotension, syncope. *GI:* Diarrhea, nausea, tooth disorder. *CNS:* Dizziness, vertigo, somnolence, insomnia, decreased libido. *Respiratory:* Rhinitis, pharyngitis, increased cough, sinusitis. *GU:* Abnormal ejaculation. *Miscellaneous:* Amblyopia.

**Drug Interactions:** Cimetidine causes significant ↓ in clearance of tamsulosin.

**How Supplied:** *Capsules:* 0.4 mg

T

---

**Dosage**
- **Capsules**
  *Benign prostatic hypertrophy.*
  **Adult males:** 0.4 mg daily given about 30 min after same meal each day. If, after 2 to 4 weeks, clients have not responded, dose can be increased to 0.8 mg daily.

## DENTAL CONCERNS
**General**
1. Monitor vital signs at every appointment because of cardiovascular side effects.
2. Have the patient sit up slowly and remain seated for at least two minutes after being supine in order to minimize the risk of orthostatic hypotension.
3. It may be necessary to place the dental chair in a semisupine position in order to minimize GI effects of the drug.

# Tazarotene
(taz-**AR**-oh-teen)
**Pregnancy Category:** X
Tazorac **(Rx)**
**Classification:** Antipsoriasis topical drug

**Action/Kinetics:** A retinoid prodrug converted by deesterification to active cognate carboxylic acid of tazarotene. Mechanism not known. Little systemic absorption. **t½, after topical use:** About 18 hr. Parent drug and metabolite are further metabolized and excreted through urine and feces.
**Uses:** Stable plaque psoriasis. Mild to moderate facial acne vulgaris.
**Contraindications:** Pregnancy. Use on eczematous skin. Use of cosmetics or skin medications that have strong drying effect.
**Special Concerns:** Use with caution during lactation. Safety and efficacy have not been determined in children less than 12 years of age. Psoriasis may worsen from month 4 to 12 compared with first 3 months of therapy. Use with caution with drugs that cause photosensitivity.
**Side Effects:** *Dermatologic:* Pruritus, photosensitivity, burning/stinging, erythema, worsening of psoriasis, skin pain, irritation, rash, desquamation, contact dermatitis, skin inflammation, fissuring, bleeding, dry skin, localized edema, skin discoloration.
**Drug Interactions:** ↑ Risk of photosensitivity when used with fluoroquinolones, phenothiazines, sulfonamides, tetracyclines, thiazides.

**Dosage**
- **Gel**
  *Acne vulgaris, Psoriasis.*
After skin is dry following cleaning, apply thin film (2 mg/cm²) on lesions once daily in evening. Cover entire affected area. For psoriasis, do not apply to more than 20% of body surface area.

## DENTAL CONCERNS
**General**
1. Lubricant may be necessary for dry lips prior to dental procedures.
**Client/Family Teaching**
1. Advise patients of the potential for increased photosensitivity if such drugs are prescribed; use sunscreens and protective clothing if exposed.

# Terazosin
(ter-**AY**-zoh-sin)
**Pregnancy Category:** C
Hytrin **(Rx)**
**Classification:** Antihypertensive, alpha-1-adrenergic receptor blocking agent

**Action/Kinetics:** Blocks postsynaptic alpha-1-adrenergic receptors, leading to a dilation of both arterioles and veins, and ultimately, a reduction in BP. Both standing and supine BPs are lowered with no reflex tachycardia. Also relaxes smooth muscle of the prostate and bladder neck. Usefulness in BPH is due to alpha-1 receptor blockade, which relaxes the smooth muscle of the prostate and bladder neck and relieves pressure on the urethra. Bioavailability is not affected by food. **Onset:** 15 min. **Peak plasma levels:** 1–2 hr. **t½:** 9–12 hr. **Duration:** 24 hr. Excreted unchanged and as inactive metabolites in both the urine and feces.

**Uses:** Alone or in combination with diuretics or beta-adrenergic blocking agents to treat hypertension. Treat symptoms of benign prostatic hyperplasia.

**Contraindications:** Hypersensitivity

**Special Concerns:** Use with caution during lactation. Safety and efficacy have not been determined in children. Geriatric clients may be more sensitive to the hypotensive and hypothermic effects of terazosin.

**Side Effects:** *First-dose effect:* Marked postural hypotension and syncope. *CV:* Palpitations, tachycardia, postural hypotension, syncope, *arrhythmias,* chest pain, vasodilation. *CNS:* Dizziness, headache, somnolence, drowsiness, nervousness, paresthesia, depression, anxiety, insomnia, vertigo. *Respiratory:* Nasal congestion, dyspnea, sinusitis, epistaxis, bronchitis, *bronchospasm,* cold or flu symptoms, increased cough, pharyngitis, rhinitis. *Oral:* Dry mouth. *GI:* Nausea, constipation, diarrhea, dyspepsia, vomiting, flatulence, abdominal discomfort or pain. *Musculoskeletal:* Asthenia, arthritis, arthralgia, myalgia, joint disorders, back pain, pain in extremities, neck and shoulder pain, muscle cramps. *Miscellaneous:* Peripheral edema, weight gain, blurred vision, impotence, chest pain, fever, gout, pruritus, rash, sweating, urinary frequency, UTI, tinnitus, conjunctivitis, abnormal vision, edema, facial edema.

**Drug Interactions**
*Indomethacin /* ↓ Effects of terazosin
*NSAIDs /* ↓ Effects of terazosin

**How Supplied:** *Capsule:* 1 mg, 2 mg, 5 mg, 10 mg

**Dosage** ─────
• **Capsules**
*Hypertension.*
**Individualized, initial:** 1 mg at bedtime (this dose is not to be exceeded); **then,** increase dose slowly to obtain desired response. **Range:**

1–5 mg/day; doses as high as 20 mg may be required in some clients. Doses greater than 20 mg daily do not provide further BP control.
*Benign prostatic hyperplasia.*
**Initial:** 1 mg/day; dose should be increased to 2 mg, 5 mg, and then 10 mg once daily to improve symptoms and/or urinary flow rates. Doses greater than 20 mg daily have not been studied.

## DENTAL CONCERNS

See also *Dental Concerns* for *Antihypertensive Agents* and *Alpha-1-Adrenergic Blocking Agents.*
**General**
1. Restrict use of sodium-containing agents such as saline IV fluids for patients with sodium restrictions.

# Terfenadine
(ter-**FEN**-ah-deen)
**Pregnancy Category:** C
Apo-Terfenadine ✦, Novo-Terfenadine ✦, Seldane **(Rx)**
**Classification:** Antihistamine, piperidine type

See also *Antihistamines.*
**Action/Kinetics:** Manifests significantly less drowsiness and anticholinergic effects than other antihistamines. **Onset:** 1–2 hr; **peak effect:** 3–4 hr; **peak plasma levels:** 2 hr. **t½:** About 20 hr. **Duration:** Over 12 hr. Metabolized in the liver and excreted in the urine and feces.
*Note:* Terfenadine has been withdrawn from the market.
**Uses:** Seasonal allergic rhinitis. *Non-FDA Approved Uses:* Histamine-induced bronchoconstriction in asthmatics; exercise and hyperventilation-induced bronchospasm.
**Contraindications:** Significant hepatic dysfunction. Use with drugs that prolong the QT interval, such as disopyramide, procainamide, quinidine, most antidepressants, and most neuroleptics. Consumption of grapefruit juice.

**Special Concerns:** Safety and efficacy in children less than 12 years of age have not been established. Hepatic insufficiency and any drug or food (e.g., grapefruit juice) that blocks the metabolism of terfenadine may cause serious CV effects (see *Side Effects* that follow).

**Additional Side Effects:** *Doses of 360 mg or more may cause serious CV effects, including death, cardiac arrest, torsades de pointes, and other ventricular arrhythmias (including QT interval prolongation).* Syncope may precede severe arrhythmias.

**Drug Interactions**

*Azole antifungal drugs* / ↑ Risk of serious CV effects, including death, cardiac arrest, torsades de pointes, and other ventricular arrhythmias

*Clarithromycin* / ↑ Risk of serious CV effects, including death, cardiac arrest, torsades de pointes, and other ventricular arrhythmias

*Erythromycins* / ↑ Risk of serious CV effects, including death, cardiac arrest, torsades de pointes, and other ventricular arrhythmias

*Itraconazole* / ↑ Risk of serious CV effects, including death, cardiac arrest, torsades de pointes, and other ventricular arrhythmias

*Ketoconazole* / ↑ Risk of serious CV effects, including death, cardiac arrest, torsades de pointes, and other ventricular arrhythmias

*Macrolide antibiotics* / ↑ Risk of serious CV effects, including death, cardiac arrest, torsades de pointes, and other ventricular arrhythmias

*Sparfloxacin* / ↑ Effect of terfenadine due to ↓ breakdown by the liver.

*Troleandomycin* / ↑ Risk of serious CV effects, including death, cardiac arrest, torsades de pointes, and other ventricular arrhythmias

**How Supplied:** *Tablet:* 60 mg

**Dosage** ─────────────
• **Tablets**
**Adults and children over 12 years:** 60 mg q 12 hr. Do not exceed this dose.

## DENTAL CONCERNS

See also *Dental Concerns* for *Antihistamines.*

**Client/Family Teaching**

1. *Do not* exceed prescribed dose or take with clarithomycin, macrolide antibiotics, azole antifungals, diltiazem, or troleandomycin because of the increased risk of side effects, especially lethal arrhythmias. Review drug information or check with pharmacist and provider for any newly added adverse effects or contraindications.

─────────────

# Tetracycline
(teh-trah-**SYE**-kleen)
**Pregnancy Category:** D
Achromycin Ophthalmic Ointment, Achromycin Ophthalmic Suspension, Actisite Periodontal Fiber **(Rx)**

# Tetracycline hydrochloride
(teh-trah-**SYE**-kleen)
**Pregnancy Category:** D (topical solution is B)
Achromycin Topical Ointment, Achromycin V, Apo-Tetra ✦, Jaa Tetra ✦, Medicycline ✦, Nor-Tet, Novo-Tetra ✦, Nu-Tetra ✦, Panmycin, Robicaps, Sumycin 250 and 500, Sumycin Syrup, Tetracap, Tetracyn ✦, Topicycline Topical Solution **(Rx)**
**Classification:** Antibiotic, tetracycline

─────────────

See also *General Information* on *Tetracyclines.*

**Action/Kinetics:** **t½:** 7–11 hr. From 40% to 70% excreted unchanged in urine; 65% bound to serum proteins. Always express dose as the hydrochloride salt.

**Uses:** See also *General Information* on *Tetracyclines.*

**Additional Uses:    Ophthalmic:** Superficial ophthalmic infections due to *Staphylococcus aureus, Streptococcus, Streptococcus pneumoniae, Escherichia coli, Neisseria,* and *Bacteroides.* Prophylaxis of *Neisseria gonorrhoeae* in newborns. With oral therapy for treatment of *Chlamydia trachomatis.* **Topical:** Acne vulgaris, prophylaxis or treatment of infection following skin abrasions, minor cuts, wounds, or burns. **Tetracycline fiber:** Adult periodontitis. *Non-FDA Approved Uses:* Pleural sclerosing agent in malignant pleural effusions (administered by chest tube); in combination with gentamicin for *Vibrio vulnificus* infections due to wound infection after trauma or by eating contaminated seafood. Mouthwash (use suspension) to treat nonspecific mouth ulcerations, canker sores, aphthous ulcers. Possible drug of choice for stage I Lyme disease.

**Contraindications:** Use of the topical ointment in or around the eyes. Ophthalmic products to treat fungal diseases of the eye, dendritic keratitis, vaccinia, varicella, mycobacterial eye infections, or following removal of a corneal foreign body. Periodontal fibers should be avoided in acutely abscessed periodontal pockets. See also *General Information* on *Tetracyclines*.

**Special Concerns:** Use tetracycline fiber with caution in clients with a history of oral candidiasis. Use of the fiber in chronic abscesses has not been evaluated. Safety and efficacy of the fiber have not been determined in children.

**Side Effects:** See also *General Information* on *Tetracyclines*.

**Additional Side Effects:** Temporary blurring of vision or stinging following administration. Dermatitis and photosensitivity following ophthalmic use. *Use of the tetracycline fiber:* Oral candidiasis, glossitis, staining of the tongue, severe gingival hyperplasia, minor throat irritation, pain following placement in an abscessed area, throbbing pain, hypersensitivity reactions.

**Drug Interactions:** See also *General Information* on *Tetracyclines*.

**How Supplied:** Tetracycline: *Syrup:* 125 mg/5 mL. Tetracycline hydrochloride: *Capsule:* 100 mg, 250 mg, 500 mg; *Ointment:* 3%; *Ophthalmic ointment:* 1%; *Solution:* 2.2 mg/mL; *Tablet:* 250 mg, 500 mg; *Periodontal fiber:* 12.7 mg/ 23 cm

## Dosage

- **Capsules, Syrup, Tablets**
  *Mild to moderate infections.*
**Adults, usual:** 500 mg b.i.d. or 250 mg q.i.d.
  *Severe infections.*
**Adult:** 500 mg q.i.d. **Children over 8 years:** 25–50 mg/kg/day in four equal doses.
  *Brucellosis.*
500 mg q.i.d. for 3 weeks with 1 g streptomycin IM b.i.d. for first week and once daily the second week.
  *Syphilis.*
Total of 30–40 g over 10–15 days.
  *Gonorrhea.*
**Initially,** 1.5 g; **then,** 500 mg q 6 hr until 9 g has been given.
  *Gonorrhea sensitive to penicillin.*
**Initially,** 1.5 g; **then,** 500 mg q 6 hr for 4 days (total: 9 g).
  *GU or rectal* Chlamydia trachomatis infections.
500 mg q.i.d. for minimum of 7 days.
  *Severe acne.*
**Initially,** 1 g/day; **then,** 125–500 mg/day (long-term).
*NOTE:* The CDC have established treatment schedules for STDs.
**Initially,** 1 g/day; **then,** 125–500 mg/day (long-term).
- **Topical**
  *Acne.*
Apply topical solution to affected areas in the morning and at night, making sure that skin is completely wet after each application.
  *Infections.*
Apply OTC ointment (3%) to affected areas 1–4 times/day. A sterile bandage may be used.
- **Tetracycline Fiber**
  *Adult periodontitis.*
Place the fiber into the periodontal pocket until the pocket is filled (amount of fiber will vary with pocket depth and contour) ensuring that the fiber is in contact with the base of the pocket. Retain the fiber in place for 10 days, after which it is to

**T**

---

be removed. The effectiveness of subsequent therapy with the fiber has not been assessed.

## DENTAL CONCERNS

See also *Dental Concerns* for *Tetracyclines* and *General Dental Concerns for All Anti-Infectives*.

**Client/Family Teaching**

1. Take PO form 1 hr before or 2 hr after meals with a full glass of water. Avoid dairy products, antacids, or iron preparations for 2 hr of ingestion of drug.

2. May cause photosensitivity reaction; avoid exposure to sunlight and wear protective clothing and sunscreen when exposed.

3. Transient blurring of vision or stinging may occur when instilled into the eye.

4. Topical ointment may stain clothing.

5. Drug may cause increased yellow-brown discoloration and softening of teeth and bones. *Not* advised for children under 8 years of age, pregnant women, or nursing mothers.

6. With oral application for gum disease, review proper care of site(s), foods to avoid, and proper cleaning while avoiding floss or toothpicks for the entire length of therapy. Symptoms that require immediate reporting include pain, abnormal discharge, fever, swelling, expulsion of fiber; return as scheduled for removal and follow-up.

7. The tetracycline fiber product consists of a monofilament of ethylene/vinyl acetate copolymer evenly dispersed with tetracycline. The fiber provides for continuous release of tetracycline for 10 days. The fiber releases about 2 mcg/cm/hr of tetracycline.

8. Avoid actions that may dislodge the fiber; i.e., chewing hard, crusty, or sticky foods; brushing or flossing near any treated areas; engaging in hygienic practices that might dislodge the fiber; probing the treated area with tongue or fingers.

9. Contact the dentist if the fiber is dislodged or falls out before the next scheduled visit or if pain or swelling occurs.

10. Dispose of any outdated tetracycline products. Fanconi-like syndrome can occur if outdated tetracycline products are ingested.

11. Document indications for therapy, type, onset, duration, and characteristics of symptoms.

---

# Theophylline
(thee-**OFF**-ih-lin)
**Pregnancy Category:** C
Immediate-release Capsules, Tablets, **Liquid Products:** Accurbron, Aquaphyllin, Asmalix, Bronkodyl, Elixomin, Elixophyllin, Lanophyllin, Lixolin, Pulmophylline ✦, Quibron-T/SR ✦, Quibron-T Dividose, Slo-Phyllin, Solu-Phyllin, Somnophyllin-T, Theo, Theoclear-80, Theolair, Theolixir ✦, Theomar, Theostat-80, Truxophyllin. **Timed-release Capsules and Tablets:** Aerolate III, Aerolate Jr., Aerolate Sr., Apo-Theo LA ✦, Quibron-T/SR Dividose, Respid, Slo-Bid Gyrocaps, Slo-Phyllin Gyrocaps, Somophyllin-CRT, Sustaire, Theo-24, Theo 250, Theobid Duracaps, Theoclear L.A.-130 Cenules, Theoclear L.A.-260 Cenules, Theocot, Theochron, Theochron-SR ✦, Theo-Dur, Theo-SR ✦, Theolair ✦, Theolair-SR, Theospan-SR, Theo-Time, Theophylline SR, Theovent Long-Acting, Uni-Dur, Uniphyl **(Rx)**
**Classification:** Antiasthmatic, bronchodilator

---

See also *Theophylline Derivatives*.
**Action/Kinetics: Time to peak serum levels, oral solution:** 1 hr; **uncoated tablets:** 2 hr; **chewable tablets:** 1–1.5 hr; **enteric-coated tablets:** 5 hr; **extended-release capsules and tablets:** 4–7 hr. In healthy adults, about 60% is bound to plasma protein whereas in neonates 36% is bound to plasma protein.

**Additional Uses: Oral liquid:** Neonatal apnea as a respiratory stimulant. Theophylline and dextrose injection: Respiratory stimulant in neonatal apnea and Cheyne-Stokes respiration.

**How Supplied:** *Capsule, extended release:* 50 mg, 65 mg, 75 mg, 100 mg, 125 mg, 130 mg, 200 mg, 260 mg, 300 mg, 400 mg; *Elixir:* 80 mg/15 mL;

*Solution:* 80 mg/15 mL; *Syrup:* 80 mg/15 mL; *Tablet:* 100 mg, 125 mg, 200 mg, 250 mg, 300 mg; *Tablet, extended release:* 100 mg, 200 mg, 250 mg, 300 mg, 400 mg, 450 mg, 500 mg, 600 mg

**Dosage** —————————————
• **Capsules, Tablets, Elixir, Oral Solution, Syrup**
See *Dosage* for *Oral Solution, Tablets,* under *Aminophylline.*
• **Extended-Release    Capsules, Extended-Release Tablets**
See *Dosage* for *Extended-Release Tablets,* under *Aminophylline.*
• **Elixir, Oral Solution, Oral Suspension, Syrup**
  *Bronchodilator, chronic therapy.*
  **9–12 years:** 20 mg/kg/day; **6–9 years:** 24 mg/kg/day.
  *Neonatal apnea.*
**Loading dose:** Using the equivalent of anhydrous theophylline administered by NGT, 5 mg/kg; **maintenance:** 2 mg/kg/day in two to three divided doses given by NGT.

---

**DENTAL CONCERNS**

See also *Dental Concerns* for *Theophylline Derivatives.*

---

# Thioridazine hydrochloride
(thigh-oh-**RID**-ah-zeen)
**Pregnancy Category:** C
Apo-Thioridazine ✽, Mellaril, Mellaril-S, Novo-Ridazine ✽, PMS-Thioridazine ✽, Thioridazine HCl Intensol Oral **(Rx)**
**Classification:** Antipsychotic, piperidine-type phenothiazine

---

See also *Antipsychotic Agents, Phenothiazines.*

**Action/Kinetics:** High incidence of hypotension; moderate incidence of sedative and anticholinergic effects and weak antiemetic and extrapyramidal effects. Can often be used in clients intolerant of other phenothiazines. **Peak plasma levels** (after PO administration): 1–4 hr. May impair its own absorption at higher doses due to the strong anticholinergic effects. **t½:** 10 hr. Metabolized in the liver to both active and inactive metabolites. **Uses:** Acute and chronic schizophrenia; moderate to marked depression with anxiety; sleep disturbances. **In children:** Treatment of hyperactivity in clients and those with retarded and behavior problems. Geriatric clients with organic brain syndrome. Alcohol withdrawal. Intractable pain.

**Special Concerns:** Safe use during pregnancy has not been established. Dosage has not been established in children less than 2 years of age. Geriatric, emaciated, or debilitated clients usually require a lower initial dose.

**Additional Side Effects:** More likely to cause pigmentary retinopathy than other phenothiazines.

**How Supplied:** *Oral concentrate:* 30 mg/mL, 100 mg/mL; *Tablet:* 10 mg, 15 mg, 25 mg, 50 mg, 100 mg, 150 mg, 200 mg

**Dosage** —————————————
• **Oral Suspension, Oral Solution, Tablets**
Highly individualized.
  *Neurosis, anxiety states, sleep disturbances, tension, alcohol withdrawal, senility.*
**Adults, range:** 20–200 mg/day; **initial:** 25 mg t.i.d. **Maintenance,** mild cases: 10 mg b.i.d.–q.i.d.; severe cases: 50 mg t.i.d.–q.i.d.
  *Psychotic, severely disturbed hospitalized clients.*
**Adults, initial,** 50–100 mg t.i.d. If necessary, increase to maximum of 200 mg q.i.d. When control is achieved, reduce gradually to minimum effective dosage. **Pediatric above 2 years:** 0.25–3.0 mg/kg/day.
  *Hospitalized psychotic children.*
**Initial:** 25 mg b.i.d.–t.i.d. *Moderate problems:* **initial,** 10 mg b.i.d.–t.i.d. Increase gradually if necessary. **Not recommended for children under 2 years of age.**

---

## DENTAL CONCERNS

See also *Dental Concerns* for *Antipsychotic Agents, Phenothiazines.*

# Tiagabine hydrochloride

(tye-**AG**-ah-been)
Pregnancy Category: C
Gabatril **(Rx)**
Classification: Anticonvulsant, miscellaneous

See also *Anticonvulsants.*
**Action/Kinetics:** Mechanism not known but activity of GABA, an inhibitory neurotransmitter, may be enhanced. Drug may block uptake of GABA into presynaptic neurons allowing more GABA to bind to postsynaptic cells. This prevents propagation of neural impulses that contribute to seizures due to GABA-ergic action. **Peak plasma levels:** About 45 min when fasting. High fat meals decrease rate but not extent of absorption. Metabolized in liver; excreted in urine and feces. **t½, elimination:** 7–9 hr. Diurnal effect occurs with levels being lower in evening compared with morning.
**Uses:** Adjunctive therapy for partial seizures.
**Contraindications:** Lactation.
**Special Concerns:** Safety and efficacy have not been determined in children less than 12 years old.
**Side Effects:** *CNS:* Dizziness, asthenia, somnolence, nervousness, tremor, insomnia, difficulty with concentration or attention, ataxia, confusion, speech disorder, difficulty with memory, paresthesia, depression, emotional lability, abnormal gait, hostility, nystagmus, problems with language, agitation. *Oral:* Dry mouth, mouth ulceration, gingivitis, stomatitis, gingival hyperplasia (uncommon). *GI:* N&V, diarrhea, increased appetite, mouth ulceration. *Respiratory:* Pharyngitis, increased cough. *Dermatologic:* Rash, pruritus. *Miscellaneous:* Abdominal pain, unspecified pain, vasodilation, myasthenia.

**Drug Interactions**
*Carbamazepine* / ↑ Clearance due to ↑ metabolism
*Phenobarbital* / ↑ Clearance due to ↑ metabolism

**Dosage**
• **Tablets**
*Partial seizures.*
**Adults and children over 18 years, initial:** 4 mg once daily. Total daily dose may be increased by 4–8 mg at weekly intervals until clinical effect is observed or daily dose is 56 mg/day. **Children, 12–18 years, initial:** 4 mg once daily. Total daily dose may be increased by 4 mg at beginning of week 2. Thereafter, dose may be increased by 4–8 mg at weekly intervals until clinical effect is seen or dose is 32 mg/day. For all ages, give total daily dose in 2–4 divided doses.

## DENTAL CONCERNS

See also *Dental Concerns* for *Anticonvulsants.*

# Ticlopidine hydrochloride

(tie-**KLOH**-pih-deen)
Pregnancy Category: B
Ticlid **(Rx)**
Classification: Platelet aggregation inhibitor

**Action/Kinetics:** Irreversibly inhibits ADP-induced platelet-fibrinogen binding and subsequent platelet-platelet interactions. This results in inhibition of both platelet aggregation and release of platelet granule constituents as well as prolongation of bleeding time. **Peak plasma levels:** 2 hr. **Maximum platelet inhibition:** 8–11 days after 250 mg b.i.d. **Steady-state plasma levels:** 14–21 days. **t½, elimination:** 4–5 days. After discontinuing therapy, bleeding time and other platelet function tests return to normal within 14 days. Rapidly absorbed; bioavailability is increased by food. Highly bound (98%) to plasma proteins. Extensively metabolized by the liver with approximately 60% excreted through the kidneys; 23% is excreted in the feces (with one-third excreted unchanged). Clearance of the drug decreases with age.

**Uses:** To reduce the risk of fatal or nonfatal thrombotic stroke in clients who have manifested precursors of stroke or who have had a completed thrombotic stroke. Due to the risk of neutropenia or agranulocytosis, use should be reserved for clients who are intolerant to aspirin therapy. *Non-FDA Approved Uses:* Chronic arterial occlusion, coronary artery bypass grafts, intermittent claudication, open heart surgery, primary glomerulonephritis, subarachnoid hemorrhage, sickle cell disease, uremic clients with AV shunts or fistulas.

**Contraindications:** In the presence of neutropenia and thrombocytopenia, hemostatic disorder, or active pathologic bleeding such as bleeding peptic ulcer or intracranial bleeding. Severe liver impairment. Lactation.

**Special Concerns:** Use with caution in clients with ulcers (i.e., where there is a propensity for bleeding). Consider reduced dosage in impaired renal function. Geriatric clients may be more sensitive to the effects of the drug. Safety and effectiveness have not been established in children less than 18 years of age.

**Side Effects:** *Hematologic:* Neutropenia, *agranulocytosis,* thrombocytopenia, pancytopenia, thrombotic thrombocytopenia purpura, immune thrombocytopenia, *hemolytic anemia with reticulocytosis. GI:* Diarrhea, N&V, GI pain, dyspepsia, flatulence, anorexia, GI fullness. *Bleeding complications:* Ecchymosis, hematuria, epistaxis, conjunctival hemorrhage, *GI bleeding,* perioperative bleeding, *intracerebral bleeding (rare). Dermatologic:* Maculopapular or urticarial rash, pruritus, urticaria. *CNS:* Dizziness, headache. *Neuromuscular:* Asthenia, SLE, peripheral neuropathy, arthropathy, myositis. *Miscellaneous:* Tinnitus, pain, allergic pneumonitis, vasculitis, hepatitis, cholestatic jaundice, nephrotic syndrome, hyponatremia, serum sickness.

**Drug Interactions**
*Antacids* / ↓ Plasma levels of ticlopidine
*Aspirin* / ↑ Effect of aspirin on collagen-induced platelet aggregation
*NSAIDs* / ↑ Risk of bleeding tendencies

**How Supplied:** *Tablet:* 250 mg

**Dosage** ⎯⎯⎯⎯⎯⎯⎯⎯⎯⎯
• **Tablets**
  *Reduce risk of thrombotic stroke.* 250 mg b.i.d.

## DENTAL CONCERNS
### General
1. Patients taking this drug require PT test prior to their dental visit because of the increased risk for prolonged bleeding.
2. Local hemostatic measures may be necessary to prevent excessive bleeding.
3. Patients taking ticlopidine for the first three months may be at a higher risk for developing blood dyscrasias. Symptoms include fever, sore throat, bleeding, and poor wound healing.

### Consultation with Primary Care Provider
1. Consultation with primary care provider may be necessary to assess patient status (disease control and ability to tolerate stress). Include patients most current PT time.
2. Patients with symptoms of blood dyscrasias should be referred to their primary care provider for complete blood counts. Treatment should be postponed until the results are known.

### Client/Family Teaching
1. Use caution when using oral hygiene aids.
2. Brush teeth with a soft-bristle tooth brush.
3. Avoid OTC agents especially aspirin and NSAIDs.
4. Report any unusual bruising or bleeding; advise others especially

**T**

---

dentist of prescribed therapy, before surgery or new meds added.

5. Drug should be discontinued 7 days prior to elective surgery (including oral surgery).

# Tiludronate disodium
(tye-**LOO**-droh-nayt)
**Pregnancy Category:** C
**Skelid (Rx)**
**Classification:** Bone growth regulator

**Action/Kinetics:** Inhibits activity of osteoclasts and decreases bone turnover. Does not interfere with bone mineralization. Poorly absorbed from GI tract when fasting and in presence of food. **Peak serum levels:** 2 hr. Not metabolized; excreted in urine. **t½:** About 150 hr.

**Uses:** Treatment of Paget's disease where level of serum alkaline phosphatase is at least twice upper limit of normal, in those who are symptomatic, or who are at risk for future complications of disease.

**Contraindications:** Not recommended for those with $C_{CR}$ less than 30 mL/min.

**Special Concerns:** Use with caution during lactation and in those with dysphagia, symptomatic esophageal disease, gastritis, duodenitis, or ulcers. Safety and efficacy have not been determined in children.

**Side Effects:** *Oral:* Dry mouth. *GI:* Diarrhea, N&V, dyspepsia, flatulence, tooth disorder, abdominal pain, constipation, gastritis. *Body as whole:* Pain, back pain, accidental injury, flu-like symptoms, chest pain, asthenia, syncope, fatigue, flushing. *CNS:* Headache, dizziness, paresthesia, vertigo, anorexia, somnolence, anxiety, nervousness, insomnia. *CV:* Dependent edema, peripheral edema, hypertension. *Musculoskeletal:* Arthralgia, arthrosis, pathological fracture, involuntary muscle contractions. *Respiratory:* Rhinitis, sinusitis, URTI, coughing, pharyngitis, bronchitis. *Dermatologic:* Rash, skin disorder, pruritus, increased sweating. *Ophthalmic:* Cataract, conjunctivitis, glaucoma. *Miscellaneous:* Hyperparathyroidism, vitamin D deficiency, UTI.

**Drug Interactions**
*Antacids, aluminum- or magnesium-containing /* ↓ Bioavailability of tiludronate when taken 1 hr before tiludronate
*Aspirin /* ↓ Bioavailability of tiludronate by 50% when taken 2 hr after tiludronate
*Calcium /* ↓ Bioavailability of tiludronate when taken at same time
*Indomethacin /* ↑ Bioavailability of tiludronate by two- to four-fold
**How Supplied:** *Tablets:* 240 mg

## Dosage
• **Tablets**
*Paget's disease.*
**Adults:** Single 400 mg dose/day taken with 6–8 oz of plain water for period of only 3 months.

## DENTAL CONCERNS
**General**
1. Evaluate the patient for oral signs of Paget's disease.
2. It may be necessary to place the dental chair in a semisupine position in order to minimize the GI effects of the drug.
3. Shorter appointments may be necessary for patient comfort.
4. Decreased saliva flow can put the patient at risk for dental caries, periodontal disease, and candidiasis.

**Consultation with Primary Care Provider**
1. Consultation may be required in order to assess extent of disease control.

**Client/Family Teaching**
1. Review the importance of good oral hygiene in order to prevent soft tissue inflammation.
2. Review the proper use of oral hygiene aids in order to prevent injury.
3. Daily home fluoride treatments for persistent dry mouth.
4. Avoid alcohol-containing mouth rinses and beverages.
5. Avoid caffeine-containing beverages.
6. Dry mouth can be treated with tart, sugarless gum or candy, water, sugar-free beverages, or with saliva substitutes if dry mouth persists.

7. Do not take aspirin, indomethacin, or calcium or mineral supplements within 2 hr before or after taking drug.

# Tizanidine hydrochloride
(tye-**ZAN**-ih-deen)
**Pregnancy Category:** C
Zanaflex **(Rx)**
**Classification:** Skeletal muscle relaxant, centrally-acting

**Action/Kinetics:** Acts on central $\alpha$-2 adrenergic receptors; reduces spasticity by increasing presynaptic inhibition of motor neurons. Greatest effects are on polysynaptic pathways. **Peak effect:** 1–2 hr. **Duration:** 3–6 hr. Extensive first pass metabolism. **t½:** About 2.5 hr. Excreted in urine and feces. Elderly clear drug more slowly.

**Uses:** Acute and intermittent management of muscle spasticity.

**Contraindications:** Use with $\alpha$-2-adrenergic agonists.

**Special Concerns:** Use with caution in renal impairment, in elderly and during laction. Use with extreme caution in hepatic insufficiency. Safety and efficacy have not been determined in children.

**Side Effects:** *Note:* Side effects listed are those with a frequency of 0.1% or greater. *Oral:* Dry mouth. *CV:* Hypotension, vasodilation, postural hypotension, syncope, migraine, arrhythmia. *GI:* Hepatotoxicity, dry mouth, constipation, pharyngitis, vomiting, abdominal pain, diarrhea, dyspepsia, dysphagia, cholelithiasis, fecal impaction, flatulence, *GI hemorrhage* hepatitis, melena. *CNS:* Dizziness, dyskinesia, nervousness, somnolence, sedation, hallucinations, psychotic-like symptoms, depression, anxiety, paresthesia, tremor, emotional lability, seizures, paralysis, abnormal thinking, vertigo, abnormal dreams, agitation, depersonalization, euphoria, stupor, dysautonomia, neuralgia. *GU:* Urinary frequency, UTI, urinary urgency, cystitis, menorrhagia, pyelonephritis, urinary retention, kidney calculus, enlarged uterine fibroids, vaginal moniliasis, vaginitis. *Hematologic:* Ecchymosis, anemia, leukopenia, leukocytosis. *Musculoskeletal:* Myasthenia, back pain, pathological fracture, arthralgia, arthritis, bursitis. *Respiratory:* Sinusitis, pneumonia, bronchitis, rhinitis. *Dermatologic:* Rash, sweating, skin ulcer, pruritus, dry skin, acne, alopecia, urticaria. *Body as a whole:* Flu syndrome, weight loss, infection, *sepsis, cellulitis, death,* allergic reaction, moniliasis, malaise, asthenia, fever, abscess, edema. *Ophthalmic:* Glaucoma, amblyopia, conjunctivitis, eye pain, optic neuritis, retinal hemorrhage, visual field defect. *Otic:* Ear pain, tinnitus, deafness, otitis media. *Miscellaneous:* Speech disorder.

**Drug Interactions**
*Alcohol /* ↑ Side effects of tizanidine; additive CNS depressant effects
*Alpha-2-Adrenergic agonists /* Additive hypotensive effects
*Oral contraceptives /* ↓ Clearance of tizanidine

**Dosage**
• **Tablets**
*Muscle spasticity.*
**Initial:** 4 mg; **then,** increase dose gradually in 2- to 4-mg steps to optimum effect. Dose can be repeated at 6- to 8-hr intervals, to maximum of 3 doses/24 hr, not to exceed 36 mg/day. There is no experience with repeated, single, daytime doses greater than 12 mg or total daily doses of 36 mg or more.

## DENTAL CONCERNS
**General**
1. Monitor vital signs at every appointment because of cardiovascular effects.
2. Have the patient sit up slowly and remain seated for at least two minutes after being supine in order to minimize the risk of orthostatic hypotension.
3. Decreased saliva flow can put the

patient at risk for dental caries, periodontal disease, and candidiasis.

4. Shorter appointments may be necessary due to the disease effects on musculature.

5. General anesthesia should be used with caution in patients requiring dental surgery.

**Consultation with Primary Care Provider**

1. Consultation with the patients health care provider may be necessary in order to determine the patient's ability to tolerate stress and the extent of disease control.

**Client/Family Teaching**

1. Do not perform activities that require mental alertness (i.e., driving a car); drug causes sedation.

2. May cause orthostatic hypotension; avoid sudden changes in position.

3. Avoid alcohol and any other CNS depressants. Antihistamines may produce an additive depressant effect.

4. Review the importance of good oral hygiene in order to prevent soft tissue inflammation.

5. Review the proper use of oral hygiene aids in order to prevent injury.

6. Daily home fluoride treatments for persistent dry mouth.

7. Avoid alcohol-containing mouth rinses.

8. Dry mouth can be treated with tart, sugarless gum or candy, sips of water, or with saliva substitutes if dry mouth persists.

# Tocainide hydrochloride
(toe-**KAY**-nyd)
**Pregnancy Category:** C
Tonocard **(Rx)**
**Classification:** Antiarrhythmic, class IB

See also *Antiarrhythmic Agents.*

**Action/Kinetics:** Similar to lidocaine. Decreases the excitability of cells in the myocardium by decreasing sodium and potassium conductance. Increases pulmonary and aortic arterial pressure and slightly increases peripheral resistance. Effective in both digitalized and nondigitalized clients. **Peak plasma levels:** 0.5–2 hr. t½: 11–15 hr. **Therapeutic serum levels:** 4–10 mcg/mL. **Duration:** 8 hr. Approximately 10% is bound to plasma protein. From 28% to 55% is excreted unchanged in the urine. Alkalinization decreases the excretion of the drug although acidification does not produce any changes in excretion.

**Uses:** Life-threatening ventricular arrhythmias, including ventricular tachycardia. Has not been shown to improve survival in clients with ventricular arrhythmias. *Non-FDA Approved Uses:* Myotonic dystrophy, trigeminal neuralgia.

**Contraindications:** Allergy to amide-type local anesthetics, second- or third-degree AV block in the absence of artificial ventricular pacemaker. Lactation.

**Special Concerns:** Increased risk of death when used in those with non-life-threatening cardiac arrhythmias. Safety and efficacy have not been established in children. Use with caution in clients with impaired renal or hepatic function (dose may have to be decreased). Geriatric clients may have an increased risk of dizziness and hypotension; the dose may have to be reduced in these clients due to age-related impaired renal function.

**Side Effects:** *CV: Increased arrhythmias,* increased ventricular rate (when given for atrial flutter or fibrillation), CHF, tachycardia, hypotension, *conduction disturbances,* bradycardia, chest pain, LV failure, palpitations. *CNS:* Dizziness, vertigo, headache, tremors, confusion, disorientation, hallucinations, ataxia, paresthesias, numbness, nervousness, altered mood, anxiety, incoordination, walking disturbances. *Oral:* Dry mouth, oral ulcerations. *GI:* N&V, anorexia, diarrhea. *Respiratory: Pulmonary fibrosis, fibrosing alveolitis,* interstitial pneumonitis, *pulmonary edema,* pneumonia. *Hematologic:* Leukopenia, *agranulocytosis,* hypoplastic anemia, *aplastic anemia,* bone marrow depression, neutropenia, *thrombocytopenia and sequelae as septicemia* *and septic shock. Musculoskeletal:* Arthritis, arthralgia, myalgia. *Dermatologic:* Rash, skin lesion, diaphoresis. *Other:* Blurred vision, visual disturbances, nystagmus, tinnitus, hearing loss, lupus-like syndrome.

**Drug Interactions:** No specific interactions have been reported with drugs that are used in dentistry. However, lowest effective dose should be used, such as a local anesthetic, vasoconstrictor, or anticholinergic, if required.

**How Supplied:** *Tablet:* 400 mg, 600 mg

**Dosage** ————————————
• **Tablets**
  *Antiarrhythmic.*
**Adults, individualized, initial:** 400 mg q 8 hr, up to a maximum of 2,400 mg/day; **maintenance:** 1,200–1,800 mg/day in divided doses. Total daily dose of 1,200 mg may be adequate in clients with liver or kidney disease.
  *Myotonic dystrophy.*
800–1,200 mg/day.
  *Trigeminal neuralgia.*
20 mg/kg/day in three divided doses.

## DENTAL CONCERNS

See also *Dental Concerns* for *Antiarrhythmic Agents.*
**General**
1. Have the patient sit up slowly and remain seated for at least two minutes after being supine in order to minimize the risk of orthostatic hypotension.
2. Patients on chronic drug therapy may develop blood dyscrasias. Symptoms include fever, sore throat, bleeding, and poor wound healing.
**Consultation with Primary Care Provider**
1. Patients with symptoms of blood dyscrasias should be referred to their primary care provider for complete blood counts. Treatment should be postponed until the results are known.

**Client/Family Teaching**
1. Review the proper use of oral hygiene aids in order to prevent injury.
2. Daily home fluoride treatments for persistent dry mouth.

# Tolazamide
(toll-**AZ**-ah-myd)
**Pregnancy Category:** C
Tolinase **(Rx)**
**Classification:** Sulfonylurea, first-generation

See also *Antidiabetic Agents: Hypoglycemic Agents.*

**Action/Kinetics:** Effective in some with a history of coma or ketoacidosis; may be effective in clients who do not respond well to other oral antidiabetics. Use with insulin is not recommended for maintenance. **Onset:** 4–6 hr. **t½:** 7 hr. **Time to peak levels:** 3–4 hr. **Duration:** 12–24 hr. Metabolized in liver to metabolites with minor hypoglycemic activity. Excreted through the kidneys (85%) and feces (7%).

**Additional Contraindications:** Renal glycosuria.

**Additional Drug Interactions:** Concomitant use of alcohol and tolazamide may → photosensitivity.

**How Supplied:** *Tablet:* 100 mg, 250 mg, 500 mg

**Dosage** ————————————
• **Tablets**
  *Diabetes.*
**Adults, initial:** 100 mg/day if fasting blood sugar is less than 200 mg/100 mL, or 250 mg/day if fasting blood sugar is greater than 200 mg/100 mL. Adjust dose to response, not to exceed 1 g/day. If more than 500 mg/day is required, it should be given in two divided doses, usually before the morning and evening meals. **Elderly, malnourished, underweight clients or those not eating properly:** 100 mg once daily with breakfast, adjusting dose by increments of 50 mg/day each week. Doses greater than 1

g/day will probably not improve control.

## DENTAL CONCERNS

See also *Dental Concerns* for *Antidiabetic Agents: Hypoglycemic Agents* and *Glipizide*.

# Tolbutamide
(toll-**BYOU**-tah-myd)
**Pregnancy Category:** C
APO-Tolbutamide ✿, Novo-Butamide
✿, Orinase **(Rx)**

# Tolbutamide sodium
(toll-**BYOU**-tah-myd)
**Pregnancy Category:** C
Orinase Diagnostic **(Rx)**
**Classification:** Sulfonylurea, first-generation

See also *Antidiabetic Agents, Hypoglycemic Agents*.
**Action/Kinetics: Onset:** 1 hr. **t½:** 4.5–6.5 hr. **Time to peak levels:** 3–4 hr. **Duration:** 6–12 hr. Changed in liver to inactive metabolites. Excreted through the kidney (75%) and feces (9%).
**Additional Uses:** Most useful for clients with poor general physical status who should receive a short-acting compound.

Tolbutamide sodium is used to diagnose pancreatic islet cell tumors. It causes blood glucose, in the presence of a tumor, to drop quickly after IV administration and remain low for 3 hr.
**Additional Side Effects:** Melena (dark, bloody stools) in some clients with a history of peptic ulcer. Relapse or secondary failure may occur a few months after therapy has been started. May cause hyponatremia and a mild goiter.
**Additional Drug Interactions**
*Alcohol* / Photosensitivity reactions
*Sulfinpyrazone* / ↑ Effect of tolbutamide due to ↓ breakdown by liver
**How Supplied:** Tolbutamide: *Tablet:* 500 mg. Tolbutamide sodium: *Powder for injection:* 1 g

## Dosage
• **Tablets**

*Diabetes mellitus.*
**Adults, initial:** 0.25–3 g/day (usually 1–2 g). Adjust dosage depending on response. **Usual maintenance:** 0.25–2 g/day). A daily dose greater than 2 g is rarely needed; maximum daily dose should not exceed 3 g.

## DENTAL CONCERNS

See also *Dental Concerns* for *Antidiabetic Agents, Oral*.

# Tolmetin sodium
(**TOLL**-met-in)
**Pregnancy Category:** C
Novo-Tolmetin ✿, Tolectin ✿, Tolectin 200, Tolectin 600, Tolectin DS **(Rx)**
**Classification:** Nonsteroidal, anti-inflammatory, analgesic

See also *Nonsteroidal Anti-Inflammatory Drugs*.
**Action/Kinetics: Peak plasma levels:** 30–60 min. **t½:** 1 hr. **Therapeutic plasma levels:** 40 mcg/mL. **Onset, anti-inflammatory effect:** within 1 week; **duration, anti-inflammatory effect:** 1–2 weeks. Inactivated in liver and excreted in urine.
**Uses:** Acute and chronic treatment of rheumatoid arthritis and osteoarthritis. Juvenile rheumatoid arthritis. *Non-FDA Approved Uses:* Sunburn.
**Special Concerns:** Use with caution during lactation. Dosage has not been determined in children less than 2 years of age.
**How Supplied:** *Capsule:* 400 mg; *Tablet:* 200 mg, 600 mg

## Dosage
• **Capsules, Tablets**
*Rheumatoid arthritis, osteoarthritis.*
**Adults:** 400 mg t.i.d. (one dose on arising and one at bedtime); adjust dosage according to client response.
**Maintenance:** *rheumatoid arthritis,* 600–1,800 mg/day in three to four divided doses; *osteoarthritis,* 600–1,600 mg/day in three to four divided doses. Doses larger than 1,800 mg/day for rheumatoid arthritis and osteoarthritis are not recommended.
*Juvenile rheumatoid arthritis.*

**2 years and older, initial:** 20 mg/kg/day in three to four divided doses to start; **then,** 15–30 mg/kg/day. Doses higher than 30 mg/kg/day are not recommended. Beneficial effects may not be observed for several days to a week.

## DENTAL CONCERNS

See also *Dental Concerns* for *Nonsteroidal Anti-Inflammatory Drugs.*

# Topiramate
(toh-**PYRE**-ah-mayt)
**Pregnancy Category:** C
Topamax **(Rx)**
**Classification:** Anticonvulsant, miscellaneous

See also *Anticonvulsants.*
**Action/Kinetics:** Precise mechanism not known. The following effects may contribute to the anticonvulsant activity. (1) Blocks repetitive action potentials. (2) Increases the frequency at which GABA activates $GABA_A$ receptors. (3) Antagonizes the ability of kainate, thus reducing the excitatory effect. Rapidly absorbed; **peak plasma levels:** About 2 hr. **t½, elimination:** 21 hr. Steady state is reached in about 4 days in those with normal renal function. Excreted mostly unchanged in the urine.
**Uses:** Adjunct to treat partial onset seizures in adults.
**Contraindications:** Lactation.
**Special Concerns:** Use with caution in impaired hepatic and renal function. Safety and efficacy have not been determined in children.
**Side Effects:** *Note:* Side effects with an incidence of 0.1% or greater are listed. *CNS:* Psychomotor slowing, including difficulty with concentration and speech or language problems. Somnolence, fatigue, dizziness, ataxia, nystagmus, paresthesia, nervousness, difficulty with memory, tremor, confusion, depression, abnormal coordination, agitation, mood problems, aggressive reaction, hypoesthesia, apathy, emotional lability, de-

personalization, hypokinesia, vertIgo, stupor, *clonic/tonic seizures,* hyperkinesia, hypertonia, insomnia, personality disorder, impotence, hallucinations, euphoria, psychosis, decreased libido, *suicide attempt,* hyporeflexia, neuropathy, migraine, apraxia, hyperesthesia, dyskinesia, hyperreflexia, dysphonia, scotoma, dystonia, coma, encephalopathy, upper motor neuron lesion, paranoid reaction, delusion, paranoia, delirium, abnormal dreaming, neuroses. *Oral:* Dry mouth, gingivitis, halitosis, gum hyperplasia, tooth caries, stomatitis, gingival bleeding, increased saliva, tongue edema. *GI:* Nausea, dyspepsia, anorexia, abdominal pain, constipation, diarrhea, vomiting, fecal incontinence, flatulence, gastroenteritis, hemorrhoids, increased appetite, dysphagia, melena, gastritis, hiccough, gastroesophageal reflux, esophagitis, gall bladder disorder. *CV:* Palpitation, hypertension, hypotension, postural hypotension, AV block, bradycardia, bundle branch block, angina pectoris, vasodilation. *Body as a whole:* Asthenia, back pain, chest pain, flulike symptoms, leg pain, hot flashes, body odor, edema, rigors, fever, malaise, syncope, enlarged abdomen. *Respiratory:* URI, pharyngitis, sinusitis, dyspnea, coughing, bronchitis, asthma, *bronchospasm, pulmonary embolism.* *Dermatologic:* Acne, alopecia, dermatitis, nail disorder, folliculitis, dry skin, urticaria, skin discoloration, eczema, photosensitivity reaction, erythematous rash, seborrhea, decreased sweating, abnormal hair texture, facial edema. *GU:* Breast pain, renal stone formation, dysmenorrhea, menstrual disorder, hematuria, intermenstrual bleeding, leukorrhea, menorrhagia, vaginitis, amenorrhea, UTI, micturition frequency, urinary incontinence, dysuria, renal calculus, ejaculation disorder, breast discharge, urinary retention, renal pain, nocturia, albuminuria, polyuria, oliguria. *Musculoskeletal:* Arthralgia, muscle weak-

**T**

*bold italic* = life-threatening side effect

ness, arthrosis, osteoporosis, myalgia, leg cramps. *Metabolic:* Increased weight, decreased weight, dehydration, xeropthalmia. *Hematologic:* Anemia, leukopenia, lymphadenopathy, eosinophilia, lymphopenia, granulocytopenia, lymphocytosis, thrombocytothemia, purpura, thrombocytopenia. *Dermatologic:* Rash, pruritus, increased sweating, flushing. *Ophthalmic:* Diplopia, abnormal vision, eye pain, conjunctivitis, abnormal accommodation, photophobia, abnormal lacrimation, strabismus, color blindness, myopia, mydriasis, ptosis, visual field defect. *Miscellaneous:* Decreased hearing, epistaxis, taste perversion, tinnitus, taste loss, parosmia, goiter, basal cell carcinoma.

**Drug Interactions**
*Alcohol* / CNS depression and cognitive and neuropsychiatric side effects
*Carbamazepine* / ↓ Plasma levels of topiramate
*CNS depressants* / CNS depression and cognitive and neuropsychiatric side effects

**How Supplied:** *Tablets:* 25 mg, 100 mg, 200 mg.

**Dosage** ————————
• **Tablets**
    *Adjunctive therapy for treatment of partial onset seizures.*
**Initial:** 50 mg/day; **then,** titrate to an effective dose of 400 mg/day in 2 divided doses. Titrate by adding 50 mg each week for 8 weeks, until the dose is 400 mg/day. Doses greater than 400 mg/day have not been shown to improve the response. If $C_{CR}$ < 70 mL/1.73 m², use one half of the usual adult dose.

---

**DENTAL CONCERNS**

See also *Dental Concerns* for *Anticonvulsants*.
1. Can cause photosensitivity. The patient may require dark glasses when the dental light is on.

---

# Tramadol hydrochloride
(**TRAM**-ah-dol)

**Pregnancy Category:** C
Ultram **(Rx)**
**Classification:** Analgesic, centrally acting

---

**Action/Kinetics:** A centrally acting analgesic not related chemically to opiates. Precise mechanism is not known. It may bind to mu-opioid receptors and inhibit reuptake of norepinephrine and serotonin. Rapidly absorbed after PO administration. Food does not affect the rate or extent of absorption. **Onset:** 1 hr. **Peak effect:** 2–3 hr. **Peak plasma levels:** 2 hr. **t½, plasma:** Approximately 7 hr after multiple doses. Extensively metabolized by one of the P-450 isoenzymes. Excreted in the urine, with about 30% excreted unchanged and 60% as metabolites. The M-metabolite is active.

**Uses:** Management of moderate to moderately severe pain.

**Contraindications:** Hypersensitivity to tramadol. In acute intoxication with alcohol, hypnotics, centrally acting analgesics, opiates, or psychotropic drugs. Use in clients with past or present addiction or opiate dependence or in those with a prior history of allergy to codeine or opiates. Use for obstetric preoperative medication or for postdelivery analgesia in nursing mothers. Use in children less than 16 years of age, as safety and efficacy have not been determined.

**Special Concerns:** Use with great caution in those taking MAO inhibitors, as tramadol inhibits norepinephrine and serotonin uptake. Dosage reduction is recommended with impaired hepatic or renal function and in clients over 75 years of age. Use with caution in increased intracranial pressure or head injury, in epilepsy, or in clients with an increased risk for seizures, including head trauma, metabolic disorders, alcohol or drug withdrawal, and CNS infections. Tramadol may complicate the assessment of acute abdominal conditions.

**Side Effects:** *CNS:* Dizziness, vertigo, headache, somnolence, CNS stimulation, anxiety, confusion, incoordination, euphoria, nervousness, sleep disorders, *seizures,* paresthesia, cognitive dysfunction, hallucinations, tremor, amnesia, concentration difficulty, abnormal gait, migraine, development of drug dependence. *Oral:* Dry mouth, stomatitis, dysgeusia. *GI:* Nausea, constipation, vomiting, dyspepsia, diarrhea, abdominal pain, anorexia, flatulence, GI bleeding, hepatitis. *CV:* Vasodilation, syncope, orthostatic hypotension, tachycardia, abnormal ECG, hypertension, myocardial ischemia, palpitations. *Dermatologic:* Pruritus, sweating, rash, urticaria, vesicles. *Body as a whole:* Asthenia, malaise, allergic reaction, accidental injury, weight loss, *suicidal tendency.* *GU:* Urinary retention, urinary frequency, menopausal symptoms, dysuria, menstrual disorder. *Miscellaneous: Anaphylaxis,* visual disturbances, cataracts, deafness, tinnitus, hypertonia, dyspnea.

**Drug Interactions**
*Alcohol* / Enhanced respiratory depression
*Anesthetics, general* / Enhanced respiratory depression
*Carbamazepine* / ↓ Effect of tramadol due to ↑ metabolism induced by carbamazepine
*CNS depressants* / Additive CNS depression
*MAO Inhibitors* / Tramadol may ↑ the risk of seizures in those taking MAO inhibitors
*Naloxone* / Use of naloxone for tramadol overdose may ↑ risk of seizures.

**How Supplied:** *Tablet:* 50 mg

**Dosage** ————————
• **Tablets**
 *Management of pain.*
**Adults:** 50–100 mg q 4–6 hr as needed, but not to exceed 400 mg/day. For moderate pain, 50 mg, initially, may be adequate, and for severe pain, 100 mg, initially, is often more effective. For clients over 75 years of age, the recommended dose is no more than 300 mg/day in divided doses. In impaired renal function

with a $C_{CR}$ less than 30 mL/min, the dosing interval should be increased to 12 hr, with a maximum daily dose of 200 mg. The recommended dose for clients with cirrhosis is 50 mg q 12 hr.

## DENTAL CONCERNS

See also *Dental Concerns* for *Opioid Analgesics.*

# Trandolapril
(tran-**DOHL**-ah-pril)
**Pregnancy Category:** C (first trimester); D (second and third trimesters)
Mavik **(Rx)**
**Classification:** Antihypertensive
————————
See also *Angiotensin Converting Enzyme (ACE) Inhibitors.*
**Action/Kinetics:** Rapidly absorbed; food slows rate, but not amount absorbed. **Peak plasma levels, trandolapril:** 30–60 min; **trandolaprilat:** 4–10 hr. **t½, trandoprilat:** 15–24 hr. Metabolized in liver to active trandolaprilat. About ⅓ trandolaprilat is excreted in urine and ⅔ in feces.
**Uses:** Hypertension, alone or in combination with other antihypertensives such as hydrochlorothiazide.
**Contraindications:** In those with history of angioedema with ACE inhibitors.
**Special Concerns:** Safety and efficacy have not been determined in children.
**Side Effects:** See also *ACE Inhibitors. Hypersensitivity: Angioedema. CNS:* Dizziness, headache, fatigue. *Oral:* Angioedema (lips, mucous membranes, tongue). *GI:* Diarrhea, dyspepsia, gastritis. *CV:* Hypotension, bradycardia, *cardiogenic shock,* intermittent claudication, stroke. *Pulmonary:* Cough, *Hepatic: Hepatic failure,* including cholestatic jaundice, *fulminant hepatic necrosis, death. Miscellaneous:* Neutropenia, syncope, myalgia, asthenia.
**Drug Interactions**
See also *Angiotensin-Converting Enzyme Inhibitors.*

**T**

————————

*Tetracyclines* / ↓ Absorption of tetracycline due to high magnesium content of quinapril tablets

**How Supplied:** *Tablet:* 1 mg, 2 mg, 4 mg

**Dosage**
- **Tablets**
  *Hypertension.*

**Initial:** 1 mg once daily in nonblack clients and 2 mg once daily in black clients. Adjust dosage according to response; usually, adjustments are made at intervals of 1 week. **Maintenance, usual:** 2–4 mg once daily. Those inadequately treated with once-daily dosing can be treated with twice-daily dosing. If BP is still not adequately controlled, diuretic may be added. If $C_{CR}$ is less than 30 mL/min or if there is hepatic cirrhosis, initial dose is 0.5 mg daily.

## DENTAL CONCERNS

See also *Dental Concerns* for *Angiotensin-Converting Enzyme Inhibitors* and *Antihypertensive Agents.*

# Tranylcypromine sulfate
(**tran**-ill-**SIP**-roh-meen)
Parnate **(Rx)**
Classification: Antidepressant, monoamine oxidase inhibitor

**Action/Kinetics:** An MAO inhibitor with a rapid onset of activity. Due to inhibition of MAO, the concentration of epinephrine, norepinephrine, and serotonin increases in storage sites throughout the nervous system. This increase has been alleged to be the basis for the antidepressant effects. MAO activity recovers in 3–5 days after drug withdrawal.

**Uses:** Treatment of major depressive episode without melancholia. Not a first line of therapy; is used when clients have failed to respond to other drug therapy. *Non-FDA Approved Uses:* Alone or as an adjunct to treat bulimia, obsessive compulsive disorder, and manifestations of psychotic disorders. Also, treatment of social phobia, seasonal affective disorders, adjunct to treat multiple sclerosis, and to treat idiopathic orthostatic hypotension (e.g., Shy-Drager syndrome), refractory to conventional therapy.

**Contraindications:** Use in those with a confirmed or suspected CV defect or in anyone with CV disease, hypertension, or history of headache. In the presence of pheochromocytoma. History of liver disease or in those with abnormal liver function. Use in combination with a large number of other drugs, especially other MAO inhibitors, tricyclic antidepressants, serotonin-reuptake inhibitors, buspirone, sympathomimetics, meperidine, CNS depressants (e.g., alcohol and narcotics), hypotensive drugs, excessive caffeine, and dextromethorphan (see *Drug Interactions*). Use with tyramine-containing foods (see *Drug Interactions*).

**Special Concerns:** Assess benefits versus risks before using during pregnancy and lactation. Use with caution in clients taking antiparkinson drugs, in impaired renal function, in those with seizure disorders, in diabetics, in hyperthyroid clients, and in those taking disulfiram. Geriatric clients may be more sensitive to the drug.

**Side Effects:** *CNS:* Anxiety, agitation, headaches (without elevation of BP), manic symptoms, restlessness, insomnia, weakness, drowsiness, dizziness, significant anorexia. *Oral:* Dry mouth. *GI:* Nausea, diarrhea, abdominal pain, constipation. *CV:* Tachycardia, edema, palpitation. *GU:* Impotence, urinary retention, impaired ejaculation. *Musculoskeletal:* Muscle spasm, tremors, myoclonic jerks, numbness, paresthesia. *Hematologic:* Anemia, leukopenia, agranulocytosis, thrombocytopenia. *Miscellaneous:* Blurred vision, chills, impotence, hepatitis, skin rash, impaired water excretion, tinnitus.

**Drug Interactions**
*Alcohol* / Possibility of excitation, seizures, delirium, hyperpyrexia, circulatory collapse, coma, death
*Anesthetics, general* / Hypotensive effect; use together with caution. Phenelzine should be discontinued

at least 10 days before elective surgery

*Anticholinergic drugs, atropine* / MAO inhibitors effect of anticholinergic drugs

*Antidepressants, tricyclic* / Comcomitant use may result in excitation, sweating, tachycardia, tachypnea, hyperpyrexia, disseminated intravascular coagulation, delirium, tremors, convulsions, death. At least 7–10 days should elapse between discontinuing an MAO inhibitor and initiating a new drug. However, such combinations have been used together successfully

*Fluoxetine* / Possibility of hyperthermia, rigidity, myoclonic movements, death. At least 10 days should elapse between discontinuation of phenelzine and initiation of fluoxetine; and, at least 5 weeks should elapse between discontinuing fluoxetine and beginning phenelzine

*MAO inhibitors* / Concomitant use of tranylcypromine with other MAO inhibitors may cause a hypertensive crisis or severe seizures

*Meperidine* / See *Opioid Analgesics*

*Opioid Analgesics* / Possibility of excitation, seizures, delirium, hyperpyrexia, circulatory collapse, coma, death

*Selective serotonin reuptake inhibitors* /See *Fluoxetine*

*Sympathomimetic drugs—amphetamine, cocaine, dopa, ephedrine, epinephrine, metaraminol, methyldopa, methylphenidate, norepinephrine, phenylephrine, phenylpropanolamine. Many OTC cold products, hay fever medications, and nasal decongestants contain one or more of these drugs* / All peripheral, metabolic, cardiac, and central effects are potentiated for up to 2 weeks after termination of MAO inhibitor therapy. Symptoms include acute hypertensive crisis with possible intracranial hemorrhage, hyperthermia, coma, and possibly death

**How Supplied:** *Tablets:* 10 mg

**Dosage** ———————————
• **Tablets**
  *Major depressive syndrome without melancholia.*
Individualize the dose. **Usual effective dose:** 30 mg/day given in divided doses. If there are no signs of improvement in 2 weeks, the dose can be increased by 10 mg/day at intervals of 1–3 weeks, up to a maximum of 60 mg/day.

## DENTAL CONCERNS

See also *Dental Concerns* for *Antidepressants, Tricyclic.*
**General**
1. Possibility of hypertensive episode with vasoconstrictors.
2. Patient should not be prescribed prescription or over-the-counter products that contain aspirin.

# Trazodone hydrochloride
(**TRAYZ**-oh-dohn)
**Pregnancy Category:** C
Alti-Trazodone ✿, Alti-Trazodone Dividose ✿, Apo-Trazodone ✿, Apo-Trazodone D ✿, Desyrel, Desyrel Dividose, Dom-Trazodone ✿, Novo-Trazodone ✿, Nu-Trazodone ✿, Nu-Trazodone-D ✿, PMS-Trazodone ✿, Trazon, Trialodine **(Rx)**
**Classification:** Antidepressant, miscellaneous

**Action/Kinetics:** A novel antidepressant that does not inhibit MAO and is also devoid of amphetamine-like effects. Response usually occurs after 2 weeks (75% of clients), with the remainder responding after 2–4 weeks. May inhibit serotonin uptake by brain cells, therefore increasing serotonin concentrations in the synapse. May also cause changes in binding of serotonin to receptors. Causes moderate sedative and orthostatic hypotensive effects and slight anticholinergic effects. **Peak plasma levels:** 1 hr (empty stomach) or 2 hr (when taken with food). **t½, initial:** 3–6 hr; **final:** 5–9 hr. **Effective plasma levels:** 800–1,600 ng/mL. **Time to reach steady state:**

3–7 days. Three-fourths of those with a therapeutic effect respond by the end of the second week of therapy. Metabolized in liver and excreted through both the urine and feces. **Uses:** Depression with or without accompanying anxiety. *Non-FDA Approved Uses:* In combination with tryptophan for treating aggressive behavior. Panic disorder or agoraphobia with panic attacks. Treatment of cocaine withdrawal. Chronic pain including diabetic neuropathy. **Contraindications:** During the initial recovery period following MI. Concurrently with electroshock therapy.

**Special Concerns:** Use with caution during lactation. Safety and efficacy in children less than 18 years of age have not been established. Geriatric clients are more prone to the sedative and hypotensive effects.

**Side Effects:** *General:* Dermatitis, edema, blurred vision, constipation, dry mouth, nasal congestion, skeletal muscle aches and pains. *CV:* Hypertension or hypotension, syncope, palpitations, tachycardia, SOB, chest pain. *Oral:* Bad taste in mouth, dry mouth, hypersalivation. *GI:* Diarrhea, N&V, bad taste in mouth, flatulence. *GU:* Delayed urine flow, priapism, hematuria, increased urinary frequency. *CNS:* Nightmares, confusion, anger, excitement, decreased ability to concentrate, dizziness, disorientation, drowsiness, lightheadedness, fatigue, insomnia, nervousness, impaired memory. Rarely, hallucinations, impaired speech, hypomania. *Other:* Incoordination, tremors, paresthesias, decreased libido, appetite disturbances, red eyes, sweating or clamminess, tinnitus, weight gain or loss, anemia. Rarely, akathisia, muscle twitching, increased libido, impotence, retrograde ejaculation, early menses, missed periods.

**Drug Interactions**
*Alcohol /* ↑ Depressant effects of alcohol
*Antihypertensives /* Additive hypotension

*Barbiturates /* ↑ Depressant effects of barbiturates
*CNS depressants /* ↑ CNS depression
*MAO inhibitors /* Initiate therapy cautiously if trazodone is to be used together with MAO inhibitors
*Phenytoin /* Trazodone may ↑ serum phenytoin levels
**How Supplied:** *Tablet:* 50 mg, 100 mg, 150 mg, 300 mg

**Dosage**
• **Tablets**
   *Antidepressant.*
**Adults and adolescents, initial:** 150 mg/day; **then,** increase by 50 mg/day every 3–4 days to maximum of 400 mg/day in divided doses (outpatients). Inpatients may require up to, but not exceeding, 600 mg/day in divided doses. **Maintenance:** Use lowest effective dose. **Geriatric clients:** 75 mg/day in divided doses; dose can then be increased, as needed and tolerated, at 3- to 4-day intervals.
   *Treat aggressive behavior.*
Trazodone, 50 mg b.i.d., with tryptophan, 500 mg b.i.d. Dosage adjustments may be required to reach a therapeutic response or if side effects develop.
   *Panic disorder or agoraphobia with panic attacks.*
300 mg/day.

## DENTAL CONCERNS

See also *Dental Concerns* for *Antidepressants, Tricyclic.*
**Client/Family Teaching**
1. Use caution when driving or when performing other hazardous tasks; may cause drowsiness or dizziness.

# Triamcinolone
(try-am-**SIN**-oh-lohn)
**Pregnancy Category:** C
**Dental Paste:** Kenalog in Orabase, Oracort, Oralone **(Rx). Tablets:** Aristocort, Atolone, Kenacort **(Rx)**

# Triamcinolone acetonide
(try-am-**SIN**-oh-lohn)
**Pregnancy Category:** C

**Dental Paste:** Oracort ✿. **Inhalation Aerosol:** Azmacort, Nasacort, Nasacort AQ **(Rx)**. **Parenteral:** Kenaject-40, Kenalog-10 and -40, Scheinpharm Triamcine-A ✿, Tac-3 and -40, Triam-A, Triamonide 40, Tri-Kort, Trilog **(Rx)**. **Topical Aerosol:** Kenalog **(Rx)**. **Topical Cream:** Aristocort, Aristocort A, Delta-Tritex, Flutex, Kenac, Kenalog, Kenalog-H, Kenonel, Triacet, Triaderm ✿, Trianide Mild, Trianide Regular, Triderm, Trymex **(Rx)**. **Topical Lotion:** Kenalog, Kenonel **(Rx)**. **Topical Ointment:** Aristocort, Aristocort A, Kenac, Kenalog, Kenonel, Triaderm ✿, Trymex, **Topical Spray:** Nasacort AQ **(Rx)**

# Triamcinolone diacetate

(try-am-**SIN**-oh-lohn)
**Pregnancy Category:** C
**Parenteral:** Amcort, Aristocort Forte, Aristocort Intralesional, Aristocort Parenteral ✿, Articulose L.A., Kenacort Diacetate, Triam-Forte, Triamolone 40, Trilone, Tristoject. **Syrup:** Aristocort Syrup ✿ **(Rx)**

# Triamcinolone hexacetonide

(try-am-**SIN**-oh-lohn)
**Pregnancy Category:** C
Aristospan Intra-Articular, Aristospan Intralesional **(Rx)**
**Classification:** Corticosteroid, synthetic

See also *Corticosteroids.*
**Action/Kinetics:** More potent than prednisone. Intermediate-acting. Has no mineralocorticoid activity. **Onset:** Several hours. **Duration:** One or more weeks. **t½:** Over 200 min.
**Additional Uses:** Pulmonary emphysema accompanied by bronchospasm or bronchial edema. Diffuse interstitial pulmonary fibrosis. With diuretics to treat refractory CHF or cirrhosis of the liver with ascites. Multiple sclerosis. Inflammation following dental procedures. Triamcinolone acetonide for PO inhalation is used for maintenance treatment of asthma. Triamcinolone hexacetonide is restricted to intra-articular or intralesional treatment of rheumatoid arthritis and osteoarthritis.
**Special Concerns:** Use during pregnancy only if benefits clearly outweigh risks. Use with special caution with decreased renal function or renal disease. Dose must be highly individualized.
**Additional Side Effects:** Intra-articular, intrasynovial, or intrabursal administration may cause transient flushing, dizziness, local depigmentation, and rarely, local irritation. Exacerbation of symptoms has also been reported. A marked increase in swelling and pain and further restricted joint movement may indicate septic arthritis. Intradermal injection may cause local vesicular ulceration and persistent scarring. *Syncope and anaphylactoid reactions* have been reported with triamcinolone regardless of route of administration.
**How Supplied:** Triamcinolone: *Tablet:* 1 mg, 2 mg, 4 mg, 8 mg. Triamcinolone acetonide: *Metered dose inhaler (nasal):* 55 mcg/inh; *Metered dose inhaler (oral)* 100 mcg/inh; *Cream:* 0.025%, 0.1%, 0.5%; *Nasal spray:* 55 mcg/inh; *Injection:* 3 mg/mL, 10 mg/mL, 40 mg/mL; *Lotion:* 0.025%, 0.1%; *Ointment:* 0.025%, 0.05%, 0.1%, 0.5%; *Paste:* 0.1%; *Topical spray:* 0.147 mg/g. Triamcinolone diacetate: *Injection:* 25 mg/mL, 40 mg/mL. Triamcinolone hexacetonide: *Injection:* 5 mg/mL, 20 mg/mL.

## Dosage
TRIAMCINOLONE
• **Tablets**
*Adrenocortical insufficiency (with mineralocorticoid therapy).*
4–12 mg/day.
*Acute leukemias (children).*
1–2 mg/kg.
*Acute leukemia or lymphoma (adults).*
16–40 mg/day (up to 100 mg/day may be necessary for leukemia).
*Edema.*
16–20 mg (up to 48 mg may be required until diuresis occurs).

*Tuberculosis meningitis.*
32–48 mg/day.
*Rheumatic disease, dermatologic disorders, bronchial asthma.*
8–16 mg/day.
*SLE.*
20–32 mg/day.
*Allergies.*
8–12 mg/day.
*Hematologic disorders.*
16–60 mg/day.
*Ophthalmologic diseases.*
12–40 mg daily.
*Respiratory diseases.*
16–48 mg/day.
TRIAMCINOLONE ACETONIDE
• **IM Only (Not for IV Use)**
2.5–60 mg/day, depending on the disease and its severity.
• **Intra-articular, Intrabursal, Tendon Sheaths**
2.5–5 mg for smaller joints and 5–15 mg for larger joints, although up to 40 mg has been used.
• **Intradermal**
1 mg/injection site (use 3 mg/mL or 10 mg/mL suspension only).
• **Topical: 0.025%, 0.1%, 0.5% Ointment or Cream; 0.025%, 0.1% Lotion; Paste: 0.1%; Aerosol—to deliver 0.2 mg)**
Apply sparingly to affected area b.i.d.–q.i.d. and rub in lightly.
• **Metered Dose Inhaler (Azmacort)**
**Adults, usual:** 2 inhalations (200 mcg) t.i.d.–q.i.d. or 4 inhalations (400 mcg) b.i.d., not to exceed 1,600 mcg/day. High initial doses (1,200–1,600 mcg/day) may be needed in some clients with severe asthma. **Pediatric, 6–12 years:** 1–2 inhalations (100–200 mcg) t.i.d.–q.i.d. or 2–4 inhalations b.i.d., not to exceed 1,200 mcg/day. Use in children less than 6 years of age has not been determined.
• **Intranasal Spray (Nasacort)**
*Seasonal and perennial allergic rhinitis.*
**Adults and children over 12 years of age:** 2 sprays (110 mcg) into each nostril once a day (i.e., for a total dose of 220 mcg/day). The dose may be increased to 440 mcg/day

given either once daily or q.i.d. (1 spray/nostril).
TRIAMCINOLONE DIACETATE
• **IM Only**
40 mg/week.
• **Intra-articular, Intrasynovial**
5–40 mg.
• **Intralesional, Sublesional**
5–48 mg (no more than 12.5 mg/injection site and 25 mg/lesion).
TRIAMCINOLONE HEXACETONIDE
**Not for IV use.**
• **Intra-articular**
2–6 mg for small joints and 10–20 mg for large joints.
• **Intralesional/Sublesional**
Up to 0.5 mg/sq. in. of affected area.

## DENTAL CONCERNS

See also *Dental Concerns* for *Corticosteroids*.
**General**
1. Monitor vital signs at every appointment because of cardiovascular and respiratory side effects.
2. The patient may require a semisupine position for the dental chair to help with breathing.
3. Dental procedures may cause the patient anxiety, which could result in an asthma attack. Make sure that the patient has his or her sympathomimetic inhaler present or have the inhaler from the office emergency kit present.
4. Morning and shorter appointments, as well as methods for addressing anxiety levels in the patient, can help reduce the amount of stress the patient is experiencing.
5. Sulfites present in vasoconstrictors can precipitate an asthma attack.
**Client/Family Teaching**
1. Daily home fluoride treatments for persistent dry mouth.
2. Avoid alcohol-containing mouth rinses and beverages.
3. Avoid caffeine-containing beverages.
4. Dry mouth can be treated with tart, sugarless gum or candy, water, sugar-free beverages, or with saliva substitutes if dry mouth persists.
5. Review use, care, and storage of in-

haler. Rinse out mouth and wash the mouth piece, spacer, sprayer and dry after each use.

6. Review technique for use and care of prescribed inhalers and respiratory equipment. Rinsing of equipment and of mouth after use is imperative in preventing oral fungal infections.

# Triamterene
(try-**AM**-ter-een)
**Pregnancy Category:** B
Dyrenium **(Rx)**
**Classification:** Diuretic, potassium-sparing

See also *Diuretics.*

**Action/Kinetics:** A mild diuretic that acts on the collecting tubule and collecting ducts to inhibit the reabsorption of sodium, chloride, and increases potassium retention. It promotes the excretion of sodium—which is exchanged for potassium or hydrogen ions—bicarbonate, chloride, and fluid. It increases urinary pH and is a weak folic acid antagonist. **Onset:** 2–4 hr. **Peak effect:** 6–8 hr. **Duration:** 7–9 hr. **t½:** 3 hr. From one-half to two-thirds of the drug is bound to plasma protein. Metabolized to hydroxytriamterene sulfate, which is also active. About 20% is excreted unchanged through the urine.

**Uses:** Edema due to CHF, hepatic cirrhosis, nephrotic syndrome, steroid therapy, secondary hyperaldosteronism, and idiopathic edema. May be used alone or with other diuretics. *Non-FDA Approved Uses:* Prophylaxis and treatment of hypokalemia, adjunct in the treatment of hypertension.

**Contraindications:** Hypersensitivity to drug, severe or progressive renal insufficiency, severe hepatic disease, anuria, hyperkalemia, hyperuricemia, gout, history of nephrolithiasis. Lactation.

**Special Concerns:** Safety and efficacy have not been determined in children.

**Side Effects:** *Electrolyte:* Hyperkalemia, electrolyte imbalance. *Oral:* Dry mouth. *GI:* Nausea, vomiting (may also be indicative of electrolyte imbalance), diarrhea. *CNS:* Dizziness, drowsiness, fatigue, weakness, headache. *Hematologic:* Megaloblastic anemia, thrombocytopenia. *Renal:* Azotemia, interstitial nephritis. *Miscellaneous:* **Anaphylaxis,** photosensitivity, hypokalemia, jaundice, muscle cramps, rash.

**Drug Interactions**
*Indomethacin and other NSAIDs* / ↑ Risk of nephrotoxicity and acute renal failure
*Indomethacin and other NSAIDs* / ↓ Antihypertensive effects

**How Supplied:** *Capsule:* 50 mg, 100 mg

**Dosage**
• **Capsules.**
 *Diuretic.*
**Adults, initial:** 100 mg b.i.d. after meals; **maximum daily dose:** 300 mg.

## DENTAL CONCERNS

See also *Dental Concerns* for *Diuretics.*

**General**
1. Patients on chronic drug therapy may develop blood dyscrasias. Symptoms include fever, sore throat, bleeding, and poor wound healing.

**Consultation with Primary Care Provider**
1. Patients with symptoms of blood dyscrasias should be referred to their primary care provider for complete blood counts. Treatment should be postponed until the results are known.

————*COMBINATION DRUG*————
# Triamterene and Hydrochlorothiazide Capsules
(try-**AM**-ter-een, hy-droh-**klor**-oh-**THIGH**-ah-zyd)
**Pregnancy Category:** C
Dyazide **(Rx)**

# Triamterene and Hydrochlorothiazide Tablets

(try-**AM**-teh-reen, hy-droh-**kloh**-roh-**THIGH**-ah-zyd)
**Pregnancy Category:** C
Apo-Triazide ✤, Dyazide, Maxide, Maxide-25 MG, Novo-Triamzide ✤, Nu-Triazide ✤, Pro-Triazide ✤ **(Rx)**
**Classification:** Diuretic, antihypertensive

---

See also *Hydrochlorothiazide* and *Triamterene*.
**Content: Capsules.** *Diuretic:* Hydrochlorothiazide, 25 or 50 mg. *Diuretic:* Triamterene, 50 or 100 mg.
**Tablets.** *Diuretic:* Hydrochlorothiazide, 25 or 50 mg. *Diuretic:* Triamterene, 37.5 or 75 mg. (In Canada the tablets contain 25 mg of hydrochlorothiazide and 50 mg triamterene.)
**Uses:** To treat hypertension or edema in clients who manifest hypokalemia on hydrochlorothiazide alone. In clients requiring a diuretic and in whom hypokalemia cannot be risked (i.e., clients with cardiac arrhythmias or those taking digitalis). Usually not the first line of therapy, except for clients in whom hypokalemia should be avoided.
**Contraindications:** Clients receiving other potassium-sparing drugs such as amiloride and spironolactone. Use in anuria, acute or chronic renal insufficiency, significant renal impairment, preexisting elevated serum potassium.
**Special Concerns:** Use with caution during lactation. Geriatric clients may be more sensitive to the hypotensive and electrolyte effects of this combination; also, age-related decreases in renal function may require a decrease in dosage.
**Side Effects:** See also *Hydrochlorothiazide* and *Triamterene*.
**Drug Interactions:** See also *Hydrochlorothiazide* and *Triamterene*.
**How Supplied:** See Content

## Dosage

- **Capsules**
  *Hypertension or edema.*
**Adults:** Triamterene/hydrochlorothiazide: 37.5 mg/25 mg—1–2 capsules given once daily with monitoring of serum potassium and clinical effect. Triamterene/hydrochlorothiazide: 50 mg/25 mg—1–2 capsules b.i.d. after meals. Some clients may be controlled using 1 capsule every day or every other day. No more than 4 capsules should be taken daily.
- **Tablets**
  *Hypertension or edema.*
**Adults:** Triamterene/hydrochlorothiazide: 37.5 mg/25 mg—1–2 tablets/day (determined by individual titration with the components). Or, triamterene/hydrochlorothiazide: 75 mg/50 mg—1 tablet daily.

---

## DENTAL CONCERNS

See also *Dental Concerns* for *Antihypertensive Agents, Triamterene,* and *Hydrochlorothiazide*.
**General**
1. Patients on chronic drug therapy may develop blood dyscrasias. Symptoms include fever, sore throat, bleeding, and poor wound healing.
**Consultation with Primary Care Provider**
1. Patients with symptoms of blood dyscrasias should be referred to their primary care provider for complete blood counts. Treatment should be postponed until the results are known.

---

# Trihexyphenidyl hydrochloride

(try-hex-ee-**FEN**-ih-dill)
**Pregnancy Category:** C
Aparkane ✤, Apo-Trihex ✤, Artane, Artane Sequels, Novo-Hexidyl ✤, PMS-Trihexyphenidyl ✤, Trihexy-2 and -5, Trihexyphen ✤ **(Rx)**
**Classification:** Antiparkinson agent, anticholinergic

---

See also *Cholinergic Blocking Agents* and *Antiparkinson Drugs*.
**Action/Kinetics:** Synthetic anticholinergic, which relieves rigidity but has little effect on tremors. Causes a direct antispasmodic effect on smooth muscle. High incidence of side effects. Small doses cause CNS

depression, whereas larger doses may result in CNS excitation. **Onset, PO:** 60 min. **Duration, PO:** 6–12 hr. **Uses:** Adjunct in the treatment of all types of parkinsonism (often used as adjunct with levodopa). Drug-induced extrapyramidal symptoms. Sustained-release medication is for maintenance dosage only. **Additional Contraindications:** Arteriosclerosis and hypersensitivity to drug. **Additional Side Effects:** Serious CNS stimulation (restlessness, insomnia, delirium, agitation) and psychotic manifestations. **Additional Drug Interactions:** ↑ Effectiveness of levodopa if used together; such combined use not recommended in clients with psychoses. **How Supplied:** *Elixir:* 2 mg/5 mL; *Tablet:* 2 mg, 5 mg

**Dosage** ————————————
• **Elixir, Tablets**
  *Parkinsonism.*
**Initial (day 1):** 1–2 mg; **then,** increase by 2 mg q 3–5 days until daily dose is 6–10 mg given in divided doses. Some clients may require 12–15 mg/day (especially those with postencephalitic parkinsonism).
  *Adjunct with levodopa.*
**Adults:** 3–6 mg/day in divided doses.
  *Drug-induced extrapyramidal reactions.*
**Initial:** 1 mg/day; **then,** increase as needed to total daily dose of 5–15 mg.

## DENTAL CONCERNS

See also *Dental Concerns* for *Cholinergic Blocking Agents* and *Antiparkinson Drugs.*

## Trimipramine maleate
(try-**MIP**-rah-meen)
**Pregnancy Category:** C
Apo-Trimip ✦, Novo-Tripramine ✦, Nu-Trimipramine ✦, Rhotrimine ✦, Surmontil **(Rx)**
**Classification:** Antidepressant, tricyclic

See also *Antidepressants, Tricyclic.*
**Action/Kinetics:** Causes moderate anticholinergic and orthostatic hypotensive effects and significant sedative effects. **Effective plasma levels:** 180 ng/mL. **Time to reach steady state:** 2–6 days. **t½:** 7–30 hr. **Uses:** Treatment of symptoms of depression. PUD. Seems more effective in endogenous depression than in other types of depression. **Contraindications:** Use in children less than 12 years of age. **How Supplied:** *Capsule:* 25 mg, 50 mg, 100 mg

**Dosage** ————————————
• **Capsules**
  *Antidepressant.*
**Adults, outpatients, initial:** 75 mg/day in divided doses up to 150 mg/day. Daily dosage should not exceed 200 mg; **maintenance:** 50–150 mg/day. Total dose can be given at bedtime. **Adults, hospitalized, initial:** 100 mg/day in divided doses up to 200 mg/day. If no improvement in 2–3 weeks, increase to 250–300 mg/day. **Adolescent/geriatric clients, initial:** 50 mg/day up to 100 mg/day. Not recommended for children.

## DENTAL CONCERNS

See also *Dental Concerns* for *Antidepressants, Tricyclic.*

## Troglitazone
(troh-**GLIH**-tah-zohn)
**Pregnancy Category:** B
Rezulin **(Rx)**
**Classification:** Oral hypoglycemic

See also *Antidiabetic Agents: Hypoglycemic Agents.*
**Action/Kinetics:** Decreases hepatic glucose output and increases insulin-dependent glucose disposal in skeletal muscle and perhaps liver and adipose tissue. Troglitazone is not an insulin secretagogue. Rapidly absorbed; **maximum plasma levels:** 2–3 hr. Steady-state plasma levels are reached in 3–5 days. Food increases the rate of absorption. **t½, elimina-**

**tion:** 16–34 hr. Metabolized in the liver and excreted mainly in the feces. **Uses:** Alone or in combination with a sulfonylurea for treatment of type II diabetes with poor glucose control despite insulin therapy. *Non-FDA Approved Uses:* Use in the productive and metabolic consequences of polycystic ovary syndrome.

**Contraindications:** Lactation. Use for type I diabetes or for the treatment of diabetic ketoacidosis.

**Special Concerns:** Use with caution in those with liver disease. Ovulation may resume in premenopausal anovulatory clients, leading to an increased risk of pregnancy. Safety and efficacy have not been determined in children.

**Side Effects:** *GI:* Nausea, diarrhea. *CNS:* Headache, dizziness. *Metabolic:* Hypoglycemia. *Hematologic:* Decreased hemoglobin, hematocrit, and white blood cell counts. *Nose/throat:* Rhinitis, pharyngitis. *Miscellaneous:* Infection, pain, accidental injury, asthenia, back pain, UTI, peripheral edema.

**Drug Interactions**
*Terfenadine* / ↓ Plasma levels of terfenadine → ↓ effect

**How Supplied:** *Tablets:* 200 mg, 400 mg

**Dosage** —————
• **Tablets**
*With insulin in type II diabetes mellitus.*
**Adults:** 200 mg daily while continuing the insulin dosage. If the response is inadequate, the dose may be increased after 2–4 weeks. **Usual daily dose:** 400 mg/day. **Maximum daily dose:** 600 mg/day. The insulin dose should be decreased by 10%–25% when fasting plasma glucose levels decrease to less than 120 mg/dL in clients receiving both insulin and troglitazone.
*Polycystic ovary syndrome.*
**Adults:** 400 mg/day.

## DENTAL CONCERNS

See also *Dental Concerns* for *Antidiabetic Agents, Hypoglycemic Agents.*

1. Place dental chair in semisupine position to help eliminate or minimize GI adverse effects of the drug.

————*COMBINATION DRUG*————
# Tylenol with Codeine Elixir or Tablets
(**TIE**-leh-noll, **KOH**-deen)
**Pregnancy Category:** C
(Tablets are C-III and Elixir is C-V) **(Rx)**
**Classification:** Analgesic
———————————————

See also *Acetaminophen* and *Opioid Analgesics.*

**Content:** *Nonopioid analgesic:* Acetaminophen, 300 mg in each tablet, and 120 mg/5 mL elixir. *Opioid analgesic:* Codeine phosphate, 15 mg (No. 2 Tablets), 30 mg (No. 3 Tablets), 60 mg (No. 4 Tablets), and 12 mg/5 mL (Elixir).

**Uses: Tablets:** Mild to moderately severe pain. **Elixir:** Mild to moderate pain.

**Special Concerns:** Use with caution during lactation. Safety has not been determined in children less than 3 years of age. May be habit-forming due to the codeine component.

**How Supplied:** See Content

**Dosage** —————
• **Tablets, Capsules**
*Analgesia.*
**Adults, individualized, usual:** 1–2 No. 2 or No. 3 Tablets or No. 3 Capsules q 2–4 hr as needed for pain. Or, 1 No. 4 Tablet or Capsule q 4 hr as required. Maximum 24-hr dose is 360 mg codeine phosphate and 4,000 mg acetaminophen. **Pediatric:** Dosage equivalent to 0.5 mg/kg codeine.
• **Elixir**
*Analgesia.*
**Adults, individualized, usual:** 15 mL q 4 hr as needed; **pediatric, 7–12 years:** 10 mL t.i.d.–q.i.d.; **3–6 years:** 5 mL t.i.d.–q.i.d.

## DENTAL CONCERNS

See also *Dental Concerns* for *Opioid Analgesics.*

# Valproic acid

(val-**PROH**-ick)
**Pregnancy Category:** D
Alti-Valproic ✦, Depakene, Gen-Valproic ✦, Novo-Valproic ✦ **(Rx)**
**Classification:** Anticonvulsant, miscellaneous

See also *Anticonvulsants.*

**Action/Kinetics:** The following information also applies to divalproex sodium (Depakote, Epival ✦). The precise anticonvulsant action is unknown, but activity is believed to be caused by increased brain levels of the neurotransmitter GABA. Absorption from the GI tract is more rapid following administration of the syrup (sodium salt) than capsules, with peak levels following administration of the syrup in 15 min–2 hr. Equivalent PO doses of divalproex sodium and valproic acid deliver equivalent amounts of valproate ion to the system. **Peak serum levels, capsules and syrup:** 1–4 hr (delayed if the drug is taken with food); **peak serum levels, enteric-coated tablet (divalproex sodium):** 3–4 hr. **t½:** 9–16 hr, with the lower time usually seen in clients taking other anticonvulsant drugs (e.g., primidone, phenytoin, phenobarbital, carbamazepine). Half-lives in children less than 10 days range 10–67 hr, compared to 7–13 hr in children over 2 months of age. The half-life may be up to 18 hr in those with cirrhosis or acute hepatitis. **Therapeutic serum levels:** 50–100 mcg/mL. Approximately 90% bound to plasma protein. Metabolized in the liver and inactive metabolites are excreted in the urine; small amounts of valproic acid are excreted in the feces.

**Uses:** Alone or in combination with other anticonvulsants for treatment of simple and complex absence seizures (petit mal). As an adjunct in multiple seizure patterns that include absence seizures. Alone or as adjunct to treat complex partial seizures that occur either in isolation or in association with other types of seizures. Divalproex sodium delayed release used for the acute treatment of manic episodes in bipolar disorder and for prophylaxis of migraine headaches. *Non-FDA Approved Uses:* Alone or in combination to treat atypical absence, myoclonic, and grand mal seizures; also, atonic, complex partial, elementary partial, and infantile spasm seizures. Prophylaxis of febrile seizures in children, to treat anxiety disorders/panic attacks, and subchronically to treat minor incontinence after ileoanal anastomosis. Management of anxiety disorders or panic attacks.

**Contraindications:** Liver disease or dysfunction.

**Special Concerns:** Use with caution during lactation. Use with caution in children 2 years of age or less as they are at greater risk for developing fatal hepatotoxicity. Geriatric clients should receive a lower daily dose because they may have increased free, unbound valproic acid levels in the serum. Safety and efficacy of divalproex sodium have not been determined for treating acute mania in children less than 18 years of age or for treating migraine in children less than 16 years of age.

**Side Effects:** *Oral:* Prolonged bleeding, delayed wound healing, gingival enlargement. *GI:* (most frequent): N&V, indigestion. Also, abdominal cramps, abdominal pain, dyspepsia, diarrhea, constipation, anorexia with weight loss or increased appetite with weight gain. *CNS:* Sedation, psychosis, depression, emotional upset, aggression, hyperactivity, deterioration of behavior, tremor, headache, dizziness, somnolence, dysarthria, incoordination, coma (rare). *Ophthalmologic:* Nystagmus, diplopia, "spots before eyes." *Hematologic:* Thrombocytopenia, leukopenia, eosinophilia, anemia, bone marrow suppression, relative lymphocytosis, hypofibrinogenemia, myelodysplastic-type syndrome. *Dermatologic:* Transient alopecia, petechiae, erythema multiforme, skin rashes. photosensitivity, pruritus, *Stevens-Johnson syndrome.* *Hepatic:* Hepatotoxicity. Also, minor increases in AST, ALT, LDH, serum bilirubin, and serum alkaline phosphatase values. *Endocrine:* Menstrual irregularities, secondary amenorrhea, breast enlargement, galactorrhea, swelling of parotid gland, abnormal thyroid function tests. *Miscellaneous:* Also asterixis, weakness, asthenia, bruising, hematoma formation, frank hemorrhage, acute pancreatitis, hyperammonemia, hyperglycinemia, hypocarnitinemia, edema of arms and legs, weakness, inappropriate ADH secretion, Fanconi's syndrome (rare and seen mostly in children), lupus erythematosus, fever, enuresis, hearing loss.

**Drug Interactions**

*Alcohol* / ↑ Incidence of CNS depression

*Carbamazepine* / Variable changes in levels of carbamazepine with possible loss of seizure control

*Chlorpromazine* / ↓ Clearance and ↑ t½ of valproic acid → ↑ pharmacologic effects

*Cimetidine* / ↓ Clearance and ↑ t½ of valproic acid → ↑ pharmacologic effects

*Clonazepam* / ↑ Chance of absence seizures (petit mal) and ↑ toxicity due to clonazepam

*CNS depressants* / ↑ Incidence of CNS depression

*Diazepam* / ↑ Effect of diazepam due to ↓ plasma binding and ↓ metabolism

*Erythromycin* / ↑ Serum valproic acid levels → valproic acid toxicity

*Phenobarbital* / ↑ Effect of phenobarbital due to ↓ breakdown by liver

*Phenytoin* / ↑ Effect of phenytoin due to ↓ breakdown by liver or ↓

effect of valproic acid due to ↑ metabolism

*Salicylates (aspirin)* / ↑ Effect of valproic acid due to ↓ plasma protein binding and ↓ metabolism

**How Supplied:** *Capsule:* 250 mg; *Syrup:* 250 mg/5 mL

**Dosage** ――――――――――

• **Capsules, Syrup, Enteric-Coated Capsules and Tablets (Divalproex)**

*Complex partial seizures.*

**Adults and children 10 years and older:** 10–15 mg/kg/day. Increase by 5–10 mg/kg/week until seizures are controlled or side effects occur, up to a maximum of 60 mg/kg/day. If the total daily dose exceeds 250 mg, the dosage should be divided. Dosage of concomitant anticonvulsant drugs can usually be reduced by about 25% every 2 weeks. Divalproex sodium may be added to the regimen at a dose of 10–15 mg/kg/day; the dose may be increased by 5–10 mg/kg/week to achieve the optimal response (usually less than 60 mg/kg/day).

*Simple and complex absence seizures.*

**Initial:** 15 mg/kg/day, increasing at 1-week intervals by 5–10 mg/kg/day until seizures are controlled or side effects occur.

*Acute manic episodes in bipolar disorder (use divalproex).*

**Initial:** 250 mg t.i.d.; **then,** increase dose q 2–3 days until a trough serum level of 50 mcg/mL is reached. The maximum dose is 60 mg/kg/day.

*Prophylaxis of migraine (divalproex sodium).*

250 mg/day b.i.d., although some may require up to 1,000 mg daily.

• **Rectal**

*Intractable status epilepticus that has not responded to other treatment.*

**Adults:** 200–1,200 mg q 6 hr rectally with phenytoin and phenobarbital. **Children:** 15–20 mg/kg.

## DENTAL CONCERNS

See also *Dental Concerns* for *Anticonvulsants.*

**General**

1. This drug may prolong bleeding time. Evaluate the patient for clotting time during gingival instrumentation.

**Client/Family Teaching**

1. Any unexplained fever, sore throat, skin rash, yellow skin discoloration, or unusual bruising or bleeding should be reported immediately.

# Valsartan

(val-**SAR**-tan)
**Pregnancy Category:** C (1st trimester), D (2nd and 3rd trimesters)
Diovan **(Rx)**
**Classification:** Antihypertensive, angiotensin II receptor blocker

See also *Antihypertensive Drugs.*

**Action/Kinetics:** Angiotensin II receptor blocker specific for $AT_1$ receptors, which are responsible for cardiovascular effects of angiotensin II. Drug blocks vasoconstrictor and aldosterone-secreting effects of angiotensin II. **Peak plasma levels:** 2–4 hr. Highly bound to plasma proteins. Eliminated mostly unchanged in feces (83%) and urine (13%).

**Uses:** Treat hypertension alone or in combination with other antihypertensive drugs.

**Contraindications:** Lactation. Hypersensitivity to the drug or any of its components.

**Special Concerns:** Use with caution in impaired hepatic and renal function. Safety and efficacy have not been determined in children. Should not be used during pregnancy.

**Side Effects:** *CNS:* Headache, dizziness, fatigue, anxiety, insomnia, paresthesia, somnolence. *Oral:* Dry mouth. *GI:* Abdominal pain, diarrhea, nausea, constipation, dyspepsia, flatulence. *Respiratory:* URI, cough, rhinitis, sinusitis, pharyngitis, dyspnea. *Body as a whole:* Viral infection, edema, asthenia, allergic reaction. *Musculoskeletal:* Arthralgia, back pain, muscle cramps, myalgia. *Der-*

*matologic:* Pruritus, rash. *Miscellaneous:* Palpitations, vertigo, neutropenia, impotence.

**Drug Interactions:** No specific interactions have been reported with drugs that are used in dentistry. However, lowest effective dose of local anesthetics, vasoconstrictors, or anticholinergics should be used if required.

**How Supplied:** *Capsules:* 80 mg, 160 mg

**Dosage**

• **Capsules**
*Hypertension.*
**Adults, initial:** 80 mg once daily as monotherapy. **Dose range:** 80–320 mg once daily. If additional antihypertensive effect is needed, dose may be increased to 160 mg or 320 mg once daily or diuretic may be added.

## DENTAL CONCERNS

See also *Dental Concerns* for *Antihypertensive Drugs.*

# Venlafaxine hydrochloride

(ven-lah-**FAX**-een)
**Pregnancy Category:** C
Effexor, Effexor XR **(Rx)**
**Classification:** Antidepressant, miscellaneous

**Action/Kinetics:** Not related chemically to any of the currently available antidepressants. A potent inhibitor of the uptake of neuronal serotonin and norepinephrine in the CNS and a weak inhibitor of the uptake of dopamine. Has no anticholinergic, sedative, or orthostatic hypotensive effects. The major metabolite—O-desmethylvenlafaxine    (ODV)—is active. The drug and metabolite are eliminated through the kidneys. **t½, venlafaxine:** 5 hr; **t½, ODV:** 11 hr. **Time to reach steady state:** 3–4 days. The half-life of the drug and metabolite are increased in clients with impaired liver or renal function. Food has no effect on the absorption of venlafaxine.

**Uses:** Treatment of depression.

**V**

---

**Contraindications:** Use with an MAO inhibitor or within 14 days of discontinuation of an MAO inhibitor. Use of alcohol.

**Special Concerns:** Use with caution with impaired hepatic or renal function, during lactation, in clients with a history of mania, and in those with diseases or conditions that could affect the hemodynamic responses or metabolism. Although it is possible for a geriatric client to be more sensitive, dosage adjustment is not necessary. Use for more than 4–6 weeks has not been evaluated.

**Side Effects:** Side effects with an incidence of 0.1% or greater are listed.

*CNS:* Anxiety, nervousness, insomnia, mania, hypomania, **seizures, suicide attempts,** dizziness, somnolence, tremors, abnormal dreams, hypertonia, paresthesia, decreased libido, agitation, confusion, abnormal thinking, depersonalization, depression, twitching, migraine, emotional lability, trismus, vertigo, apathy, ataxia, circumoral paresthesia, CNS stimulation, euphoria, hallucinations, hostility, hyperesthesia, hyperkinesia, hypertonia, hypotonia, incoordination, increased libido, myoclonus, neuralgia, neuropathy, paranoid reaction, psychosis, psychotic depression, sleep disturbance, abnormal speech, stupor, torticollis. *CV:* Sustained increase in BP (hypertension), vasodilation, tachycardia, postural hypotension, angina pectoris, extrasystoles, hypotension, peripheral vascular disorder, syncope, thrombophlebitis, peripheral edema. *Oral:* Dry mouth, glossitis, cheilitis, gingivitis, candidiasis, edema of the tongue. *GI:* Anorexia, N&V, constipation, diarrhea, dyspepsia, flatulence, dysphagia, eructation, colitis, esophagitis, gastroenteritis, gastritis, hemorrhoids, **rectal hemorrhage,** melena, stomach ulcer. *Body as a whole:* Headache, asthenia, infection, chills, chest pain, trauma, yawn, weight loss, accidental injury, malaise, neck pain, enlarged abdomen, allergic reaction, cyst, facial edema, generalized edema, hangover effect, hernia, intentional injury,

neck rigidity, moniliasis, substernal chest pain, pelvic pain, photosensitivity reaction. *Respiratory:* Bronchitis, dyspnea, asthma, chest congestion, epistaxis, hyperventilation, laryngismus, laryngitis, pneumonia, voice alteration. *Dermatologic:* Acne, alopecia, brittle nails, contact dermatitis, dry skin, herpes simplex, herpes zoster, maculopapular rash, urticaria. *Hematologic:* Ecchymosis, anemia, leukocytosis, leukopenia, lymphadenopathy, lymphocytosis, thrombocytopenia, thrombocythemia, abnormal WBCs. *Endocrine:* Hypothyroidism, hyperthyroidism, goiter. *Musculoskeletal:* Arthritis, arthrosis, bone pain, bone spurs, bursitis, joint disorder, myasthenia, tenosynovitis. *Ophthalmic:* Blurred vision, mydriasis, abnormal accommodation, abnormal vision, cataract, conjunctivitis, corneal lesion, diplopia, dry eyes, exophthalmos, eye pain, photophobia, subconjunctival hemorrhage, visual field defect. *GU:* Urinary retention, abnormal ejaculation, impotence, urinary frequency, impaired urination, disturbed orgasm, menstrual disorder, anorgasmia, dysuria, hematuria, metrorrhagia, vaginitis, amenorrhea, kidney calculus, cystitis, leukorrhea, menorrhagia, nocturia, bladder pain, breast pain, kidney pain, polyuria, prostatitis, pyelonephritis, pyuria, urinary incontinence, urinary urgency, enlarged uterine fibroids, **uterine hemorrhage, vaginal hemorrhage,** vaginal moniliasis. *Miscellaneous:* Sweating, tinnitus, taste perversion, thirst, diabetes mellitus, alcohol intolerance, gout, hypoglycemic reaction, hemochromatosis, ear pain, otitis media.

**Drug Interactions**
*Cimetidine* / ↓ First-pass metabolism of venlafaxine
*MAO inhibitors* / Serious and possibly fatal reaction, including hyperthermia, rigidity, myoclonus, autonomic instability with rapid changes in VS, extreme agitation, coma

**How Supplied:** *Tablet:* 25 mg, 37.5 mg, 50 mg, 75 mg, 100 mg

## Dosage
- **Tablets**

*Depression.*

**Adults, initial:** 75 mg/day given in two or three divided doses. Depending on the response, the dose can be increased to 150–225 mg/day in divided doses. Dosage increments should be made up to 75 mg/day at intervals of 4 or more days. Severely depressed clients may require 375 mg/day in divided doses. **Maintenance:** Sufficient studies have not been undertaken to determine how long a client should continue to take venlafaxine.

- **Tablets, Extended-Release**

*Depression.*

**Adults, initial:** 75 mg once daily. Dose can be increased by up to 75 mg no more often than every 4 days, to a maximum of 225 mg/day.

## DENTAL CONCERNS

See also *Dental Concerns* for *Antidepressants, Tricyclic.*

# Verapamil

(ver-**AP**-ah-mil)
**Pregnancy Category:** C
Alti-Verapamil I ICI ✽, Apo-Verap ✽, Calan, Calan SR, Covera HS, Gen-Verapamil SR ✽, Isoptin, Isoptin I.V. ✽, Isoptin SR, Novo-Veramil ✽, Novo-Veramil SR ✽, Nu-Verap ✽, Taro-Verapamil ✽, Verelan **(Rx)**
**Classification:** Calcium channel blocking agent

See also *Calcium Channel Blocking Agents.*

**Action/Kinetics:** Slows AV conduction and prolongs effective refractory period. IV doses may slightly increase LV filling pressure. Moderately decreases myocardial contractility and peripheral vascular resistance. Worsening of heart failure may result if verapamil is given to clients with moderate to severe cardiac dysfunction. **Onset: PO,** 30 min; **IV,** 3–5 min. **Time to peak plasma levels (PO):** 1–2 hr (5–7 hr for extended-release). **t½, PO:** 4.5–12 hr with repet-

itive dosing; **IV, initial:** 4 min; **final:** 2–5 hr. **Therapeutic serum levels:** 0.08–0.3 mcg/mL. **Duration, PO:** 8–10 hr (24 hr for extended-release); **IV:** 10–20 min for hemodynamic effect and 2 hr for antiarrhythmic effect. Verapamil is metabolized to norverapamil, which possesses 20% of the activity of verapamil.

*NOTE:* Covera HS is designed to deliver verapamil in concert with the 24-hr circadian variations in BP.

**Uses: PO:** Angina pectoris due to coronary artery spasm (Prinzmetal's variant), chronic stable angina including angina due to increased effort, unstable angina (preinfarction, crescendo). With digitalis to control rapid ventricular rate at rest and during stress in chronic atrial flutter or atrial fibrillation. Prophylaxis of repetitive paroxysmal supraventricular tachycardia. Essential hypertension. Sustained-release tablets are used to treat essential hypertension (Step I therapy). **IV:** Supraventricular tachyarrhythmias. Atrial flutter or fibrillation *Non-FDA Approved Uses:* PO for prophylaxis of migraine, manic depression (alternate therapy), exercise-induced asthma, recumbent nocturnal leg cramps, hypertrophic cardiomyopathy, cluster headaches.

**Contraindications:** Severe hypotension, second- or third-degree AV block, cardiogenic shock, severe CHF, sick sinus syndrome (unless client has artificial pacemaker), severe LV dysfunction. Cardiogenic shock and severe CHF unless secondary to SVT that can be treated with verapamil. Lactation. Use of verapamil, IV, with beta-adrenergic blocking agents (as both depress myocardial contractility and AV conduction). Ventricular tachycardia.

**Special Concerns:** Infants less than 6 months of age may not respond to verapamil. Use with caution in hypertrophic cardiomyopathy, impaired hepatic and renal function, and in the elderly.

**Side Effects:** *CV:* CHF, bradycardia, *AV block, asystole,* premature ventric-

**V**

---

ular contractions and tachycardia (after IV use), peripheral and pulmonary edema, hypotension, syncope, palpitations, AV dissociation, *MI, CVA. Oral:* Dry mouth, gingival hyperplasia. *GI:* Nausea, constipation, abdominal discomfort or cramps, dyspepsia, diarrhea. *CNS:* Dizziness, headache, sleep disturbances, depression, amnesia, paranoia, psychoses, hallucinations, jitteriness, confusion, drowsiness, vertigo. IV verapamil may increase intracranial pressure in clients with supratentorial tumors at the time of induction of anesthesia. *Dermatologic:* Rash, dermatitis, alopecia, urticaria, pruritus, erythema multiforme, *Stevens-Johnson syndrome. Respiratory:* Nasal or chest congestion, dyspnea, SOB, wheezing. *Musculoskeletal:* Paresthesia, asthenia, muscle cramps or inflammation, decreased neuromuscular transmission in Duchenne's muscular dystrophy. *Other:* Blurred vision, equilibrium disturbances, sexual difficulties, spotty menstruation, sweating, rotary nystagmus, flushing, polyuria, nocturia, gynecomastia, claudication, hyperkeratosis, purpura, petechiae, bruising, hematomas, tachyphylaxis.

**Drug Interactions**
*Anesthetics /* ↑ Effect of verapamil
*Barbiturates /* ↓ Effect of verapamil
*Carbamazepine /* ↑ Effect of verapamil due to ↓ breakdown by liver
*Fentanyl /* Possible severe hypotension or ↑ fluid volume
*Indomethacin /* ↓ Effect of verapamil
*Muscle relaxants, nondepolarizing /* ↑ Neuromuscular blockade due to effect of verapamil on calcium channels
*NSAIDs /* ↓ Possible effect of verapamil
*Phenobarbital /* ↓ Effect of verapamil
*Other drugs with hypotensive effects /* ↑ Effect of verapamil

**How Supplied:** *Capsule, extended release:* 120 mg, 180 mg, 240 mg, 360 mg; *Injection:* 2.5 mg/mL; *Tablet:* 40 mg, 80 mg, 120 mg; *Tablet, extended release:* 120 mg, 180 mg, 240 mg

**Dosage** ⎯⎯⎯⎯⎯⎯⎯⎯⎯⎯
• **Tablets**
*Angina at rest and chronic stable angina.*
**Individualized.  Adults,  initial:** 80–120 mg t.i.d. (40 mg t.i.d. if client is sensitive to verapamil); **then,** increase dose to total of 240–480 mg/day. Covera HS is given once daily at bedtime in doses of either 180 or 240 mg.
*Arrhythmias.*
Dosage range in digitalized clients with chronic atrial fibrillation: 240–320 mg/day in divided doses t.i.d.–q.i.d. For prophylaxis of nondigitalized clients: 240–480 mg/day in divided doses t.i.d.–q.i.d. Maximum effects are seen within 48 hr.
*Essential hypertension.*
**Initial, when used alone:** 80 mg t.i.d. Doses up to 360 mg daily may be used. Effects are seen in the first week of therapy. In the elderly or in people of small stature, initial dose should be 40 mg t.i.d.
• **Extended-Release    Capsules and Tablets**
*Essential hypertension.*
**Initial:** 240 mg/day in the a.m. (120 mg/day in the elderly or people of small stature). If response is inadequate, increase dose to 240 mg in the a.m. and 120 mg in the evening and then 240 mg q 12 hr. Covera HS is given once daily at bedtime in doses of either 180 or 240 mg.
• **IV, Slow**
*Supraventricular tachyarrhythmias.*
**Adults, initial:** 5–10 mg (0.075–0.15 mg/kg) given over 2 min (over 3 min in older clients); **then,** 10 mg (0.15 mg/kg) 30 min later if response is not adequate. **Infants, up to 1 year:** 0.1–0.2 mg/kg (0.75–2 mg) given as an IV bolus over 2 min; **1–15 years:** 0.1–0.3 mg/kg (2–5 mg, not to exceed 5 mg total dose) over 2 min. If response to initial dose is inadequate, it may be repeated after 30 min, but not more than a total of 10 mg should be given to clients from 1 to 15 years of age.

**V**

## DENTAL CONCERNS

See also *Dental Concerns* for *Calcium Channel Blocking Agents.*
**General**
1. Frequent visits to assess for gingival hyperplasia.
2. Vasoconstrictors should be used with caution, in low doses, and with careful aspiration. Epinephrine-impregnated gingival retraction cords should be avoided.
3. Patients on chronic drug therapy may develop blood dyscrasias. Symptoms include fever, sore throat, bleeding, and poor wound healing.

**Consultation with Primary Care Provider**
1. Patients with symptoms of blood dyscrasias should be referred to their primary care provider for complete blood counts. Treatment should be postponed until the results are known.

**Client/Family Teaching**
1. Practice frequent careful oral hygiene to minimize the incidence and severity of drug-induced gingival hyperplasia.
2. Need for frequent visits with a dental health professional if hyperplasia occurs.

# Z

# Zafirlukast
(zah-**FIR**-loo-kast)
**Pregnancy Category:** B
Accolate **(Rx)**
**Classification:** Antiasthmatic

**Action/Kinetics:** A selective and competitive antagonist of leukotriene receptors $D_4$ and $E_4$, inhibits bronchospasm and airway edema. Rapidly absorbed after PO use; bioavailabilty may be decreased when taken with food. **Peak plasma levels:** 3 hr. **t½, terminal:** About 10 hr. Over 99% bound to plasma proteins. Extensively metabolized in the liver, with about 90% excreted in the feces and 10% in the urine. Inhibits certain cytochrome P450 isoenzymes.

**Uses:** Prophylaxis and chronic treatment of asthma in adults and children 12 years of age and older.

**Contraindications:** Use to terminate an acute asthma attack, including status asthmaticus. Lactation.

**Special Concerns:** The clearance is reduced in clients 65 years of age and older. Safety and efficacy have not been determined in children less than 12 years of age.

**Side Effects:** *GI:* N&V, diarrhea, abdominal pain, dyspepsia. *CNS:* Headache, dizziness. *Miscellaneous:* Infection, generalized pain, asthenia, accidental injury, myalgia, fever, back pain.

**Drug Interactions**
*Aspirin* / ↑ Plasma levels of zafirlukast
*Erythromycin* / ↓ Plasma levels of zafirlukast
*Terfenadine* / ↓ Plasma levels of zafirlukast
*Theophylline* / ↓ Plasma levels of zafirlukast
*Warfarin* / Significant ↑ PT
**How Supplied:** *Tablet:* 20 mg

**Dosage**
• **Tablets**
*Asthma.*
**Adults and children aged 12 and older:** 20 mg b.i.d.

## DENTAL CONCERNS

See also *Dental Concerns* for *Theophylline Derivatives.*
**Client/Family Teaching**
1. Remember to provide your dental health professional with updated information regarding your breathing status and medications.

# Zalcitabine
# (Dideoxycytidine, ddC)
(zal-**SIGH**-tah-been)
**Pregnancy Category:** C
Hivid **(Rx)**
**Classification:** Antiviral

See also *Antiviral Drugs* and *Anti-Infectives.*

**Action/Kinetics:** Converted in cells to the active metabolite by cellular enzymes and inhibits replication of the HIV virus in vitro. Food reduces the rate of absorption. Does not appear to undergo significant metabolism by the liver. **Elimination t½:** 1–3 hr. Approximately 70% of a PO dose is excreted through the kidneys and 10% in the feces. Prolonged elimination (t½ up to 8.5 hr) is observed in clients with impaired renal function.

**Uses:** In combination with AZT in advanced HIV infections (CD$_4$ cell count of 300/mm$^3$ or less and who have shown significant clinical or immunologic deterioration). Alone for HIV-infected adults with advanced disease who are intolerant to AZT or where the disease has progressed while taking AZT.

**Contraindications:** Hypersensitivity to zalcitabine or any components of the product. Use in clients with moderate or severe peripheral neuropathy or with drugs that have the potential to cause peripheral neuropathy (see *Drug Interactions*). Concomitant use with didanosine. Lactation.

**Special Concerns:** Use with extreme caution in clients with low CD$_4$ cell counts (< 50/mm$^3$). Use with caution in clients with a history of pancreatitis or known risk factors for the development of pancreatitis. Clients with a creatinine clearance less than 55 mL/min may be at a greater risk for toxicity due to decreased clearance. Clients may continue to develop opportunistic infections and other complications of HIV infection. Safety and efficacy have not been determined in HIV-infected children less than 13 years of age.

**Side Effects:** The incidence of certain side effects is dependent on the duration of use and the dose of the drug. *Neurologic:* Peripheral neuropathy (may be severe) characterized by numbness and burning dysesthesia involving the distal extremities; this may be followed by sharp shooting pains or severe continuous burning pain if the drug is not withdrawn. The neuropathy may progress to severe pain requiring narcotic analgesics and may be irreversible. *Oral:* oral ulcers, ulcerative stomatitis, aphthous stomatitis, dry mouth, glossitis, gum disorders, tongue ulceration, salivary gland enlargement, painful swallowing, mouth lesion, dental abscess, gagging with pills, gingivitis, increased salivation, painful sore gums, sore tongue, tongue disorder, toothache. *GI:* **Fatal pancreatitis** when given alone or with AZT. Esophageal ulcers, nausea, dysphagia, anorexia, abdominal pain, vomiting, constipation, diarrhea, dyspepsia, **rectal hemorrhage,** hemorrhoids, enlarged abdomen, flatulence, anorexia, dysphagia, eructation, gastritis, **GI hemorrhage,** left quadrant pain, esophageal pain, esophagitis, rectal ulcers, melena, acute pharyngitis, abdominal bloating or cramps, anal/rectal pain, colitis, epigastric pain, heartburn, **hemorrhagic pancreatitis,** odynophagia, rectal mass, sore throat, unformed/loose stools. *Dermatologic:* Rash (including erythematous, maculopapular, follicular), pruritus, night sweats, dermatitis, skin lesions, acne, alopecia, bullous eruptions, increased sweating, urticaria, hot flashes, lip blister or lesions, carbuncle/furuncle, cellulitis, dry skin, dry rash desquamation, exfoliative dermatitis, finger inflammation, impetigo, infection, itchy rash, moniliasis, mucocutaneous/skin disorder, nail disorder, photosensitivity, skin fissure, skin ulcer. *CNS:* Headache, dizziness, seizures, ataxia, abnormal coordination, Bell's palsy, dysphonia, hyperkinesia, hypokinesia, migraine, neuralgia, neuritis, stupor, aphasia, decreased neurologic function, disequilibrium, facial nerve palsy, focal motor seizures, memory loss, paralysis, speech disorder, *status epilepticus,* tremor, vertigo, hypertonia, hand tremor, twitching, confusion, impaired concentration, insomnia, agitation, depersonalization, hallucinations, emotional lability, nervousness, anxiety, depression, euphoria, manic reaction, dementia, amnesia, somnolence, abnormal thinking, crying, loss of memory, decreased concentration, acute psychotic disorder, acute stress reaction, decreased motivation, decreased sexual desire, mood swings, paranoid states, *suicide attempt. Respiratory:* Coughing, dyspnea, respiratory distress, rales/rhonchi, nasal discharge, flulike symptoms, cyanosis, acute nasopharyngitis, chest congestion, dry nasal mucosa, hemoptysis, sinus congestion, sinus pain, sinusitis, wheezing. *Musculoskeletal:* Myalgia, arthralgia, arthritis, arthropathy, cold extremities, leg cramps, myositis, joint pain or inflammation, weakness in leg muscle, generalized muscle weakness, back pain, backache, bone aches and pains, bursitis, pain in extremities, joint swelling, muscle disorder, muscle stiffness, muscle cramps, arthrosis, myopathy, neck pain, rib pain, stiff neck. *Hepatic:* Exacerbation of hepatic dysfunction, especially in those with preexisting liver disease or with a history of alcohol abuse. Abnormal hepatic function, hepatitis, jaundice, hepatocellular damage, hepatomegaly with steatosis, cholecystitis. *CV: **Cardiomyopathy,*** CHF, abnormal cardiac movement arrhythmia, atrial fibrillation, *cardiac failure,* cardiac dysrhythmias, heart racing, hypertension, palpitations, ***subarachnoid hemorrhage,*** syncope, tachycardia, ventricular ectopy, epistaxis. *Hematologic:* Anemia, leukopenia, thrombocytopenia, alteration of absolute neutrophil count, granulocytosis, eosinophilia, neutropenia, hemoglobinemia, neutrophilia, platelet alteration, purpura, throm-

bus, unspecified hematologic toxicity, alteration of WBCs. *Hypersensitivity:* Urticaria, ***anaphylaxis*** (rare). *Endocrine:* Diabetes mellitus, gout, hot flushes, hypoglycemia, hyperglycemia, hypocalcemia, hypophosphatemia, hypernatremia, hyponatremia, hypomagnesemia, hyperkalemia, hypokalemia, hyperlipidemia, polydipsia. *GU:* Dysuria, toxic nephropathy, polyuria, renal calculi, ***acute renal failure,*** hyperuricemia, increased frequency of micturition, abnormal renal function, renal cyst, albuminuria, bladder pain, genital lesion/ulcer, nocturia, painful/sore penis, penile edema, testicular swelling, urinary retention, vaginal itch/ulcer/pain, vaginal/cervix disorder. *Ophthalmologic:* Abnormal vision, burning or itching eyes, xerophthalmia, eye pain or abnormality, blurred or decreased vision, eye inflammation/irritation, eye redness/hemorrhage, increased tears, mucopurulent conjunctivitis, photophobia, dry eyes, unequal sized pupils, yellow sclera. *Otic:* Ear pain/blockage, fluid in ears, hearing loss, tinnitus. *Body as a whole:* Fatigue, fever, rigors, chest pain or tightness, weight decrease, pain, malaise, asthenia, generalized edema, general debilitation, chills, difficulty moving, facial pain or swelling, flank pain, flushing, pelvic/groin pain. *Miscellaneous:* Lymphadenopathy, taste perversion, decreased taste, parosmia, lactic acidosis.

**Drug Interactions**
*Antacids (Mg/Al-containing)* / ↓ Absorption of zalcitabine
*Cimetidine* / ↓ Elimination of zalcitabine by ↓ renal tubular secretion
*Dapsone* / ↑ Peripheral neuropathy
*Metronidazole* / ↑ Peripheral neuropathy
*Pentamidine* / ↑ Risk of fulminant pancreatitis
*Probenecid* / ↓ Elimination of zalcitabine by ↓ renal tubular secretion
**How Supplied:** *Tablet:* 0.375 mg, 0.75 mg

---

## Dosage
### • Tablets
*In combination with AZT in advanced HIV infection.*

**Adults:** 0.75 mg given at the same time with 200 mg AZT q 8 hr for a total daily dose of 2.25 mg zalcitabine and 600 mg AZT.
*Alone in advanced HIV infection.* 0.75 mg q 8 hr (2.25 mg/day).

## DENTAL CONCERNS

See also *Dental Concerns* for *Antiviral Drugs.*

### General
1. Examine patient for oral signs and symptoms of long-term therapy.
2. Decreased saliva flow can put the patient at risk for dental caries, periodontal disease, and candidiasis.
3. Frequent recall in order to evaluate healing of infection.
4. Prophylactic antibiotics may be necessary if surgery or deep scaling is necessary.
5. Patients may be more susceptible to infection and poor wound healing.
6. Medication may be necessary to treat oral adverse effects.
7. Check vital signs at each appointment because of cardiovascular adverse effects.

### Consultation with Primary Care Provider
1. Medical consultation may be necessary in order to assess patient's ability to tolerate stress.
2. Medical consultation may be necessary in order to assess patient's level of disease control.

### Client/Family Teaching
1. Review the importance of good oral hygiene in order to prevent soft tissue inflammation.
2. Review the proper use of oral hygiene aids in order to prevent injury.
3. Daily home fluoride treatments for persistent dry mouth.
4. Avoid alcohol-containing mouth rinses and beverages.
5. Avoid caffeine-containing beverages.
6. Dry mouth can be treated with tart, sugarless gum or candy, water, sugar-free beverages, or with saliva substitutes if dry mouth persists.

7. Report oral sores, lesions, or bleeding to the dentist.
8. Update patient's dental record (medication/health history) as needed.

# Zidovudine (Azidothymidine, AZT)
(zye-**DOH**-vyou-deen, ah-**zee**-doh-**THIGH**-mih-deen)
**Pregnancy Category:** C
Apo-Zidovudine ✸, Novo-AZT ✸, Retrovir **(Rx)**
**Classification:** Antiviral

See also *Antiviral Drugs* and *Anti-Infectives.*

**Action/Kinetics:** Inhibits the replication of viral DNA. Rapidly absorbed from the·GI tract and is distributed to both plasma and CSF. **Peak serum levels:** 0.1–1.5 hr. t½: approximately 1 hr. Metabolized rapidly by the liver and excreted through the urine.

**Uses: PO:** Initial treatment of HIV-infected adults who have a $CD_4$ cell count of 500/$mm^3$ or less. Has been found superior to either didanosine or zalcitabine monotherapy for initial treatment of HIV-infected clients who have not had previous antiretroviral therapy. To prevent HIV transmission from pregnant women to their fetuses. For HIV-infected children over 3 months of age who have HIV-related symptoms or are asymptomatic with abnormal laboratory values indicating significant immunosuppression. In combination with zalcitabine in selected clients with advanced HIV disease ($CD_4$ cell count of 300 cells/$mm^3$ or less).

**IV:** Selected adults with symptomatic HIV infections who have a history of confirmed *Pneumocystis carinii* pneumonia or an absolute $CD_4$ ($T_4$ helper/inducer) lymphocyte count of less than 200 cells/$mm^3$ in the peripheral blood prior to therapy.

**Contraindications:** Allergy to AZT or its components. Lactation.

**Special Concerns:** Use with caution in clients who have a hemoglobin level of less than 9.5 g/dL or a granulocyte count less than 1,000/$mm^3$.

AZT is not a cure for HIV; thus, clients may continue to acquire opportunistic infections and other illnesses associated with ARC or HIV. AZT has not been shown to reduce the risk of HIV transmission to others through sexual contact or blood contamination.

**Side Effects: Adults.** *Hematologic:* Anemia (severe), granulocytopenia. *Body as a whole:* Headache, asthenia, fever, diaphoresis, malaise, body odor, chills, edema of the lip, flu-like syndrome, hyperalgesia, abdominal/chest/back pain, lymphadenopathy. *Oral:* Edema of the tongue, bleeding gums, mouth ulcers, taste changes, delayed healing, opportunistic infections. *GI:* Nausea, GI pain, diarrhea, anorexia, vomiting, dyspepsia, constipation, dysphagia, eructation, flatulence, *rectal hemorrhage. CNS:* Somnolence, dizziness, paresthesia, insomnia, anxiety, confusion, emotional lability, depression, nervousness, vertigo, loss of mental acuity. *CV:* Vasodilation, syncope, vasculitis (rare). *Musculoskeletal:* Myalgia, myopathy, myositis, arthralgia, tremor, twitch, muscle spasm. *Respiratory:* Dyspnea, cough, epistaxis, rhinitis, pharyngitis, sinusitis, hoarseness. *Dermatologic:* Rash, pruritus, urticaria, acne, pigmentation changes of the skin and nails. *GU:* Dysuria, polyuria, urinary hesitancy or frequency. *Other:* Amblyopia, hearing loss, photophobia, ***severe hepatomegaly with steatosis,*** lactic acidosis, change in taste perception, hepatitis, pancreatitis, hypersensitivity reactions, including ***anaphylaxis,*** hyperbilirubinemia (rare), ***seizures.***

**Children.** The following side effects have been observed in children, although any of the side effects reported for adults can also occur in children. *Body as a whole:* Granulocytopenia, anemia, fever, headache, phlebitis, bacteremia. *GI:* N&V, abdominal pain, diarrhea, weight loss. *CNS:* Decreased reflexes, nervousness, irritability, insomnia,

***seizures. CV:*** Abnormalities in ECG, left ventricular dilation, CHF, generalized edema, ***cardiomyopathy,*** S$_3$ gallop. *GU:* Hematuria, viral cystitis

**Drug Interactions**
*Acetaminophen* / ↑ Risk of granulocytopenia
*Clarithromycin* / ↓ Peak serum levels of clarithromcyin
*Fluconazole* / ↑ Levels of AZT
*Indomethacin* / ↑ Risk of granulocytopenia
*Phenytoin* / Levels of phenytoin may ↑ , ↓ , or remain unchanged; also, ↓ excretion of AZT
*Probenecid* / ↓ Biotransformation or renal excretion of AZT → flu-like symptoms, including myalgia, malaise or fever, and maculopapular rash
*Trimethoprim* / ↑ Serum levels of AZT

**How Supplied:** *Capsule:* 100 mg; *Injection:* 10 mg/mL; *Syrup:* 50 mg/5 mL; *Tablet:* 300 mg

**Dosage** ─────────────
• **Capsules, Syrup**
*Symptomatic HIV infections.*
**Adults:** 100 mg (one 100-mg capsule or 10 mL syrup) q 4 hr around the clock (i.e., total of 600 mg daily).
*Asymptomatic HIV infections.*
**Adults:** 100 mg q 4 hr while awake (500 mg/day); **Pediatric, 3 months–12 years, initial:** 180 mg/m$^2$ q 6 hr (720 mg/m$^2$/day, not to exceed 200 mg q 6 hr).
*Prevent transmission of HIV from mothers to their fetuses (after week 14 of pregnancy).*
**Maternal dosing:** 100 mg 5 times a day until the start of labor. During labor and delivery, AZT IV at 2 mg/kg over 1 hr followed by continuous IV infusion of 1 mg/kg/hr until clamping of the umbilical cord. **Infant dosing:** 2 mg/kg PO q 6 hr beginning within 12 hr after birth and continuing through 6 weeks of age. Infants unable to take the drug PO may be given AZT IV at 1.5 mg/kg, infused over 30 min q 6 hr.
*In combination with zalcitabine.*

Zidovudine, 200 mg, with zalcitabine, 0.75 mg, q 8 hr.
• **IV**
1–2 mg/kg infused over 1 hr. The IV dose is given q 4 hr around the clock only until PO therapy can be instituted. Dosage adjustment may be necessary due to hematologic toxicity.

## DENTAL CONCERNS

See also *Dental Concerns* for *Antiviral Agents.*
**General**
1. Examine patient for signs and symptoms of oral opportunistic infections
2. Patients on chronic drug therapy may develop blood dyscrasias. Symptoms include fever, sore throat, and bleeding, and poor wound healing.
3. Avoid direct dental light in the patient's eyes. Keep dark glasses available for patient comfort.
4. Patients may require frequent recall because of oral adverse effects.
**Consultation with Primary Care Provider**
1. Patients with symptoms of blood dyscrasias should be referred to their primary care provider for complete blood counts. Treatment should be postponed until the results are known.
2. Medical consultation may be necessary in order to assess disease control.
**Client/Family Teaching**
1. Review the importance of good oral hygiene in order to prevent soft tissue inflammation.
2. Review the proper use of oral hygiene aids in order to prevent injury.
3. Report oral sores, lesions, or bleeding to the dentist.
4. Update patient's dental record (medication/health history) as needed.

## Zileuton

(zye-**LOO**-ton)
**Pregnancy Category:** C
Zyflo **(Rx)**
**Classification:** Antiasthmatic, leukotriene receptor inhibitor

**Action/Kinetics:** As a specific inhibitor of 5-lipoxygenase, zileuton inhibits the formation of leukotrienes. By inhibiting leukotriene formation, zileuton reduces bronchoconstriction due to cold air challenge in asthmatics. Rapidly absorbed from the GI tract; **peak plasma levels:** 1.7 hr. Metabolized in liver and mainly excreted through the urine. t½: 2.5 hr.
**Uses:** Prophylaxis and chronic treatment of asthma in adults and children over 12 years of age.
**Contraindications:** Active liver disease or transaminase elevations greater than or equal to three times the upper limit of normal. Hypersenstivity to zileuton. Treatment of bronchoconstriction in acute asthma attacks, including status asthmaticus. Lactation.
**Special Concerns:** Use with caution in clients who ingest large quantities of alcohol or who have a past history of liver disease. Safety and efficacy have not been determined in children less than 12 years of age.
**Side Effects:** *Oral:* Dry mouth, taste alterations. *GI:* Dyspepsia, nausea, constipation, flatulence, vomiting. *CNS:* Headache, dizziness, insomnia, malaise, nervousness, somnolence. *Body as a whole:* Unspecified pain, abdominal pain, chest pain, asthenia, accidental injury, fever. *Musculoskeletal:* Myalgia, arthralgia, neck pain/rigidity. *GU:* Urinary tract infection, vaginitis. *Miscellaneous:* Conjunctivitis, hypertonia, lymphadenopathy, pruritus.
**Drug Interactions**
*Propranolol* / ↑ Effect of propranolol
*Terfenadine* / ↑ Effect of terfenadine due to ↓ clearance
*Theophylline* / Doubling of serum theophylline levels → ↑ effect
*Warfarin* / ↑ Prothrombin time
**How Supplied:** *Tablets:* 600 mg.

## Dosage
• **Tablets**
*Symptomatic treatment of asthma.*
**Adults and children over 12 years of age:** 600 mg q.i.d.

## DENTAL CONCERNS

See also *Dental Concerns* for *Theophylline Derivatives*.

**Client/Family Teaching**

1. Remember to provide your dental health professional with updated information regarding your breathing status and medications.

---

# Zolmitriptan
(zohl-mih-**TRIP**-tin)
**Pregnancy Category:** C
Zomig **(Rx)**
**Classification:** Antimigraine drug

**Action/Kinetics:** Binds to serotonin 5-$HT_{1B/1D}$ receptors on intracranial blood vessels and in sensory nerves of trigeminal system. This results in cranial vessel constriction and inhibition of pro-inflammatory neuropeptide release. Well absorbed after PO use. **Peak plasma levels:** 2 hr. **t½, elimination:** 3 hr (for zolmitriptan and active metabolite). Excreted in feces and urine.

**Uses:** Treatment of acute migraine in adults with or without aura. Use only when there is clear diagnosis of migraine.

**Contraindications:** Prophylaxis of migraine or management of hemiplegic or basilar migraine. Use in angina pectoris, history of MI, documented or silent ischemia, ischemic heart disease, coronary artery vasospasm (including Prinzmetal's variant angina), other significant underlying CV disease. Also use in uncontrolled hypertension, within 24 hr of treatment with another serotonin $HT_1$ agonist or an ergotamine-containing or ergot-type drug (e.g., dihydroergotamine, methysergide). Concurrent use with MAO A inhibitor or within 2 weeks of discontinuing MAO A inhibitor.

**Special Concerns:** Use with caution in liver disease. Safety and efficacy have not been determined for cluster headache.

**Side Effects:** *Oral:* Dry mouth, tongue edema. *GI:* Dyspepsia, dysphagia, nausea, increased appetite, esophagitis, gastroenteritis, abnormal liver function, thirst. *CV:* Palpitations, arrhythmias, hypertension, syncope. *Atypical sensations:* Hypesthesia, paresthesia, warm/cold sensation. *CNS:* Dizziness, somnolence, vertigo, agitation, anxiety, depression, emotional lability, insomnia. *Pain pressure sensations:* Chest pain, tightness, pressure and/or heaviness. Pain, tightness, or heaviness in the neck, throat, or jaw. Heaviness, pressure, tightness other than in the chest or neck. *Musculoskeletal:* Myalgia, myasthenia, back pain, leg cramps, tenosynovitis. *Respiratory:* Bronchitis, **bronchospasm,** epistaxis, hiccup, laryngitis, yawn. *Dermatologic:* Sweating, pruritus, rash, urticaria, ecchymosis, photosensitivity. *GU:* Hematuria, cystitis, polyuria, urinary frequency or urgency. *Body as a whole:* Asthenia, allergic reaction, chills, facial edema, edema, fever, malaise. *Miscellaneous:* Dry eye, eye pain, hyperacusis, ear pain, parosmia, tinnitus.

**Drug Interactions**

*Cimetidine* / Half life of zolmitriptan is doubled

**How Supplied:** *Tablets:* 2.5 mg, 5 mg

**Dosage** ————
• **Tablets**

  *Migraine headaches.*

**Adults, initial:** 2.5 mg or lower. Dose of 5 mg may be required. If headache returns, repeat dose after 2 hr, not to exceed 10 mg in 24-hr period.

---

## DENTAL CONCERNS

**General**

1. This drug is for acute migraine headaches. Patients are usually not in the office if they are having a migraine headache.

2. Inform patient if dental drugs are photosensitive.

**Consultation with Primary Care Provider**

1. Consultation with appropriate health care provider may be necessary in order to evaluate level of disease

---

control and the patient's ability to tolerate stress.

**Client/Family Teaching**

1. Avoid alcohol-containing mouth rinses and beverages.

2. Avoid caffeine-containing beverages.

3. Dry mouth can be treated with tart, sugarless gum or candy, water, sugar-free beverages, or with saliva substitutes if dry mouth persists.

---

# Zolpidem tartrate

(**ZOL**-pih-dem)

**Pregnancy Category:** B

Ambien **(Rx) (C-IV)**

**Classification:** Nonbarbiturate, non-benzodiazepine sedative-hypnotic

**Action/Kinetics:** May act by subunit modulation of the GABA receptor. Specifically, it binds the omega-1 receptor preferentially. No evidence of residual next-day effects or rebound insomnia at usual doses; little evidence for memory impairment. Sleep time spent in stage 3 to 4 (deep sleep) was comparable to placebo with only inconsistent, minor changes in REM sleep at recommended doses. Rapidly absorbed from the GI tract. **t½:** About 2.5 hr (increased in geriatric clients and those with impaired hepatic function). Bound significantly (92.5%) to plasma proteins. Food decreases the bioavailability of zolpidem. Metabolized in the liver; inactive metabolites are excreted primarily through the urine.

**Uses:** Short-term treatment of insomnia.

**Contraindications:** Lactation.

**Special Concerns:** Use with caution and at reduced dosage in clients with impaired hepatic function, in compromised respiratory function, in those with impaired renal function, and in clients with S&S of depression. Impaired motor or cognitive performance after repeated use or unusual sensitivity to hypnotic drugs may be noted in geriatric or debilitated clients. Closely observe individuals with a history of dependence on

or abuse of drugs or alcohol. Safety and efficacy have not been determined in children less than 18 years of age.

**Side Effects:** *Symptoms of withdrawal:* Although there is no clear evidence of a withdrawal syndrome, the following symptoms were noted with zolpidem following placebo substitution: fatigue, nausea, flushing, lightheadedness, uncontrolled crying, emesis, stomach cramps, panic attack, nervousness, abdominal discomfort.

The most common side effects following use for up to 10 nights included drowsiness, dizziness, and diarrhea. The side effects listed in the following are for an incidence of 1% or greater. *CNS:* Headache, drowsiness, dizziness, lethargy, drugged feeling, lightheadedness, depression, abnormal dreams, amnesia, anxiety, nervousness, sleep disorder, ataxia, confusion, euphoria, insomnia, vertigo. *Oral:* Dry mouth, taste alteration. *GI:* Nausea, diarrhea, dyspepsia, abdominal pain, constipation, anorexia, vomiting. *Musculoskeletal:* Myalgia, arthralgia. *Respiratory:* Upper respiratory infection, sinusitis, pharyngitis, rhinitis. *Body as a whole:* Allergy, back pain, flu-like symptoms, chest pain, fatigue. *Ophthalmologic:* Diplopia, abnormal vision. *Miscellaneous:* Rash, UTI, palpitations, infection.

**Drug Interactions:** Additive CNS depressant effects are possible when combined with alcohol and other drugs with CNS depressant effects.

**How Supplied:** *Tablet:* 5 mg, 10 mg

---

**Dosage**

• **Tablets**

*Hypnotic.*

**Adults, individualized, usual:** 10 mg just before bedtime. An initial dose of 5 mg is recommended in clients with hepatic insufficiency.

---

## DENTAL CONCERNS

See also *Dental Concerns* for *Sedative-Hypnotics, (Anti-anxiety)/Antimanic Drugs, and Hypnotics.*

**Z**

# APPENDIX 1
# Controlled Substances in the United States and Canada

### Controlled Substances Act—United States

The U.S. Federal Controlled Substances Act of 1970 placed drugs controlled by the Act into five categories or schedules based on their potential to cause psychologic and/or physical dependence as well as on their potential for abuse. The schedules are defined as follows:

**Schedule (C-I):** Includes substances for which there is a high abuse potential and no current approved medical use (e.g., heroin, marijuana, LSD, other hallucinogens, certain opiates and opium derivatives).

**Schedule (C-II):** Includes drugs that have a high abuse potential and a high ability to produce physical and/or psychologic dependence and for which there is a current approved or acceptable medical use.

**Schedule (C-III):** Includes drugs for which there is less potential for abuse than drugs in Schedule II and for which there is a current approved medical use. Certain drugs in this category are preparations containing limited quantities of codeine. Also, anabolic steroids are classified in Schedule III.

**Schedule (C-IV):** Includes drugs for which there is a relatively low abuse potential and for which there is a current approved medical use.

**Schedule (C-V):** Drugs in this category consist mainly of preparations containing limited amounts of certain narcotic drugs for use as antitussives and antidiarrheals. Federal law provides that limited quantities of these drugs (e.g., codeine) may be bought without a prescription by an individual at least 18 years of age. The product must be purchased from a pharmacist who must keep appropriate records. However, state laws vary, and in many states such products require a prescription.

### Controlled Substances—Canada

In Canada, narcotics are governed by the Narcotics Control regulations and are designated by the letter N. Drugs that are

441

considered subject to abuse, have an approved medical use, and are not narcotics are designated by the letter C.

Generally prescriptions for Schedule II (high-abuse-potential) drugs cannot be transmitted over the phone and they cannot be refilled. Prescriptions for Schedule III, IV, and V drugs may be refilled up to five times within 6 months. Schedule II drugs are not necessarily "stronger" than drugs in Schedules III, IV, or V; Schedule II drugs are classified as such due to their high abuse potential.

| | Drug Schedule | |
| Drug | United States | Canada |
| --- | --- | --- |
| Alfentanil | II | N |
| Alprazolam | IV | * |
| Amobarbital | II | C |
| Amphetamine | II | Not available |
| Aprobarbital | III | * |
| Benzphetamine | III | Not available |
| Buprenorphine | V | * |
| Butabarbital | III | C |
| Butorphanol | * | C |
| Chloral hydrate | IV | * |
| Chlordiazepoxide | IV | * |
| Clonazepam | IV | * |
| Clorazepate | IV | * |
| Codeine | II | N |
| Dextroamphetamine | II | C |
| Diazepam | IV | * |
| Diethylpropion | IV | C |
| Estazolam | IV | * |
| Ethchlorvynol | IV | * |
| Fenfluramine | IV | * |
| Fentanyl | II | N |
| Fluoxymesterone | III | * |
| Flurazepam | IV | * |
| Glutethimide | III | * |
| Halazepam | IV | Not available |
| Hydrocodone | Not available | N |
| Hydromorphone | II | N |
| Levomethadyl acetate HCl | II | Not available |
| Levorphanol | II | N |
| Lorazepam | IV | * |
| Mazindol | IV | * |
| Meperidine | II | N |
| Mephobarbital | IV | C |
| Meprobamate | IV | * |
| Methadone | II | N |
| Methamphetamine | II | Not available |
| Metharbital | III | C |
| Methylphenidate | II | C |
| Methyltestosterone | III | * |
| Methyprylon | III | * |
| Midazolam | IV | * |
| Morphine | II | N |
| Nalbuphine | * | C |

| Drug | Drug Schedule United States | Canada |
|------|------|--------|
| Nandrolone decanote | III | * |
| Nandrolone phenpropionate | III | * |
| Opium | II | N |
| Oxandrolone | III | * |
| Oxazepam | IV | * |
| Oxycodone | II | N |
| Oxymetholone | III | * |
| Oxymorphone | II | N |
| Paraldehyde | IV | * |
| Paregoric | III | N |
| Pemoline | IV | * |
| Pentazocine | IV | N |
| Pentobarbital | | |
|    PO, parenteral | II | C |
|    Rectal | III | C |
| Phendimetrazine | III | Not available |
| Phenmetrazine | II | Not available |
| Phenobarbital | IV | C |
| Phentermine | IV | C |
| Prazepam | IV | Not available |
| Propoxyphene | IV | N |
| Quazepam | IV | Not available |
| Secobarbital | | |
|    PO | II | C |
|    Parenteral | II | * |
|    Rectal | III | * |
| Stanozolol | III | * |
| Sulfentanil | II | N |
| Talbutal | III | * |
| Temazepam | IV | * |
| Testosterone cypionate in oil | III | * |
| Testosterone enanthante in oil | III | * |
| Testosterone in aqueous suspension | III | * |
| Testosterone propionate in oil | III | * |
| Testosterone transdermal system | III | * |
| Triazolam | IV | * |
| Zolpidem tartrate | IV | * |

*Not controlled

# APPENDIX 2
# Elements of a Prescription

In order to safely communicate the exact elements desired on a prescription, the following items should be addressed:

**A.** The prescriber: Name, address, and phone number and associated practice/speciality

**B.** The client: Name, age, address and social security number

**C.** The prescription itself: Name of the medication (generic or trade); quantity to be dispensed (e.g., tablets or capsules, 1 vial, 1 tube, volume of liquid); the strength of the medication (e.g., 125-mg tablets, 250 mg/5 mL, 80 mg/1 mL, 10%); and directions for use (e.g., 1 tablet po t.i.d.; 2 gtt to each eye q.i.d.; 1 teaspoonful po q 8 hr for 10 days; apply a thin film to lesions b.i.d. for 14 days)

**D.** Other elements: Date prescription is written, signature of the provider, number of refills; provider number: state license number and Drug Enforcement Agency (DEA) number (when applicable); and brand-product-only indication (when applicable)

A typical prescription is depicted as follows:

---

**A.**          **Julia Bryan, DDS**
                **Dental Care Associates**
                **1611 Kirkwood Highway**
                **Wilmington, DE 19805**
                **555-645-8261**

                                    **Date: July 10, 2000**

**B.  For: Kathryn Woods, Age 8**
        **27 East Parkway**
        **Lewes, DE 19958**
        **123-555-1234**

**C.    Rx        Amoxicillin 500 mg**
                **Disp. 30**
                **Sig: Take 1 cap 3x/day**

**D.  Refills: 0**
☐ **Dispense as Written**                **Provider signature**
☐ **Substitution Allowed**        **Provider/State license number**

---

*Interpretation of prescription:* The above prescription is written by Dentist Julia Bryan for Kathryn Woods and is for amoxicillin suspension. The concentration desired is 500 mg. The directions for taking the medication are 1 cap by mouth every 8 hr for 10 days. The prescriber wants 30 capsules dispensed and there are no refills allowed.

# APPENDIX 3
# Pregnancy Categories: FDA Assigned

The U.S. Food and Drug Administration's use-in-pregnancy rating system weighs the degree to which available information has ruled out risk to the fetus against the drug's potential benefit to the patient. The ratings, and their interpretation, are as follows:

| Category | Interpetation |
|---|---|
| A | **CONTROLLED STUDIES SHOW NO RISK.** Adequate, well-controlled studies in pregnant women have failed to demonstrate a risk to the fetus in any trimester of pregnancy. |
| B | **NO EVIDENCE OF RISK IN HUMANS.** Adequate, well-controlled studies in pregnant women have not shown increased risk of fetal abnormalities despite adverse findings in animals, or, in the absence of adequate human studies, animal studies show no fetal risk. The chance of fetal harm is remote, but remains a possibility. |
| C | **RISK CANNOT BE RULED OUT.** Adequate, well-controlled human studies are lacking, and animal studies have shown a risk to the fetus or are lacking as well. There is a chance of fetal harm if the drug is administered during pregnancy; but the potential benefits may outweigh the potential risk. |
| D | **POSITIVE EVIDENCE OF RISK.** Studies in humans, or investigational or post-marketing data, have demonstrated fetal risk. Nevertheless, potential benefits from the use of the drug may outweigh the potential risk. For example, the drug may be acceptable if needed in a life-threatening situation or serious disease for which safer drugs cannot be used or are ineffective. |
| X | **CONTRAINDICATED IN PREGNANCY.** Studies in animals or humans, or investigational or post-marketing reports, have demonstrated positive evidence of fetal abnormalities or risk which clearly outweighs any possible benefit to the patient. |

# APPENDIX 4
# Drugs Causing Dry Mouth by Class

| Drug Class | Generic Name | Trade Name |
|---|---|---|
| Anorexiants | Diethylpropion | Tennuate, Tepanil |
| | Mazindol | Mazanor, Sanorex |
| | Phendimetrazine | Anorex |
| | Phentermine | Adipex-P, Fastin |
| Antiacne | Isotretinoin | Accutane |
| Antianxiety | Alprazolam | Xanax |
| | Chlordiazepoxide | Librium |
| | Diazepam | Valium |
| | Halazepam | Paxipam |
| | Hydroxyzine | Atarax, Vistaril |
| | Lorazepam | Ativan |
| | Meprobamate | Equanil, Miltown |
| | Oxazepam | Serax |
| | Prazepam | Centrax |
| Anticholinergic/ Antispasmodic | Atropine | Atropisol |
| | Belladonna alkaloids | Bellergal |
| | Dicyclomine | Bentyl |
| | Hyoscyamine | Anaspraz |
| | Methantheline | Banthine |
| | Oxybutynin | Ditropan |
| | Propantheline | Pro-Banthine |
| | Scopolamine | Transderm-Scōp |
| Anticonvulsants | Carbamazepine | Tegretol |
| | Felbamate | Felbatol |
| | Gabapentin | Neurontin |
| | Lamotrigine | Lamictal |
| Antidepressants | Amitriptyline | Elavil |
| | Amoxapine | Ascendin |
| | Buproprion | Wellbutrin |
| | Clomipramine | Anafranil |
| | Desipramine | Norpramin |

| Drug Class | Generic Name | Trade Name |
|---|---|---|
| | Doxepin | Sinequan |
| | Fluoxetine | Prozac |
| | Fluvoxamine | Luvox |
| Antidiarrheal | Diphenoxylate, atropine | Lomotil |
| | Loperamide | Imodium AD |
| Antihistamines | Astemizole | Hismanal |
| | Brompheniramine | Dimetane |
| | Brompheniramine/ phenylpropanolamine | Dimetapp |
| | Chlorpheniramine | Chlor-Trimeton |
| | Diphenhydramine | Benadryl |
| | Loratidine | Claritin |
| | Promethazine | Phenergan |
| | Tripelennamine | Pyrbenzamine (PBZ) |
| | Terfenadine | Seldane |
| | Tripolidine/ pseudoephedrine | Actifed |
| Antihypertensives | Captopril | Capoten |
| | Carvedilol | Coreg |
| | Clonidine | Catapress |
| | Guanabenz | Wytensin |
| | Guanethidine | Ismelin |
| | Prazosin | Minipress |
| | Reserpine | Serpasil |
| Antinauseants | Cyclizine | Marezine |
| | Diphenhydramine | Dramamine |
| | Meclizine | Antivert |
| Antiparkinson Drugs | Benztropine mesylate | Cogentin |
| | Biperiden | Akineton |
| | Carbidopa/levodopa | Sinemet |
| | Ethopropazine | Parsidol |
| | Levodopa | Larodopa |
| | Orphenadrine HCl | Marflex |
| | Trihexyphenidyl | Artane |
| Antipsychotics | Amitriptyline/ perphenazine | Triavil |
| | Chlorpromazine | Thorazine |
| | Clozapine | Clozaril |
| | Fluphenazine | Prolixin |
| | Haloperidol | Haldol |
| | Lithium | Eskalith |

| Drug Class | Generic Name | Trade Name |
|---|---|---|
| | Pimozide | Orap |
| | Prochlorperazine | Compazine |
| | Thioridazine | Mellaril |
| | Thiothixene | Navane |
| | Trifluoperazine | Stelazine |
| Decongestants | Phenylpropanolamine/ chlorpheniramine | Ornade |
| | Pseudoephedrine | Sudafed |
| Diuretics | Amiloride | Midamor |
| | Chlorothiazide | Diuril |
| | Furosemide | Lasix |
| | Hydrochlorothiazide | HydroDIURIL, Esidrix |
| | Triamterene/ hydrochlorothiazide | Dyazide |
| Muscle Relaxants | Baclofen | Lioresal |
| | Cyclobenzaprine | Flexeril |
| | Orphenadrine | Norflex |
| NSAIDs | Diflunisal | Dolobid |
| | Fenoprofen | Nalfon |
| | Ibuprofen | Motrin |
| | Naproxen | Naprosyn |
| | Piroxicam | Feldene |
| Opioid Analgesics | Meperidine | Demerol |
| | Morphine | MS-Contin |
| Sedative-Hypnotics | Flurazepam | Dalmane |
| | Temazepam | Restoril |
| | Triazolam | Halcion |
| Sympathomimetics | Albuterol | Proventil, Ventolin |
| | Isoproterenol | Isuprel |

# APPENDIX 5
# Classes of Drugs Altering Sense of Taste

Anesthetics, Local
Anesthetics, General
Anorexiants
Antacids
Anticholinergics
Anticonvulsants
Antidepressants
Antidiabetics
Antidiarrheals
Antiemetics
Antigout
Antihistamines ($H_1$ and $H_2$)
Antihyperlipidemics
Anti-Infectives
Anti-Inflammatory (arthritis)
Antiparkinson
Antipsychotics
Antithyroid
Antivirals
Calcium Affecting Drugs
Cancer Chemotherapy
Cardiovascular Drugs
CNS Stimulants
Decongestants
Diuretics
Glucocorticoids
Immunomodulators
Immunosuppressants
Methylxanthines
Nicotine Cessation Therapy
NSAIDs
Ophthalmic
Retinoid, Systemic
Salivary Stimulants
Sedative-Hypnotics
Skeletal Muscle Relaxants
Sympathomimetics

# APPENDIX 6
# Common Drug-Drug and Drug-Food Interactions

**Drug-Drug Interactions**

Antibiotics - Oral Contraceptives
Tetracycline - Antacids
Tetracycline - Penicillin
Erythromycin - Penicillin
Erythromycin - Theophylline
Erythromycin - Astemizole
Erythromycin - Terfenadine
Erythromycin - Carbamazepine
Erythromycin - Triazolam
Ibuprofen - Oral Anticoagulants
Ibuprofen - Lithium
Aspirin - Anticoagulants
Naproxen - Anticoagulants
Ketoprofen - Anticoagulants
Aspirin - Probenecid
Epinephrine - Tricyclic Antidepressants
Epinephrine - Monoamine Oxidase Inhibitors
Opioid Analgesics - Cimetidine
Benzodiazepines - Alcohol
Opioid Analgesics - Alcohol

**Drug-Food Interactions**

Tetracycline — Antacids — Sodium bicarbonate, milk and milk products, iron
Erythromycin and Penicillin G — Fruit, fruit juices, tomatoes, vegetable juices
Monoamine Oxidase Inhibitors — Tyramine-rich foods
Levodopa — High-protein foods, pyridoxine
Digoxin — Chocolate , oxalic acid (spinach), phytic acid (cereal grains, nuts, legumes), bran
Calcium Channel Blockers — Grape fruit juice
Quinolones — Antacids

# Antibiotics Used to Treat Periodental Disease

Amoxicillin
Clindamycin
Doxycycline
Metronidazole
Tetracycline

# APPENDIX 8

# Prophylactic Regimens for Bacterial Endocarditis for Dental Procedures

| Situation | Agent | Regimen* |
|---|---|---|
| Standard general prophylaxis | Amoxicillin | **Adults:** 2 g orally 1 hr prior to procedure<br>**Children:** 50 mg/kg orally 1 hr prior to procedure |
| Unable to take oral medications | Ampicillin | **Adults:** 2 g IM or IV within 30 min of starting the procedure<br>**Children:** 50 mg/kg IM or IV within minutes of starting the procedure |
| Allergic to penicillin | Clindamycin | **Adults:** 600 mg orally 1 hr prior to procedure<br>**Children:** 20 mg/kg orally 1 hr prior to procedure |
| | Cephalexin** or Cefadroxil** | **Adults:** 2 g orally 1 hr prior to procedure<br>**Children:** 50 mg/kg orally 1 hr prior to procedure |
| | Azithromycin or Clarithromycin | **Adults:** 500 mg orally 1 hr prior to procedure<br>**Children:** 15 mg/kg orally 1 hr prior to procedure |
| Allergic to penicillin and unable to take oral medications | Clindamycin | **Adults:** 600 mg IV within 30 min of starting the procedure<br>**Children:** 20 mg/kg IV within 30 min of starting the procedure |
| | Cefazolin** | **Adults:** 1 g IM or IV within 30 min of starting the procedure<br>**Children:** 25 mg/kg IM or IV within 30 min of starting the procedure |

*Children's dose should not exceed adult dose.
**Cephalosporins should not be used in those with immediate type (anaphylaxis) hypersensitivity reactions to penicillins.

**Antibiotic Prophylaxis Is Recommended for the Following Cardiovascular Conditions:**

- Prosthetic Cardiac Valves*
- Previous Bacterial Endocarditis*
- Complex Cyanotic Congenital Heart Disease*
- Surgically Constructed Systemic Pulmonary Shunts or Conduits*
- Most other Congenital Cardiac Malformations (other than those listed)†
- Acquired Valvar Dysfunction†
- Hypertrophic Cardiomyopathy†
- Mitral Valve Prolapse with Valvar Regurgitation or thickened leaflets

* = High risk for endocarditis; † = Moderate risk for endocarditis

**Dental Procedures**

- Dental Extractions
- Periodontal Procedures (surgery, scaling and root planing, probing, recall maintenance)
- Dental Implant Replacement and Reimplantation of Avulsed Teeth
- Endodontic Instrumentation or Surgery only Beyond the Apex
- Subgingival Placement of Antibiotic Fibers or Strips
- Initial Placement of Orthodontic Bands but not Brackets
- Intraligamentary Local Anesthetic Injections
- Prophylactic Cleaning of Teeth or Implants when Bleeding is Anticipated

# APPENDIX 9

# Example Calculations— Drugs Administered Per Dental Cartridge

| Drug Name | Cartridges (1.8 mL) N | Drug mg | Vasoconstrictor mg (µg) |
|---|---|---|---|
| Bupivacaine | 1 | 9 | 0.009 (9) |
| 0.5% with | 2 | 18 | 0.018 (18) |
| 1:200,000 | 4 | 36 | 0.036 (36) |
| vasoconstrictor | 6 | 54 | 0.054 (54) |
| | 10 | 90 | 0.090 (90) |
| Etidocaine 1.5% | 1 | 27 | 0.009 (9) |
| with 1:200,000 | 2 | 54 | 0.018 (18) |
| vasoconstrictor | 4 | 108 | 0.036 (36) |
| | 6 | 162 | 0.054 (54) |
| Lidocaine 2% | 1 | 36 | |
| without a | 2 | 72 | |
| vasoconstrictor | 4 | 144 | |
| Lidocaine 2% | 1 | 36 | 0.036 (36) |
| with 1:50,000 | 2 | 72 | 0.072 (72) |
| vasoconstrictor | 3 | 108 | 0.108 (108) |
| | 4 | 144 | 0.144 (144) |
| | 5 | 180 | 0.180 (180) |
| | 5.5 | 198 | 0.198 (198) |
| Lidocaine 2% | 1 | 36 | 0.018 (18) |
| with 1:100,000 | 2 | 72 | 0.036 (36) |
| vasoconstrictor | 3 | 108 | 0.054 (54) |
| | 6 | 216 | 0.108 (108) |
| | 8 | 288 | 0.144 (144) |
| | 10 | 360 | 0.180 (180) |
| Mepivacaine 3% | 1 | 54 | |
| without a | 2 | 108 | |
| vasoconstrictor | 4 | 216 | |
| Mepivacaine 2% | 1 | 36 | 0.090 (90) |
| 1:20,000 | 2 | 72 | 0.180 (180) |
| vasoconstrictor | 3 | 108 | 0.270 (270) |
| | 5 | 180 | 0.450 (450) |
| | 8 | 288 | 0.720 (720) |
| | 10 | 360 | 0.900 (900) |

| Drug Name | Cartridges (1.8 mL) N | Drug mg | Vasoconstrictor mg (µg) |
|---|---|---|---|
| Prilocaine(4%) | 1 | 72 | |
| without a | 2 | 144 | |
| vasoconstrictor | 3 | 216 | |
| | 4 | 288 | |
| Prilocaine 4% | 1 | 72 | 0.009 (9) |
| with a 1:200,000 | 2 | 144 | 0.018 (18) |
| vasoconstrictor | 4 | 288 | 0.036 (36) |

# APPENDIX 10
# Typical Local Anesthetic and Vasoconstrictor Concentrations

| Agent | Strength | mg/mL (µg/mL) Equivalent |
|---|---|---|
| Local Anesthetic | 0.5% | 5 |
| | 1.5% | 15 |
| | 2% | 20 |
| | 3% | 30 |
| | 4% | 40 |
| Vasoconstrictor | 1:20,000 | 0.05 (50) |
| | 1:50,000 | 0.02 (20) |
| | 1:100,000 | 0.01 (10) |
| | 1:200,000 | 0.005 (5) |

# Index

---

**Boldface** = generic drug name
*italics* = therapeutic drug class

Regular type = trade names
CAPITALS = combination drugs

---

**Boldface** = generic drug name    Regular type = trade names
*italics* = therapeutic drug class    CAPITALS = combination drugs

---

**Boldface** = generic drug name
*italics* = therapeutic drug class

Regular type = trade names
CAPITALS = combination drugs

---

**Boldface** = generic drug name
*italics* = therapeutic drug class

Regular type = trade names
CAPITALS = combination drugs

---

**Boldface** = generic drug name
*italics* = therapeutic drug class

Regular type = trade names
CAPITALS = combination drugs

---

**Boldface** = generic drug name
*italics* = therapeutic drug class

Regular type = trade names
CAPITALS = combination drugs

5-FU (Adrucil), **233**
Fungizone ✿ **(Amphotericin B)**, 104
Fungizone Intravenous **(Amphotericin B)**, 104
**Furosemide** (Lasix), **244**
Furoside ✿ **(Furosemide)**, 244

**Gabapentin** (Neurontin), 245
Gabatril **(Tiagabine hydrochloride)**, 408
Garamycin **(Gentamicin sulfate)**, 247
Garamycin Cream or Ointment **(Gentamicin sulfate)**, 247
Garamycin Intrathecal **(Gentamicin sulfate)**, 247
Garamycin IV Piggyback **(Gentamicin sulfate)**, 247
Garamycin Ophthalmic Ointment **(Gentamicin sulfate)**, 247
Garamycin Ophthalmic Solution **(Gentamicin sulfate)**, 247
Garamycin Pediatric **(Gentamicin sulfate)**, 247
Garatec ✿ **(Gentamicin sulfate)**, 247
Gastrocrom **(Cromolyn sodium)**, 182
Gee-Gee **(Guaifenesin)**, 251
Gemcor **(Gemfibrozil)**, 246
**Gemfibrozil** (Lopid), **246**
Genahist **(Diphenhydramine hydrochloride)**, 201
Gen-Alprazolam ✿ **(Alprazolam)**, 96
Gen-Amantadine ✿ **(Amantadine hydrochloride)**, 97
Genapap **(Acetaminophen)**, 83
Genapap Children's **(Acetaminophen)**, 83
Genapap Extra Strength **(Acetaminophen)**, 83
Genapap Infants' Drops **(Acetaminophen)**, 83
Genaphed **(Pseudoephedrine hydrochloride)**, 373
Gen-Atenolol ✿ **(Atenolol)**, 112
Genatuss **(Guaifenesin)**, 251
Gen-Beclo Aq. ✿ **(Beclomethasone dipropionate)**, 119
Gencalc 600 **(Calcium carbonate)**, 135
Gen-Captopril ✿ **(Captopril)**, 135
Gen-Clomipramine ✿ **(Clomipramine hydrochloride)**, 173
Gen-Diltiazem ✿ **(Diltiazem hydrochloride)**, 199
Genebs **(Acetaminophen)**, 83
Genebs Extra Strength **(Acetaminophen)**, 83
Genebs Extra Strength Caplets **(Acetaminophen)**, 83
Gen-Famotidine ✿ **(Famotidine)**, 223

Gen-Glybe ✿ **(Glyburide)**, 251
Gen-Indapamide ✿ **(Indapamide hemihydrate)**, 260
Gen-Metformin ✿ **(Metformin hydrochloride)**, 302
Gen-Metoprolol ✿ **(Metoprolol tartrate)**, 306
Gen-Nifedipine ✿ **(Nifedipine)**, 335
Genoptic Ophthalmic Liquifilm **(Gentamicin sulfate)**, 247
Genoptic S.O.P. Ophthalmic **(Gentamicin sulfate)**, 247
Genora 0.5/35, 64
Genora 1/35, 64
Genora 1/50, 64
Gen-Piroxicam ✿ **(Piroxicam)**, 365
Genpril Caplets and Tablets **(Ibuprofen)**, 259
Genprin **(Acetylsalicylic acid)**, 86
Gen-Salbutamol Sterinebs P.F. ✿ **(Albuterol)**, 92
Gentacidin Ophthalmic **(Gentamicin sulfate)**, 247
Gentafair **(Gentamicin sulfate)**, 247
Gentak Ophthalmic **(Gentamicin sulfate)**, 247
Gentamicin **(Gentamicin sulfate)**, 247
Gentamicin Ophthalmic **(Gentamicin sulfate)**, 247
**Gentamicin sulfate** (Garamycin), **247**
Gentamicin Sulfate IV Piggyback **(Gentamicin sulfate)**, 247
Gen-Tamoxifen **(Tamoxifen)**, 400
Gentrasul Ophthalmic **(Gentamicin sulfate)**, 247
Genuine Bayer Aspirin Caplets and Tablets **(Acetylsalicylic acid)**, 86
Gen-Valproic ✿ **(Valproic acid)**, 427
Gen-Verapamil SR ✿ **(Verapamil)**, 431
GG-Cen **(Guaifenesin)**, 251
Glaucon **(Epinephrine hydrochloride)**, 214
**Glimepiride** (Amaryl), **249**
**Glipizide** (Glucotrol), **250**
Glucophage **(Metformin hydrochloride)**, 302
Glucotrol **(Glipizide)**, 250
Glucotrol XL **(Glipizide)**, 250
Glyate **(Guaifenesin)**, 251
**Glyburide** (Gen-Glybe, Glynase PresTab, Micronase), **251**
**Glyceryl guaiacolate** (Robitussin), **251**
Gly-Cort **(Hydrocortisone)**, 257
Glycotuss **(Guaifenesin)**, 251
Glynase PresTab **(Glyburide)**, 251
Glyset **(Miglitol)**, 312
Glytuss **(Guaifenesin)**, 251
G-myticin Cream or Ointment **(Gentamicin sulfate)**, 247

---

**Boldface** = generic drug name
*italics* = therapeutic drug class

Regular type = trade names
CAPITALS = combination drugs

---

**Boldface** = generic drug name        Regular type = trade names
*italics* = therapeutic drug class        CAPITALS = combination drugs

---

**Boldface** = generic drug name
*italics* = therapeutic drug class

Regular type = trade names
CAPITALS = combination drugs

---

**Boldface** = generic drug name
*italics* = therapeutic drug class

Regular type = trade names
CAPITALS = combination drugs

---

**Boldface** = generic drug name
*italics* = therapeutic drug class

Regular type = trade names
CAPITALS = combination drugs

---

**Boldface** = generic drug name

*italics* = therapeutic drug class

Regular type = trade names

CAPITALS = combination drugs

---

**Boldface** = generic drug name
*italics* = therapeutic drug class

Regular type = trade names
CAPITALS = combination drugs

---

**Boldface** = generic drug name
*italics* = therapeutic drug class

Regular type = trade names
CAPITALS = combination drugs

---

**Boldface** = generic drug name
*italics* = therapeutic drug class

Regular type = trade names
CAPITALS = combination drugs

---

**Boldface** = generic drug name    Regular type = trade names
*italics* = therapeutic drug class    CAPITALS = combination drugs